NHS The Leeds Teaching Hospitals NHS Trust

This book must be returned by the date shown
below or a fine will be charged.

1 6 JUN 2021	

The NHS Staff Library at the L.G.I.
☎ 0113 39 26445

D1337321

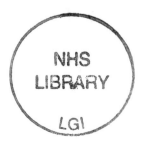

Spinal and Epidural Anesthesia

NOTICE

Spinal and Epidural Anesthesia

Cynthia A. Wong, MD
Chief, Obstetrical Anesthesia
Director, Obstetrical Anesthesia Fellowship Program
Associate Professor of Anesthesiology
Department of Anesthesiology
Feinberg School of Medicine
Northwestern University
Chicago, Illinois

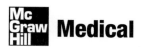 **Medical**

New York   Chicago   San Francisco   Lisbon   London   Madrid
Mexico City   Milan   New Delhi   San Juan   Seoul   Singapore   Sydney   Toronto

The McGraw·Hill Companies

Spinal and Epidural Anesthesia

1 2 3 4 5 6 7 8 9 0   DOC/DOC   0 9 8 7 6

ISBN-13: 978-0-07-143772-1
ISBN-10: 0-07-143772-X

This book was set in Minion by International Typesetting and Composition.

The editors were Joseph Rusko and Lester A. Sheinis.

The production supervisor was Catherine H. Saggese.

The cover designer was Cathleen Elliott.

The design was coordinated by Charissa Baker; the text designer was Alan Barnett.

Cover photo credit: LADA/Photo Researchers, Inc.

The indexer was Susan Hunter.

RR Donnelley was printer and binder.

This book is printed on acid-free paper.

Cataloging-in-Publication Data are on file for this book at the Library of Congress.

CONTENTS

CONTRIBUTORS

Honorio T. Benzon, MD
Professor of Anesthesiology
Chief, Section of Pain Medicine
Department of Anesthesiology
Feinberg School of Medicine
Northwestern University
Chicago, Illinois
Chapter 16

David J. Birnbach, MD
Professor, Executive Vice Chair
Department of Anesthesiology
Chief, Women's Anesthesia Department of Anesthesiology
University of Miami School of Medicine
Miami, Florida
Chapter 13

Lynn Broadman, MD
Professor of Anesthesiology and Pediatrics
West Virginia University School of Medicine
Morgantown, West Virginia
Chapter 11

Kenneth D. Candido, MD
Chief, Section of Acute Pain Management
Associate Professor
Northwestern University
Chicago, Illinois
Chapter 16

Eric Cappiello, MD
Department of Anesthesia
Brigham and Women's Hospital
Boston, Massachusetts
Chapter 6

Dominic Cottrell, MD
Clinical Assistant Professor
Pediatric and Cardiothoracic Anesthesia
Department of Anesthesiology
West Virginia University
Morgantown, West Virginia
Chapter 11

Nathaniel Diaz, MD
Department of Anesthesiology
Feinberg School of Medicine
Northwestern University
Chicago, Illinois
Chapter 9

Robert Doty, Jr., MD
Assistant Professor, Department of Anesthesiology
Feinberg School of Medicine
Northwestern University
Chicago, Illinois
Chapter 7

David L. Hepner, MD
Assistant Professor of Anesthesia
Harvard Medical School
Staff Anesthesiologist
Brigham and Women's Hospital
Department of Anesthesia
Perioperative, and Pain Medicine
Boston, Massachusetts
Chapter 5

Marcelle Hernandez, MD
Department of Anesthesiology
University of Miami School of Medicine
Miami, Florida
Chapter 13

Quinn Hogan, MD
Professor, Department of Anesthesiology
Medical College of Wisconsin
Milwaukee, Wisconsin
Chapter 1

Khadija Khan, MD
Instructor in Anesthesia
Harvard Medical School
Staff Anesthesiologist
Brigham and Women's Hospital
Boston, Massachusetts
Chapter 5

Joon Kim, MD
Instructor in Anesthesiology
Weill Medical College of Cornell University
Assistant Attending Anesthesiologist
New York Presbyterian Hospital
New York, New York
Chapter 12

Klaus Kjaer, MD
Assistant Professor of Anesthesiology
Weill Medical College of Cornell University
Assistant Attending Anesthesiologist
New York Presbyterian Weill Cornell Medical Center
New York, New York
Chapter 12

Philipp Lirk, MD, MSc
Department of Anesthesiology and Critical Care Medicine
Medical University of Innsbruck
Innsbruck, Austria
Chapter 1

Robert E. Molloy, MD
Associate Chair, Department of Anesthesiology
Feinberg School of Medicine
Northwestern University
Chicago, Illinois
Chapter 17

Antoun M. Nader, MD
Assistant Professor, Director, Regional Anesthesiology
Feinberg School of Medicine
Northwestern University
Chicago, Illinois
Chapter 17

John Ratliff, MD
Department of Anesthesiology
Feinberg School of Medicine
Northwestern University
Chicago, Illinois
Chapter 4

Nollag O'Rourke, MD
Fellow in Anesthesiology
Harvard Medical School
Obstetric Anesthesia Fellow
Brigham and Women's Hospital
Harvard Medical School
Boston, Massachusetts
Chapter 5

Francis V. Salinas, MD
Clinical Assistant Professor
Department of Anesthesiology
University of Washington
Staff Anesthesiologist
Department of Anesthesiology
Virginia Mason Medical Center
Seattle, Washington
Chapter 3

Barbara M. Scavone, MD
Assistant Professor of Anesthesiology
Feinberg School of Medicine
Northwestern University
Department of Anesthesiology
Staff Anesthesiologist
Department of Anesthesiology
Northwestern Memorial Hospital
Chicago, Illinois
Chapter 4

Michele Sproviero, MD
Instructor, Department of Anesthesiology
Northwestern University
Northwestern Memorial Hospital
Chicago, Illinois
Chapter 10

Radha Sukhani, MD
Associate Professor, Department of Anesthesiology
Northwestern University
Chicago, Illinois
Chapter 7

John T. Sullivan, MD
Assistant Professor, Associate Chair for Education
Department of Anesthesiology
Feinberg School of Medicine
Northwestern University
Chicago, Illinois
Chapter 14

Santhanam Suresh, MD, FAAP
Associate Professor of Anesthesiology and Pediatrics
Children's Memorial Medical Center
Feinberg School of Medicine
Northwestern University
Chicago, Illinois
Chapter 15

Lawrence C. Tsen, MD
Associate Professor in Anesthesia
Harvard Medical School
Director of Anesthesia
Center for Reproductive Medicine
Brigham and Women's Hospital
Boston, Massachusetts
Chapter 6

Tetsu Uejima, MD, FAAP
Assistant Professor of Anesthesiology
Children's Memorial Medical Center
Feinberg School of Medicine
Northwestern University
Chicago, Illinois
Chapter 15

Cynthia A. Wong, MD
Chief, Obstetrical Anesthesia
Director, Obstetrical Anesthesia Fellowship Program
Associate Professor of Anesthesiology
Department of Anesthesiology
Feinberg School of Medicine
Northwestern University
Chicago, Illinois
Chapters 2, 4, 9, 16

Hak Yui Wong, MBBS
Assistant Professor of Anesthesiology
Feinberg School of Medicine
Northwestern University
Chicago, Illinois
Chapter 8

Meltem Yilmaz, MD
Department of Anesthesiology
Feinberg School of Medicine
Northwestern University
Chicago, Illinois
Chapter 2

PREFACE

This textbook is devoted to the practice of neuraxial anesthesia and analgesia, that is, spinal and epidural anesthesia/ analgesia. These important anesthetic techniques have contributed to the health and well-being of many patients since spinal anesthesia was first described by August Bier in 1899. The ability to take away or block pain with a relatively simple and safe injection often seems near miraculous to patients. Think of the woman whose excruciating labor pains are gone within minutes or the child who wakes from an anesthetic without pain or emergence delirium. The knowledge contained within this book is a tribute to physicians and scientists whose research for the past century has contributed to the art and science of neuraxial anesthesia.

Although the word *regional* (anesthesia) is often used when the writer/speaker means spinal/epidural anesthesia, the word *neuraxial* (anesthesia) is more specific and correct, as regional anesthesia can refer to other blocks of major nerve groupings such as a brachial plexus block. Therefore, throughout the text, the word *neuraxial* refers to *spinal/epidural* anesthesia or analgesia.

There are several outstanding major textbooks covering the practice of anesthesiology as a whole that include one or two chapters devoted to neuraxial anesthesia. There are several major textbooks devoted to regional anesthesia and pain management that include chapters devoted to neuraxial anesthesia. There are, however, no textbooks devoted solely to the clinical practice of spinal and epidural anesthesia/ analgesia. This textbook was designed to fill that void. Our intent was to give the practitioner of neuraxial anesthesia (a skill required of all competent anesthesiologists) a global review of the theory and practice of neuraxial anesthesia/ analgesia, the detail of which is lacking in major

anesthesiology textbooks. Often major textbooks do not contain "clinical pearls," and handbooks do not contain enough information to thoroughly understand and learn the theory behind the practice. This book attempts to bridge this gap and contains information necessary to the safe and skillful practice of neuraxial anesthesia.

The book is organized into two major sections. The first six chapters cover general aspects of neuraxial anesthesiology and include discussions of vertebral anatomy, neuraxial block technique, pharmacology of drugs utilized for neuraxial anesthesia, physiologic changes associated with neuraxial anesthesia, as well as contraindications and complications of spinal and epidural anesthesia. The second part of the book is organized into chapters of all the major surgical subspecialties. Each chapter discusses the clinical application of neuraxial anesthesia relative to the type of surgery. There may be some overlap among these chapters and the first part of the book; however, this allows the reader with a basic understanding of neuraxial anesthesia to read each subspecialty chapter and come away with a solid understanding of how neuraxial anesthesia fits into the practice of anesthesiology in each surgical specialty. The last two chapters of the book deal with the use of neuraxial techniques in the management of acute postoperative and chronic pain.

This book would not have been possible without the work of the contributors, each of whom has a passion for neuraxial anesthesia. They have put much effort into sharing their knowledge with you, the reader. My hope is that our attempts to communicate this knowledge with you will make you a better practitioner of neuraxial anesthesia/ analgesia, ultimately to the benefit of our patients.

Spinal and Epidural Anatomy

CHAPTER 1

Philipp Lirk
Quinn Hogan

Peripheral and neuraxial anesthesia are most important exercises in applied anatomy. The ability of the anesthesiologist to visualize relevant anatomy three-dimensionally during needle manipulation, and the appreciation of potential anatomic variations, remain paramount in the safe and effective conduct of regional, and specifically neuraxial anesthesia.

SURFACE ANATOMY AND LOCALIZATION OF VERTEBRAL INTERSPACES

Identification of the spinal level is the first anatomic consideration during initiation of spinal or epidural anesthesia. The spinal level at which anesthetic is injected substantially contributes to the extent of blockade in both types of anesthesia. The level of injection is customarily determined prior to puncture by means of inspection and palpation of anatomic landmarks.

The most prominent spinous process is usually the seventh cervical spinous process, but in subjects with scoliosis, the first thoracic spinous process may be most prominent in up to a third of patients[1] (Fig. 1-1). Attempting to locate the seventh cervical vertebra by palpating downward from the nuchal furrow can similarly lead to confusion with the sixth cervical spinous process in about half of cases.[1] This variability is even more pronounced in cases where degenerative processes further distort underlying anatomy.

The inferior angle of the scapula is assumed to indicate the level of the seventh thoracic spinous process, while the line connecting the left and right iliac crests (Tuffier's line) most commonly crosses the vertebral column at the L4-L5 intervertebral disc. There is, however, considerable inherent variability, and the line may actually cross the vertebral column anywhere between the intervertebral discs of L3-L4 and L5-S1.[2] Thus, we must recognize the limits of the ability

of landmarks to predict lumbar interspaces. Even though bony landmarks are most often used to determine vertebral level, the results are not always in concordance with the vertebral level as determined by vertebral column imaging. The result is a high rate of incorrectly determining a given lumbar interspace when using the usual palpable bony landmarks[3,4] even in the absence of factors obscuring these landmarks.[5]

Imaging studies in both human volunteers and cadavers have demonstrated that the identified interspace is actually more cephalad than estimated by experienced anesthesiologists.[5–8] This is undesirable since moving up only two

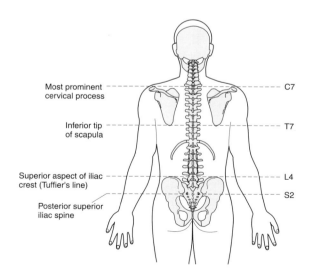

FIGURE 1-1. Frequently used skeletal landmarks used to determine level of puncture, respective vertebral level given on the right. *Used with permission from Kleinman W, Mikhail M. Spinal, epidural, and caudal blocks. In: Morgan GE, Mikhail MS, Murray M, eds, Clinical Anesthesiology, 4th ed. New York: McGraw-Hill, 2006, pp. 289–323.*

interspaces from the classical L3-L4 interspace to administer spinal anesthesia would locate the puncture site in the vicinity of the spinal cord. In general, the accuracy of predicting the vertebral level of needle insertion is, at best, about 50% when unaided by radiologic imaging.[8–10] As yet, aids in the accurate determination of vertebral level have not proven helpful in the clinical arena.[11]

ANATOMY OF THE VERTEBRAL COLUMN

The vertebral column serves as reference for various blocks used in surgery, obstetrics, and pain management, including spinal and epidural anesthetics, blocks of paravertebral and prevertebral sympathetic structures, blocks of segmental nerves emerging from the vertebral column, and facet joint blockade. Knowledge of the anatomy of the vertebral col-

umn is important to the successful execution of all these blocks, as well as to understanding the complications and side effects of the blocks.

► Composition of the Vertebral Column

The vertebral column is a sinuous and flexible[12] column consisting of 7 cervical, 12 thoracic, 5 lumbar, 5 sacral, and 4 coccygeal vertebrae. During development, however, only the cervical, thoracic, and lumbar vertebrae normally remain movable, while the sacral and coccygeal vertebrae fuse to form the sacrum, and coccyx or terminal bone, respectively.

The representative vertebra consists of the anterior vertebral body (corpus) and posterior elements forming the vertebral arch (arcus) (Fig. 1-2). The arch consists of a flattened portion (lamina) and seven processes, the paired superior

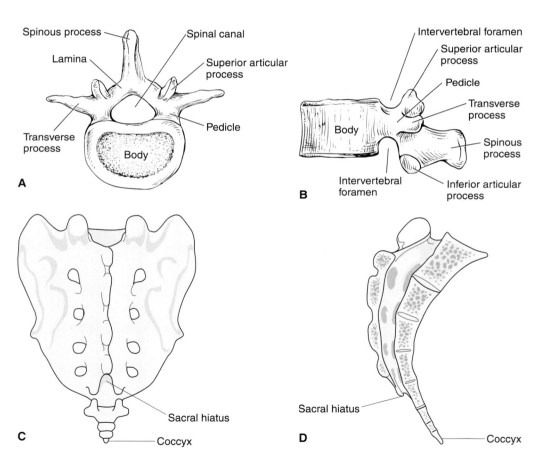

FIGURE 1-2. Schematic representation of vertebra at various levels. (A) Lumbar vertebra (superior view). (B) Lumbar vertebra (lateral view). (C) Sacrum and coccyx (posterior view). (D) Sacrum and coccyx (lateral view). *Used with permission from Kleinman W, Mikhail M. Spinal, epidural, and caudal blocks. In: Morgan GE, Mikhail MS, Murray M, eds, Clinical Anesthesiology, 4th ed. New York: McGraw-Hill, 2006, pp. 289–323.*

and inferior articular processes, the paired transverse processes, and the midline spinous process.[12] The vertebral body and arch together enclose the vertebral foramen. The vertebral foramina of each vertebra combine to enclose the longitudinal spinal canal. In the cervical and lumbar regions, where the column is most flexible, the canal approaches a triangular shape, but is circular and smaller in the thoracic region. The width of the spinal canal is approximately 25 mm throughout the cervical canal, approximately 17 mm in the thoracic region, 22 mm at L1, and widens to approximately 27 mm towards the lower lumbar levels.[13-17] The anterior/posterior diameter of the vertebral canal is uniform at 15 to 16 mm throughout the vertebral column.[18] The spinal canal communicates with the paravertebral space through intervertebral foramina, which are delineated by concavities on the superior and inferior aspect of the pedicle (Fig. 1-2). These foramina, also referred to as nerve root canals, transmit segmental nerves as well as the spinal rami of segmental arteries and veins.

The transverse process is based at the junction of the pedicle and lamina and passes laterally at cervical and thoracic levels. The lumbar transverse process is, correctly speaking, rudimentary, and instead the lumbar process, homologous to the ribs, takes its place. The spinous process projects posteriorly from the laminae. It is typically bifid at the 2nd and 6th cervical levels. Degenerative changes can lead to deviation of the spinous process from the midline.

Cervical Spine

Cervical vertebrae (with the exception of the atlas [C1] and axis [C2] [epistropheus]) have small vertebral bodies. The pedicles, facing laterally and posteriorly, support the laminae, which are flat. The spinous processes of the second to sixth vertebrae are typically bifurcated posteriorly, while the seventh vertebra features a long, horizontal spinous process, which is not bifurcated. Its easy palpability has given rise to its designation as the "vertebra prominens." The vertebral foramen is large compared to the vertebral body.

Cervical transverse processes feature a spinal nerve sulcus, a groove for the spinal nerve as it emerges from the interspinal foramen, and the transverse foramen, which allows for the passage of the vertebral artery (usually from C6 to C1), vein (usually from C7 to C1), and sympathetic plexus. The spinal nerve sulcus is delineated by the posterior and anterior tubercles, but the latter is absent in the case of the seventh vertebra.

Thoracic Spine

The thoracic vertebrae are larger than the cervical, but smaller than the lumbar vertebrae. Most notably, their bodies and transverse processes (except for T11 and T12) both feature facets for articulation with the ribs. The body has a larger

posterior compared to anterior vertical dimension, giving rise to the thoracic kyphosis. The laminae are supported by pedicles directed backward and upward, and are more solid than the cervical laminae. Furthermore, laminae of adjacent thoracic vertebrae overlap. The vertebral foramen is relatively small compared to the body and round in shape.

Lumbar Spine

Lumbar vertebrae are the largest movable segments, and feature strong pedicles, laminae, and spinous processes. Two small processes, the accessory and mamillary, are present on the articular process. The anterior aspect of the body of the fifth lumbar vertebra is substantially higher than the posterior aspect, emphasizing the lumbar lordosis. Lastly, the lumbar vertebral bodies are hourglass shaped, with a diameter 15% less at the middle than at the end plates.[19]

Lumbosacral Segmentation

In contrast to the stability of cervical and thoracic vertebrae during development, the lumbosacral spine frequently features anatomical variations.[20] Similarly, investigations in primates have demonstrated that lumbar vertebral variations are most common.[21] The most important variations are a partial or bilateral fusion of the last lumbar vertebra to the sacral bone ("sacralization"), or incomplete fusion between the segments S1 and S2 ("lumbarization").[20] Moreover, the lumbar vertebral arch may exhibit fusion defects in approximately 4% of the general population.

Sacral Anatomy

Childhood sacral vertebrae are connected by cartilage but progress to bony fusion after puberty. In the adult, only a narrow residue of the sacral discs persists (Fig. 1-2). An abrupt increase in the lumbar lordotic curve occurs at the L5-S1 junction (Fig. 1-3), accentuating the prominence of the anterior S1 vertebral body. Sacral anatomy is even more variable than at

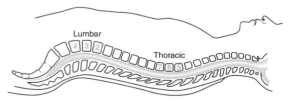

FIGURE 1-3. Lordosis and kyphosis of the vertebral column. Note that in the supine position, the lowest spot is found approximately at thoracic levels 5–7. *Used with permission from Kleinman W, Mikhail M. Spinal, epidural, and caudal blocks. In: Morgan GE, Mikhail MS, Murray M, eds, Clinical Anesthesiology, 4th ed. New York: McGraw-Hill, 2006, pp. 289–323.*

lumbar levels, which is unfortunate since anatomic variation may substantially impede success of caudal epidural blockade.[22] The volume of the adult sacral canal ranges between 12 mL and 65 mL.[23] Even though the vertebral arches of sacral vertebrae typically fuse to form a posterior roof, partial or total failure of fusion is frequently observed. Similarly, the anterior/posterior diameter of the sacral canal exhibits substantial inter-individual variation, and diameters of 2 mm or less at the level of the hiatus are found in 5% of adults.[23] This contrasts with usual diameters of approximately 6–12 mm.[24] A recent anatomic study demonstrated that sacral cornua are not present in half of adults, whereas the hiatus itself may be absent in 4%.[24] Fortunately, access through the sacral hiatus is consistent enough in children to allow for safe performance of caudal epidural blockade. The coccyx, or terminal bone, is a fusion of the last four to seven rudimentary vertebrae (Fig. 1-2).

JOINTS AND LIGAMENTS OF THE VERTEBRAL COLUMN

Movement of the vertebral column is determined by interactions between several types of articulations and the spinal ligaments. Whereas the vertebral bodies are joined by a series of amphiarthrodial joints, "true" diarthrodial joints link the vertebral arches. Furthermore, the vertebral column is supported by the anterior and posterior longitudinal ligaments (Fig. 1-4).

The endplates of the vertebral bodies are connected by fibrocartilaginous intervertebral discs. The latter are comprised of the annular ligament and the nucleus pulposus. The annular ligament is composed of concentric lamellae of collagenous fibers, and surrounds the colloidal nucleus pulposus. The nucleus is not vascularized in the adult, since blood vessels retract soon after birth. Since it is predominantly composed of fluid, it acts as a shock absorber. When the nucleus pulposus is compressed it exerts pressure on the annular ligament. The longitudinal ligaments of the vertebral column link the intervertebral discs, the anterior aspect being supported by the broad anterior longitudinal ligament. The posterior longitudinal ligament is less broad, and widens only where it merges with the intervertebral disc. This is of considerable clinical relevance, since with age, degenerative processes may cause the disc to herniate, and this occurs predominantly in the paramedian sections of the posterior disc. Moreover, ossification of the ligament may cause spinal stenosis.[25] Extruded nuclear material may compress the spinal cord or nerves in the vertebral canal. Disc herniation produces pathogenic effects not only by mechanical compression of affected nerve roots,

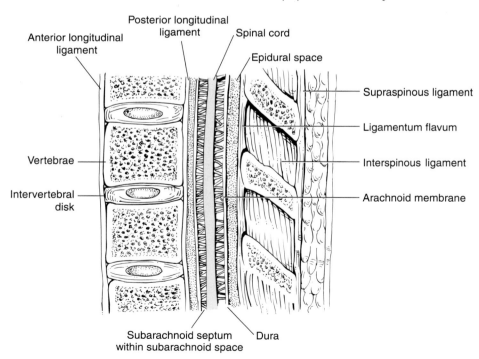

FIGURE 1-4. Vertebral ligaments: lateral view and sagittal section through the vertebral canal. The epidural space is in reality thought to be discontinuous and compartmented (Fig. 1-6). *Used with permission from Kleinman W, Mikhail M. Spinal, epidural, and caudal blocks. In: Morgan GE, Mikhail MS, Murray M, eds, Clinical Anesthesiology, 4th ed. New York: McGraw-Hill, 2006, pp. 289–323.*

but also because nucleus pulposus material per se directly elicits neural inflammation. In contrast, the posterior vertebral elements are connected by the zygapophyseal (facet) joints, which link the inferior articular process of one vertebra, and the superior articular process of the next most caudal vertebra. The facet joints are localized posterior to the transverse process at cervical and lumbar levels, and anterior to the transverse process at the thoracic level. Their three-dimensional arrangement determines the possible range of movements. Specifically, the plane of cervical facet joint is approximately midway between the axial and coronal plane, while it is almost coronal and more vertical at thoracic levels.[26] The lumbar facet joints are almost parallel to the sagittal plane, and the superior articular processes of one vertebra clasp around the inferior articular processes of the next cranial vertebra. The transition from the typical thoracic to the lumbar facet joint orientation is variable, with about half of adults showing a gradual transition, and the other half exhibiting an abrupt change in morphology.[27]

As mentioned above, the transverse process discernible on cervical and thoracic vertebrae is, correctly speaking, not apparent as such in lumbar vertebrae. These feature a lumbar process, perhaps more appropriately referred to as a costal process, since it represents rudimentary costal tissue. The superior articular process at lumbar levels instead features the accessory process and the mammillary process as remnants of the transverse process, the latter of which contributes to articular stability by encircling the inferior articular process of the adjacent vertebra.[28,29] The thoracolumbar transition zone represents a most important access route for neuraxial anesthesia.

The orientation of facet joints described above governs which movements are possible in segments of the vertebral column. The cervical spine is most flexible, with flexion and extension of the head, and bending and turning as possible motions. Uncinate processes of the cervical vertebrae have a dynamic function as lateral guide rails.[26] Thoracic facet joints are arranged to allow for rotation, but flexion and bending are limited. Retroflexion of the thoracic spine is also inhibited by the overlapping spinous processes, while the ribs and intercostal tissue inhibit excessive lateral bending. The lumbar spine is responsible for flexion and extension. In addition to their dynamic function in determining range of movement, facet joints in the cervical and lumbar region are weight bearing.[30–32]

The capsule of facet joints is distinctly different at various levels. It is most flaccid at cervical levels and becomes increasingly firm in more caudad segments. Frequently, injection of joints leads to capsule rupture, and leakage of injectate into the epidural space.[33,34] The superior and inferior articular process are covered by cartilage, and supported by synovial folds, and by menisci in young subjects.[35] Facet joints and their menisci are innervated by the dorsal rami of segmental nerves,[36,37] and limited evidence suggests that their

entrapment may contribute to the genesis of chronic back pain.[35] It should be noted, however, that in general, mechanical failure of the intervertebral disc precedes facet disease.[38] Degeneration of the disc then brings about loss of disc height, and subsequently increased pressure on facet joints. Facet joints may feature periarticular exostoses, and these can compress adjacent neural structures.[39] Protrusion of exostoses may also interfere with needle placement during spinal or epidural anesthesia.

Ligaments with both static and dynamic functions further connect the vertebral arches. Most superficially, the supraspinous ligament connects the tips of the spinous processes. It is most prominent in the upper thoracic region, but becomes frail towards the lower lumbar region (Fig. 1-4).[40] The spinous processes are joined by the interspinous ligament, which may feature a slit-like midline cavity filled with fat.[40] Since the latter ligaments are composed of collagenous fibers, a traversing needle creates a distinct crackle as the individual fiber bundles are penetrated.

In contrast to the supra- and interspinous ligaments, the ligamentum flavum, a key landmark in neuraxial anesthesia, is composed mainly of elastic fibers (80%), providing a unique tactile clue for epidural needle placement using the loss-of-resistance technique. The ligamentum flavum is under considerable elastic tension. The teleologic reasons for the ligament's elasticity are twofold. In addition to its static stabilizing function, the ligamentum flavum is extended as the vertebral column is flexed, and this tension facilitates subsequent erecting. The ligamentum flavum stretches between the anterior laminar surface of the cephalad vertebra, and the posterior lamina of the more caudad vertebra. It spans the vertebral arch from the roots of the articular processes to the midline. The anterior aspect of the facet joint capsule is strengthened by the ligamentum flavum.

Ossification of the ligamentum flavum may occur to varying degrees, even at a young age.[41,42] Interestingly, this occurs commonly at inferior thoracic levels, while it is less frequent at lumbar levels. Since the inferior thoracic level with its coronally oriented facet joints is the most frequent site of ossification, it has been proposed that this process may reflect amplified rotary strain.[43] The clinical relevance of these ingrowing bone spikes is that they may impede needle advancement. In macerated thoracic and lumbar vertebrae, these bony protuberances are often clearly discernible. They may also be of interest following spinal trauma, when bony spikes may constitute a differential diagnosis to fracture fragments.

Between the left and right half of the ligamentum flavum, intervals for the passage of veins connecting the posterior external vertebral venous plexus with the posterior internal vertebral venous plexus have been described.[12] The right and left halves meet at an angle of less than 90 degrees, and depending on the vertebral level, up to 74% of cervical, and up to 22% of lumbar ligamenta flava are discontinuous in the midline.[44] Overall, the incidence of gaps is highest in the cervical region, and decreases in the thoracic and lumbar regions.[45] Absence of a continuous ligamentous arch formed by the ligamenta flava may result in a blunted or absent "loss-of-resistance" when entering the epidural space with an epidural needle. Because the supra- and interspinous ligaments[46,47] are composed of collagenous fibers, the same "pop" feel may not result when the needle emerges from the interspinous ligament into the epidural space. Midline gaps exceeding sizes of 1 mm could be responsible for a failure to recognize a loss-of-resistance in some patients, such that one cannot always rely on the ligamentum flavum to provide a tactile clue during epidural needle placement. It is not known how often "midline" punctures are actually midline, rather than actually slightly paramedian.

LORDOSIS AND KYPHOSIS

The vertebral column features typical physiologic curves. Whereas the thoracic and sacral segments are naturally concave anteriorly (*kyphosis*), the cervical and lumbar segments are concave posteriorly (*lordosis*) (Fig. 1-3). This vertebral column configuration provides longitudinal elasticity and acts as a suspension for the cranium and its contents. During pregnancy, the lumbar lordosis and compensatory thoracic kyphosis are especially pronounced. For the patient in the supine position, the two highest points in the curvature are at the level of L3 and C5. Conversely, the two most dependent points are at T5 and S2. Clinically, the consequence is that hyperbaric local anesthetics injected at lumbar levels will most likely ascend toward the level of T5.

EPIDURAL SPACE ANATOMY

The conformation of the epidural space and its contents is of utmost importance to any physician performing a neuraxial intervention. The epidural space can be defined as the area outside the dural sac but inside the spinal canal, and extends from the foramen magnum to the sacrococcygeal ligament (Figs. 1-5 and 1-6). Understanding these structures and their exact interplay is limited by the fact that studies into epidural anatomy face methodological difficulties. For example, epiduroscopy[48] probably distorts relevant anatomy to a substantial degree. Similarly, direct dissection may not give a true representation of epidural anatomy directly relevant to needle advancement and placement in vivo. Investigations using cryomicrotome sections are probably the most useful, as this technique does not distort anatomic structures, and leaves the epidural space undisturbed. These investigations have primarily shown that the dural sac and its contents occupy a large part of the spinal canal. Most of the remainder of the canal is occupied by fatty and fibrous tissues, and blood vessels. These are organized into discontinuous compartments, which are separated by regions where the dura is in contact with the border of the spinal canal (Fig. 1-6).[49] Most often, the dura only touches the border of the spinal

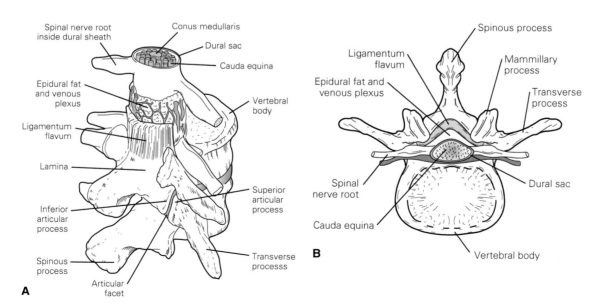

FIGURE 1-5. Lumbar vertebral column. (A) Posterolateral view. (B) Superior view, cross-section. *Used with permission from Cousins MJ, Veering BT. Epidural neural blockade. In: Cousins MJ, Bridenbaugh PO, eds, Neural Blockade in Clinical Anesthesia and Management of Pain, 3rd ed. Philadelphia, PA: Lippincott-Raven, 1998, pp. 243–321.*

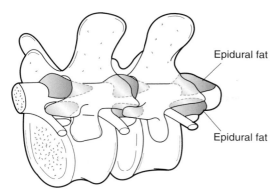

Epidural fat

Epidural fat

FIGURE 1-6. Discontinuous compartments of the epidural space. Note areas where the dura is directly adjacent to the bony canal, although not adherent to it. *Used with permission from Hogan QH. Lumbar epidural anatomy. A new look by cryomicrotome section. Anesthesiology 75:767–775, 1991.*

canal, but does not adhere to it. This permits the passage of catheters and solutions across segments. Only in rare cases, most probably following surgery or inflammation, the dura may be tethered to the bony spinal canal. This may explain some occurrences of inadvertent dural perforation during epidural needle placement or patchy epidural blockade.

The epidural space is discontinuous and is divided into posterior, lateral, and anterior compartments (Figs. 1-5 and 1-6). The posterior epidural space is of greatest relevance to the anesthesiologist because this is where the epidural needle is placed during epidural anesthesia. It is bordered posteriorly by the ligamentum flavum. The space between the two halves of the ligamentum flavum is filled by epidural fat, which is notable in that it is practically devoid of fibrous content.[50] The fat is connected to the ligamentum flavum and the dura by frail and incomplete membrane attachments only in the midline,[49] and encloses minute vessels that may penetrate the ligamentum flavum through small gaps in the midline.[44] The anterior-posterior dimension of the posterior epidural space is largest at midlumbar levels, decreases at thoracic levels, and disappears above C7.[46] Many investigators have attempted to define how far one can advance a lumbar epidural needle that has just perforated the ligamentum flavum before puncturing the dura. Studies suggest this distance ranges from 2 to 20 mm among individuals.[49] Furthermore, it is important to consider that the "physiologic safety margin" is substantially decreased should the needle traverse the epidural space parallel to the midline, but off to the left or right side. Some investigators have alluded to a midline barrier, or membrane, within the posterior epidural space, but this has not been confirmed using refined techniques such as cryomicrotome sections.[51]

The lateral epidural space is occupied by the spinal nerves, fat, and vessels, and is characterized by widely open intervertebral foramina (Fig. 1-5), which serve to connect the epidural space with the paravertebral space. Increased intra-abdominal pressure is transmitted to the epidural and subarachnoid space through this open passage, and this may explain the enhanced extent of cephalad blockade in cases of increased abdominal pressure. The anterior internal venous vertebral plexus predominantly occupies the anterior epidural space.

▶ Epidural Space Pressure

Several factors contribute to the generation of subatmospheric pressure in the epidural space. The natural effects of Starling forces across capillary walls produce a low fluid pressure in all tissues on the basis of oncotic pressure. This results in subatmospheric pressure and tissue collapse in the spaces of the opposing surfaces of the spinal canal, including the planes where dura opposes epidural fat or the canal wall, and between epidural fat and the canal wall. Entry of a needle into these planes is signaled by the entry of a hanging drop into the needle hub. Additionally, dural tenting during needle advancement may also contribute to subatmospheric pressure. Finally, subatmospheric intrathoracic pressure is thought to contribute to the occurrence of subatmospheric epidural pressure at thoracic levels. Under conditions of severe obstructive lung disease, the subatmospheric pressure in the thoracic epidural space may be considerably attenuated.[47]

The pressure in the epidural space is important for several reasons. First, the *hanging-drop technique* used to identify entry into the epidural space directly relies on recognition of subatmospheric pressure in the spinal canal. In this respect, it is imperative to consider that subatmospheric pressure is most pronounced at cervical and thoracic levels, but is less reliable at lumbar levels. Secondly, recent reports indicate that presence of epidural pressure waveforms will reliably confirm needle position in the epidural space.[52] Lastly, increases in epidural pressure above its natural subatmospheric level by infusion of solutions may cause adverse effects by displacing cerebrospinal fluid (CSF), and thereby raising intracranial pressure.[53] This rise may be associated with impaired ocular venous outflow and subsequent retinal extravasation or hemorrhage.[54] The latter effects may be even more pronounced under conditions of diagnostic[55] and surgical[56] epiduroscopy, when high fluid pressures are used to distend the epidural space.

Impaired ocular venous outflow may explain recently reported cases of vision loss associated with epidural drug injection and epiduroscopy.[54–59] These reports, however, were associated with a wide range of fluid volumes injected into the epidural space, ranging from epidural test doses to artificial distention of the epidural space during epiduroscopy. The direct relationship among epidural anesthesia, epiduroscopy, and retinal hemodynamics has not been investigated. Finally, epidural pressure rises much more abruptly in infants during epidural injection; therefore a slower injection speed is recommended in this patient population.[60]

AGE-RELATED CHANGES OF SPINAL ANATOMY

Effects of age on bony anatomy are considerable, and these changes influence spinal canal puncture and spread of local anesthetics. Epiduroscopy has revealed that the epidural fat content is smaller in aged individuals,[48] although distortion of the epidural space by epiduroscopy may bias such observations. The loss of epidural fat with age is of special importance, since the latter is assumed to act as a separate compartment for local anesthetic and other drugs during epidural anesthesia.[47] Significant negative effects of fat volume on degree and onset of motor block have been reported.[61]

SPINAL CANAL CONTENTS

▶ Spinal Cord

The *spinal cord* is an extension of the central nervous system (CNS) into the vertebral canal, and is the conduit between the periphery (via spinal nerves) and the brain. For a given patient, it is approximately as wide as the individual's little finger, and, in adults, extends from the atlas to the first or second lumbar vertebral level (Fig. 1-7). In the embryo, the spinal cord spans the entire length of the vertebral column, and spinal nerves emerge at the level of their corresponding intervertebral foramen. Subsequent growth of the vertebral column, however, is faster than that of the spinal cord, and by the sixth month of gestation, the spinal cord only extends caudad to the first sacral vertebra, and at birth it reaches the third lumbar vertebra. Therefore, lumbar and sacral spinal nerves of the adult, after emerging from the spinal cord, follow a steep downward trajectory before reaching their respective intervertebral foramen (Fig. 1-7). The anterior and posterior roots of the most caudal spinal nerves emerge from the conical terminus of the spinal cord (the *conus medullaris*) and form a bundle of nerves referred to as the *cauda equina*. The pia mater continues caudally from the conus medullaris as a rudimentary neuron-free structure, the *filum terminale*.[12]

Developmentally, the spinal cord is derived from the neural tube. Primordial sensory neurons responsible for deep sensory perception extend into the developing sclerotomes. New neural connections are later established with the dermatome, and these neurons later become the surface mechanoreceptors and nociceptors. Other fibers arising from

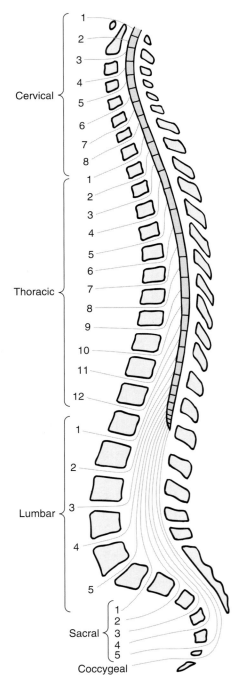

FIGURE 1-7. Schematic longitudinal section of the vertebral canal, spinal cord, and spinal nerve roots. *Used with permission from Waxman SG. Clinical Neuroanatomy, 25th ed. New York: McGraw-Hill, 2003, p. 47.*

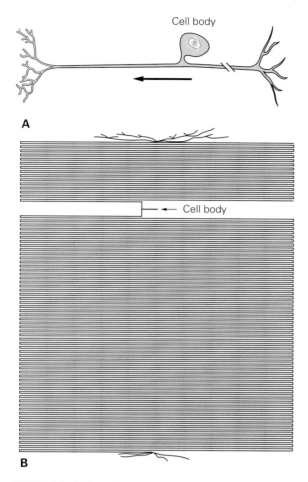

A

B

Cell body

Cell body

FIGURE 1-8. (A) Conventional view of the dorsal root ganglion, the direction of impulse propagation being indicated by an arrow. (B) Actual relationship in size between neuronal cell body and axon. *Used with permission Devor M. Unexplained peculiarities of the dorsal root ganglion. Pain Suppl 6:S27, 1999.*

the ventral part of the spinal cord follow the developing muscles, and these functional units later correspond to the myotomes. Sensory fibers providing proprioceptive innervation to the musculature accompany these fibers.[62]

The primary sensory neurons of the dorsal root ganglia are initially bipolar, but later become pseudounipolar with a single process that branches into a peripheral and central axon. This T-branch has been implicated in filtering afferent information.[63–64] Neuroepithelial cells surround the dorsal root ganglion neurons as satellite cells. The dorsal root ganglion has received attention as a potential pathogenic site for chronic neuropathic pain.[65] Its peculiar location in the intervertebral foramen and its distinct morphology are not fully understood.[66] For example, it is not clear whether

impulse propagation up the T-branch into the neuronal soma has any physiologic role (Fig. 1-8).

Macroscopically, the spinal cord features two portions with enlarged diameters, the cervical (C3 to T2) and lumbosacral (T9 to L2) enlargements, corresponding approximately to the origin of the nerves supplying the arm and leg, respectively.

In transverse section, the gray center of the spinal cord resembles a butterfly, with ventral and dorsal horns on either side corresponding to sites of motor and sensory regulation. In the midline, the spinal cord is largely divided by the ventral median fissure and dorsal median sulcus (Fig. 1-9).

Spinal Nerves

The spinal cord connects with the periphery by way of 31 pairs of spinal nerves, each composed of several radicular filaments (Figs. 1-7 and 1-9). The human spinal nerve pairs are subdivided into 8 cervical, 12 thoracic, 5 lumbar, 5 sacral, and 1 coccygeal pair of nerves. The ventral root of the spinal nerve emerges from the ventral horn of the gray substance in the *radicular area*, whereas the dorsal roots emerge in the *radicular line*. They join to form the spinal nerve before dividing into the anterior (ventral) and posterior (ventral) rami (Fig. 1-10). The spinal nerves supply the meninges by way of the *meningeal ramus*, and feature communicating rami with the sympathetic trunk (from spinal nerve to sympathetic trunk: white communicating ramus, from sympathetic trunk to spinal nerve: gray communicating ramus) (see "Anatomy of the Autonomous Nervous System," below).

Myelin

Peripheral and central neurons are ensheathed to a variable extent by Schwann cells and oligodendrocytes, respectively. The sheath is collectively referred to as myelin, and consists of cytoplasmic processes wrapped spirally around the axon

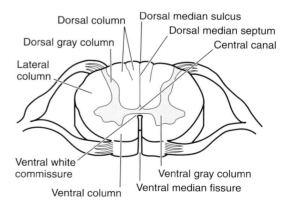

FIGURE 1-9. Cross-section of the spinal cord. *Used with permission from Waxman SG. Clinical Neuroanatomy, 25th ed. New York: McGraw-Hill, 2003, p. 48.*

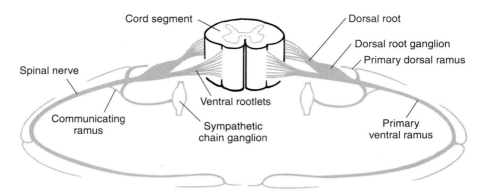

FIGURE 1-10. Cross-section of spinal cord with spinal nerve roots, ganglia, and its branches. Note communicating circuit between spinal nerve and sympathetic chain ganglion. *Used with permission from Waxman SG. Clinical Neuroanatomy, 25th ed. New York: McGraw-Hill, 2006, p. 49.*

(Fig. 1-11 and Fig. 1-12). It is important to note that several Schwann cells accompany a single axon, each covering a circumscribed portion. Axons are designated as unmyelinated when the Schwann cell simultaneously ensheathes segments of several axons at once. In myelinated axons, each Schwann cell ensheathes only one neuron (Fig. 1-11). The process by which the complex geometrical myelin structure is formed begins when a Schwann cell encloses part of an axon. Subsequently, an active process (myelogenesis) leads to the formation of lamellae around the neuron. Finally, the myelin matures, and the cytoplasm is largely extruded from these lamellae, leaving behind a membrane complex rich in lipids and proteins. This membrane complex is interrupted at so-called *nodes of Ranvier* (Fig. 1-12). These are essential to impulse propagation, and Na^+ and K^+ channels are abundant in these areas (see Chap. 3).

The most obvious function of the myelin sheath is to enhance the propagation of action potentials along the axon. Whereas unmyelinated neurons propagate action potentials continuously along the axon, myelinated nerves are capable of accelerated saltatory (*jumping*) propagation, which occurs at the nodes of Ranvier.

The simplistic view of the myelin sheath as a mere insulator has been largely revised, and Schwann cells appear to be more versatile and essential than previously assumed.[67–69] For example, the Schwann cell depends on neuronal signals for its survival. In turn, Schwann cells influence the specific localization of ion channels in and around nodes of Ranvier. Furthermore, axonal transport and diameter depend on supporting glia cells. Lastly, recent evidence implicates glial activation as a major causative factor in the generation of chronic neuropathic pain.[70]

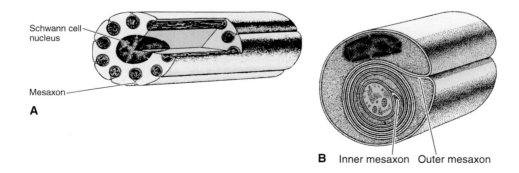

FIGURE 1-11. Nerve fibers. (A) Unmyelinated nerve fibers: the most frequent type of unmyelinated nerve fiber in which isolated axons are surrounded by a Schwann cell. (B) Myelinated nerve fiber: the Schwann cell forms lamellae around the axon. *Used with permission from Junqueira LC, Carneiro J. Basic Histology, 11th ed. New York: McGraw-Hill, 2005.*

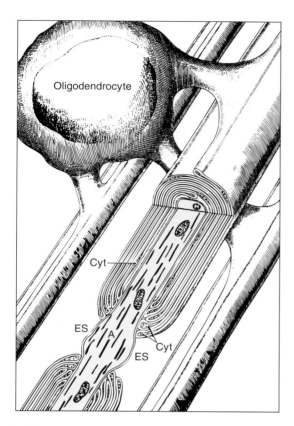

FIGURE 1-12. Nerve in the central nervous system. A single oligodendrocyte myelinates an entire family of axons. The myelin is periodically interrupted at nodes of Ranvier where the axon (A) is exposed to extracellular space (ES). Cyt: oligodendrocyte cytoplasm. *Used with permission from Junqueira LC, Carneiro J. Basic Histology, 11th ed. New York: McGraw-Hill, 2005 (redrawn with permission from Bunge M, Bunge R, Pappas G. J Biophys Biochem Cytol 10:67, 1961).*

▶ Dermatomes and Myotomes

A *dermatome* is defined as the cutaneous area supplied by a single spinal nerve (Fig. 1-13 and Table 1-1). In contrast, a *myotome* is defined as the muscles developmentally stemming from one somite, supplied by one spinal nerve (Table 1-2). Knowledge of cutaneous and motor neuronal projections is essential to preoperatively plan the necessary extent of neuraxial anesthesia for a specific operation. It is important to note that internal organs are innervated differently, and anesthesia of a cutaneous region does not necessarily confer anesthesia to underlying viscera (Table 1-3). Moreover, there is considerable overlap in spinal nerve innervation of adjacent dermatomes.

Table 1-1

Surface Anatomy and Dermatome Levels

Surface Anatomy	Sensory Dermatome
Perineum	S2-S4
Lateral foot	S1
Inguinal ligament	T12
Umbilicus	T10
Tip of xiphoid process	T7
Nipple	T4
Inner aspect of arm and forearm	T1-T2
Fifth finger	C8
Thumb	C6
Clavicle	C5

▶ Meninges

The dura mater encloses the CNS. It is composed of collagen fibers, which form a dense and solid membrane that typically yields to some degree to an advancing epidural needle (Fig. 1-5). On the inner aspect of the dura mater, the arachnoid mater is loosely attached. The latter is a fine membrane that ensheathes the subarachnoid space and the cerebrospinal fluid (CSF) (Fig. 1-14). A physiologically active barrier is maintained by arachnoid cells and the basal lamina, which feature tight intracellular junctions, and the pia mater.[71] Because the dura mater is mostly composed of collagen fibers, it can be easily punctured like a sheet of paper. In contrast, the arachnoid layer is more flexible, and may tent when a needle is advanced beyond the dural membrane to achieve spinal anesthesia.[47] The potential space between the dura and arachnoid mater is called the subdural space. This space can expand when small veins traversing the arachnoid rupture in response to shear stress, resulting in subdural hemorrhage.

Recent evidence, however, suggests that subsequent to mechanical stress, a cleft forms more easily between layers of arachnoid than between the arachnoid and dura.[72,73] Therefore, the term subdural space may need to be redefined, or replaced by a more appropriate name. Few studies exist as to the subsequent spread of solutions injected subdurally. While some have proposed that subdural solution does not propagate laterally, a study of intentional subdural injection has demonstrated spread along nerve roots.[74]

Recent literature has moved away from the concept of a potential subdural space containing minute amounts of fluid[75] toward the notion that accumulation of fluid in the "subdural" space only occurs after tissue damage.[76] The interface between the dura and arachnoid is unique, and the fibroblasts

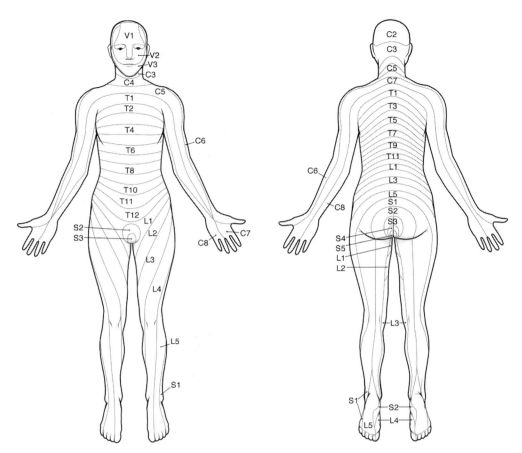

FIGURE 1-13. Distribution of dermatomes. *Used with permission from Cunningham FG, Leveno KL, Bloom SL, et al. Williams Obstetrics, 22nd ed. New York: McGraw-Hill, 2005.*

Table 1-2

Myotomes

Spinal Nerve	Peripheral Nerve(s)	Innervated Muscle(s)	Function
C5-C6	Musculocutaneous	Biceps, brachialis	Elbow flexion
C7-C8	Radial	Triceps	Elbow extension
L2-L3	Lumbar plexus branches	Iliopsoas	Hip flexion
L4-L5	Inferior/superior gluteal	Gluteal muscles	Hip extension
L5-S1	Tibial Common peroneal	Hamstring	Knee flexion
L2-L4	Femoral	Quadriceps femoris	Knee extension
L4-S1	Deep peroneal	Anterior tibial Digital extensors	Ankle flexion
S1-S2	Tibial	Triceps surae	Ankle extension

Table 1-3

Dermatome Level of Visceral Innervation

Type of Operation	Upper Dermatomal Level of Blockade	Anatomic Landmark
Esophagus, lung	T1	Below clavicle
Upper abdomen	T1	Below clavicle
Lower abdomen	T6	Distal sternum
Cesarean delivery	T4	Nipples
Knee/foot	L1-L2	Inguinal crease

located at this interface have been described as *dural border cells*, featuring intracellular spaces, decreased collagen content, and few cell junctions (Fig. 1-15).[76,77] Therefore, this region is prone to injury, and may readily shear open following, for example, needle penetration.[76] This hypothesis has been further supported by experiments showing that injection of blood into the layer of dural border cells separated dura and arachnoid membranes at this weakest point of the meninges.[76,78]

When compared with the anterior subarachnoid space, which is practically devoid of connective tissue, the posterior subarachnoid compartment comprises a variety of fibrous tissues forming membrane-like structures.[79] They are thought to constitute residues of embryologic connective tissue, which gradually degenerates, and loses cellular content. This process begins in the anterior subarachnoid space and progresses posteriorly.[80] Rudimentary trabeculae may persist as a random mesh, and connect the pia and arachnoid mater.

The pia mater is the third meningeal layer. It encases the spinal cord and its blood vessels, and nerve roots and blood vessels in the subarachnoid space. Since arachnoid and pia mater share a common embryologic origin (the inner lamella of the primitive meninx) and are similar in ultrastructure, they are often summarized as leptomeninges. Depending upon the exact site, the pia mater may consist of a single layer, or be arranged in multiple layers.[76]

The spinal cord is suspended within the dural sac by denticulate ligaments. These are stronger than trabeculae and extend from the lateral surface of the spinal cord (Fig. 1-14). This suspension is further supported by the brain stem and connective tissue, and facilitated by the CSF. Nerve roots can not participate in fastening the spinal cord, since they are very sensitive to stretch. The *subarachnoid septum* or *septum posticum* is a membrane that spans the subarachnoid space from the posterior midline of the cord to the arachnoid. It is often discontinuous and has been demonstrated in cadaver dissection in about one third of cases at lumbar levels, and very commonly at thoracic and cervical levels.[46,49,51] These membranes may be responsible for the asymmetric spread of anesthetics, although no studies exist to prove this hypothesis. The spread of myelogram dye injected in high volumes is usually not substantially confined by membranous subarachnoid elements.

Among the variations encountered in the subarachnoid space, cysts may pose considerable problems to the anesthesiologist. These cysts are recesses within the subarachnoid septum that communicate with the subarachnoid space. Mixture of fluids is typically dependent upon body posture. Cysts, as such, rarely cause symptoms, but may be a cause of inadequate spinal anesthesia. The anesthetic solution injected into CSF in the cyst may only slowly equilibrate with CSF outside the cyst in the subarachnoid space. In asymptomatic subjects, cysts have been demonstrated in 45%[81] to 84%[82] of upright films when large amounts of oily contrast medium were used. When modern contrast agents are employed, cysts are thought to opacify very rapidly, such that they are now rarely seen in routine imaging.

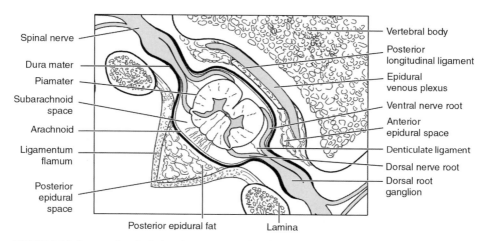

Spinal nerve
Dura mater
Piamater
Subarachnoid space
Arachnoid
Ligamentum flamum
Posterior epidural space
Posterior epidural fat
Lamina
Vertebral body
Posterior longitudinal ligament
Epidural venous plexus
Ventral nerve root
Anterior epidural space
Denticulate ligament
Dorsal nerve root
Dorsal root ganglion

FIGURE 1-14. Cross-section of spinal cord, nerve roots, and meninges.

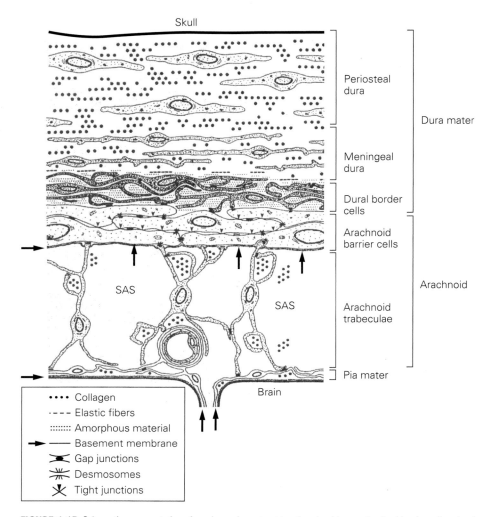

Skull

Periosteal
dura

Meningeal
dura

Dura mater

Dural border
cells

Arachnoid
barrier cells

SAS

SAS

Arachnoid
trabeculae

Arachnoid

Pia mater

Brain

```
•••• Collagen
- - - Elastic fibers
::::::: Amorphous material
——— Basement membrane
⋈ Gap junctions
⋇ Desmosomes
⋏ Tight junctions
```

FIGURE 1-15. Schematic representation of meninges. In contrast to other dural layers, the dural border cell region features fibroblasts, but no collagen, enlarged extracellular spaces, and few cell junctions. SAS: subarachnoid space. *Used with permission from Haines DE. On the question of a subdural space. Anat Rec 230:3, 1991.*

Similar to the fashion in which the subarachnoid nerves and blood vessels are ensheathed in pia mater, the dura and arachnoid membranes continue to ensheathe the spinal nerves as they exit the dural sac and enter the intervertebral foramena. This meningeal covering extends as far laterally as the dorsal root ganglion (Fig. 1-14).[83] The lateral dural extensions serve to fix the dural sac within the spinal column. This suspension is additionally reinforced by epidural ligaments connecting the dura to the periosteum of the vertebrae. Here, the arachnoid folds back along the nerve root, and forms a cul-de-sac. This dead end is approximately 6 mm wide at lumbar levels, and up to 15 mm at sacral levels.[84] In this lateral area the dural membrane is eroded by arachnoid villi. The villi may be filled with CSF and herniate outside the dural cuff. These protrusions have been likened to arachnoid granulations in the cranium.[85,86] When ink was injected into the CSF, lateral pouches were stained, as was epidural fat and lymphatics, suggesting that villi may be a source of CSF loss.[87]

It is assumed, however, that in addition to villous protrusions, other passageways must exist to explain the transport of material out of the CSF in the lateral nerve root cuff region. It should be noted that however tempting it is to compare spinal arachnoid protrusions with their intracranial counterparts, the former do not drain into a vein, and lack the connective tissue geometry necessary for a controlled flow of liquid.[88] The nerve root cuff laterally is filled with cellular debris and macrophages,[89] and could therefore play an important role in the cleansing of the subarachnoid space. Finally, it has been suggested that these cuffs may facilitate the entry of epidural local anesthetic into the subarachnoid space, although there is little evidence to support this mechanism. Moreover, the nerve roots are very close to the dura mater, and the amount of CSF present in nerve root cuffs to dilute the anesthetic is minimal. This may, at least in part, explain the segmental onset of epidural anesthesia, with the nerve roots at the site of injection being more rapidly blocked than those in the subarachnoid space exiting via more caudal intervertebral foramina.

As mentioned previously, nerve root cuff arachnoid granulations may herniate outside the dural sac.[90] Of clinical importance, these recesses can expand into the spinal canal, typically at lower thoracic levels.[91] Referred to as arachnoid or perineural cysts depending upon their exact location, their exact prevalence in asymptomatic individuals is not agreed upon in literature, and reported incidences range between 9 and 37%.[92] Unfortunately, in some patients these cysts may erode bony structures and cause substantial symptoms. One particularly severe form of arachnoid cyst, Tarlov cysts, originate at sacral levels and can destroy the os sacrum. The term anterior sacral meningocele is reserved for those cases in which the cyst protrudes into the pelvic cavity.[93] Tarlov cysts may be inherited.[94] Next to genetic predisposition, age seems to be an important risk factor, since small cysts (less than 7 mm in size) are observed in a third of aged subjects at cervical levels.[95]

Theoretically, injection of local anesthetic into the nerve root cuff may occur during paravertebral anesthesia. It should be noted, however, that the farthest lateral extension of the nerve root cuff occurs at the sacral level, while at more cranial levels, the sheath typically ends more proximally.[96] For this reason, the risk of injecting local anesthetic into the sheath during paravertebral anesthesia is virtually nonexistent, unless the needle is driven into the intervertebral foramen.

Degenerating and facet joint capsules are another type of cystic structure that may potentially impede neuraxial anesthesia. Most commonly these are found at lumbar levels and can cause compression of the dural sac or nerve roots.[97] These cysts are called synovial cysts when synovia is demonstrated upon histological examination, or ganglion cysts. Very infrequently these cysts may arise from spinal ligaments or the dura mater. Since the cysts constitute separate cavities and do not communicate with the subarachnoid or epidural space, they may be an explanation for failed spinal or epidural anesthesia.

▶ Cerebrospinal Fluid

The CNS is surrounded by CSF, which is essentially an ultrafiltrate of the blood. About 500 mL of CSF is formed each day,[98,99] mostly by choroid plexuses of the cerebral ventricles, and possibly by ependyma, pia mater, and brain parenchyma.[100,101] Formation of CSF is achieved by active secretion from the choroid epithelium, and filtration of plasma across the endothelial wall of the choroid capillary.[102] The production of CSF is age-dependent, and production rate decreases by about half in the elderly.[103] CSF appears to be in substantial contact with the cerebral interstitial fluid.[104] The main functions of CSF are to provide a fluid cushion for the CNS, to drain products of cerebral metabolism, and possibly to serve as a pathway to distribute mediators within the CNS.[105]

Developmentally, the choroid plexus forms as tortuous arteries covered by pia mater begin to protrude into the ventricle during development, and are then covered by plexus epithelium. Therefore, the blood-CSF barrier consists of blood vessels covered by pia mater connective tissue, and plexus epithelium (ependyma). It is connected to the pia mater on the outer surface of the brain by a rudimentary cleft, the choroid fissure.[62]

The choroid plexus is found exclusively within the ventricles. It is attached to the roof of the third ventricle (two layers of choroid plexus overlap in what is commonly referred to as the *tela choroidea*), the central and temporal portion of the lateral ventricle, and the fourth ventricle. The plexus sometimes protrudes out of the ventricular system through the lateral foramen (of Luschka) of the fourth ventricle.

CSF begins to circulate in the fifth post-conceptual week.[62] In the adult, unidirectional bulk flow fueled by the arteriovenous pressure gradient distributes the fluid from the cerebral ventricular system to the cisterns at the base of the brain (Fig. 1-16). Most CSF flows along the convexities of the brain toward the arachnoid granulations (also called *Pacchionian bodies*) along the sagittal sinus. Arachnoid granulations are macroscopic defects in the dura through which arachnoid membrane herniates, and probably account for much of the CSF absorption back into the venous circulation, although other mechanisms are also present. In particular, the spinal nerve sheaths with their dense venous and lymphatic vascularization contribute to CSF resorption. A minority of CSF leaves the cranial cavity and enters the spinal subarachnoid space to circulate. It has been estimated that less than 10% of newly produced CSF actually follows this pathway.[49]

Superimposed on bulk CSF flow is a longitudinal oscillation of the CSF column in synchrony with the pulsations of the arteries in the skull.[106] Pulsations of the CSF are most prominent just below the foramen magnum, where they compensate for arterial filling of large intracranial vessels.[107,108]

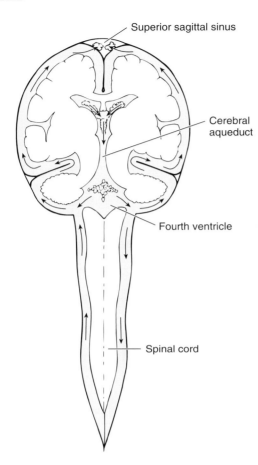

FIGURE 1-16. Cranial and spinal circulation of CSF, coronal section. *Used with permission from Waxman SG. Clinical Neuroanatomy, 25th ed. New York: McGraw-Hill, 2003, p 160.*

The amplitude of this movement is approximately 9 mm per cycle in the cervical CSF and 4 mm at the thoracolumbar junction, with minimal movement being observed in the distal lumbar sac. Oscillatory CSF pulsation is a possible, but unexplored, mechanism for local anesthetic distribution after subarachnoid injection, and its dependence on intra-abdominal pressure may explain the prolonged duration of spinal anesthesia in pregnant and obese patients.[49] However, other mechanisms are likely to contribute to spinal CSF circulation, such as respiration and slow-frequency flow waves.[107] Material injected into the lumbar CSF ascends to the basal cisterns within an hour.[109]

Without imaging techniques such as magnetic resonance tomography, the volume of spinal CSF in a given patient cannot be estimated, although a correlation with body mass index has been described.[110] This is unfortunate, since CSF volume is a key factor in the dilution of subarachnoid anesthetic solutions, and hence its concentration in the CSF. When considering the total CSF volume of 2 mL/kg body weight (approximately 140 mL), the estimates for the spinal subarachnoid volume range between 30 and 80 mL, and imaging studies show large inter-individual variation. Lumbar CSF volume has been estimated at 30 to 40 mL, critically depending upon respiratory changes and abdominal compression.[111]

Other CSF characteristics, however, contribute to the extent and duration of spinal anesthesia. For example, CSF velocity and density may substantially influence extent and duration of spinal anesthesia.

Cerebrospinal Fluid Composition

The composition of CSF is similar to serum, but with a lower pH, potassium and glucose (about half to two-thirds of concurrent serum concentration) content, and a higher PCO_2, magnesium, sodium, and chloride content (Table 1-4). CSF protein concentration is much less than serum concentration (approximately 5%), with a higher concentration in the lumbar CSF compared to ventricular CSF. The concentration of protein is lowest in the ventricular system. Specific gravity of lumbar CSF is about 1.006, with decreased density in pregnant women and the immediate postpartum period (see Chap. 3).[112] This has relevance during spinal anesthesia, since even changes in CSF density as small as 0.0006 g/mL may profoundly influence intrathecal drug distribution.[113,114]

The lower CSF protein concentration makes it more susceptible to changes in acid-base parameters. This is beneficial, since intracranial chemoreceptors (e.g., those located on the floor of the fourth ventricle) can rapidly respond to changes. In contrast, lumbar CSF does not reflect systemic acid-base changes as quickly, probably due to its site off the main CSF flow pathways. Proteins in the CSF are largely derived from blood (e.g., albumin, which accounts for up to 80% of CSF protein[115]), but there is also substantial brain-derived protein in the CSF. These proteins are not, however,

Table 1-4	
CSF Composition	
pH	7.32
PCO_2	47 mmHg
Na	142–150 meq/L
K	2.2–3.2 meq/L
Cl	120–130 meq/L
Glucose*	45–80 mg/dL
Protein	5–45 mg/dL
Specific gravity at body temperature	1.003–1.007

*Usually about 20 mg/dL less than blood glucose.
†Specific gravity varies with patient population (see Chap. 3).

brain-specific. Furthermore, pathologic conditions, such as multiple sclerosis, may be associated with modulated CSF protein composition. In particular, the previously accepted notion that CSF proteins were a simple function of blood protein content and blood-CSF barrier leakage has been dismissed. It has become evident that CSF proteins can traverse the blood-brain barrier and can be detected in the systemic circulation.[101]

Particulate matter as large as 7μ may pass through the granulations from CSF into venous blood[116] and electron microscopy has confirmed widened intracellular spaces[117] and transcellular fenestrations[118] in arachnoid granulations. These passages open only when exposed to CSF pressure in excess of venous pressure, which assures that flow will only be from CSF to veins. The pressure-sensing feature of arachnoid granulations regulates CSF pressure to about 10–20 cm H_2O in the lateral position.[119]

▶ Blood Supply

Arteries

Arteries supplying the spinal cord are covered by the pia mater. They are supplied by the vertebral and segmental arteries.

The vertebral arteries, near their convergence into the basilar artery, give rise to the anterior and posterior spinal arteries (Fig. 1-17). The anterior spinal arteries join at the lower border of the olives to form one single anterior spinal artery, which lies in the ventral sulcus of the spinal cord and descends to the cauda equina (Fig. 1-18). The posterior spinal arteries divide on each side to give rise to arteries dorsal and ventral to the dorsal root, which then form an arterial network on the posterior aspect of the spinal cord. The anterior spinal artery supplies approximately the anterior two thirds of the spinal cord, while the posterior arteries and the arterial network of the pia mater supply the remainder of the cord. The circular anastomoses between the spinal arteries are commonly referred to as the *vasocorona medullaris*. The anterior spinal artery is thinnest at the midthoracic level, and this area represents the watershed area between the cranial and caudal blood supply areas. Relatively few thoracic segmental arteries feed the arterial network at this level and therefore, the midthoracic spinal cord is particularly vulnerable to ischemia.

The longitudinal arteries are further supplied by segmental anastomoses (*rami spinales*) along the entire axis, arising from the dorsal branches of vessels such as the deep and ascending cervical artery, the vertebral artery, and intercostal and iliac arteries (Fig. 1-17). These spinal rami enter the spinal canal via the intervertebral foramen, and supply the vertebral canal via an anterior and a posterior (peridural) ramus, and the meninges. Only a third of the

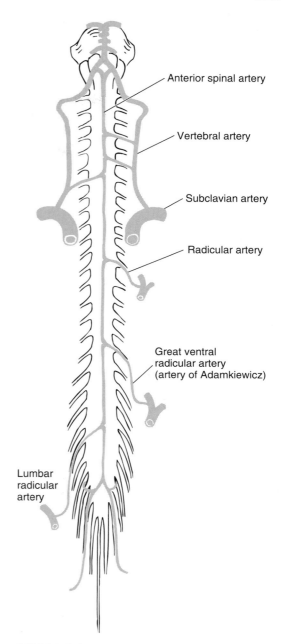

FIGURE 1-17. Arterial blood supply of the spinal cord, ventral view. *Used with permission from Waxman SG. Clinical Neuroanatomy, 25th ed. New York: McGraw-Hill, 2003, p. 73.*

Anterior spinal artery

Vertebral artery

Subclavian artery

Radicular artery

Great ventral radicular artery (artery of Adamkiewicz)

Lumbar radicular artery

segmental arteries reach the spinal arteries, but many are assumed to reach the spinal cord via small branches. In the vertebral canal the medullary artery continues as the nervomedullar artery. This gives rise to anterior and posterior *radicular* rami, which reach the spinal cord following along

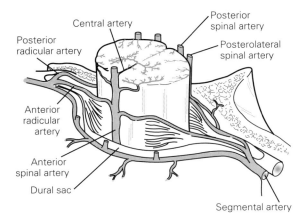

FIGURE 1-18. Arterial blood supply of the spinal cord, cross-section of single vertebral level. *Used with permission from Bridenbraugh PO, Greene NM, Brull SJ. Spinal (subarachnoid) neural blockade. In: Cousins MJ, Bridenbaugh PO, eds, Neural Blockade in Clinical Anesthesia and Management of Pain, 3rd ed. Philadelphia, PA: Lippincott-Raven, 1998, pp. 203–241.*

the ventral and dorsal root. The radicular rami of the entire vertebral column form longitudinal anastomoses in continuation of the anterior and posterior spinal arteries.

The most important caudal vessel supplying the longitudinal network is the *arteria radicularis magna* (artery of Adamkiewicz), which is a unilateral segmental branch, most often on the left side (Fig. 1-17).[120] Controversy exists as to whether the artery more frequently reaches the dural sac at one of the lower thoracic levels or at the first or second lumbar level.[120] In cases of a high radicularis magna artery, the lower segmental arteries are of larger diameter to accommodate blood flow to the lower spinal cord.

Veins

Spinal veins usually drain into the vertebral venous plexuses. Intramedullary veins join to form a plexus of anterior and posterior spinal veins within the pia mater. The anterior spinal vein drains the central spinal cord and ventral two-thirds of the gray matter, whereas the posterior spinal veins drain the posterior areas. Spinal veins form radicular veins, and join the internal venous vertebral plexuses situated within the epidural space. These veins are wide and lack venous valves. Furthermore, they anastomose with the basal intracranial sinuses. Intervertebral veins conduct blood from the internal venous plexuses to segmental veins (azygos, hemiazygos, ascending lumbar, and internal iliac vein). Because the thoracic intercostal veins drain into the azygos vein, and the lumbar veins drain into both the azygos vein, and the iliac vein and inferior vena cava, the

vertebral venous system may serve as an anastomosis between the superior and inferior venae cavae.

Lymphatics

No lymphatic vessels exist within the CNS. Rather, the CSF and the adventitial perivascular tissue perform this function. This fluid reaches the subarachnoid space via spaces of Virchow-Robin at the surface of the pia mater. There are lymphatic vessels outside the dura accompanying segmental nerves and vessels, which drain into segmental lymphatic vessels. These in turn drain into the intercostal lymphatics. This system is thought to contribute to the absorption of the CSF. However, direct data about lymphatic kinetics in the epidural space remain scarce. Epidural ink injection in rabbits shows that lymphatics begin draining particulate matter from the epidural space within 5 min.[121] Lymphatics appear to play a minor role in the uptake of epidural drugs,[122] but the dissipation of extruded disc material[123] and blood injected for the treatment of postlumbar puncture headache[124] indicate an active lymphatic system.

ANATOMY OF THE AUTONOMOUS NERVOUS SYSTEM

The vegetative or autonomous nervous system controls organ function and internal homeostasis, and reacts to endogenous and exogenous stressors. Visceral somatic afferents from nociceptors, mechanoreceptors, and chemoreceptors supply the afferent information, while efferent vegetative fibers innervate smooth muscle cells, and glands, and control reflexes such as coughing and vomiting. Complex autonomous reflexes necessitate processing in higher integration centers such as the hypothalamus or the cortex. It is notable that major regulatory centers are located outside of the CNS, that is, in ganglia and plexuses.

The sympathetic system arises from thoracic and lumbar centers, whereas the parasympathetic system is carried by the 3rd, 7th, 9th, and 10th cranial nerves, and sacral splanchnic nerves (from segments S2 to S4). Most target organs, such as the heart, are innervated by both sympathetic and parasympathetic fibers; however, there are obvious exceptions such as vessels supplying skin and skeletal musculature, that are solely innervated by sympathetic fibers. Preganglionic autonomic neurons arise from various regions within the CNS, such as the intermediolateral tract (sympathetic), nuclei of cranial nerves (parasympathetic), or the spinal cord (both sympathetic and parasympathetic), and are, in general, thinly myelinated. Postganglionic axons arising from vegetative ganglia are not myelinated. The intricate connections of the autonomic nervous system and subsequent reactions in response to neuraxial blockade make it essential to be aware of the autonomic nervous system anatomy. In general, autonomic sequelae of neuraxial block, whether desired or accidental, are almost exclusively due to sympathetic blockade.[125]

Parasympathetic Nervous System

The parasympathetic nervous system consists of cranial and sacral components (Fig. 1-19). The cranial parasympathetic system is associated with the oculomotor, facial, glossopharyngeal, and vagal nerves. It is relayed to postganglionic fibers in the parasympathetic cranial ganglia (ciliary, pterygopalatine, otic, and submandibular), or ganglia of cervical, thoracic, or abdominal viscera. While the oculomotor, facial, and glossopharyngeal nerves supply organs of the head and neck, the vagus nerve holds a unique position among the cranial nerves, in that its parasympathetic supply area comprises head, neck, the thoracic organs, and the parts of the digestive system supplied by the celiac and superior mesenteric arteries. In detail, it originates from the medulla oblongata to exit the cranium via the jugular foramen. From here, the vagus nerve runs caudally as the most posterior structure within the carotid sheath, behind the internal and common carotid arteries, and the internal jugular vein.

The left and right vagus nerves differ in their topographic relationships with surrounding structures. Specifically, the right vagus nerve passes between the subclavian artery and the innominate vein. Here, the right recurrent nerve branches off, wraps around the subclavian artery to reach its posterior surface, and subsequently runs cranially in the groove between trachea and esophagus to supply all laryngeal muscles except the cricothyroid muscle, and the laryngeal mucosa below the vocal cords. On the left side, the vagus nerve passes between the subclavian and common carotid artery, behind the innominate vein. Here, the left recurrent nerve originates, and winds around the aortic arch, subsequently following a cranial course similar to the right recurrent nerve, in the groove between trachea and esophagus. The reason for this rather strange difference in nerve topography between the right and the left side is explained by the fact that embryologically, the subclavian artery and the aortic arch arise from the arteries of the fourth branchial arch.

In the thoracic cavity, the vagus nerve surrounds the esophagus, forming the esophageal plexus, and supplies the cardiac and bronchial plexuses. In the abdomen, the left and right vagus nerves supply the anterior and posterior portion of the stomach, and consequently distribute into three main branches: hepatic, gastric, and celiac. Its supply area comprises the stomach, spleen, liver, pancreas, small intestine, and the large intestine as far as the left curvature.

The splanchnic component of the parasympathetic system is associated with the ventral rami of spinal nerves S2 to S4

(inferior hypogastric plexus, pelvic splanchnic nerves). It supplies the organs of the small pelvic cavity, and the descending and rectal part of the large intestine. Parasympathetic ganglia are found both in the connective tissue around organs, as well as within the walls of hollow viscera.

Sympathetic Nervous System

Preganglionic sympathetic fibers arise from the intermediolateral tract of the spinal cord from the eighth cervical to second lumbar segments (Fig. 1-20). Axons leave the spinal cord via the anterior root of the spinal nerve (Fig. 1-21). As a bundle, these myelinated axons form the white communicating ramus (ramus communicans albus). They synapse with cell bodies in the sympathetic ganglion of the *sympathetic trunk* or with cell bodies in one of several prevertebral ganglia. The sympathetic trunk is a bilateral chain of ganglia and connecting fibers, consisting of cervical, thoracic, lumbar, and sacral components, and the median ganglion impar. Most of the unmyelinated postsynaptic fibers leave the sympathetic ganglion via the gray communicating ramus (ramus communicans griseus). They rejoin the spinal nerve and supply sympathetic innervation to blood vessels, glands, and the erector pili muscle. Splanchnic nerves arise from the sympathetic chain, supply the viscera, and do not pass through a grey ramus. Some preganglionic axons travel up or down in the sympathetic trunk before synapsing. The postganglionic fibers of the prevertebral ganglia form the hypogastric, splanchnic, and mesenteric plexuses, and supply sympathetic innervation to the glands, smooth muscles, and blood vessels of the pelvic and abdominal viscera.

The adrenal gland is the only organ innervated by the sympathetic nervous system that is directly innervated by preganglionic, rather than postganglionic fibers (T9 to T10). Sympathetic stimulation of the adrenal gland causes the direct release of epinephrine and norepinephrine into the blood stream, rather than mediating the release of these neurotransmitters from postganglionic nerve endings.

Knowledge of the intricate relationships between the spinal nerves and the autonomous nervous system is essential to understand the consequences of both spinal and epidural anesthesia and analgesia. As a rule of thumb, sympathetic blockade during spinal anesthesia extends two segments beyond the sensory block, whereas the sympathetic block during epidural anesthesia is similar to the height of the sensory block (see Chap. 4).[125] Internal organs are shifted and rotated relative to their embryonic position; therefore, sensory dermatome innervation does not necessarily correspond to the innervation of the viscera deep to the skin (Table 1-3).

Two areas are of obvious interest in the performance of spinal and epidural anesthesia: the autonomic innervation of bladder and bowel. Sympathetic, parasympathetic, and

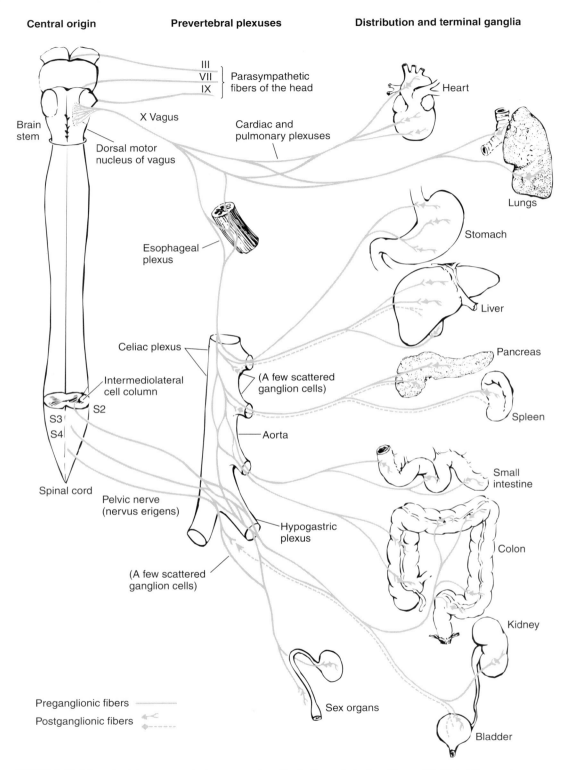

Central origin

Prevertebral plexuses

Distribution and terminal ganglia

III
VII
IX — Parasympathetic fibers of the head

Brain stem

X Vagus

Dorsal motor nucleus of vagus

Cardiac and pulmonary plexuses

Heart

Lungs

Esophageal plexus

Stomach

Liver

Celiac plexus

(A few scattered ganglion cells)

Pancreas

Intermediolateral cell column

S2

Aorta

Spleen

S3
S4

Small intestine

Spinal cord

Pelvic nerve (nervus erigens)

Hypogastric plexus

Colon

(A few scattered ganglion cells)

Kidney

Sex organs

Bladder

Preganglionic fibers
Postganglionic fibers

FIGURE 1-19. Schematic of the parasympathetic nervous system. *Used with permission from Waxman SG. Clinical Neuroanatomy, 25th ed. New York: McGraw-Hill, 2003, p. 255.*

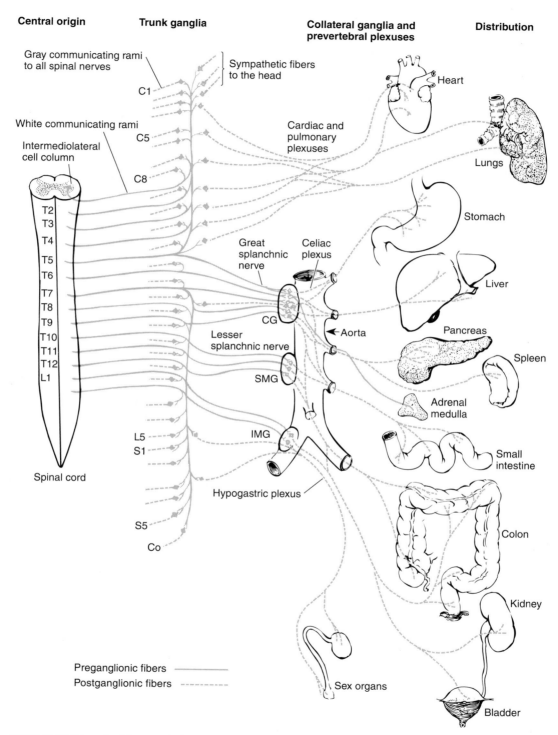

FIGURE 1-20. Schematic of the sympathetic nervous system. CG: celiac ganglion, SMG: superior mesenteric ganglion, IMG: inferior mesenteric ganglion. *Used with permission from Waxman SG. Clinical Neuroanatomy, 25th ed. New York: McGraw-Hill, 2003, p. 252.*

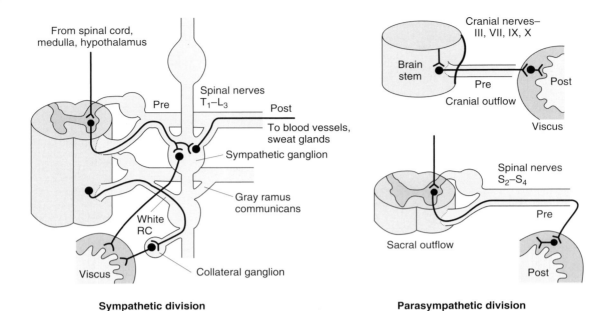

Sympathetic division

Parasympathetic division

FIGURE 1-21. Schematic of autonomic outflow from the central nervous system. RC: ramus communicans. *Used with permission from Waxman SG. Clinical Neuroanatomy, 25th ed. New York: McGraw-Hill, 2003, p. 253.*

somatic nerves innervate the bladder. Bladder preganglionic parasympathetic fibers originate at spinal cord levels S2 to S4, and reach the bladder via the inferior hypogastric plexus. Their function is to relax the internal sphincter and contract the detrusor muscle, culminating in micturition. Blockade of these fibers results in urinary retention, which may outlast sensory block duration. Sympathetic nerves to the bladder originate in the intermediolateral tract of the spinal segments T11 to L2. Preganglionic fibers pass through the sympathetic paravertebral ganglia, and reach the inferior mesenteric ganglion. Postganglionic fibers innervate the bladder to relax the detrusor muscle, and contract the internal sphincter, with the net effect of urinary retention. It is notable that blockade of thoracic sympathetic nerves may reduce the likelihood of acute urinary retention due to reflex sympathetic activity.[47] Somatic supply to the striated external urinary sphincter originates from the spinal cord levels S2 to S4.

Parasympathetic innervation to the bowel is via the vagus nerve to the stomach, the small intestine, and the ascending and transverse segments of the large intestine, whereas the pelvic splanchnic nerves supply the descending segment of the large intestine, the sigmoid, and the rectum. Sympathetic supply is achieved via the celiac, superior mesenteric, and inferior mesenteric ganglia. The latter is blocked during thoracic anesthesia, resulting in increased gastrointestinal motility. Mid- to low-thoracic sympathetic blockade may be associated with a dilation of splanchnic vascular beds and a marked decrease in preload to the right heart.

Neuraxial anesthesia and analgesia have been repeatedly shown to improve aspects of outcome following major surgery,[126] presumably by blocking the systemic stress response to surgery more reliably than general anesthesia. These effects may, at least in part, be explained by blockade of the sympathetic nervous system.

SUMMARY

Thorough knowledge of human anatomy is indispensable in performing regional anesthesia, especially in the case of neuraxial techniques. Even though imaging techniques such as ultrasound, and guidance devices such as nerve stimulators provide visual support to the anesthesiologist during nerve block procedures, neuraxial blockade techniques depend critically on three-dimensional anatomic understanding. This is even more so in cases where age-related degenerative disease complicates needle placement. Skeletal landmarks aid in determining the approximate level of injection. Next, the anatomic structures encountered during spinal or epidural puncture must be considered. The epidural space is organized into discontinuous compartments, occupied by blood vessels, fatty and fibrous tissues. The subarachnoid space is filled with CSF, the individual volume of which is impossible to predict without advanced imaging techniques. Blockade of somatic nerves is accompanied by autonomic nervous system blockade. During neuraxial blockade, effects on the sympathetic nervous system are largely responsible for undesirable side effects.

Even though anatomy is an ancient science, our perception of certain anatomic aspects has changed over time with the advent of new anesthetic and surgical techniques, and more sophisticated visualization of relevant structures. Therefore, anatomical research is not outdated; rather it constitutes a major contributor to guide development of new invasive procedures and to implement advanced imaging technology into clinical practice.

REFERENCES

1. Stonelake PS, Burwell RG, Webb JK. Variation in vertebral levels of the vertebra prominens and sacral dimples in subjects with scoliosis. *J Anat* 159:165, 1988.
2. Quinnell RC, Stockdale HR. The use of in vivo lumbar discography to assess the clinical significance of the position of the intercrestal line. *Spine* 8:305, 1983.
3. Render CA. The reproducibility of the iliac crest as a marker of lumbar spine level. *Anaesthesia* 51:1070, 1996.
4. Thavasothy M. The reproducibility of the iliac crest as a marker of lumbar spinal level. *Anaesthesia* 52:811, 1997.
5. Broadbent CR, Maxwell WB, Ferrie R, et al. Ability of anaesthetists to identify a marked lumbar interspace. *Anaesthesia* 55:1122, 2000.
6. Hogan Q. Epidural catheter tip position and distribution of injectate evaluated by computed tomography. *Anesthesiology* 90:964, 1999.
7. Lirk P, Messner H, Deibl M, et al. Accuracy in estimating the correct intervertebral space level during lumbar, thoracic and cervical epidural anaesthesia. *Acta Anaesthesiol Scand* 48:347, 2004.
8. Van Gessel EF, Forster A, Gamulin Z. Continuous spinal anesthesia: Where do spinal catheters go? *Anesth Analg* 76:1004, 1993.
9. Sjogren P, Gefke K, Banning AM, et al. Lumbar epidurography and epidural analgesia in cancer patients. *Pain* 36:305, 1989.
10. Gielen M, Slappendel R, Merx J. Asymmetric onset of sympathetic blockade in epidural anaesthesia shows no relation to epidural catheter position. *Acta Anaesthesiol Scand* 35:81, 1991.
11. Ievins FA. Accuracy of placement of extradural needles in the L3-4 interspace: Comparison of two methods of identifying L4. *Br J Anaesth* 66:381, 1991.
12. Gray H. In: Lewis WH, ed, *Gray's Anatomy*, 20th ed. New York: Bartleby, 2000.
13. Berry J, Moran J, Berg W, et al. A morphometric study of human lumbar and selected thoracic vertebrae. *Spine* 12:362, 1987.
14. Scoles P, Linton A, Latimer B, et al. Vertebral body and posterior element morphology: The normal spine in middle life. *Spine* 10:1082, 1988.
15. Hurme M, Alaranta H, Aalto T, et al. Lumbar spinal canal size of sciatica patients. *Acta Radiol* 30:353, 1989.
16. Panjabi M, Duranceau J, Goel V, et al. Cervical human vertebrae: Quantitative three-dimensional anatomy of the middle and lower region. *Spine* 16:861, 1991.
17. Panjabi M, Takata K, Goel V, et al. Thoracic human vertebrae: Quantitative three-dimensional anatomy. *Spine* 16:889, 1991.
18. Amonoo-Kuofi H. The sagittal diameter of the lumbar vertebral canal in normal adult Nigerians. *J Anat* 140:69, 1985.
19. Ericksen M. Some aspects of aging in the lumbar spine. *Am J Phys Anthropol* 45:575, 1976.
20. Willis T. An analysis of vertebral anomalies. *Am J Surg* 6:163, 1929.
21. Todd T. Numerical significance in the thoracolumbar vertebrae of the mammalia. *Anat Rec* 24:261, 1922.
22. Crighton I, Barry B, Hobbs G. A study of the anatomy of the caudal space using magnetic resonance imaging. *Br J Anaesth* 78:391, 1997.
23. Trotter M. Variations of the sacral canal: Their significance in the administration of caudal analgesia. *Anesth Analg* 26:192, 1947.
24. Sekiguchi M, Yabuki S, Satoh K, et al. An anatomic study of the sacral hiatus: A basis for successful caudal epidural block. *Clin J Pain* 20:51, 2004.
25. Miyasaka K, Kaneda K, Ito T, et al. Ossification of spinal ligaments causing thoracic radiculomyelopathy. *Radiology* 143:463, 1982.
26. Milne N. The role of zygapophysial joint orientation and uncinate processes in controlling motion in the cervical spine. *J Anat* 178:189, 1991.
27. Singer K, Breidahl P, Day R. Variations in zygapophyseal joint orientation and level of transition at the thoracolumbar junction. *Surg Radiol Anat* 10:291, 1988.
28. Davis P. The thoraco-lumbar mortice joint. *J Anat* 89:370, 1955.
29. Singer K. Thoracolumbar mortice joint: Radiological and histological observations. *Clin Biomech* (Bristol, Avon) 4:137, 1989.
30. Pal G, Routal R. A study of weight transmission through the cervical and upper thoracic regions of the vertebral column in man. *J Anat* 148:245, 1986.
31. Davis P. Human lower lumbar vertebrae: Some mechanical and osteological considerations. *J Anat* 95:337, 1961.
32. Yang K, King A. Mechanism of facet load transmission as a hypothesis for low-back pain. *Spine* 9:557, 1984.
33. Dory M. Arthrography of the lumbar facet joints. *Radiology* 140:23, 1981.
34. Moran R, O'Connell D, Walsh M. The diagnostic value of facet injections. *Spine* 13:1407, 1988.
35. Bogduk N, Engel R. The menisci of the lumbar zygapophyseal joints. *Spine* 9:454, 1984.
36. Wang Z, Yu S, Haughton V. Age-related changes in the lumbar facet joints. *Clin Anat* 2:55, 1989.
37. Giles L, Taylor J, Cockson A. Human zygapophyseal joint synovial folds. *Acta Anat* (Basel) 126:110, 1986.
38. Butler D, Trafimow J, Andersson G, et al. Discs degenerate before facets. *Spine* 15:111, 1990.
39. Epstein J, Epstein B, Lavine L, et al. Lumbar nerve root compression at the intervertebral foramina caused by arthritis of the posterior facets. *J Neurosurg* 39:362, 1973.
40. Heylings J. Supraspinous and intraspinous ligaments of the human lumbar spine. *J Anat* 125:127, 1978.
41. Williams D, Gabrielsen T, Latack J. Ossification in the caudal attachments of the ligamentum flavum. *Radiology* 145:693, 1982.
42. Williams D, Gabrielsen T, Latack J, et al. Ossification in the cephalic attachment of the ligamentum flavum. *Radiology* 150:423, 1984.
43. Maigne J, Ayral X, Guerin-Surville H. Frequency and size of ossifications in the caudal attachments of the ligamentum flavum of the thoracic spine. Role of rotatory strains in their development. *Surg Radiol Anat* 14:119, 1992.
44. Lirk P, Kolbitsch C, Putz G, et al. Cervical and high thoracic ligamentum flavum frequently fails to fuse in the midline. *Anesthesiology* 99:1387, 2003.

45. Lirk P, Moriggl B, Colvin J, et al. The incidence of lumbar ligamentum flavum midline gaps. *Anesth Analg* 98:1178, 2004.

46. Hogan QH. Epidural anatomy examined by cryomicrotome section. Influence of age, vertebral level, and disease. *Reg Anesth* 21:395, 1996.

47. Cousins M, Bridenbaugh P. *Neural Blockade in Clinical Anesthesia and Management of Pain*, 3rd ed. Philadelphia, PA: Lippincott Williams & Wilkins, 1998.

48. Igarashi T, Hirabayashi Y, Shimizu R, et al. The lumbar extradural structure changes with increasing age. *Br J Anaesth* 78:149, 1997.

49. Hogan QH. Epidural anatomy: New observations. *Can J Anaesth* 45:R40, 1998.

50. Ramsey RH. The anatomy of the ligamenta flava. *Clin Orthop* 44:129, 1966.

51. Hogan QH. Lumbar epidural anatomy. A new look by cryomicrotome section. *Anesthesiology* 75:767, 1991.

52. Ghia J, Arora S, Castillo M, et al. Confirmation of location of epidural catheters by epidural pressure waveform and computed tomography cathetergram. *Reg Anesth Pain Med* 26:337, 2001.

53. Hilt H, Gramm HJ, Link J. Changes in intracranial pressure associated with extradural anaesthesia. *Br J Anaesth* 58:676, 1986.

54. Day CJ, Shutt LE. Auditory, ocular, and facial complications of central neural block. A review of possible mechanisms. *Reg Anesth* 21:197, 1996.

55. Amirikia A, Scott IU, Murray TG, et al. Acute bilateral visual loss associated with retinal hemorrhages following epiduroscopy. *Arch Ophthalmol* 118:287, 2000.

56. Tabandeh H. Intraocular hemorrhages associated with endoscopic spinal surgery. *Am J Ophthalmol* 129:688, 2000.

57. Young WF. Transient blindness after lumbar epidural steroid injection: A case report and literature review. *Spine* 27:E476, 2002.

58. Gupta M, Puri P, Rennie IG. Anterior ischemic optic neuropathy after emergency caesarean section under epidural anesthesia. *Acta Anaesthesiol Scand* 46:751, 2002.

59. Purdy EP, Ajimal GS. Vision loss after lumbar epidural steroid injection. *Anesth Analg* 86:119, 1998.

60. Vas L, Raghavendran S, Hosalkar H, et al. A study of epidural pressures in infants. *Paediatr Anaesth* 11:575, 2001.

61. Higushi H, Adachi Y, Kazama T. Factors affecting the spread and duration of epidural anesthesia with ropivacaine. *Anesthesiology* 101:451, 2004.

62. Moore K, Persaud T. *The Developing Human. Clinically Oriented Embryology*, 5th ed. Philadelphia, PA: W.B. Saunders, 1993.

63. Luscher C, Streit J, Lipp P, et al. Action potential propagation through embryonic dorsal root ganglion cells in culture. II. Decrease of conduction reliability during repetitive stimulation. *J Neurophysiol* 72:634, 1994.

64. Luscher C, Streit J, Quadroni R, et al. Action potential propagation through embryonic dorsal root ganglion cells in culture. I. Influence of the cell morphology on propagation properties. *J Neurophysiol* 72:622, 1994.

65. Devor M, Seltzer Z. Pathophysiology of damaged nerves in relation to chronic pain. In: Wall PD, Melzack R, eds, *Textbook of Pain*. Edinburgh: Churchill Livingstone, 1999.

66. Devor M. Unexplained peculiarities of the dorsal root ganglion. *Pain* Suppl 6:S27, 1999.

67. Edgar J, Garbern J. The myelinated axon is dependent on the myelinating cell for support and maintenance: Molecules involved. *J Neurosci Res* 76:593, 2004.

68. Barres B, Barde Y. Neuronal and glial cell biology. *Curr Opin Neurobiol* 10:642, 2000.

69. Arroyo E, Xu Y, Zhou L, et al. Myelinating Schwann cells determine the internodal localization of Kv1.1, Kv1.2, Kvb2, and Caspr. *J Neurocytol* 28:333, 1999.

70. Wieseler-Frank J, Maier SF, Watkins LR. Glial activation and pathological pain. *Neurochem Int* 45:389, 2004.

71. Shanthaveerappa TR, Bourne GH. The "perineural epithelium," a metabolically active, continuous, protoplasmic cell barrier surrounding peripheral nerve fasciculi. *J Anat* 96:527, 1962.

72. Shantha TR. Subdural space: What is it? Does it exist? *Reg Anesth* 17:S85, 1992.

73. Collier CB. Accidental subdural injection during attempted lumbar epidural block may present as a failed or inadequate block: Radiographic evidence. *Reg Anesth Pain Med* 29:45, 2004.

74. Mehta M, Maher R. Injection into the extra-arachnoid subdural space. Experience in the treatment of intractable cervical pain and in the conduct of extradural (epidural) analgesia. *Anaesthesia* 32:760, 1977.

75. Collier CB. Accidental subdural block: Four more cases and a radiographic review. *Anaesth Intensive Care* 20:215, 1992.

76. Haines DE, Harkey HL, al-Mefty O. The "subdural" space: A new look at an outdated concept. *Neurosurgery* 32:111, 1993.

77. Nabeshima S, Reese TS, Landis DM, et al. Junctions in the meninges and marginal glia. *J Comp Neurol* 164:127, 1975.

78. Orlin JR, Osen KK, Hovig T. Subdural compartment in pig: A morphologic study with blood and horseradish peroxidase infused subdurally. *Anat Rec* 230:22, 1991.

79. Di Chiro G, Timins EL. Supine myelography and the septum posticum. *Radiology* 111:319, 1974.

80. Osaka K, Handa H, Matsumoto S, et al. Development of the cerebrospinal fluid pathway in the normal and abnormal human embryos. *Childs Brain* 6:26, 1980.

81. Teng P, Papatheodorou C. Spinal arachnoid diverticula. *Br J Radiol* 39:249, 1966.

82. Teng P, Rudner N. Multiple arachnoid diverticula. *AMA Arch Neurol* 2:348, 1960.

83. Brierley J. The penetration of particulate matter from the cerebrospinal fluid into the spinal ganglia, peripheral nerves, and perivascular spaces of the central nervous system. *J Neurol Neurosurg Psychiatr* 13:203, 1950.

84. Cohen M, Wall E, Brown R, et al. Cauda equina anatomy: II. Extrathecal nerve roots and dorsal root ganglia. *Spine* 15:1248, 1990.

85. Shantha T, Evans J. The relationship of epidural anesthesia to neural membranes and arachnoid villi. *Anesthesiology* 37:543, 1972.

86. Basmajian J. The depressions for the arachnoid granulations as a criterion of age. *Anat Rec* 112:843, 1952.

87. Brierley J, Field E. The connections of the spinal sub-arachnoid space with the lymphatic system. *J Anat* 82:153, 1948.

88. Hassin G. Villi (Pacchionian bodies) of the spinal arachnoid. *Arch Neurol Psychiatry* 23:65, 1930.

89. Himango W, Low F. The fine structure of a lateral recess of the subarachnoid space in the rat. *Anat Rec* 171:1, 1971.

90. Nabors M, Pait T, Byrd E, et al. Updated assessment and current classification of spinal meningeal cysts. *J Neurosurg* 68:366, 1988.

91. Gortvai P. Extradural cysts of the spinal canal. *J Neurol Neurosurg Psychiatr* 26:223, 1963.

92. Rexed B, Wennstrom K. Arachnoid proliferation and cystic formation in the spinal nerve-root pouches of man. *J Neurosurg* 16:73, 1959.

93. North R, Kidd D, Wang H. Occult, bilateral anterior sacral and intrasacral meningeal and perineural cysts: Case report and review of literature. *Neurosurgery* 27:981, 1990.

94. Thomas M, Halaby F, Hirschauer J. Hereditary occurrence of anterior sacral meningocele: Report of ten cases. *Spine* 12:351, 1987.

95. Holt S, Yates P. Cervical nerve root "cysts." *Brain* 87:481, 1964.

96. Lindblom K. The subarachnoid spaces of the root sheaths in the lumbar region. *Acta Radiol* 30:419, 1948.

97. Hemminghytt S, Daniels D, Williams A, et al. Intraspinal synovial cysts: Natural history and diagnosis by CT. *Radiology* 145:375, 1982.

98. Cuttler RW, Page L, Galicich P, et al. Formation and absorption of cerebrospinal fluid in man. *Brain* 91:707, 1968.

99. Rubin RC, Henderson ES, Ommaya A, et al. The production of cerebrospinal fluid in man and its modification by acetazolamide. *J Neurosurg* 25:430, 1966.

100. Oreskovic D, Whitton PS, Lupret V. Effect of intracranial pressure on cerebrospinal fluid formation in isolated brain ventricles. *Neuroscience* 41:773, 1991.

101. Milhorat TH. The third circulation revisited. *J Neurosurg* 42:628, 1975.

102. Reiber H. Proteins in cerebrospinal fluid and blood: Barriers, CSF flow rate and source-related dynamics. *Restor Neurol Neurosci* 21:79, 2003.

103. May C, Kaye JA, Atack JR, et al. Cerebrospinal fluid production is reduced in healthy aging. *Neurology* 40:500, 1990.

104. Abbott NJ. Evidence for bulk flow of brain interstitial fluid: Significance for physiology and pathology. *Neurochem Int* 45:545, 2004.

105. Segal MB. The choroid plexuses and the barriers between the blood and the cerebrospinal fluid. *Cell Mol Neurobiol* 20:183, 2000.

106. Enzmann DR, Pelc NJ. Normal flow patterns of intracranial and spinal cerebrospinal fluid defined with phase-contrast cine MR imaging. *Radiology* 178:467, 1991.

107. Friese S, Hamhaber U, Erb M, et al. The influence of pulse and respiration on spinal cerebrospinal fluid pulsation. *Invest Radiol* 39:120, 2004.

108. Henry-Feugeas MC, Idy-Peretti I, Baledent O, et al. Origin of subarachnoid cerebrospinal fluid pulsations: A phase-contrast MR analysis. *Magn Reson Imaging* 18:387, 2000.

109. Di Chiro G, Grove AS Jr. Evaluation of surgical and spontaneous cerebrospinal fluid shunts by isotope scanning. *J Neurosurg* 24:743, 1966.

110. Carpenter RL, Hogan QH, Liu SS, et al. Lumbosacral cerebrospinal fluid volume is the primary determinant of sensory block extent and duration during spinal anesthesia. *Anesthesiology* 89:24, 1998.

111. Lee RR, Abraham RA, Quinn CB. Dynamic physiologic changes in lumbar CSF volume quantitatively measured by three-dimensional fast spin-echo MRI. *Spine* 26:1172, 2001.

112. Richardson MG, Wissler RN. Density of lumbar cerebrospinal fluid in pregnant and nonpregnant humans. *Anesthesiology* 85:326, 1996.

113. Stienstra R, van Poorten JF. The temperature of bupivacaine 0.5% affects the sensory level of spinal anesthesia. *Anesth Analg* 67:272, 1988.

114. Stienstra R, Gielen M, Kroon JW, et al. The influence of temperature and speed of injection on the distribution of a solution containing bupivacaine and methylene blue in a spinal canal model. *Reg Anesth* 15:6, 1990.

115. Reiber H, Peter JB. Cerebrospinal fluid analysis: Disease-related data patterns and evaluation programs. *J Neurol Sci* 184:101, 2001.

116. Welch K, Pollay M. Perfusion of particles through arachnoid villi of the monkey. *Am J Physiol* 201:651, 1961.

117. Gomez DG, Potts DG. The surface characteristics of arachnoid granulations. *Arch Neurol* 31:88, 1974.

118. Levine JE, Povlishock JT, Becker DP. The morphological correlates of primate cerebrospinal fluid absorption. *Brain Res* 241:31, 1982.

119. Gilland O. Normal cerebrospinal-fluid pressure. *N Engl J Med* 280:904, 1969.

120. Biglioli P, Roberto M, Cannata A, et al. Upper and lower spinal cord blood supply: The continuity of the anterior spinal artery and the relevance of the lumbar arteries. *J Thorac Cardiovasc Surg* 127:1188, 2004.

121. Nohara Y, Brown MD, Eurell JC. Lymphatic drainage of epidural space in rabbits. *Orthop Clin North Am* 22:189, 1991.

122. Durant PA, Yaksh TL. Distribution in cerebrospinal fluid, blood, and lymph of epidurally injected morphine and inulin in dogs. *Anesth Analg* 65:583, 1986.

123. Saal JA, Saal JS, Herzog RJ. The natural history of lumbar intervertebral disc extrusions treated nonoperatively. *Spine* 15:683, 1990.

124. DiGiovanni AJ, Galbert MW, Wahle WM. Epidural injection of autologous blood for postlumbar-puncture headache. II. Additional clinical experiences and laboratory investigation. *Anesth Analg* 51:226, 1972.

125. Hogan Q. Cardiovascular response to sympathetic block by regional anesthesia. *Reg Anesth* 21:26, 1996.

126. Rigg JR, Jamrozik K, Myles PS, et al. Epidural anaesthesia and analgesia and outcome of major surgery: A randomised trial. *Lancet* 359:1276, 2002.

Technique of Neuraxial Anesthesia

Meltem Yilmaz
Cynthia A. Wong

CHAPTER 2

INTRODUCTION

The success of any neuraxial anesthetic depends on multiple factors. These factors include extensive knowledge of anatomy of the vertebral column and its contents, selection and preparation of patients, optimal patient positioning, appropriate monitoring, knowledge of the details and duration of the planned surgical procedure, appropriate choice of anesthetics, and finally the technique of neuraxial anesthesia. The technique of neuraxial anesthesia, including preparation, equipment, and monitoring, is the scope of this chapter. Without using the appropriate technique(s) one cannot provide safe, effective, and efficient anesthesia.

One of the more important factors to the success of neuraxial blockade is efficiency. Induction of anesthesia should not unnecessarily delay the surgical procedure, or surgeons and nurses will not be proponents of the technique. Neuraxial blockade can be performed in the operating room or a preoperative area while the preceding operative procedure is being completed or the operating room is being prepared for the patient. Regardless of where the actual procedure is performed, adequate space, proper lighting, equipment, and monitoring are of utmost importance to provide safe and efficient care of the patient. The designated area for performance of the neuraxial block procedure should have enough space for the physical comfort of the anesthesiologist, his or her assistant, and patient, as well as be equipped for resuscitation, should an emergency arise.

PREPARATION FOR NEURAXIAL ANESTHESIA

▶ Emergency Drugs and Supplies

Adverse events are fortunately relatively infrequent; however, immediate action must be taken when they occur in order to mitigate or prevent severe complications. The area where the block is to be performed must be equipped with an oxygen source, a means to administer positive pressure ventilation, suction, equipment for airway management, as well as emergency drugs (Box 2-1). The drugs should be placed in a drawer or a box which is immediately accessible and they should be checked on a regular basis for availability and expiration dates. Standardization of emergency equipment and resuscitation drugs in each anesthetizing location is recommended, as this will increase efficiency and decrease errors in an emergency situation. Finally, the physical space should be large enough to allow for ready access and resuscitation of the patient.

Box 2-1

Emergency Equipment and Drugs

Airway equipment

- ▶ Ambu bag with mask
- ▶ Oral and nasal airways (various sizes)
- ▶ Laryngoscope handles and blades
- ▶ Endotracheal tubes (various sizes)
- ▶ Endotracheal tube stylet
- ▶ Eschmann stylet
- ▶ Syringes (10 mL)

Emergency drugs

- ▶ Ephedrine
- ▶ Phenylephrine
- ▶ Epinephrine
- ▶ Atropine
- ▶ Sedative/hypnotic
- ▶ Succinylcholine

Syringes and needles

Patient Preparation

Patient preparation procedures that apply to general anesthesia apply to neuraxial anesthesia as well. Patients' last solid intake should have occurred more than 6 h, and clear liquids more than 2 h, prior to the induction of anesthesia. A thorough preoperative evaluation should be performed, followed by a discussion with the patient regarding the anesthetic plan and alternatives. Finally, informed, written consent should be obtained. One can argue that this is particularly important before the initiation of neuraxial anesthesia, as the patient will be awake and needs to know what to expect during the course of the anesthetic and operative procedure. A back-up plan in the event of neuraxial anesthesia failure should be discussed.

Monitoring

The majority of neuraxial blocks are performed smoothly and without any complications. However, there is a finite risk of total spinal anesthesia or symptomatic hypotension, and in the case of epidural or caudal blockade, inadvertent intrathecal or intravascular injection. For this reason, all patients undergoing neuraxial blockade should have vascular access and be monitored for the timely detection of any adverse effects.

Monitoring during the performance of neuraxial blockade should include recording the baseline level of consciousness, continuous pulse oximetry and heart rate (HR) monitoring, and intermittent noninvasive blood pressure measurement, as well as the availability of ECG monitoring. Intraoperative monitoring of patients should include the American Society of Anesthesiologists' standard monitoring, including the availability of temperature measurement.

Sedation

Light sedation may be administered before initiation of neuraxial blockade, if this is desired by the patient and deemed appropriate by the anesthesiologist. Generally, the patient should not be heavily sedated because successful spinal and epidural anesthesia requires patient participation to maintain good body position. In addition, the ability to effectively communicate is an essential part of the safe conduct of neuraxial anesthesia in older children and adults. Patients should be able to communicate the presence of paresthesias, and two-way communication is essential to properly evaluate the epidural test dose and degree of sensory blockade. On questioning, an awake and cooperative patient may be able to alert the anesthesiologist that the needle is not in the midline, thus assisting with correct needle placement. Once adequate anesthesia is assured, the patient can be sedated as

deemed appropriate. If the spinal or epidural block is performed in the preoperative holding area and neuraxial drugs have been injected, or sedation has been administered, the patient should not be left alone or unmonitored. Medical personnel, not a family member, should be present until the patient is transported to the operating room.

Patient Positioning

Careful attention to patient positioning is critical to successful spinal or epidural blockade. Spinal or epidural anesthesia can be performed in the sitting, lateral decubitus, or jackknife prone positions. Each position has advantages in specific situations. A number of factors should be considered when deciding the position of the patient for performing the neuraxial block procedure.

Neither the sitting nor the lateral position is consistently more comfortable for patients. The most comfortable position is likely to be the position in which the anesthesiologist can perform the procedure in the smoothest and fastest fashion. The sitting position allows for easier recognition of the midline, especially in obese patients, or those with scoliosis. Minimal sedation and analgesia may allow elderly patients with hip fractures to assume the sitting position. Heavily sedated patients, however, or those who are very ill, are better suited for the lateral decubitus position. Medical reasons to choose the lateral decubitus position include avoidance of the upright position in pregnant patients with an incompetent cervix or umbilical cord prolapse, or patients with hip fractures. The incidence of orthostatic hypotension or vasovagal syncope may be higher in the sitting position. Baricity of the intrathecal solution and site of surgery also play an important role in determining the optimal patient position. The left lateral recumbent position is preferred for right-handed physicians and right lateral recumbent position for left-handed physicians.

The jackknife prone position is used less often, but may be used when the planned surgical procedure is to be performed in this position. The use of intrathecal hypobaric local anesthetic solutions with the patient in jackknife position produces sacral anesthesia for perirectal surgery. The following discussion of patient positioning describes patient positioning for spinal anesthesia or lumbar epidural blockade. Patient positioning for cervical, thoracic, and caudal epidural anesthesia is discussed later in the chapter.

It is useful to have an assistant who can help the patient maintain the correct position for initiation of all neuraxial blocks. The assistant should not be a family member. The authors prefer to ask family and friends to step out of the procedure room for the duration of the procedure. This allows the anesthesiologist to focus on the patient and vice versa. If the anesthesiologist cannot easily communicate verbally with the patient because of a language barrier or other issues, arrangements should be made for an interpreter to be present. Again, if at all possible, this should not be a family member. Finally, the duration of time the patient needs to maintain the block position after completion of the procedure (e.g., remain in the lateral or sitting position) depends on whether this is critical to the development of sensory blockade (e.g., unilateral blockade or saddle blockade).

Lateral Position

The patient's back should be positioned at and parallel to the edge of the bed or operating table so that the patient is within easy reach of the anesthesiologist (Fig. 2-1). The knees should be drawn toward the chest, and the neck should be in the neutral or flexed position. The head and shoulders may need to be slightly raised on a blanket or pillow, particularly if the hips are broad. The patient should be asked to actively curve the lower back toward the anesthesiologist in order to flex the lumbar spine. The anesthesiologist may wish to place his or her hand on the patient's lower back and ask him or her to push against the hand. This overcomes the lumbar lordosis that narrows the interspace between adjacent spinous processes and laminae. The hips should be aligned exactly one above the other to keep the coronal plane of the spine perpendicular to the floor, thus preventing the spine from rotating. Patients tend to rotate forward when asked to flex their backs. In particular, the nondependent shoulder rotates forward and down, thus rotating the spine. Often, the dependent shoulder may

need to be pulled forward slightly. Women with broad hips may require support under or between their legs to prevent forward rotation of the nondependent hip.

Sitting Position

The sitting position patient should be seated with the legs hanging off the side of the bed or operating table, with the backs of the knees touching the edge of the bed and the feet supported by a stool (Fig. 2-2). The patient should sit squarely on both buttocks. Patients should be asked to flex the lumbar spine as much as possible. This request often causes patients to hunch their shoulders, or lean forward, rather than flex the lumbar spine. The authors find it useful to ask patients to "slouch" and assume a position of "bad posture." The patient should not be allowed to slump to either side or twist one shoulder forward relative to the other. The shoulders should remain over the hips. Depending on the anticipated or desired degree of sensory blockade, patients may need to be placed supine relatively quickly after the initiation of spinal anesthesia

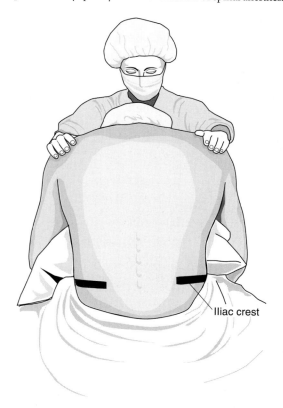

FIGURE 2-2. Spinal or lumbar epidural anesthesia in the sitting position. *Used with permission from Kleinman W, Mikhail M. Spinal, epidural, and caudal blocks. In: Morgan GE, Mikhail MS, Murray M, eds, Clinical Anesthesiology, 4th ed. New York: McGraw-Hill, 2006, p. 289.*

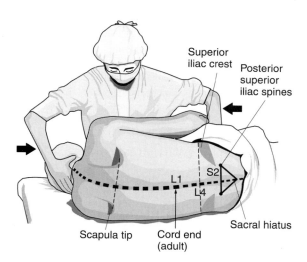

FIGURE 2-1. Spinal or lumbar epidural anesthesia in the lateral position. *Used with permission from Kleinman W, Mikhail M. Spinal, epidural, and caudal blocks. In: Morgan GE, Mikhail MS, Murray M, eds, Clinical Anesthesiology, 4th ed. New York: McGraw-Hill, 2006, p. 289.*

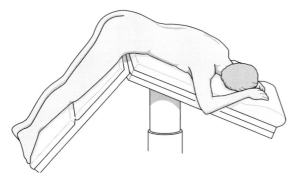

FIGURE 2-3. Spinal or lumbar epidural anesthesia in the prone jack-knife position. *Used with permission from Lambert DH, Covino BG. Hyperbaric, hypobaric, and isobaric spinal anesthesia. Resid Staff Physician 10:84, 1987.*

in order to avoid profound hypotension secondary to pooling of blood in the legs and subsequent decreased venous return.

Prone Position

The prone patient is positioned facedown on the bed or operating table. The hips should be placed over the break in the table to facilitate placing the patient in the jackknife position. A pillow under the abdomen helps flex the lower spine (Fig. 2-3).

▶ Supplies and Equipment

The ability to efficiently and safely initiate neuraxial blockade depends on having the right equipment immediately available. It is useful to have a neuraxial block cart(s) that is routinely stocked with the necessary supplies, equipment, and drugs, and can be easily wheeled to the location where the block is to be performed (Fig. 2-4). Suggested cart supplies and equipment are listed in Box 2-2. This list should be modified based on individual institution practice and practice settings.

Prepackaged Disposable Spinal and Epidural Trays

There has been progressive improvement in the quality and reliability of disposable, commercially prepared spinal and epidural trays. These commercially produced kits can be customized to the specific needs and preferences of an institution. The convenience of the prepackaged tray, improvements in the quality of disposable needles and other tray components, and advantages in terms of sterility and patient safety, have virtually eliminated the use of reusable regional anesthesia trays in the United States. Although industrially prepared disposable anesthesia trays are convenient, they have some minor drawbacks. Disposable trays are more expensive, less adaptable to local preferences, add to hospital waste, and may be more difficult to supply to remote areas.

Box 2-2

Equipment and Supplies for a Neuraxial Anesthesia Block Cart

Spinal and epidural trays

Sterile gloves of different sizes

Syringes of different sizes (1, 3, 5, 10, 20 mL)

Alcohol wipes

Filter needles

Extra spinal needles of varying gauge (22-, 24-, 25-, and 27-gauge) and length

Extra epidural needles (9, 13, and 15 cm)

Drug labels

Transparent occlusive dressing

Tape (including latex-free type)

Adhesive spray or solution

Emergency drugs*

Local anesthetics for spinal use

Local anesthetics for epidural use

Other drugs (epinephrine, sodium bicarbonate, preservative-free saline)

*See Box 2-1.

The minimum equipment required to initiate spinal or epidural anesthesia includes antiseptic solution and application swab(s), sterile gauze, a sterile drape, local anesthetic for the skin and subcutaneous tissue, and a small-gauge needle and syringe to administer the local anesthetic. Most tray manufacturers supply a fenestrated drape with adhesive that allows easy placement of the drape over the back. A clear, plastic drape allows easier identification of anatomic landmarks and the ability to assess whether the patient is in the correct position. Other supplies particular to spinal and epidural anesthesia are discussed later.

▶ Setting Up the Work Area

The work area should be organized so that the anesthesiologist is comfortable and does not have to move or turn his or her back to the patient once the procedure has begun. The patient's bed or cart should be placed at a height that is comfortable for the anesthesiologist, so that he or she does not have to bend over, or stand on tiptoes to reach the patient. The anesthesia tray and drugs should be set on the side of the anesthesiologist's dominant hand. This allows the anesthesiologist to pick up objects without reaching across his or her own body. The risk of contamination is decreased and the anesthesiologist can keep one hand on the

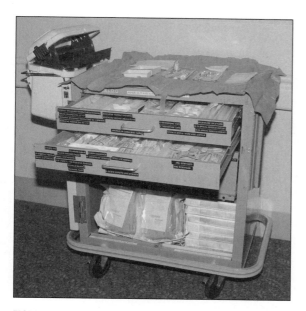

FIGURE 2-4. Neuraxial block cart. *Note that all the supplies are in a single, mobile cart and that the top of the cart is used as a work surface.*

patient, or needle in the patient's back, while setting down or reaching for supplies with the dominant hand.

▶ Aseptic Technique

Adherence to aseptic technique is critically important to the safe practice of neuraxial anesthesia. Fortunately, the incidence of bacterial meningitis following spinal anesthesia is rare due to the use of disposable trays and needles, and attention to aseptic technique. Puncture of skin during administration of neuraxial anesthesia damages the most important barrier of the human body against infection of the central nervous system. Although large retrospective and prospective studies have found spinal and epidural anesthesia safe with regard to infectious complications, serious infections after neuraxial blocks have been described (see Chap. 6). Skin disinfection according to aseptic guidelines, and sterile handling of invasive devices, are a routine and accepted part of standard practice, although clinical data on the efficacy of these guidelines are lacking. The American Society of Regional Anesthesia and Pain Medicine held a consensus conference in the spring of 2004 addressing infection and neural blockade. Consensus statements generated during this conference are due to be published in 2006.

Face Masks

Observational and case-controlled studies have implicated health-care providers, including anesthesiologists, as the source of iatrogenic infections after the initiation of neuraxial blockade.[1] An epidural abscess was caused by a staphylococcus phage that was cultured from the nares of the anesthesiologist who had inserted the epidural catheter.[2] Moreover, laboratory evidence appears to corroborate the clinical value of preventing the transmission of infectious agents from the upper airway by wearing a face mask.[3] Face masks have been shown to reduce the number of bacteria cultured in plates placed in front of speaking persons.[4] Nonwoven tissue or glass fibers are superior to linen or paper masks. Although the use of surgical masks during placement of neuraxial techniques is not uniformly accepted,[5,6] given the available evidence on the relationship between oral commensal bacteria and iatrogenic infection, the use of surgical masks is strongly recommended by the authors of this chapter.[7]

Hand Washing

Hand washing is the single most cost-effective component of aseptic techniques.[8] Careful hand washing should precede gloving for a neuraxial procedure as microperforations of gloves may occur. Polyvinyl pyrrolidone-iodine (PVPI) and chlorhexidine provide similar efficacy in decreasing bacterial skin counts on the practitioners' hands. Both solutions should remain on the skin for at least 1 min before drying. During hand washing and before drying, fingers should remain above the elbow and only nails and subungual regions should be brushed.

Waterless soaps are an alternatives to hand washing, and their use is increasing. The Centers for Disease Control and Prevention (CDC) published guidelines for surgical hand washing and hand antisepsis in 2002.[9] The CDC currently recommends hygienic hand disinfection with an alcohol-based hand rub, rather than traditional hand washing. It also recommends treating hands before contact with patients, before donning sterile gloves, and when inserting devices such as indwelling catheters.

Cap, Gown, and Gloves

The combined use of cap and mask was shown to reduce bacterial shedding 22-fold in procedure rooms with laminar flow.[10] Most anesthesiologists in the United States wear a cap, but not a sterile gown during the initiation of neuraxial anesthesia. Surgical scrubs are usually worn. There are no data as to whether wearing a surgical gown decreases the incidence of iatrogenic infection. Given that the incidence of infection associated with neuraxial anesthesia is rare, a very large study would be necessary, and the numbers needed to treat would likely be quite high. Similarly, there are no data as to whether wearing a cap (either the patient or the anesthesiologist) decreases the incidence of infection. The wearing of sterile gloves is an accepted part of aseptic technique for initiating neuraxial anesthesia.

Skin Disinfection

Skin preparation is the accepted standard before initiating neuraxial anesthesia. In their 1998 Recommendations for Infection Control for the Practice of Anesthesiology, the ASA recommended PVPI, chlorhexidine, iodine tincture, or ethanol 70% for skin antisepsis.[11] Ethyl alcohol or isopropyl alcohol 60–90% have the most rapid bactericidal effect, but skin contact for at least 2 min is required. For practical purposes, no solution is sporicidal. Many studies have shown that exposure of microorganisms to povidone-iodine (PI) solution for 60 s or longer reduces bacterial colony count by greater than 95%. However, PI is not effective for bacteria deep within the skin. Culture of skin biopsies from the lumbar region obtained after aseptic application were positive in 32% of cases with aqueous PI compared to 5.7% after application of chlorhexidine in alcohol.[12]

Epidural catheter contamination rates from 22 to 65% have been reported.[13,14] Yentur et al. investigated the incidence of epidural needle and catheter contamination in the general adult population after skin disinfection with 10% PI solution and found rates for contamination of needles and catheters during epidural catheterization to be 34 and 46%, respectively.[15] *Staphylococcus epidermidis,* followed by *Staphylococcus aureus*, were the organisms most often isolated. In the obstetric population the most common bacterial isolate was also *S. epidermidis* (87%).[14] Other isolated organisms included other coagulase-negative staphylococci, enterococcus species, Bacillus species, α- and β-hemolytic streptococci, *Escherichia coli,* diphtheroids, *S. aureus, Acinetobacter calcoaceticus,* and Citrobacter species.

An in vitro study compared the effectiveness of 0.5% chlorhexidine in 80% ethanol (chlorhexidine-alcohol) solution to 10% PI solution.[16] Chlorhexidine in alcohol was more potent and more rapidly bacteriocidal against methicillin-susceptible and methicillin-resistant strains of *S. aureus.* A concern with chlorhexidine-alcohol solutions is the lack of color. This makes the uniform application of the solution to a broad area of skin more difficult, since the practitioner cannot see which areas might have been missed. The absence of color may increase the chance of glove, needle, and ampule content chemical contamination, which may cause aseptic meningitis. Stained PI solution or DuraPrep (iodophor in isopropyl alcohol solution) may be safer for these reasons, although this has not been studied.

Birnbach et al. compared PI and DuraPrep for skin preparation prior to epidural labor analgesia.[14] DuraPrep solution provided a greater decrease in the number of positive skin cultures immediately after disinfection, as well as bacterial regrowth and colonization of epidural catheters. Since one of the proposed mechanisms for catheter infection is the contamination of the catheter by skin flora, the presence of bacteria at the insertion site would be expected to correlate with an increased risk of catheter contamination. The mechanism by which DuraPrep protects against bacterial growth is thought to be the formation of protective film on the skin.

If PI is chosen as the disinfectant, it is preferable to use sterile single-use PI packages. Multidose bottles of PI can have decreased activity against skin flora and may support bacterial growth.[17] To minimize the risk of contamination and maximize convenience, manufacturers are supplying single-use PI packages in epidural trays.

Epidural catheters can be contaminated at both the skin insertion site (32%) and the catheter hub (40%).[18] Theoretically, because the catheter hub appears to represent the main route of catheter colonization, the use of bacterial filters at the catheter hub should decrease the rate of epidural catheter colonization. However, cases of epidural infection exist despite the use of bacterial filters, suggesting that filters may lose their efficacy after prolonged use or that catheter hubs are directly contaminated. Investigators found a direct correlation between the frequency of catheter hub colonization and filter change.[19] There are no data to support the use of filters to decrease the incidence of epidural catheter-related infection. It should be noted that catheter colonization did not result in infection in any of the patients included in these studies. This is not surprising since estimates of the incidence of infections related to epidural catheters are very low.

No matter the solution, skin should be disinfected before the sterile drape is applied to the back. The patient's entire back should be exposed as this facilitates identification of anatomic landmarks and decreases the risk of contamination from the patient's gown. An area with a radius of approximately 6 in. (15 cm) should be disinfected around the presumed skin puncture site. Prepping a large area is preferred as it allows one to readily move to another interspace if this becomes necessary. Excess disinfectant should be allowed to dry on the skin. All antiseptic solutions are neurotoxic, and care must be taken not to contaminate spinal needles or local anesthetics with the disinfectant solution.

Other Sources of Contaminants

In the last decade, the addition of opioid or other adjuvants to local anesthetics has increased and aspiration of drugs from nonsterile ampules has been blamed for infectious complications after neuraxial blockade. Small glass fragments produced during ampule opening may contaminate its contents.[20] Routine use of 0.2 μm bacterial filter for aspirating drugs from glass ampules is recommended.[21] Wiping vials and ampules intended for intravenous use with alcohol is recommended by the ASA.[11] Although there are no specific recommendations for drugs intended for intrathecal use, this practice would seem to make sense. The ideal practice would be to use drugs in sterilely packed ampules, thereby avoiding contamination during opening, and decreasing the risk of injection of drugs not intended for spinal use. However, this is often not practical.

SPINAL ANESTHESIA

Spinal anesthesia should be in the armamentarium of all anesthesiologists. The technique is relatively simple to learn, but repetition is necessary to refine one's technique and gain experience so that spinal anesthesia is almost always successful and both the surgeon and patient have confidence in the technique. Successful spinal anesthesia is initiated in a facile manner with minimal patient discomfort. It provides excellent surgical anesthesia with minimal side effects and complications. It may also contribute to postoperative analgesia.

▶ Spinal Needles

The most important piece of equipment necessary for successful spinal anesthesia is the spinal needle. Spinal needles have evolved over the past several decades. The current practice is to use small-gauge, noncutting bevel needles (Fig. 2-5). Almost all spinal needles currently used in the United States are onetime use, disposable needles. Spinal needles have a close-fitting stylet that prevents coring of the skin and possible contamination of the intrathecal space with epidermis.

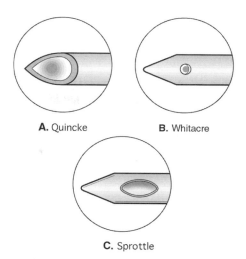

A. Quincke   **B.** Whitacre

C. Sprottle

FIGURE 2-5. Spinal needles. (A) Quincke (cutting bevel). (B) Whitacre (pencil-point). (C) Sprotte (pencil-point).

Small-gauge, noncutting needles are associated with an acceptably low incidence of postdural puncture headache (PDPH) after spinal anesthesia. Studies with cutting and noncutting needles have documented a lower incidence of

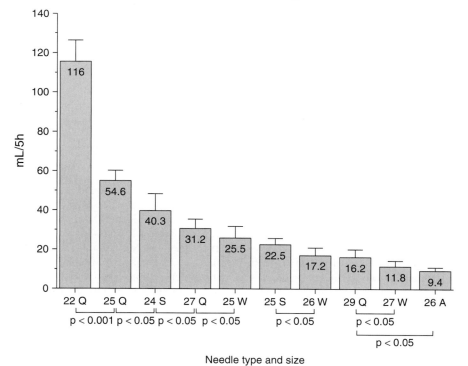

FIGURE 2-6. Relationship between needle size and bevel and leakage of CSF (mL/5 h) after puncture of cadaver dura. Q = Quincke, S = Sprotte, W = Whitacre, A = Atraucan. *Used with permission from Holst D, Mollmann M, Ebel C, et al. In vitro investigation of cerebrospinal fluid leakage after dural puncture with various spinal needles. Anesth Analg 87:1331, 1998.*

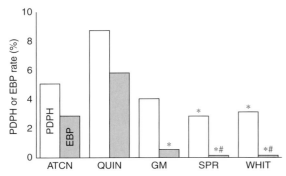

FIGURE 2-7. Incidence of PDPH (white bar) or epidural blood patch (gray bar) with different spinal needle tips. ATCN (Atraucan), QUIN (Quincke), GM (Gertie Marx), SPR (Sprotte), and WHIT (Whitacre). *Significantly different from the Quincke group, $P <0.05$. Significantly# different than the Atraucan group, $P <0.05$. *Used with permission from Vallejo MC, Mandell GL, Sabo DP, et al. Postdural puncture headache: A randomized comparison of five spinal needles in obstetric patients. Anesth Analg 91:916, 2000.*

PDPH associated with smaller-gauge spinal needles compared to larger needles. An in vitro study using cadaver dura found progressively less cerebrospinal fluid (CSF) leak with smaller needles (Fig. 2-6).[22] Noncutting needles are associated with a lower incidence of PDPH compared to cutting needles (Fig. 2-7).[23] The advantage of a noncutting needle is still present with small-gauge needles. In two separate studies, patients were randomized to spinal anesthesia with a 27-gauge noncutting needle and a 27-gauge cutting needle (Atraucan or Quincke). The incidence of PDPH in both studies was lower with the noncutting needle.[24,25] Electron microscopy showed that 26- or 27-gauge noncutting needles caused blunt penetration of the dura. It was impossible to trace a channel through this hole in the dura.[22] Conversely, puncture with a 29-gauge Quincke needle resulted in a sharply delineated hole and channel through which more CSF leaked.

Other factors may contribute to the decreased incidence of PDPH observed with noncutting needles. Microscopic analysis of cutting and noncutting needle tips used for spinal anesthesia showed that cutting needles were more susceptible to tip damage when bony contact occurred, compared to noncutting needles.[26]

Noncutting bevel needles have been referred to as "pencil-point" or "atraumatic" needles. However, using fresh cadaver dura and scanning electron microscopy, investigators demonstrated that dural punctures made with noncutting needles produced significantly coarser lesions with more destruction of the dural fibers compared to lesions made with a cutting needle.[27] The investigators suggested that dural puncture with noncutting needles results in an inflammatory reaction that causes tissue edema around the puncture site. This serves to plug the hole, thus limiting the leakage of CSF and occurrence of PDPH.

There are several disadvantages of small-gauge needles. They must be used with an introducer and have less directional stability, and are, therefore, more difficult to manipulate. Backflow of CSF is slower with smaller needles. In general, for most patients anesthesiologists should be able to initiate spinal anesthesia with 25-gauge noncutting needles. The incidence of PDPH with these needles is acceptably low for most patients. An even lower incidence of PDPH can be achieved with 27- or 29-gauge needles, but these are harder to use and the success rate may be lower.[28]

There are several different types of noncutting spinal needles available to the anesthesiologist. Noncutting needles differ in the conical angle and shape of the tip, the size and location of the orifice, and the internal diameter of the needle (Fig. 2-5). There are minor differences among the noncutting needles in the "feel" during dural puncture and differences in the rate of CSF return. The Atraucan needle has a modified cutting bevel that is associated with a low risk of PDPH.[23] The ball-pen needle has a conical tip formed by the stylet, and a symmetrical end hole when the stylet is withdrawn. A multi-center study in 700 patients comparing the 25-gauge ball-pen needle to a 25-gauge Sprotte needle found no difference in the ease of use, failure rate, or incidence of PDPH.[29]

▶ Other Supplies and Equipment and Set Up for Spinal Anesthesia

The anesthesiologist should use aseptic technique to open the spinal tray, glove, and prepare the patient's back as described earlier in the chapter. Local anesthetic (usually several milliliters of lidocaine 1%) should be drawn up in a syringe attached to a small-gauge (25- or 27-gauge) needle. The drug(s) for intrathecal injection should be drawn up through a filter needle into a non-Luer-locking syringe. Luer-locking syringes are more difficult to attach to the spinal needle without moving the needle. Typical contents of a spinal anesthesia tray are listed in Box 2-3.

The manner in which drug mixtures are prepared for intrathecal injection has been shown to influence the final concentrations of drugs.[30] When using a filter needle or straw the final concentration of a tracer drug varied by four- to fivefold, depending on the order in which the drugs were aspirated into the syringe. There was less variation in drug concentration when small doses of drugs were drawn into a 1-mL tuberculin syringe through the attached needle (27-gauge, 0.5 in.) and added to the mixture. This study showed the importance of attention to technical details when preparing spinal adjuvants with potential for dose-related adverse side effects, such as opioids. At the authors' institution, adjuvants such as epinephrine, fentanyl, and morphine are drawn up into an insulin (0.5 or 1.0 mL) or tuberculin (1 mL) syringe under

`Box 2-3

Typical Contents of Neuraxial Anesthesia Trays*

General contents

    Antiseptic solution and applicator

    Fenestrated sterile drape, preferably clear plastic

    Sterile gauze

    Sterile sheet

    Tuberculin syringe (1 mL)—for measuring small volumes accurately

    Filter straw or needle (5 μ)—to draw up drugs from glass vials

    Needles (18-, 22-, 25-gauge)

    Syringe (3 mL)—for skin infiltration

    1% lidocaine (5 mL)—for skin infiltration

    Needle guard for sharps disposal

Spinal Tray	Epidural Tray	CSE Tray
Spinal needle (24- to 27-gauge)	Epidural needle (17-, 18-gauge)	Epidural tray contents
Spinal needle introducer needle	LOR syringe	Syringe with slip connector for spinal drug(s), 5 mL
Syringe with slip connector for spinal drug(s) (5 mL)	Epidural catheter with connector	Long spinal needle, 12.7 cm (24-, 25-, 27-gauge)
	Epidural catheter label	
	1.5% lidocaine with epinephrine 1:200,000 (5 mL)—for test dose	
	Syringe (20 mL)	

*The tray content list does not include drugs (local anesthetics, opioids, and epinephrine) intended for neuraxial injection. Contents of trays may vary depending on specific technique or patient population.

Once preparations are complete, the patient should be asked to assume the optimal position and instructed to remain still until the procedure is complete.

▶ Technique of Spinal Anesthesia

Spinal anesthesia is always performed in the mid-lower lumbar subarachnoid space, usually through the L4-L5 or L3-L4 interspace. Interspaces above L2-L3 should be avoided to decrease the risk of injuring the spinal cord with the needle. Although the conus medullaris ends at the lower part of the vertebral body of L1 in most patients, it ends more caudal in a small percentage of patients (see Chap. 1). Both the iliac crests and the 12th rib margins are used to help pinpoint the appropriate intervertebral space (Fig. 1-1 and Figs. 2-1 and 2-2).

Either a midline or paramedian approach can be used. The midline approach is easier to teach and learn and is less painful for the patient. The paramedian approach is useful when patients cannot assume a flexed position or in the elderly when the spinal ligaments are calcified. The paramedian approach requires mental triangulation in three planes, instead of two, and this requires the anesthesiologist to estimate the skin to subarachnoid space depth. Occasionally, the anesthesiologist intends to use a midline approach, but because of difficulty identifying the midline, is actually using a paramedian approach.

Various methods are used to locate the midline, usually using the nondominant hand. These include palpation with a single index finger or thumb, palpation between the index finger and thumb, or index and middle fingers. The authors prefer locating the interspinous space with the index finger, pressing the skin to produce a temporary imprint, and raising a local anesthetic skin wheal in the middle of the imprint. Other anesthesiologists mark the space with a nail imprint. Anesthesiologists who use the two-digit technique raise a skin wheal between the two digits. If this technique is used, care must be taken to avoid accidental needle puncture of the practitioner's fingers with a contaminated needle if the patient moves with the initial needle insertion.

Midline Approach

Skin and subcutaneous tissue over the interspinous process should be anesthetized to the depth of the supraspinous ligament. Needle penetration of the ligament is not painful and the spinal ligaments need not be anesthetized. A skin wheal is raised with a 25- or 27-gauge, 1.6-cm needle. The needle used to inject the local anesthetic should puncture the skin in the midline at the site at which the anesthesiologist anticipates insertion of the spinal needle (Fig. 2-8). In thin patients, the supraspinous ligament can be penetrated with this short needle. In heavier patients, a 2–3-cm 22- or 25-gauge needle is used to inject additional local anesthetic to the depth of the

sterile conditions, and the contents of the syringe(s) are injected into the syringe containing the local anesthetic intended for the spinal block. A separate syringe should be used for each drug. This prevents inaccurate measurement of drug volume (and mass) because of the extra drug contained in the dead space of the needle.

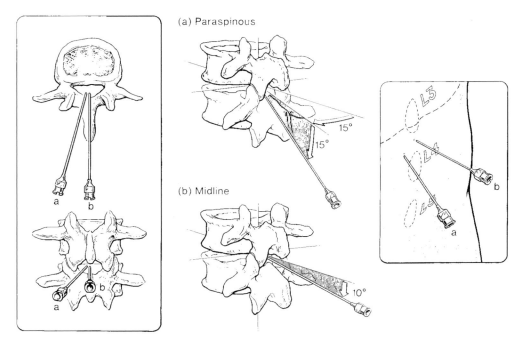

FIGURE 2-8. Angle of spinal needle insertion for the paramedian (paraspinous) (a) and midline (b) lumbar approaches to the vertebral canal. Note the needle in the paramedian approach is angled 10–15 degrees off the midline (sagittal plane) and 15 degrees down from the transverse plane. *Used with permission from Bridenbaugh PO, Greene NM, Brull SJ. Spinal (subarachnoid) neural blockade. In: Cousins MJ, Bridenbaugh PO, eds, Neural Blockade in Clinical Anesthesia and Management of Pain, 3rd ed. Philadelphia, PA: Lippincott-Raven, 1998, p. 203.*

supraspinous ligament. This needle can also function as a "seeker" needle to verify that the anesthesiologist has correctly located the interspinous space. If bone is encountered with the seeker needle, the appropriate maneuvers can be undertaken to relocate the needle to the proper place and more local anesthetic is injected (see "Troubleshooting," later). Care should be taken not to insert the seeker needle too deeply in thin patients, as the needle tip may pierce the dura-arachnoid, leaving a dural puncture with a cutting needle bevel, and increasing the risk of PDPH.

Small-gauge spinal needles (25-gauge and smaller) are easier to use with an introducer needle. Twenty-two-gauge spinal needles are usually used without an introducer. In a randomized study of introducer compared to no-introducer with a 24-gauge noncutting needle (Sprotte), investigators found that the number of redirections of the spinal needle was significantly higher in the no-introducer compared to the introducer group.[31]

The introducer (or spinal) needle is inserted through the skin at the puncture site used for the local anesthetic and directed cephalad about 10–15° (Fig. 2-8). In the lumbar area the spinous processes point slightly downward at the tips and the interlaminar space is slightly cephalad to the interspinous space. The introducer needle is advanced into the supraspinous ligament (Figs. 2-9 and 2-10). If the introducer needle does not reach the ligament, a longer introducer needle should be substituted. When the practitioner releases the introducer needle, the needle should assume the proper direction. If it points laterally, it is likely that the needle is not in the interspinous space, but instead lateral to a spinous process. In this case, the introducer needle should be repositioned (see "Troubleshooting," later).

After the introducer needle is correctly positioned, the practitioner should stabilize the needle by grasping the hub between the thumb and index finger of the nondominant hand. Additional stability is provided if the practitioner places the back of his hand against the patient's back (Fig. 2-10). The hub of the spinal needle is grasped like a dart with the dominant hand. The fourth and fifth fingers can be used like a tripod against the patient's back to further stabilize the needle and control movement. The bevel of a cutting spinal needle should face laterally, as this has been shown to be associated with a decreased incidence of PDPH. The spinal needle is advanced slowly. There is usually a characteristic

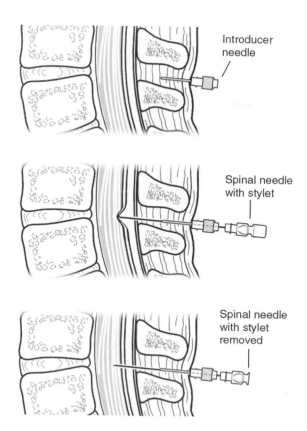

Introducer needle

Spinal needle with stylet

Spinal needle with stylet removed

FIGURE 2-9. Sagittal view of spinal anesthesia. (A) Introducer needle is introduced through the skin and advanced into the interspinous ligament. (B) The spinal needle is advanced through the introducer needle through the interspinous ligament, ligamentum flavum, and epidural space to tent the dura. (C) The spinal needle is advanced through the dura into the subarachnoid space.

change in "feel" as the needle traverses the tougher ligamentum flavum and "pops" through the dura-arachnoid membranes. Needle advancement should stop as soon as the pop is felt. Noncutting needles "tent" the dura (Fig. 2-9). The dura springs back after the needle pops into the subarachnoid space, leaving the needle tip and orifice wholly within the subarachnoid space. Advancing the needle further increases the risk of paresthesias and neuronal injury. In the majority of the adult population the distance from the skin to the subarachnoid space is 4–6 cm.

After the pop is felt, the nondominant hand releases the introducer needle hub and grasps the spinal needle hub in a similar fashion. The stylet is removed with the dominant hand to allow free flow of CSF. CSF appears within 1 or 2 s in patients in the sitting position. The backflow

may be slightly slower for patients in the lateral position. Occasionally, there will be no flow for patients in the prone position and gentle aspiration is necessary to document correct placement of the needle tip in the subarachnoid space.

If CSF does not appear in the hub of the spinal needle, the stylet should be reinserted and the spinal needle once again slowly advanced. There is sometimes a false "pop" as the spinal needle enters the epidural space and advancement of the spinal needle through the dura-arachnoid is necessary. Occasionally, the anesthesiologist "misses" the subarachnoid space and the spinal needle "pops" out the anterior dura-arachnoid membrane. The tip of the spinal needle is located in the anterior epidural space; hence no CSF will be noted in the spinal needle. When the practitioner advances the spinal needle, bone (the posterior surface of the vertebral body) is encountered. In this case, the anesthesiologist should slowly withdraw the spinal needle until CSF is noted in the needle hub.

The syringe containing the spinal anesthetic solution is attached to the hub of the spinal needle while immobilizing the spinal needle with the nondominant hand using the technique described earlier. The syringe should be free of air. Position of the needle orifice in the subarachnoid space is once again verified by gentle aspiration on the syringe plunger. CSF should aspirate freely into the syringe. Care should be taken not to allow needle movement during aspiration and to keep the syringe attached tightly to the spinal needle.

Needle Bevel Orientation and Speed of Injection The degree and direction of anesthetic dispersion as it exits the spinal needle is dependent on type of spinal needle, speed of injection, and orifice area.[32,33] Anesthetic solution exits from the tip of a cutting needle as an undeviated stream; therefore, needle bevel direction during the injection of the anesthetic solution does not change distribution of the anesthetic within the spinal canal.[32] In contrast, the anesthetic stream exits at an angle to the longitudinal axis of noncutting spinal needles (Fig. 2-11)[32] and dispersion is less with slower injections rates.[33] Whether or not injection rate through noncutting needles affects sensory level likely depends on the baricity of the anesthetic solution, as well as patient position and spinal needle orifice. For example, median peak thoracic sensory blockade was higher with administration of isobaric solution after spinal anesthesia initiated in the lateral position with the bevel of the noncutting needle oriented cephalad, compared to injection of the spinal solution with the needle orifice oriented in the caudad direction.[34] In addition, resolution of lumbar blockade was faster.

Using a spinal cord model, investigators demonstrated maldistribution of dye solution injected at a rate of 2 mL/60 s though a Whitacre needle.[33] This did not occur after a faster

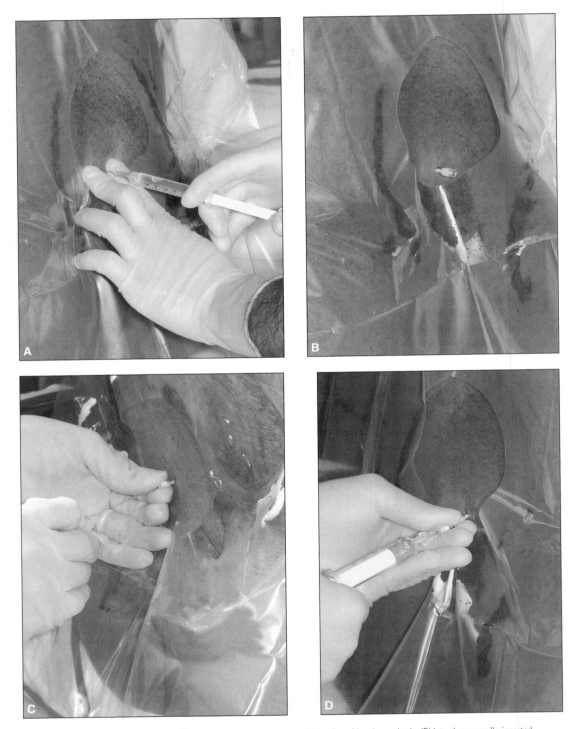

FIGURE 2-10. Spinal anesthesia. (A) Palpation of the spinous process and injection of local anesthetic. (B) Introducer needle inserted. (C) Spinal needle inserted through introducer needle. (D) Syringe attached to spinal needle. Note triangulation of hand against the patient's back and thumb and index finger grasping hub of spinal needle. This position should also be used when removing the spinal needle stylet.

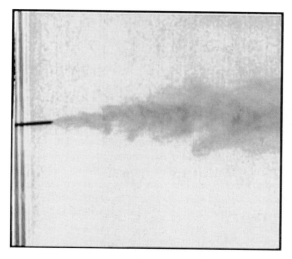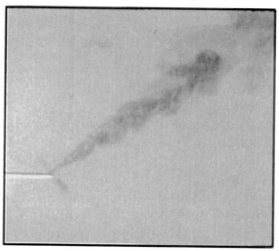

FIGURE 2-11. Dye solution injected at a rate of 15 mL/min exiting a 25-gauge Whitacre spinal needle into an open tank. (A) Overhead view. (B) Lateral view. The dye exits through the aperture at a mean angle of 40 degrees to the shaft of the needle. *Used with permission from Serpell MG, Gray WM. Flow dynamics through spinal needles. Anaesthesia 52:229, 1997.*

injection through the Whitacre needle (2 mL/10 s) or after slow or fast injection through the cutting (Quincke) needle. Maldistribution was also more likely to occur with a smaller orifice. Holman et al. suggested that anesthetic maldistribution can be minimized by using injection rates greater than 2 mL/20 s through noncutting, side-port needles (Fig. 2-12).[33]

Some practitioners aspirate midway through the injection or at the end of the injection to verify needle orifice position in the subarachnoid space. Whether this practice improves the success rate of spinal anesthesia is not known. Once the injection is complete the spinal needle and introducer are removed together as a unit.

Paramedian Approach

As with the midline approach, the midline, spinous processes and interspinous space are identified by the practitioner's palpating finger(s). A skin wheal is raised approximately 1 cm lateral to the midline at the cephalad border of the inferior spinous process (Fig. 2-8). A longer 22-gauge needle is usually necessary to anesthetize the soft tissue to the depth of the lamina or ligamentum flavum. The introducer needle is introduced at an angle of 10–15 degrees to the midline (with the goal of puncturing the dural-arachnoid in the midline), in a slightly cephalad direction (100–105 degrees to the skin in the sagittal plane). The introducer and spinal needles are stabilized as described for the midline technique. The spinal needle is introduced through the introducer needle and advanced until a "pop" is perceived as the needle pierces the dura-arachnoid. The

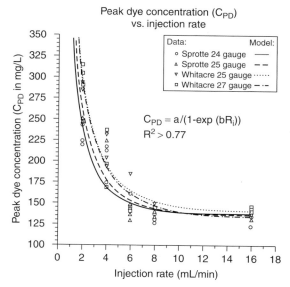

FIGURE 2-12. Relation between peak dye concentration, C_{pd} (mg/L), and injection rate (mL/min) for caudally directed injections through 24-gauge Sprotte (circle), 25-gauge Sprotte (up triangle), 25-gauge Whitacre (inverted triangle), and 27-gauge Whitacre (square) needles. Injection via the 24-gauge Sprotte needle, which has a larger orifice area and internal diameter, resulted in significantly lower peak dye concentrations than via the smaller Whitacre needles tested ($P<0.05$). *Used with permission from Holman SJ, Robinson RA, Beardsley D, et al. Hyperbaric dye solution distribution characteristics after pencil-point needle injection in a spinal cord model. Anesthesiology 86:966, 1997.*

stylet is removed to ascertain free flow of CSF. The remainder of the procedure mimics that for the midline approach described earlier. If bone is encountered, the introducer and needle should be redirected as described in the troubleshooting section later.

Taylor Approach

The Taylor approach is a special paramedian approach at the L5-S1 interspace. This interspace boasts the largest interlaminar space. The patient is positioned in the sitting or lateral position. A skin wheal is raised 1 cm caudad and 1 cm medial to the posterior superior iliac crest. A 12-cm (5-in.) spinal needle is introduced through the skin wheal and directed medial and cephalad (Fig. 2-13).

Testing for Adequate Spinal Anesthesia

Patients usually perceive warmth in their low extremities within 1 min of the intrathecal injection of local anesthetic. Inability to discriminate temperature is an early indication of neuraxial blockade, and should be tested first, before testing with a painful stimulus. Metal (the grip of a hemostat or barrel of a laryngoscope handle), or an alcohol wipe can be used as a cold stimulus. The patient is exposed to the cold

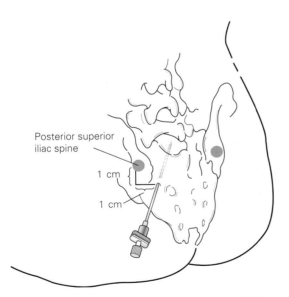

Posterior superior iliac spine

1 cm

1 cm

FIGURE 2-13. Taylor approach to neuraxial anesthesia. A 12.5-cm spinal needle is inserted 1 cm caudad and 1 cm medial to the posterior superior iliac spine and walked off the sacrum in a cephalad and medial direction into the L5-S1 interlaminar space. *Used with permission from Brown DL. Spinal, epidural, and caudal anesthesia. In: Miller RD (ed). Miller's Anesthesia, 6th ed. Philadelphia, PA: Churchill Livingstone, 2005, p. 1665.*

stimulus on an unblocked area, for example, the cheek or shoulder. The anesthesiologist should place the stimulus on the skin at the dermatome level at which the spinal injection occurred, for example, lateral thigh for L3, and "walk" the stimulus cephalad, asking the patient to indicate when he or she perceives the same degree of coldness as the control. Convenient surface structures and their dermatome correlations are listed in Table 1-1. For perineal procedures, the testing should proceed in the caudad direction to assess sacral dermatomes. The dermatomal level of temperature discrimination corresponds to the sympathetic level of blockade.

Sensory testing with a noxious stimulus should occur after sympathetic blockade has been ascertained. If testing with a painful stimulus begins too early, and there is minimal sensory blockade, the patient will lose confidence in the anesthetic and the anesthesiologist, and anxiety levels may be needlessly increased. Sensory blockade can be ascertained by moving the noxious stimulus cephalad and asking the patient to state when the stimulus becomes painful (as opposed to the perception of touch). A dull, large bore needle or a pinch with a hemostat can be used to produce a sharp stimulus. Small-gauge needles should not be used, as they puncture the skin and leave "track" marks on the skin surface.

Motor blockade is tested by asking the patient to dorsiflex the foot (S1 to S2), bend the knees (L2 to L3), or tense the rectus abdominis (T6 to T12). Weakness of hand grasp indicates cervical motor blockade and high spinal anesthesia.

Troubleshooting

Troubleshooting a neuraxial procedure when the anesthesiologist fails to identify the subarachnoid (or epidural) space on the initial attempt involves constructing a three-dimensional image of vertebral column anatomy and using surface anatomy, and information from the patient and the needle tip to ascertain the current location of the needle, and the path the needle needs to follow to access the central canal. The patient's position should be reassessed to ascertain that an optimal position has been attained. Care should be taken to withdraw the spinal needle into the shaft of the introducer needle before the direction of the introducer needle is changed. To do otherwise is to risk bending and breaking the spinal needle. The spinal needle should not be advanced with force if resistance is encountered, as this is likely to damage the tip of the spinal needle. Small changes in hub position and the angle of the introducer needle will result in proportionally larger changes in the spinal needle tip position.

Paresthesias During Needle Insertion Before initiating the procedure, the patient should be warned of the possibility of a paresthesia. The authors usually tell the patients that they may feel a "zing" or "a funny bone sensation" in their buttocks or legs, and if this occurs they should inform the anesthesiologist. If the patient experiences a paresthesia, it is important to identify the side, and to attempt to ascertain whether the needle tip has encountered a nerve root in the epidural space or subarachnoid space. Needle advancement should stop immediately and the stylet removed to look for CSF in the needle hub. The presence of CSF confirms the subarachnoid position of the needle tip, in which case the needle has contacted part of the cauda equina. If the paresthesia has resolved and does not recur, the intrathecal anesthetic can be safely injected at this point. If the paresthesia recurs with aspiration or injection, the needle should be repositioned. If CSF is not visible at the hub, then the paresthesia probably resulted from contact with a spinal nerve root traversing the epidural space. This is especially true if the paresthesia occurs in the dermatome corresponding to the nerve root that exits the vertebral canal at the same level that the spinal needle is inserted. In this case, the needle has most likely deviated from midline and should be redirected to the side opposite the paresthesia. Occasionally, pain experienced when the needle contacts bone may be misinterpreted by the patient as a paresthesia.

Midline Approach If the local anesthetic, seeker needle, or introducer needle encounters bone at a superficial level, the needle tip has probably contacted a spinous process. This information should tell the practitioner that he or she is in the midline, but needs to move the needle up or down into the next cephalad or caudad interspinous space (Fig 2-14). If the needle tip is near the cephalad or caudad aspect of the tip of the spinous process, changing the angle of the needle up or down may suffice for the needle to slip into the interspinous space. Alternatively, the needle may be withdrawn back to skin and the skin moved cephalad or caudad on the back with the nondominant fingers, relative to the spinous process, to allow the needle to enter the interspinous space at a less acute angle. If the spinous process is encountered directly at the midpoint (in the sagittal plane), the needle may need to be withdrawn from the skin and reinserted more cephalad or caudad to the original insertion side. If the angle necessary to "bounce off" the superior or inferior surface of the spinous process is too acute, the needle will contact the inferior or superior aspect of the next spinous process deep to the skin before the ligamentum flavum is encountered (Fig. 2-14).

If bone is encountered several centimeters deep to the skin, the needle tip is probably impinging on the cephalad surface of the inferior spinous process, or the caudad surface of the superior spinous process (Fig. 2-14). Withdrawing the needle slightly and changing the up-down angle in the midline may allow the needle to advance in the interspinous space.

If bone is encountered yet deeper (3–4 cm from the skin in patients with normal body habitus), the needle tip is probably impinging on lamina (Fig. 2-14). The needle may have been deflected off the midline, the insertion site was not in the midline, or the patient has scoliosis (see "Scoliosis," later). Often the patient can feel whether the needle tip is right, left, or midline. The anesthesiologist can gain some useful information by questioning the patient and following his or her cue. For example, if the patient states that he or she feels the needle on the left, the anesthesiologist should withdraw the needle slightly, and then "walk" the needle cephalad and to the right until the needle slips off the cephalad surface of the lamina and pierces the ligamentum flavum and dura-arachnoid membrane. The opposite changes are indicated if the patient perceives the needle on the right. Occasionally, the needle will have contacted the inferior aspect of the lamina. A very steep cephalad angle may be necessary to access the interlaminar space, or the needle may need to be withdrawn to skin and redirected.

Occasionally, the introducer and spinal needle are advanced without encountering any resistance. A "pop" is sometimes appreciated, but no CSF appears after the stylet is withdrawn. In this case, the needle tip is probably located in the lateral epidural space. It has either deviated from the midline, or was not in the midline at the skin. Again, the patient should be questioned and needle direction changes should be guided by whether the needle is likely on the right or left side.

If the anesthesiologist has difficulty locating the subarachnoid space after several attempts, it is better to choose a different interspace, rather than continue attempts at the same interspace. Although local anesthetic will have to be reinjected, the patient will appreciate the decreased trauma associated with a smooth insertion, rather than continued attempts at the initial site.

Paramedian Approach The ipsilateral lamina is often encountered using the paramedian approach. In this case, the needle should be walked in a cephalad direction until it slips off the superior surface of the lamina. A slightly more medial direction may also be needed. Occasionally, the practitioner angles the needle too much and the tip of the needle encounters the spinous process or even traverses the interspinous ligament to end up in the contralateral epidural space (Fig. 2-14). In this case, the needle should be withdrawn and angled less acutely.

Obesity The obese patient provides a technical challenge as surface anatomy is obscured and the neuraxial canal is deeper to the skin. Neuraxial anesthesia for obese patients is more easily initiated in the sitting position. This allows adipose tissue to fall to either side of the midline symmetrically, so that the midline is easier to identify. The practitioner should

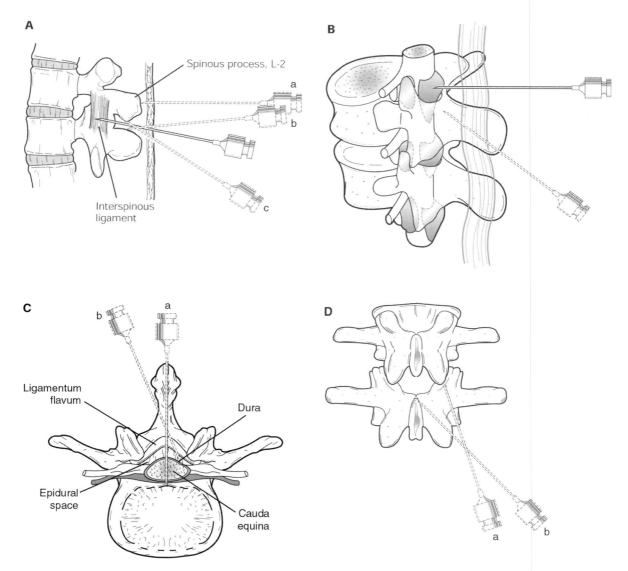

FIGURE 2-14. Techniques for troubleshooting initiating of neuraxial anesthesia. The dotted needle is the misplaced needle. The solid needle is in the correct position. Midline approach. (A) If the spinal needle contacts bone superficially, it is probably the tip of the spinous process (a). If bone is encountered several centimeters deep to the skin, the needle tip is probably impinging on the cephalad surface of the inferior spinous process (b), or the caudad surface of the superior spinous process (c). (B) If bone is encountered yet deeper, the needle tip is probably impinging on lamina and the tip may be off the midline. (C) If bone is encountered even deeper, the needle may have passed through the subarachnoid space and anterior dura and is impinging on the posterior aspect of the vertebral body (a). Occasionally, the introducer and spinal needle are advanced without encountering any resistance and a "pop" is perceived, but no CSF appears after the stylet is withdrawn. In this case, the needle tip is probably located in the lateral epidural space (b). If advanced further, the needle may contact the interior lateral wall of the vertebral canal. (D) Paramedian approach. The ipsilateral lamina is often encountered using the paramedian approach (a). Occasionally, the practitioner angles the needle too much and the tip of the needle encounters the lateral aspect or root of the spinous process (b). *Used with permission from Kleinman W, Mikhail M. Spinal, epidural, and caudal blocks. In: Morgan GE, Mikhail MS, Murray M, eds. Clinical Anesthesiology, 4th ed. New York: McGraw-Hill, 2005, pp. 289-323.*

anticipate the necessity for longer needles, although this is usually not necessary. In very heavy people there is often a "crater" in the midline between the adipose tissue of the hips and lower abdomen, and adipose tissue of the chest. The corresponding interspinous spaces, however, are likely to be high lumbar and therefore, unsuitable for spinal anesthesia.

Several options may be used to increase success rate for neuraxial anesthesia for obese patients. A longer introducer needle is often needed, as the introducer needle tip should be implanted in the interspinous ligament. Alternatively, a larger-gauge spinal needle may be chosen (e.g., 22-gauge) as this can be used without an introducer and is easier to manipulate and "walk." Obese patients may be at a lower risk for PDPH after dural puncture.[36] The epidural space is often easier to locate using the larger-gauge and stiffer epidural needle and location of the needle tip off the midline is recognized because of the typically "soft" feel of the paraspinous tissue (compared to the ligaments). In addition, epidural anesthesia may be preferred to spinal anesthesia for other reasons for the morbidly obese patient, including the observation that the upper lumbar central canal is located more superficially and the spinous processes at this level are often easier to palpate. When redirecting the spinal needle, it may be necessary to withdraw the needle to the subcutaneous tissue before changing the angle of the needle in order to avoid bowing of the needle. Finally, an epidural needle may be used as an introducer needle for the spinal needle, or alternatively, combined spinal-epidural anesthesia (CSE) can be initiated (see "Combined Spinal-Epidural Anesthesia," below).

Scoliosis Scoliosis is a lateral deviation of the spine from the vertical axis (Fig. 2-15). More severe curves are often associated with rotation of the spine, so that the spinous processes are rotated toward the concave side of the curve, or the anatomic midline. The vertebral bodies are deformed, as is the vertebral canal. The shorter and thinner pedicles, and narrower canal, are located on the concave side of the curve. The degree of scoliosis is measured by calculating the Cobb angle (Fig. 2-15). A rib hump is often present on the convex side of a thoracic curve, and the shoulder appears "higher" on this side. This may help identify the presence of scoliosis, even when the spinous processes cannot be palpated because of body habitus.

Neuraxial anesthesia is technically more difficult and the success rate is lower for patients with scoliosis.[37] Local anesthetic requirements are less predictable and inadequate blockade may result from inadequate dispersion and pooling of intrathecal drug.

The interspinous space should be identified, as with spinal anesthesia in a patient with normal vertebral anatomy. Interspaces at the distal aspects of the curve are easier to access. Since the interlaminar space is deviated toward the convexity of the curve (away from the patient's

midline), the needle should be directed laterally; the more severe the curve, the more lateral the direction of the needle. The practitioner can often track the interspinous ligament with the tip of the spinal needle and thus maintain a needle course parallel to the direction of the spinous process. The patient is often helpful in this regard, as he or she can state whether the needle tip is on the right or left side and appropriate needle adjustments can be made. For patients with Cobb angles less than 20 degrees, there is minimal rotation and therefore minimal lateral correction is necessary.

Failed Spinal Anesthesia Spinal anesthesia fails if the resulting blockade is not adequate to block the painful surgical stimulus or provide necessary motor blockade. There may be no sensory blockade, partial sensory blockade, or inadequate blockade of all the necessary dermatomes. Possible reasons for failed block include intrathecal drug error, inadequate dose or intrathecal dispersion of local anesthetic, subdural injection, movement of the needle during injection, and injection into the spinal nerve dural cuff. Management options include induction of general anesthesia, administration of supplemental sedation and analgesia short of general anesthesia, a peripheral nerve block, or supplemental injection of local anesthetic at the surgical site. Finally, neuraxial block (epidural or spinal) may be repeated. The choice will depend on individual patient circumstances and preferences, and the degree to which the block has failed. If a neuraxial technique is chosen, the dose of local anesthetic may need to be altered, depending on whether no or partial blockade is present. The anesthesiologist should bear in mind that the procedure is being initiated in a partially anesthetized patient (i.e., the patient may not be able to complain of symptoms should the needle be irritating nerve tissue). If at all possible, a different lumbar interspace should be chosen for the second block.

Predicting the Difficulty of Spinal Anesthesia

Several groups of investigators have studied variables that predict difficulty in locating the epidural or subarachnoid space. In a study of almost 1500 patients undergoing spinal or epidural anesthesia, anesthesiologist experience, patient position (ability to flex spine judged adequate or inadequate before attempting the block), and quality of anatomic landmarks were independent predictors of the number of attempts necessary to attain successful neuraxial blockade.[38] An attempt was defined as *one skin puncture.*

Ultrasonography

The use of ultrasonography to facilitate neuraxial anesthesia by improving the correct identification of vertebral level, aiding in spinal and epidural needle insertion, and redirection if necessary, has been suggested. Correct identification of

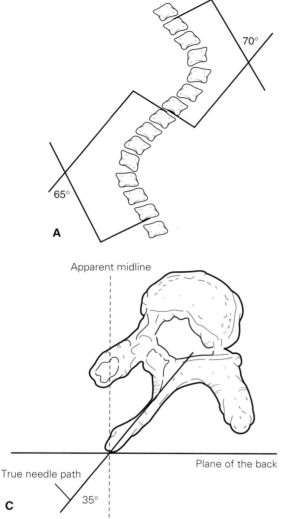

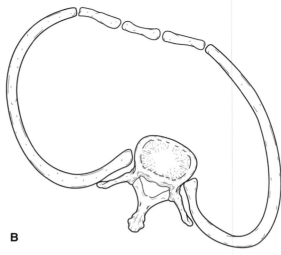

FIGURE 2-15. Scoliosis. (A) Schematic drawing of the Cobb angle. A line is drawn parallel to the superior cortical plate of the proximal end vertebrae and the inferior cortical plate of the distal end vertebrae. A perpendicular line is erected to each line and the angle of intersection of these lines determines the Cobb angle of the curve. (B) Schematic drawing of a transverse section of the rib cage. As a result of the rotation of the vertebrae the ribs on the convex side of the curve are pulled backward (posterior), producing the rib hump and raised shoulder. (C) Schematic drawing of the vertebral rotation. The vertebral body is deviated from the midline while the tip of the spinous process remains closer to the true midline (line drawn from C7 to sacrum). The interlaminar space is also deviated away from the midline. A needle inserted between the tips of the spinous processes should be directed into the curve. The angle of the needle path is dependent on the magnitude of the curve. *Used with permission from Crosby ET. Musculoskeletal disorders. In: Chestnut DH, ed,* Obstetric Anesthesia Principles and Practice, *3rd ed. Philadelphia, PA: Elsevier, 2004, p. 856; Crosby ET. Scoliosis and major spinal surgery. In: Gambling DR, Douglas MJ, eds,* Obstetric Anesthesia and Uncommon Disorders. *Philadelphia, PA: W.B. Saunders, 1998, p. 195.*

lumbar epidural spaces was successful 71% of the time after ultrasonic imaging, but only 30% of the time after palpation by an anesthesiologist.[39] In a small study, real-time ultrasonography facilitated the performance of CSE anesthesia.[40]

▶ Continuous Spinal Anesthesia

Inserting a catheter into the subarachnoid space increases the utility of spinal anesthesia by permitting continuous or repeated drug delivery in order to extend the level or duration of spinal blockade. A common and reasonable recommendation for subsequent dosing of continuous spinal anesthesia is to administer half the initial dose of local anesthetic when the

block duration is two-thirds of its expected duration. The technique is useful after inadvertent dural puncture with an epidural needle during attempted epidural anesthesia.

The technique is similar to that described for spinal anesthesia except that a needle large enough to accommodate the desired catheter must be used. After the subarachnoid placement of this needle, and ascertaining free flow of CSF, the catheter is threaded 2–3 cm into the subarachnoid space. It is often easier to insert the catheter if the needle bevel is directed cephalad or caudad instead of lateral. If the catheter does not easily pass beyond the needle tip, rotating the shaft of the needle 180 degrees may be helpful or another interspace can be used. The catheter should never be pulled back into the needle shaft because of the risk of shearing the catheter off into the subarachnoid space. If the catheter needs to be removed while it resides in the needle, the catheter and the needle should be removed as a unit.

There are no catheters currently marketed in the United States that have specifically been approved by the United States Food and Drug Administration (FDA) for continuous spinal anesthesia. Commonly, 18-gauge epidural needles and 20-gauge epidural catheters are used. Unfortunately, needles and catheters of this size carry a high risk of PDPH, especially in young patients. Because of this risk, smaller needle/catheter combinations have been developed with catheters ranging from 24- to 32-gauge. Although smaller catheters have decreased the incidence of PDPH, they have been associated with reports of neurologic injury, specifically cauda equina syndrome (see Chap. 6).

LUMBAR EPIDURAL ANESTHESIA

Epidural anesthesia is often initiated in the lumbar space for lower extremity orthopedic procedures (see Chap. 7), gynecologic pelvic procedures (see Chap. 12), and labor analgesia and cesarean delivery (see Chaps. 13 and 14). Because the vertebral spinous processes are relatively straight and do not overlap (see Chap. 1), the procedure is technically easier than thoracic epidural anesthesia. There is a greater margin for error if the procedure is performed caudad to the termination of the spinal cord. Approaches to the lumbar epidural space mimic those described for spinal anesthesia.

▶ Equipment

Commercial epidural trays are, in general, used in many parts of the world. The equipment in these trays is disposable, negating the need to sterilize needles and syringes. Usually, epidural anesthesia involves the placement of an epidural catheter in the epidural space, allowing for continuous anesthesia or analgesia. However, single-shot epidural anesthesia may be appropriate in some circumstances.

Epidural Needles

Epidural needles used in conjunction with epidural catheters are usually 17- or 18-gauge, allowing a 19- or 20-gauge catheter to be threaded through them. Standard epidural needles are 9-cm long. Most current needles have external centimeter markings so that the anesthesiologist can more precisely define the depth of the epidural space. This facilitates threading of the epidural catheter at a known distance into the epidural space. Smaller epidural needles have been advocated for single-shot techniques, for example, epidural steroid injections.

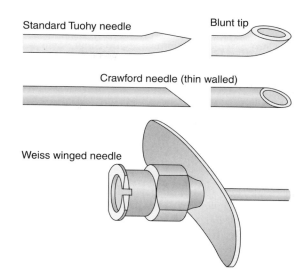

FIGURE 2-16. Epidural needle tips. *Used with permission from Kleinman W, Mikhail M. Spinal, epidural, and caudal blocks. In: Morgan GE, Mikhail MS, Murray M, eds, Clinical Anesthesiology, 4th ed. New York: McGraw-Hill, 2006, p. 289.*

Epidural needles have different tip designs (Fig. 2-16). All have a close-fitting stylet to prevent plugging of the needle during insertion through the skin and subcutaneous tissue. Most epidural needles (e.g., Tuohy and Husted designs) have a curved tip with a lateral facing orifice. This allows threading of an epidural catheter through the needle into the epidural space. The Crawford needle has a forward facing opening, which may be useful for facilitating threading of the epidural catheter if the needle is expected to enter the epidural space at a more acute angle (e.g., during the Taylor approach).

The sharpness of the tip of the epidural needle varies. Blunter needles permit easier identification of tissue along the path of the needle to the epidural space. The anesthesiologist has a better "feel" for the position of the tip of the needle as it is advanced through soft tissue, the intraspinous ligament, and the tougher ligamentum flavum. Many epidural needles have winged hubs (Fig. 2-16). This is particularly advantageous when using the hanging-drop method of identifying the epidural space, as the fingers should be well away from hub when using this technique. The wings are especially useful for cervical epidural injections. Disposable needles often have detachable plastic wings.

Epidural Catheters

Epidural catheters are made from plastic materials. There are two types of epidural catheters: single and multiorifice

Comparison of Multiorifice and Single-orifice Epidural Catheters

Single-orifice catheters

   Orifice in single compartment

Multi-orifice catheters

   Lower incidence of patchy or unilateral blocks

   Easy to aspirate blood or CSF

(Box 2-4). The *single-orifice* catheter has one opening at the tip, whereas the *multiorifice* catheter has a closed, bullet tip and several (usually 3) openings 0.5–1.5 cm from tip (Fig. 2-17). Current evidence suggests that the multiorifice catheter results in fewer patchy or unilateral blocks.[41–43] A theoretical disadvantage of multiorifice catheters is that the catheter openings may be located in more than one anatomic site (e.g., one orifice in the subarachnoid space with the others in the epidural space). However, there is no evidence that this is a clinical problem. The ability to aspirate blood should the catheter tip be located in a vessel is much easier with multiorifice compared to single-orifice catheters. Norris et al. found aspiration identified 47 of 48 intravascular catheters and suggested that an epinephrine containing test dose is unnecessary when using a multiorifice catheter.[44]

Epidural catheters made from different materials have different degrees of "stiffness."[45] The wire-embedded Arrow epidural catheter (FlexTip Plus™) is a single-orifice catheter that is very flimsy (Fig. 2-17). Banwell et al. found that use of this catheter compared to a stiffer epidural catheter resulted in fewer paresthesias and intravascular cannulations.[46] The authors of this chapter have noted a decreased incidence of paresthesias and intravascular catheters, as well as a markedly decreased incidence of patchy blocks compared to the stiffer catheters. Presumably, the flimsy catheter tends to coil near the entrance site in the epidural space instead of snaking off to one side, or through a vertebral foramen.

Modern epidural catheters have centimeter markings along the catheter, usually between 5 and 20 cm from the tip (Fig. 2-17). This aids in leaving a known length of catheter in the epidural space. In addition, the catheter has a darkened tip for confirmation of complete, intact removal of the catheter from the patient. An adapter attaches to the proximal end of the epidural catheter to allow attachment of a syringe or infusion tubing. The use of a Luer-lock tubing-catheter interface is recommended. A bacterial filter may be attached to the injection port to filter glass particles or bacterial contamination although there is no evidence that filters decrease the rate of infection or injection of undesirable foreign substances.[47] Westphal et al. demonstrated that a standard epidural catheter filter adsorbs sufentanil and suggested that filters be primed with the anesthetic solution before infusing into the patient.[48] Epidural catheters with stylets are no longer in common use. Although insertion may be easier, styleted catheters have been associated with higher incidence of paresthesias, intravascular catheters, and dural puncture.

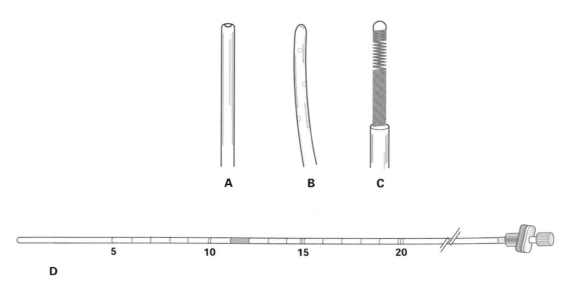

FIGURE 2-17. Epidural catheters. (A) Standard open-tipped catheter. (B) Multiorifice, bullet-tipped catheter. (C) Wire-embedded open-tipped catheter. (D) Centimeter markings are between 5 and 20 cm starting at distal tip. The distal tip is darkened so that complete withdrawal of the catheter can be ascertained. The proximal end of the catheter has a Luer-lock connector.

Syringes for Loss-of-Resistance

Syringes used for the loss-of-resistance (LOR) technique to identify the epidural space were traditionally made of glass with a Luer-lock connector. Currently, preassembled epidural trays with disposable contents contain either plastic or glass syringes. The type of syringe is largely a matter of personal preference. There are no data to support the superiority of one type compared to another.

▶ Technique of Epidural Anesthesia

Patient monitoring, positioning, and preparation for lumbar epidural anesthesia mimic that for spinal anesthesia. Patient position during and after injection of the anesthetic plays less of a role in determining the final extent of sensory blockade, as gravity has a little effect on the distribution of epidural anesthetic solution(s). Block onset was faster and motor blockade was denser on the dependent side when epidural lumbar anesthesia was initiated in the lateral position.[49] This suggests that the operative side should be placed down when initiating lumbar epidural anesthesia for lower extremity surgical procedures in the lateral position.

Lumbar epidural anesthesia is most often initiated at L2-L3, L3-L4, L4-L5, and sometimes at L5-S1. There is inherently added safety in performing the procedure below L1, as the spinal cord terminates at this level in most adults (see Chap. 1). It is easier to learn a midline approach to lumbar epidural anesthesia. Once the midline approach has been mastered, the paravertebral approach should also be learned. In both cases, the epidural needle should enter the epidural space in the midline (Fig. 2-8).

Two methods are used to identify entrance of the epidural needle into the epidural space: LOR and hanging-drop. The *LOR* technique is the most popular, particularly for lumbar epidural anesthesia. The *hanging-drop* method is described in the Cervical Epidural Anesthesia section.

Midline Approach

The interspinous space is identified as for spinal anesthesia and local anesthetic is infiltrated to the depth of the supraspinous ligament. If the epidural needle is very blunt, the anesthesiologist may wish to puncture the skin with a sharper needle of similar gauge. The epidural needle with stylet is placed through the skin wheal and subcutaneous tissue to the depth of the interspinous ligament (Fig. 2-18). The authors prefer to puncture the skin in the middle of the interspinous space. Others have recommended puncturing the skin in the top third of the interspinous space, as the interlaminar space is slightly cephalad to the interspinous space. Such an approach allows the needle to be advanced perpendicular to the long axis of the spine in the sagittal plane.

Epidural Needle Bevel Orientation In general, if *bilateral blockade* is desired, the epidural needle bevel should be facing cephalad. Analgesia is more symmetric[50] and the catheter is easier to thread[51] when the bevel is oriented cephalad compared to lateral. Rotation of the needle after identification of the epidural space increases the likelihood of inadvertent dural puncture.[52] If a *unilateral block* is desired (e.g., lower extremity surgery), threading the epidural catheter with the needle bevel oriented 45 degrees toward the right or left from the cephalad position is associated with unilateral sensory blockade and shorter latency and greater density of motor blockade on the side toward which the bevel is oriented.[53]

After the epidural needle is advanced into the interspinous ligament, the stylet is removed. When the anesthesiologist removes his or her hand from the needle, the needle should remain in the midline (in the sagittal plane), and remain at the desired angle to the skin in all planes. If the needle tip is correctly anchored in the ligament, the needle shaft will not fall downward when released. If the needle shaft falls, the tip is still in subcutaneous tissue, and not in the ligament. If the needle deviates laterally, it should be withdrawn, repositioned, and readvanced. Lateral deviation of the needle implies that the needle may not be in the interspinous space, but rather is being deflected off a spinous process.

Loss-of-Resistance to Air Versus Saline The LOR syringe is filled with either air or saline. Air and saline have a slightly different "feel" and whether an individual anesthesiologist uses air or saline may largely be a matter of habit or training. Recent evidence suggests several reasons for the superiority of saline compared to air.[54] These include a lower incidence of patchy epidural blockade, pneumocephalus (causing headache and neurologic symptoms), and PDPH should the dura be inadvertently punctured with the epidural needle. Reported complications of LOR to air include venous air embolism, subcutaneous emphysema, and nerve root compression. Evidence suggests that the LOR to saline technique is gaining acceptance among anesthesiologists.

Some anesthesiologists prefer not to use LOR to saline when performing a combined spinal-epidural technique (see "Combined Spinal-Epidural Anesthesia," later), as the saline may be confused with CSF. Many anesthesiologists who use saline (several milliliters) intentionally fill the syringe with a small air bubble (0.25–0.5 mL). This air bubble will compress if the saline is injected into a space other than the epidural space, but will not compress if the saline is injected into the epidural space. There is greater resistance to plunger movement when glass syringes are lubricated with saline compared to a dry plunger.[55]

Advancement of the Epidural Needle After removal of the stylet, the anesthesiologist should attach the LOR syringe, filled with 2–4 mL of air or saline, to the needle with the

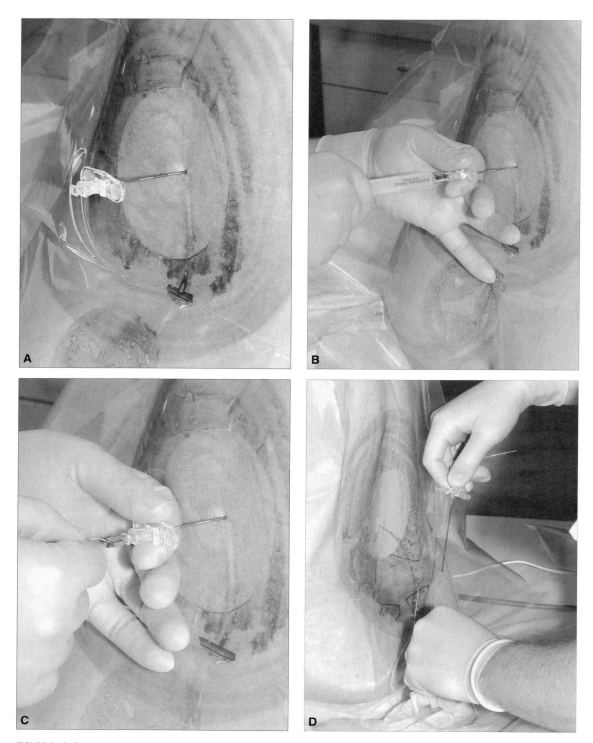

FIGURE 2-18. Epidural anesthesia. (A) Epidural needle inserted to depth of interspinous ligament. Note that the needle is supported by the ligament. (B) The stylet is removed and the LOR syringe is attached to the needle. (C) The epidural catheter is threaded through the epidural needle. (D) The needle is removed and the epidural catheter remains in the epidural space.

dominant hand while anchoring the epidural needle with the nondominant hand (Fig. 2-18). There are several techniques for advancing the epidural needle-syringe ensemble, and several hand positions for controlling the advancement of the epidural needle. Again, the chosen technique is largely a matter of training and personal preference. Of importance is control of the epidural needle. The anesthesiologist should be able to stop needle advancement immediately if it is evident that the tip is in the epidural space. Needle advancement can be controlled at the needle shaft near the skin, at the hub, or both. Anesthesiologists may place their fingers on the shaft or hub, or wings of the needle, or some combination of these (Fig. 2-19).

The epidural needle may be advanced with continuous or intermittent pressure on the plunger of the syringe. Light pressure to the syringe plunger is usually applied with the dominant hand. Heavy pressure may allow the injection of air or saline into tissue that is not the epidural space. Using an intermittent advancement technique, the dominant (plunger) hand may be moved back and forth between the needle and syringe plunger, as the needle is advanced, or it may remain on the plunger. The needle is advanced several millimeters and then pressure is applied to the syringe

plunger (usually with the thumb) to test for LOR. If resistance is encountered, the needle is advanced several more millimeters and again the plunger is depressed. This sequence is repeated until LOR is encountered.

Anesthesiologists who advance the needle-syringe ensemble continuously must keep one thumb on the syringe plunger while advancing the needle with the other hand. Most skilled practitioners of epidural anesthesia can "feel" as the needle tip advances into the ligamentum flavum. This is particularly true if a dull needle is being used. The ligamentum flavum is tougher than the interspinous ligament; therefore, advancement of the needle tip through the ligamentum flavum requires slightly more pressure. Sometimes crepitation is felt, or even heard, as the ligamentum flavum is encountered. Typically, the lumbar ligamentum flavum is 5–6 mm thick in the midline.

As the epidural needle tip encounters the epidural space, LOR occurs. The plunger suddenly depresses and the air or saline is easily injected into the epidural space. The entire contents of the LOR syringe need not be injected into the epidural space. This may result in a significant amount of air or saline in the epidural space, both of which may contribute to patchy anesthesia.

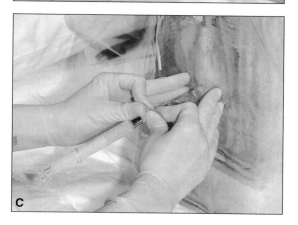

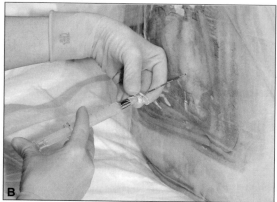

FIGURE 2-19. Hand positions for advancement of an epidural needle. (A) Triangulation of nondominant hand: back of hand is against the patient's back and thumb and index finger grasp the shaft of the epidural needle near the back. The needle is moved incrementally or continuously. The thumb of the dominant hand exerts a small amount of pressure on the syringe barrel, either continuously or intermittently. (B) Triangulation of nondominant hand: back of hand is against the patient's back and thumb and index finger grasp the hub of the epidural needle near the back. The needle is moved incrementally or continuously. The thumb of the dominant hand exerts a small amount of pressure on the syringe barrel, either continuously or intermittently. (C) Triangulation using the third through fifth fingers of both hands. The thumb and index finger grasp the epidural needle wings. Between incremental needle advancements the thumb of the dominant hand exerts a small amount of pressure on the syringe barrel. This technique is also used with the hanging-drop method of identifying the epidural space.

The depth of the epidural space from the skin can often be estimated based on experience and inspection of body habitus. Epidural space depth in the average adult ranges from 4 to 6 cm,[56,57] but can be less than 3 cm in thin patients. The depth is usually greater in obese individuals,[58] although many obese individuals have a midline concavity so that the epidural space depth is not markedly increased compared to nonobese individuals. Individual anatomy, however, varies widely, and some individuals have a convex tissue curve over the lumbar spine, rather than a concave curve. This may add several centimeters of soft tissue to the skin-epidural space depth. The skin to epidural space distance is greater in patients placed in the lateral compared to sitting position.[58]

The anteroposterior depth of the epidural space is greatest in the midline and varies from 2 to 20 mm, but is usually 5–6 mm in the lumbar region (see Chap. 1). The anesthesiologist should aim to puncture the epidural space in the midline, no matter the angle of approach, as the epidural space depth is significantly decreased at the lateral aspects of the posterior epidural space (Fig. 1-5). The perceived depth of the epidural space (the distance the epidural needle must traverse from the ligamentum flavum until the dura is punctured) varies, depending on individual anatomy, the point of puncture of the epidural space, and the angle of the needle. The smallest ligamentum flavum-dura distance will be encountered if the epidural needle is parallel, but lateral to the midline.

If a single-shot epidural technique is planned, the entire anesthetic dose is injected through the epidural needle, and the needle is removed. The authors prefer not to aspirate through the epidural needle. Rather, to increase the margin of safety, the total dose should be injected incrementally over several minutes, following a test dose to rule out intrathecal or intravascular needle placement. Even when planning to insert an epidural catheter, all or part of the initial epidural dose may be injected through the epidural needle before placement of the epidural catheter. The incidence of one-sided epidural blockade may be less if the entire dose is injected through the needle. There are several disadvantages to this technique, however. The patient must not move for several minutes while the dose is injected slowly and incrementally. Correct catheter placement cannot be verified and a nonfunctioning epidural catheter may not be identified until an additional epidural dose is necessary. At this point in time it may be impossible to replace the catheter.

Insertion of the Epidural Catheter   In most circumstances, after the epidural space is identified, an epidural catheter is threaded through the epidural needle. Although the injection of 5–10 mL of saline through the epidural needle may decrease the incidence of epidural vein puncture with the epidural catheter, injection of 3 mL offers no advantage.[59] The authors do not routinely inject saline, as this may increase the incidence of inadequate anesthesia and may also be confused with CSF.

The epidural catheter is usually threaded with the assistance of a threading device that fits into the hub of the epidural needle (Fig. 2-18). This centers the catheter in the needle hub. The needle is anchored with the nondominant hand, by placing the back of the hand against the patient's back and holding the needle hub between the index finger and thumb. The catheter is threaded in short increments (approximately 1 cm at a time) by grasping the catheter 1 cm proximal to the needle hub and advancing it to the hub. Once the catheter has passed the 12-cm mark at the hub of the needle, the catheter is advancing past the tip of the epidural needle into the epidural space. The catheter is usually advanced 4–6 cm into the space. Although the length of epidural needle hubs and threading devices vary slightly, this usually means the catheter is threaded to a depth of 16–18 cm at the hub of the 9-cm epidural needle before removal.

Before removing the epidural needle, the epidural space depth should be noted by counting the visible centimeter markings on the shaft of the epidural needle. The epidural needle is then withdrawn slowly with one hand, while the other hand continues to "thread" the epidural catheter through the epidural needle (in reality holding the catheter in place relative to the skin while the needle is withdrawn over the catheter). The epidural needle is withdrawn over the entirety of the epidural catheter. Finally, the connector (and filter, if it is used) is attached to the epidural catheter. The length of epidural catheter in the epidural space may need to be adjusted by withdrawing the catheter until an appropriate depth is reached by noting the markings on the catheter relative to the skin.

Length of Epidural Catheter in the Epidural Space   The optimal length of epidural catheter in the epidural space may depend on the type of catheter, surgical procedure, patient body habitus, duration of catheterization, and expected patient movement. Although it is advisable to err on the side of too much catheter threaded into the epidural space, rather than too little, threading too much catheter increases the risk that the catheter will advance off the midline or through an intervertebral foramen, resulting in an inadequate block.[60] This problem is less likely with flexible catheters, as they tend to coil in the epidural space, rather than advance.[61] In addition, redundant catheter in the epidural space may increase the risk of intravenous catheter placement, paresthesia, or dural puncture with the catheter.

Catheters "move" relative to the skin, and relative to the epidural space if the catheter is anchored to the skin when patients move. Asking the patient to straightened his or her back after having assumed the sitting flexed spine position for insertion of the epidural catheter will cause the catheter to move in (relative to the skin). Catheters are advanced inward at an average of 7–10 mm (range 0–42 mm) when patients move from sitting flexed, to sitting straight, to a lateral decubitus position.[62] This "movement" was more pronounced in obese individuals. Repetitive position changes in an active patient may eventually cause the epidural catheter to become dislodged.

For limited duration surgical procedures with planned removal of the epidural catheter immediately after the procedure, 2–3 cm catheter length in the epidural space is sufficient. The patient will not move during the procedure, and this length decreases the risk of a one-sided or patchy block.[60] In contrast, if the epidural catheter will be used for labor analgesia, or postoperative analgesia, or other circumstances in which significant patient movement is anticipated, the catheter should be inserted 4–6 cm into the epidural space. This will decrease the risk of catheter dislodgment, but at the cost of a higher incidence of one-sided blockade.

Securing the Epidural Catheter Prior to securing the epidural catheter, or injecting drugs through the catheter, the epidural connector cap should be removed and the proximal end of the catheter lowered below the level of the epidural catheter tip. Often, if the catheter tip is malpositioned in the intrathecal space, or in a blood vessel, CSF or blood will spontaneously drip from the end of the catheter. This allows identification of a misplaced catheter before any drug is injected.

The epidural catheter should be secured at the puncture site with a transparent dressing. This allows inspection of the catheter and puncture site. If prolonged catheterization or patient movement is anticipated, an adhesive skin preparation should be applied to the skin before affixing the dressing. The edges of the dressing can be further secured with tape. The proximal catheter is usually taped to the patient's back so that it is easily assessable from the shoulder.

Paramedian (Paraspinous) Approach

The preparation for a paramedian approach to the epidural space mimics that for spinal anesthesia (Fig. 2-8). It may be helpful to infiltrate local anesthetic with a 22-gauge 9-cm spinal needle inserted at a 90-degree angle to all planes to the depth of the lamina. This will give an estimate of the depth of the ligamentum flavum. The epidural needle is inserted close to the spinal process. This avoids extreme angulation of the needle and the needle is more likely to penetrate the ligamentum flavum in the midline. The epidural needle is usually advanced to the depth of the ligamentum flavum before attachment of the LOR syringe as the paraspinous soft tissue does not offer "resistance." If the lamina is encountered, the needle should be redirected or "walked" in a more cephalad and medial direction. If the lateral aspect of the spinous process is encountered, a more cephalad and lateral direction may be necessary.

Injection of Epidural Anesthetic Solutions

Injection of drugs through an epidural catheter should also be made with the thought that the catheter tip may not be in the epidural space. Even catheters known to have been in the epidural space (because injection through them has produced successful epidural anesthesia) can migrate. Therefore, unless the risk outweighs the benefit (e.g., emergency cesarean delivery), drugs should be injected slowly and incrementally, usually after administration of an epidural test dose. The identity of the drug should be checked, and rechecked before injection.

Gentle aspiration should be performed prior to each injection, although negative aspiration, particularly through a single-orifice catheter, does not reliably rule out intravascular or intrathecal placement of the epidural catheter tip.[63] In contrast, aspiration identified 60 of 62 intravenous multiorifice catheters.[64] Free, easy aspiration of clear fluid almost always indicates location of the catheter tip in the intrathecal space. If aspiration of clear fluid is slow, or "stop and go," the anesthesiologist must differentiate between CSF and previously injected anesthetic solution/saline. Several tests differentiate CSF from anesthetic solutions. CSF is warm (body temperature), whereas recently injected anesthetic solution feels cooler (room temperature). CSF contains glucose, whereas epidural anesthetic solutions do not. A urine dipstick test can verify the presence or absence of glucose. If CSF is identified, a decision should be made as to whether to continue with continuous spinal anesthesia, or replace the epidural catheter. No attempt should be made to withdraw the catheter tip into the epidural space, as subdural placement of the catheter tip may result. Aspiration of blood indicates that the catheter tip is located in a blood vessel. Recommendations for further management are discussed later.

Epidural Test Dose The traditional epidural test dose tests whether the epidural catheter tip is malpositioned in a blood vessel or the intrathecal space. The intravascular and intrathecal test doses may either be combined (to test for both intravascular and intrathecal placement with a single injection) or divided. *A negative response to an epidural test dose does not guarantee the correct placement of the epidural catheter in the epidural space*, but rather decreases the likelihood that the catheter tip is in a blood vessel or the subarachnoid space.

The inadvertent intrathecal placement of a catheter is tested by injecting a small, subanesthetic bolus dose of local anesthetic (Table 2-1). The dose should be low enough so that there is minimal risk of total spinal anesthesia. Patients usually perceive warmth in their legs within 1 min of the intrathecal injection. Impaired straight leg raise 4 min after an intrathecal test dose injection, however, was the only test that had a sensitivity of 100%, whereas the sensitivity for warmth and impaired pinprick was only 93%.[65] Ropivacaine 15 mg was not a useful intrathecal test dose because of the slow onset of motor blockade.[66]

The intravascular placement of a catheter is traditionally tested by injecting epinephrine or subtoxic doses of local anesthetic (Table 2-1). Moore and Batra first described the

Table 2-1		
Epidural Test Doses		
Test Dose Components	Positive Intravascular Test Dose	Positive Intrathecal Test Dose
Combined Intrathecal and Intravenous Test Dose		
Lidocaine 1.5% with epinephrine 1:200,000, 3 mL Bupivacaine 0.25% with epinephrine 1:200,000, 3 mL	Increase HR 20 bpm	Motor blockade at 3–5 min*
Intravenous Test Dose		
Lidocaine 100 mg	Tinnitus, circumoral numbness, "dizziness"	
Bupivacaine 25 mg		
Chloroprocaine 90 mg		
Fentanyl 100 μg	Dizziness, drowsiness	
Air 1 mL	Mill-wheel murmur over right heart	
Intrathecal Test Dose		
Lidocaine 40–60 mg Bupivacaine 7.5 mg		Motor blockade at 3–5 min*

*Weakness in hip flexion. Test doses may be less sensitive in premedicated patients, patients treated with beta-blockers, pregnant patients, and anesthetized patients.

injection of epinephrine 15 μg.[67] An increase in HR of 20 bpm within 45 s was 100% sensitive and specific for intravascular injection in unpremedicated patients.[68] An increase in systolic blood pressure between 15 and 25 mmHg was also observed. The test is less sensitive for patients with pharmacologic beta-blockade,[68] sedated patients,[69] and during general[70] or high-thoracic[71] anesthesia; and may be less specific in laboring women.[72] The epinephrine bolus should be injected quickly through the epidural catheter, as slow injection results in more equivocal responses. Typically, 3-mL of a premixed local anesthetic-epinephrine solution (epinephrine 1:200,000 dilution, or 5 μg/mL) is injected.

Subtoxic doses of local anesthetics may be used to detect an intravascular catheter. For example, the intravascular injection of lidocaine 100 mg (2% lidocaine 5 mL) will usually cause symptoms of central nervous system irritability, including tinnitus, circumoral paresthesias, and dizziness.[73] Unpremedicated patients were able to recognize the intravenous injection of 2-chloroprocaine 90 mg and bupivacaine 25 mg, but patients premedicated with fentanyl and midazolam were not.[74]

Other markers of intravascular injection have been investigated. Leighton et al. found the injection of 1–2 mL of air (monitored by placing the external fetal HR Doppler probe over the parturient's heart) was a sensitive and specific indicator of intravascular injection for single-orifice catheters,[75] but not for multiorifice catheters.[76] Isoproterenol has also been investigated in a small number of patients,[77] as has fentanyl 100 μg.[78,79] Finally, electrical stimulation of a wire-embedded epidural catheter has been suggested as a possible technique to identify correct placement of the epidural catheter in the epidural space.[80]

No matter what "test dose" is used, or whether one is used, incremental dosing of epidural catheters is essential. No test has a sensitivity of 100% and catheters may migrate during use.

Anesthetic Bolus Dose Epidural anesthetic solutions should be injected slowly and incrementally following aspiration. The rate of injection does not influence the distribution of solution within the epidural space unless the solution is injected extremely slowly, over many minutes. The total estimated dose is usually injected in 3–5 mL increments over 5 min. If precise control of the level of blockade is important for patient well-being (e.g., avoidance of an extensive blockade and associated hypotension), the initial dose should be conservative. The mass (volume and concentration) of drug influences the extent and density of blockade (see Chap. 3).

If time permits a small increment of the planned total dose (approximately 3–5 mL, including the test dose) should be injected and the anesthesiologist should wait to inject the remaining dose until there is evidence of successful epidural anesthesia (e.g., blockade to temperature at and near the dermatome of injection). This allows replacement of the epidural catheter, if necessary, before the maximum allowable dose is injected. If a large dose of local anesthetic has been injected before the diagnosis of failed blockade is made, the block cannot be immediately repeated.

Epidural anesthesia is maintained by either intermittent injection or a continuous infusion. Intermittent injection of 50% of the initial dose as the blockade begins to regress, or at the time of expected blockade regression, will maintain blockade at the initial sensory level. Waiting for blockade regression may cause an anesthetic "window," particularly with short-acting local anesthetics such as 2-chloroprocaine.

Twenty to twenty–five percent of the initial epidural dose is often injected 20–25 min after the initial dose. This effectively results in denser blockade without extending dermatomal distribution, and is particularly useful for intra-abdominal procedures with extensive visceral surgical stimulation.

Continuous Epidural Infusion Epidural anesthesia can be maintained with a continuous infusion of local anesthetic. The requirement for an infusion pump is a disadvantage of this technique. However, this technique may be inherently safer, as no concentrated local anesthetic bolus injection is required after the initial injection.

Epidural Catheter Removal

Removal of the epidural catheter is usually a simple process of removing the dressing and pulling the catheter out using steady traction. Less force may be required to remove the epidural catheter if the patient is placed in the same position as catheter insertion.[81] The catheter tip should be checked to ensure that the catheter has been removed in its entirety. Techniques to remove a recalcitrant catheter are discussed later.

Troubleshooting Epidural Anesthesia

Difficulty Locating the Epidural Space Techniques used to locate the lumbar epidural space closely mimic those used to locate the subarachnoid space during initiation of spinal anesthesia. It is usually easier to make small adjustments and "walk" the relatively rigid epidural needle off bone compared to the flimsier spinal needle. In contrast to a spinal needle, for which a change in needle direction necessitates withdrawal to subcutaneous tissue before redirecting, the epidural needle may be withdrawn several millimeters and then readvanced with a small change in needle direction. The needle tip may become occluded with bony debris, particularly, if pressure was applied to the needle during bone contact. If the needle tip is occluded, LOR may not be appreciated,

even if the needle tip is in the epidural space, thus increasing the risk of dural puncture. Therefore, it may be advisable to replace and remove the stylet, or flush the needle with a small amount of saline, if a bone plug is likely.

False Loss-of-Resistance A LOR sensation may be perceived, even though the epidural needle tip is not located in the epidural space. In particular, this may occur if the needle enters the interspinous ligament at an oblique angle. The needle tip will exit the ligament into the soft tissue on the opposite side with a LOR feel. It is usually more difficult to thread an epidural catheter into a false "space," but it is certainly not impossible. This is the probable explanation for many failed epidural blocks.

It is often possible to ascertain whether the LOR is due to entry into the epidural or false space by injecting several milliliters of saline, and then gently tapping the plunger of the air- or saline-filled LOR syringe. If the saline was injected into soft tissue, the plunger will again encounter "resistance." If the saline was injected into the epidural space, the plunger will easily depress.

Another method to differentiate between soft tissue and the epidural space is to inject saline with a small air bubble in the syringe (about 0.5 mL). If the saline is being injected into the epidural space the bubble will not compress. In contrast, the bubble will compress if the saline is being injected into soft tissue. Some anesthesiologists have suggested passing a long spinal needle through the epidural needle, in an attempt to puncture the dura, even if a combined spinal-epidural technique is not planned. The presence of CSF in the hub of the spinal needle is a good indication that the epidural needle is correctly placed in the epidural space (see "Combined Spinal-Epidural Anesthesia," below).

If the connection between the LOR syringe and epidural needle is not tight, there will be an air or saline leak as resistance is checked. This may result in a false LOR sensation. Finally, if the epidural catheter does not advance smoothly, particularly after the tip of the catheter has passed the tip of the epidural needle, the anesthesiologist should suspect that a false space has been identified.

Difficulty Threading the Epidural Catheter into the Epidural Space Occasionally, the epidural catheter will meet resistance as catheter advancement through the epidural needle is attempted. This may be a sign that the epidural needle tip is not in the epidural space and the needle should be withdrawn and repositioned. However, if the anesthesiologist is convinced that the needle tip is located in the epidural space, several "tricks" may help overcome this problem. Asking the patient to take a deep breath during attempted advancement of the epidural catheter may facilitate threading of the epidural catheter. Epiduroscopy demonstrated that this maneuver opened up space at the needle tip.[82] The injection of saline 10 mL did not facilitate advancement of epidural catheters;[83] however, changing the angle of needle insertion did.[84] Lumbar and thoracic epidural catheters inserted through needles angled 50–60 degrees to the plane of the skin, compared to 90 degrees, were more likely to advance in the midline. The authors do not recommend rotating the epidural needle, as this may increase the risk of inadvertent dural puncture. Instead, the epidural needle should be withdrawn several millimeters and downward pressure applied to the hub of the epidural needle. This may slightly change the angle of the tip of the needle and move it away from the dura.

If the epidural catheter has been advanced beyond the tip of the epidural needle (as indicated by the centimeter markings on the catheter), and the catheter needs to be withdrawn, the epidural needle and catheter *must always be withdrawn together*. There is a risk of shearing off the catheter tip if the catheter is withdrawn through the needle.

Paresthesias During Needle or Catheter Advancement
Needle or catheter advancement should cease if the patients complains of paresthesias. Paresthesias with needle advancement should prompt the withdrawal and repositioning of the epidural needle at a different angle (toward the midline). The side of the paresthesia (left or right) should direct the anesthesiologist toward the correct side. If the paresthesia is transient during epidural catheter advancement, a further attempt at catheter advancement can be made. However, if the paresthesia recurs, the needle and catheter should be withdrawn and repositioned. The injection of a small amount of saline (3–4 mL) through the epidural needle before attempted catheter advancement did not decrease the incidence of paresthesia.[85]

Blood in the Epidural Needle or Catheter   The epidural needle may puncture a blood vessel in soft tissue as the needle is advanced toward the epidural space, or puncture a blood vessel in the epidural space. The needle should be withdrawn, flushed with saline, and readvanced through a different puncture site, or at a different angle through the same puncture site. If blood fills the epidural needle, but is not removed by flushing, the blood may clot in the needle and the anesthesiologist will fail to recognize the LOR as the epidural needle traverses the epidural space, thus increasing the risk of an inadvertent dural puncture.

The authors advocate removal and replacement of the epidural catheter after blood vessel puncture, particularly if the catheter has multiple orifices. Norris et al. withdrew eight multiorifice intravascular catheters until aspiration was negative for blood.[44] Six of the eight catheters, however, subsequently tested positive for intravascular placement when tested with a lidocaine/epinephrine test dose. In contrast, D'Angelo et al. were able to "rescue" approximately 50% of single-orifice catheters by withdrawing the catheter until blood could no longer be aspirated.[60] The catheter tips of the remaining 50% were no longer in the epidural space (as assessed by location of the catheter markings relative to skin). If the anesthesiologist plans on attempting to use the epidural catheter, the blood should be flushed from the catheter immediately, as it will otherwise quickly clot and occlude the catheter.

Inadvertent Dural Puncture   Experienced anesthesiologists have all experienced the sinking feeling that accompanies the sight of CSF pouring into the LOR syringe. The reflex reaction of an inexperienced anesthesiologist is to immediately withdraw the epidural needle. This reflex reaction should be suppressed. The stylet should be replaced in the needle, or a finger placed over the hub to stop the CSF leak while management options are considered (Table 2-2). If locating the epidural space has been difficult, the anesthesiologist may

Table 2-2

Advantages and Disadvantages of Management Options after Inadvertent Dural Puncture during Attempted Epidural Anesthesia

Option	Advantages	Disadvantages
Continuous spinal analgesia	1. Avoid risk of second dural puncture	1. Risk of total spinal if an "epidural" dose is inadvertently injected into the catheter
	2. Reliable continuous anesthesia	2. Possible increased risk of infection
	3. Possible decreased risk of PDPH*	
Place/replace catheter at different interspace	1. May use for a prophylactic blood patch*	1. Risk of second dural puncture
	2. Higher margin of safety relative to local anesthetic injection	2. Risk of high spinal anesthesia with epidural bolus injection of local anesthetic

*See Chap. 6 for discussion of risk and treatment of PDPH and prophylactic blood patch.

wish to consider continuous spinal anesthesia or analgesia. Other alternatives include attempting epidural anesthesia at a different interspace. Intrathecal anesthetics can be administered through the epidural needle before it is removed and repositioned. If a dural puncture occurs during attempted combined spinal-epidural labor analgesia, the authors often inject the intrathecal analgesia dose through the epidural needle before withdrawing it from the intrathecal space, and then place an epidural catheter at a different interspace. It is controversial whether the placement of an intrathecal catheter after inadvertent dural puncture decreases the incidence of PDPH (see Chap. 6).

The presence of a large hole in the dura may facilitate the passage of anesthetic agents from the epidural to intrathecal space, resulting in higher than intended anesthetic concentrations in the CSF. This may be particularly true during epidural bolus injections (compared to continuous infusions). The clinical affect is also likely to be greater for hydrophilic as compared to lipophilic substances.[86] Therefore, care should be taken when injecting epidural morphine or large volumes of local anesthetics after dural puncture with an epidural needle.

Patchy or Unilateral Epidural Blockade   The treatment of "patchy" or unilateral epidural blockade depends on several factors, including a risk/benefit analysis of alternative anesthetic options compared to attempted "rescue" of the current epidural anesthetic or repeating a new neuraxial anesthetic. Other factors include the likely cause of inadequate anesthesia/analgesia. For example, the dermatomal extent of sensory blockade may be inadequate. In this case, additional local anesthetic should be administered. In contrast, the caudal and cephalad extend of blockade may be adequate, but there may be "missed" segments, or the blockade may not be dense enough to block visceral pain during abdominal surgery. In this case, 20–25% of the initial anesthetic dose should be injected 20–25 min after the initial dose. This will increase the density of blockade without increasing the extent of blockade. The injection of opioids into the epidural space is also an option (see Chap. 3).

Particularly when some block is present, and the maximum local anesthetic dose has not been injected, it may be reasonable to inject more local anesthetic in an attempt to increase the distribution of local anesthetic to "missed" dermatomes. Patient position has little effect on the distribution of an epidural bolus dose of anesthetic solution; however, it may be reasonable to perform the supplemental injection with the less blocked side in the dependent position.

Patchy anesthesia may result if the epidural catheter tip has migrated into the lateral epidural space or into an intervertebral foramen. This situation is more likely to occur when longer lengths of catheter are advanced into the epidural space. Beilin et al. randomized parturients with inadequate epidural analgesia to one of two rescue techniques: women in one group received an additional 5 mL bolus of local anesthetic without catheter manipulation.[87] The epidural catheter was withdrawn 1 cm before the additional 5 mL of local anesthetic was injected in women in the second group. Twenty-gauge multiorifice catheters were originally secured 5 cm in the epidural space. The ability to achieve satisfactory analgesia was not different between the two techniques. These results suggest that manipulation of multiorifice epidural catheters does not reliably improve the ability to "rescue" inadequate epidural anesthesia/analgesia.

The authors believe that one attempt to rescue inadequate epidural anesthesia/analgesia may be justified, depending on the circumstances. However, if this is unsuccessful, an alternative plan of action should be undertaken. It is often difficult to admit failure, and easy for the anesthesiologist to convince himself or herself that the block is adequate, when in fact, it is not. The anesthesiologist, surgeon, and patient will rue this decision. The surgical procedure should not be allowed to commence with inadequate anesthesia. Inadequate epidural anesthesia may be rescued with systemic analgesia/sedation, or even general anesthesia, but this may not be desirable or advisable in certain circumstances.

Failed Epidural Anesthesia   Several options exist for failed epidural anesthesia (Box 2-5). These include abandonment of a neuraxial technique or repeating neuraxial anesthesia. It is best to diagnose failed epidural anesthesia before the entire planned dose has been injected. This is particularly important when large doses of local anesthetic are necessary for adequate anesthesia (e.g., when a lumbar epidural

---

Box 2-5

Options for Failed Epidural Anesthesia

Nonneuraxial anesthetic technique

General anesthesia

Peripheral nerve block*

Local anesthesia*

Neuraxial techniques

Epidural anesthesia*

Spinal anesthesia[†]

CSE anesthesia

*Care should be taken to monitor total dose of local anesthetic (from failed epidural anesthesia attempt and second rescue anesthetic) in order to avoid systemic local anesthetic toxicity.

[†]Increased risk of high or total spinal anesthesia (see text).

catheter is used for abdominal surgery). In these situations, the total dose of local anesthetic approaches the maximum suggested dose (Table 3-6). In addition, the injection of a large volume of local anesthetic into tissue other than the epidural space may distort vertebral anatomy and make subsequent attempts at neuraxial anesthesia more difficult.

If the initial "failed" dose was such that additional epidural local anesthetic injection is safe, epidural anesthesia can be repeated. A different vertebral interspace should be chosen. A second alternative is spinal anesthesia. However, there have been several reports of high or total spinal anesthesia when spinal anesthesia is performed after failed epidural anesthesia.[88,89] Particularly if some degree of neuraxial blockade is present at the time of initiation of spinal anesthesia, it is advisable to reduce the intrathecal dose of local anesthetic. A final neuraxial anesthetic alternative is CSE. This offers the advantage of a small initial intrathecal dose of local anesthetic, which decreases the risk of both systemic local anesthetic toxicity and high spinal anesthesia, with the ability to titrate additional local anesthetic into the epidural space should the extent of dermatomal blockade be inadequate. Supplemental doses of local anesthetic can be administered to extend the duration of blockade, if necessary.

Epidural Catheter Connector Disconnection Epidural catheter connectors occasionally become disconnected from the catheter. Several options exist, including discontinuing the epidural catheter or reconnecting the catheter to a connector. Langevin et al. used an in vitro model to address the question of catheter microbial contamination and whether reconnection after cutting the catheter is safe. They demonstrated that the exterior of the catheter can be decontaminated by immersing the catheter in PI for 2 min and then air drying for 3 min.[90] In addition, they found that there may be an area of catheter distal to the disconnected end where the interior remains sterile for a least 8 h, provided the fluid column in the catheter is static. Therefore, it may be safe to decontaminate a segment of the catheter more than 8 cm distal to the connector end, followed by cutting with a sterile instrument and reconnecting to a new connector. This technique is not possible with wire-embedded catheters.

Inability to Remove the Epidural Catheter Occasionally, the catheter will be difficult to remove and will merely "stretch" with traction. Change in patient position (e.g., flexion or extension of the spine, or lateral rotation), may aid in the smooth removal of the catheter. If these maneuvers are not successful, a short length of epidural catheter, immediately adjacent to the insertion site, should be taped to the skin under traction. The patient and epidural catheter

should be reevaluated after several hours. Usually, the catheter will have worked its way loose and will be easy to remove. If this fails, catheter injection with radiopaque material and radiography may be necessary to visualize the reason for catheter resistance to removal.

Rarely, catheters may sheer and break under the skin. A neurosurgical consult should be obtained; however, if the patient is asymptomatic, most experts recommend that the catheter segment be left in situ. In fact, the catheter fragment may be difficult to locate, even with attempted surgical exposure.

THORACIC EPIDURAL ANESTHESIA

Thoracic epidural anesthesia has become widely accepted for anesthesia and analgesia, with or without general anesthesia, for thoracic, abdominal, and retroperitoneal (nephrectomy, adrenalectomy, and thoracoabdominal aneurysm) procedures (see Chaps. 8–10). The improvements in the respiratory mechanics and the superiority of pain relief, as well as decreased incidence of postoperative ileus, have made the intra- and postoperative thoracic epidural anesthesia/analgesia common practice. Therefore, proficiency in the technique of thoracic epidural anesthesia is a useful skill. While removal of chest wall masses and mastectomy can be performed under a thoracic epidural blockade with sedation, thoracic epidural anesthesia combined with general anesthesia is preferred for intrathoracic, mediastinal, upper and lower abdominal, and retroperitoneal procedures.

▶ Preparation, Equipment, and Patient Positioning

Placement of a thoracic epidural catheter commonly occurs outside of the operating room, in the preoperative holding area, while the patient is awake. This facilitates operating room turnover. In addition, there have been several reports of neurologic complications attributed to the placement of thoracic epidural catheters in anesthetized adult patients. Unlike the lumbar epidural space, the spinal cord is but a short distance from the thoracic epidural space and it would seem wise to initiate thoracic epidural anesthesia in awake patients who are able to verbalize symptoms of pain and paresthesias, unless the benefit to placement of the catheter while the patient is anesthetized far outweighs the risks.[91]

In general, equipment and supplies for thoracic epidural anesthesia mimic those for lumbar epidural anesthesia discussed earlier in the chapter (Box 2-2). Patients may be positioned sitting or lateral and the advantages and disadvantages of each position are similar to those for lumbar epidural anesthesia. The sitting position with the back curved in an extreme slouching position helps accentuate the normal thoracic kyphosis, thus widening the posterior interlaminar space. In addition, the midline may be easier to identify in the sitting compared to lateral position, particularly in obese individuals.

▶ Technique

Discussion with the surgeon is necessary to determine the precise nature of the planned operative approach and therefore the level of blockade required. The vertebral level of epidural catheter placement should correspond to the level of maximal surgical stimulus, usually at the level of incision. Insertion of a thoracic epidural catheter is technically more challenging than lumbar epidural placement, and therefore detailed knowledge of anatomic structures is necessary. For the novice, prior experience with initiation of lumbar epidural anesthesia is helpful before attempting to learn the thoracic epidural technique.

Midline Approach

The landmark for high thoracic epidural placement is the C7 spinous process, the most prominent spinous process (see Chap. 1) (Fig. 1-1). At midthoracic levels, landmarks include the T3 spinous process, which lies at the level of the root of the scapula with the arm at the side of the body, and the T7 spinous process, which lies at the level of the inferior angle of the scapula. The lower rib margin 10 cm from midline corresponds to the L1 spinous process. Using a cadaver model, Lirk et al. found that anesthesiologists are more likely to correctly identify low thoracic-lumbar interspaces compared to cervical-high thoracic interspaces.[92] Although there is a tendency for anesthesiologists to perform epidural anesthesia more cranially than estimated, the vast majority of punctures (93.7%) were performed within one interspace of the predicted level.

The C7 to T1 interlaminar spaces can be accessed directly from the midline (Fig. 2-20). This is also the case for punctures below T7 as the spinous processes become progressively less angled. In contrast, access to the T2 to T7 interlaminar spaces is more difficult because of the angled and overlapping spinous processes, as well as overlap of adjacent laminae. Therefore, the midline approach can be attempted from T7 to T12, but the paramedian approach is the preferred technique for the T3 to T7 interspaces. The thoracic spine is more superficial than the lumbar spine.

Thoracic epidural anesthesia/analgesia may be initiated in either the sitting or lateral position. The midline and chosen interspace should be located in a manner similar to that for lumbar epidural anesthesia (Fig. 2-21A and D). Using sterile technique and following appropriate skin preparation, a skin wheal is raised with 1% lidocaine with a

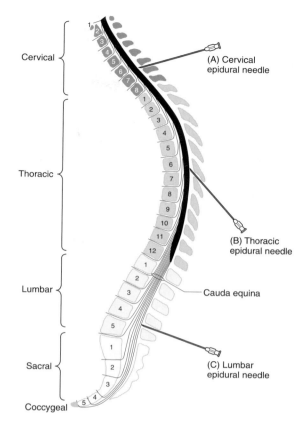

FIGURE 2-20. Lateral diagram of the vertebral column indicating the angulation of the epidural needle necessary to access the interlaminar space in the midline at the cervical, thoracic, and lumbar levels. *Used with permission from Kleinman W, Mikhail M. Spinal, epidural, and caudal blocks. In: Morgan GE, Mikhail MS, Murray M, eds, Clinical Anesthesiology, 4th ed. New York: McGraw-Hill, 2006, p. 289.*

25-gauge needle. Deep infiltration with a 3.8 cm 22-gauge needle is important to "explore" the anatomy, including identification of the spinous processes and the angle at which the needle is able to advance in the interspace. The skin may be punctured with a large bore (18-gauge) needle to avoid "drag" on the epidural needle. The epidural needle is advanced through this puncture site and advanced to 2.5 cm with the needle bevel oriented cephalad. Once the epidural needle is "engaged" in the interspinous ligament the epidural needle will stay firmly at midline without support, thus indicating correct placement into the interspinous ligament. If the needle is displaced to the side and appears to have no support, the needle is completely off midline and is located lateral to the interspinous ligament.

The epidural needle is grasped and advanced as described for lumbar epidural anesthesia (Figs. 2-18 and 2-19). The

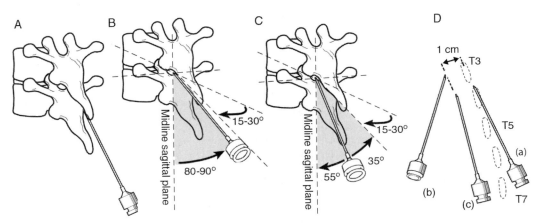

FIGURE 2-21. Thoracic epidural anesthesia. (A) Midline approach. (B) Paramedian (paraspinous) approach. (C) Alternative paramedian (paraspinous) approach. (D) Site of skin wheal for three techniques: (a) midline, (b) paramedian, and (c) alternative paramedian. Note that the landmark for the insertion site for (b) is the interspinous space one level higher than the intended interlaminar space. *Used with permission from Cousins MJ, Veering BT. Epidural neural blockade. In: Cousins MJ, Bridenbaugh PO, eds, Neural Blockade in Clinical Anesthesia and Management of Pain, 3rd ed. Philadelphia, PA: Lippincott-Raven, 1998, pp. 243–321.*

needle is usually controlled with the nondominant hand, placed on either the needle shaft or hub. The dorsal surface of the hand is placed against the patient's back in order to stabilize and "brake" the needle. This position also allows one's hand to move with the patient. The dominant hand connects the saline- or air-filled epidural syringe to the hub of the epidural needle. Gentle pressure in the form of an intermittent tap, or constant pressure, should be applied to the plunger with the thumb. As the needle is advanced, the tissues feel firmer upon needle tip entry into the ligamentum flavum. The epidural needle is advanced slowly until LOR is felt (the plunger moves freely into the syringe) indicating entry into the epidural space. It may be helpful to verify needle tip location in the epidural space by filling the syringe with 2–3 mL of preservative free saline and a small air bubble. If the saline can be injected with ease, and the air bubble does not compress, the needle tip is probably in the epidural space.

The epidural catheter should be advanced into the thoracic epidural space as described for lumbar epidural anesthesia (Fig. 2-18). Although excessive length of epidural catheter in the epidural space may promote knot formation, there is no consensus with regard to the optimal length of insertion. The optimal length may depend on catheter type and vertebral level of insertion. It has been postulated that thoracic epidural catheters can be advanced a greater length without kinking compared to lumbar catheters. This difference may be due to the incomplete segmentation of the posterior epidural space at thoracic levels as compared to the compartmentalized nature of the posterior lumbar space.[93]

Troubleshooting   If resistance is encountered superficially, the needle has probably made contact with the spinous process. It should be withdrawn and the interspace relocated, using the 22-gauge seeker needle, if necessary. Usually at this depth the epidural needle is not engaged in the ligament, and the unsupported needle will not stay firmly in the skin at the angle it was inserted. Once the interspace is located and the needle is advanced into the interspinous ligament, the tissue will have a clear-cut resistance and the needle will sit firmly at midline. Lateral angulation of the needle at this point indicates needle entry to the side of the interspinous ligament and the need to redirect or reposition the needle.

If resistance is encountered as the needle is advanced, indicating contact with bone, the needle tip is most likely too close to the superior aspect of the inferior spinous process or the superior aspect of the lamina. The needle should be withdrawn and readvanced at a steeper angle with the needle tip directed more cephalad. Contact with bone when the angle of the needle is steep indicates contact with the inferior aspect of the superior spinous process. The needle should be withdrawn and the tip directed slightly inferiorly. If contact is made with bone and coring of the tissue is suspected, the stylet of the epidural needle should be reinserted to clear any possible plug that may give a false sense of resistance.

False LOR should be managed as described for lumbar epidural anesthesia. Some patients have ligaments that feel particularly "spongy" while testing for resistance. The injection of 1–3 mL saline "tightens" the tissue and gives a better feeling of resistance.

If a sudden unisegmental paresthesia is felt by the patient, advancement of the needle should be halted and the patient queried as to which side it was noted, as this indicates lateral placement of the needle. The needle should be withdrawn and redirected appropriately. This may require reidentification of the midline and a new puncture site.

If sudden pain or muscle spasm is felt on one side of the back, the spinal needle has most likely come in contact with the articular process of the vertebra. The needle should be withdrawn and redirected accordingly.

The presence of blood in the syringe or at the hub of the epidural needle indicates probable puncture of an epidural vein. These are more prominent in the lateral epidural space. Again the needle should be withdrawn and repositioned. Care must be taken to ensure that a blood clot does not form at the tip of the epidural needle, creating a false sense of resistance, or that the syringe plunger does not become "sticky." The needle and syringe should be flushed with saline to prevent this situation.

If LOR occurs, followed by free flow of fluid into the syringe, or constant dripping of fluid is observed when the syringe is removed, the dura mater has been punctured. The needle should be removed and a decision made whether to proceed with further attempt at epidural catheter placement or abandonment of the technique.

If, despite redirecting the epidural needle, the epidural space cannot be located, landmarks should be rechecked to assure midline placement. Cooperative patients can often assist in the identification of the midline. If the epidural space cannot be located after several attempts, another interspace or a paramedian approach should be attempted. The risk of any procedure increases as the number of attempts are increased; therefore one should not persist with the same technique and the same interspace. In experienced hands, if this approach was unsuccessful the first time, it is likely to be unsuccessful on further attempts. One should remember to "do no harm" and not persist if epidural catheter placement is not possible after several attempts.

Paramedian (Paraspinous) Approach

The paramedian approach differs from the midline approach in that little resistance is encountered until the needle tip reaches the ligamentum flavum. Therefore, a small-gauge seeker needle is often used to ascertain the depth of the lamina from the skin before the epidural needle is inserted.

Skin infiltration is made with local anesthetic 1–1.5 cm lateral and 1 cm inferior to the interspinous space one level higher than the intended interlaminar space C. A longer infiltration needle (22-gauge, 3.8 cm) is inserted 90 degrees to the skin and local anesthetic injected into the deeper tissues while "seeking" the lamina or the transverse process. The depth of the lamina is noted. The epidural needle is inserted along the same track, again at a 90-degree angle to the skin, and advanced until the periosteum of the lamina is encountered. The needle is then withdrawn approximately 1 cm, and angled toward the midline 15–30 degrees to the sagittal plane and slightly superiorly until the needle is walked off the lamina. The stylet of the epidural needle is removed and LOR syringe is connected with air or saline. The needle is then advanced until there is LOR. If bone is encountered the stylet should be inserted to clear any plug at the tip of the needle prior to proceeding with the LOR technique. The epidural catheter is inserted as described in the midline approach above.

A variation of this technique is to raise a skin wheal 1 cm lateral to the interspinous space one level higher than the intended interlaminar space. The epidural needle is inserted through the skin wheal and aimed directly toward the midline (15–30 degrees in the sagittal plane), without first seeking the lamina or transverse process. If bone is encountered, the needle is aimed cephalad until the tip slips off the lamina into the ligamentum flavum.

Alternative Paramedian Approach

Another paramedian technique accesses the interlaminar space from the skin at the level of the corresponding interspinous space (Fig. 2-21). The skin is infiltrated with local anesthetic 0.5–1 cm lateral to the caudad edge of the superior spinous process. A seeker needle (22-gauge, 3.8 cm) is inserted at 90 degrees to the skin down to the lamina to assess the depth. The epidural needle is then inserted through the skin wheal and aimed cephalad toward the midline at a 10–15-degree angle to the sagittal plane and 55 degrees to the long axis of the spine (coronal plane). The stylet is removed from the epidural needle and the LOR syringe is attached. The needle is advanced until there is LOR. Although the skin to epidural space depth is less in the thoracic area, the steeper angle of the needle increases the perceived depth of the epidural space from the skin. Care must be taken to prevent any bowing of the needle by withdrawing before changing the angle of the needle.

CAUDAL EPIDURAL ANESTHESIA

Caudal anesthesia in adults appears to be a dying art. It is still, however, a useful technique. Single-shot caudal anesthesia is appropriate for anal surgery, procedures of the vulva and vagina, scrotal skin, and penis. A catheter can be placed if a long procedure is anticipated. In the pain clinic and labor and delivery unit the caudal technique provides useful access to the epidural space in patients with lumbar spine pathology. For example, continuous caudal labor analgesia is useful for women with spinal cord injuries and fused thoracolumbar vertebra. Caudal anesthesia/analgesia in children is frequently combined with general anesthesia for lower extremity and lower abdominal procedures (see Chap. 15). This allows lower doses of systemic agents, thus decreasing the incidence of side effects, and provides post-operative analgesia.

▶ Equipment and Patient Positioning

Equipment necessary for caudal anesthesia is similar to that described for spinal and epidural anesthetic. For a single-shot procedure, a 22-gauge, short-beveled needle is preferable. The short-beveled needle gives a better "feel" as the ligament is penetrated and the entire bevel is more likely to enter the caudal canal when the canal is very shallow. A standard or short (5–7 cm) Crawford tip epidural needle is often used if a catheter technique is planned (Fig. 2-16). In contrast to a Tuohy needle, in which the bevel opens to the side of the long axis of the needle, the bevel of the Crawford needle faces forward, along the long axis of the canal. This allows direction of the epidural catheter along the axis, instead of into the wall of the canal. A standard epidural catheter is used for the continuous caudal technique.

Positioning for caudal anesthesia may be prone or lateral in adults (Fig. 2-22). The knee-chest position has been used for pregnant women. The lateral decubitus position is chosen in children because it is easier to maintain a patent airway in this position than in the prone position, and landmarks are more easily palpable than in adults. Caudal anesthesia is usually performed in awake adults, but children are usually anesthetized. Details of pediatric caudal anesthesia are discussed in Chap. 15.

When positioning an adult patient for a caudal block in the prone position, a pillow should be inserted beneath the iliac crests to rotate the pelvis and make cannulation of the caudal canal easier. Additionally, the lower extremities can be spread about 20 degrees with the heels rotated laterally. This position minimizes gluteal muscle contraction and eases needle insertion.

The right-handed anesthesiologist should place the patient in the left lateral position. The lower thigh and leg are slightly flexed at the hip and knee. The upper thigh and leg are more flexed and lay over the lower thigh with the knee touching the bed. If the gluteal fold sags and obscures the midline, an assistant stands facing the patient and holds the upper buttock forward.

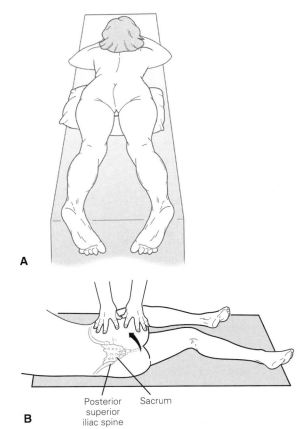

A

B

Posterior superior iliac spine   Sacrum

FIGURE 2-22. Patient positioning for caudal anesthesia. (A) Prone: A pillow is placed under the anterior iliac crests to tilt the pelvis and the hips are internally rotated with the toes together. *Used with permission from Brown DL. Spinal, epidural, and caudal anesthesia. In: Miller RD (ed). Miller's Anesthesia, 6th ed. Philadelphia, PA: Churchill Livingstone, 2005, pp. 1672,1674.* (B) Lateral position: The left lateral position is usually more comfortable for a right-handed practitioner, and the right lateral position for a left-handed practitioner. This allows the practitioner to palpate the sacral cornu with the nondominant hand and insert the needle with the dominant hand. The dependent leg is slightly flexed at the hip and knee. The upper thigh and leg are more flexed so that the knee is rotated over the dependent leg and makes contact with the bed. An assistant can stand in front of the patient and reposition the upper buttock so that the gluteal fold is in the midline. *Used with permission from Cousins MJ, Bridenbaugh PO (eds). Neural Blockade in Clinical Anesthesia, 3rd ed. Philadelphia, PA: Lippincott Williams & Wilkins, 1998, p. 333.*

▶ Technique

A wide skin area should be prepared so that all the landmarks are visible and can be palpated. Alternatively, a clear plastic drape facilitates landmark identification. A folded gauze pad should be placed deep in the gluteal fold before the antiseptic solution is applied, so the solution does not run down into the sensitive perineal area and cause discomfort or irritation.

Although some practitioners intentionally advance the needle until bone is contacted (the dorsal aspect of the ventral plate of the sacrum), this practice may increase the risk of vascular trauma as the venous plexus tends to lie against the ventral wall. If bone is contacted, the needle is slightly withdrawn and redirected so that the angle of insertion relative to the skin surface is decreased. If bone is not contacted, the needle is similarly redirected by depressing the hub and shaft so that they are aligned with the axis of the caudal canal (Fig. 2-23 inset). In the male patient, this angle is almost parallel to the axis of the spinal column; in female patients, a slightly steeper angle (15 degrees) is necessary. After redirection, the needle is advanced approximately 1–2 cm into the sacral canal. Further advance should not be attempted as this increases the risk of inadvertent dural puncture and intravascular cannulation.

Correct needle placement in the caudal canal can be surmised by several observations and maneuvers (Box 2-6).[94] In particular, the caudal needle tip should be surrounded by

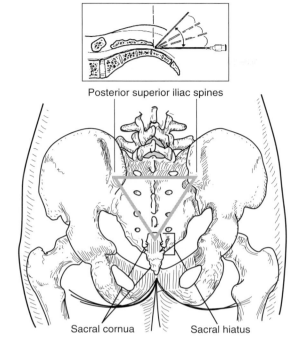

Posterior superior iliac spines

Sacral cornua   Sacral hiatus

FIGURE 2-23. Caudal anesthesia. The sacral hiatus is located between cornu, at the apex of an equilateral triangle whose base is a line connecting the posterior superior iliac crests. The S2 vertebral body is located under this line and approximates the termination of the dural sac. Inset: The needle penetrates the sacrococcygeal ligament at approximately 90 degrees to the skin (1) and then is angled downward (2, 3) until it is aligned with the axis of the sacral canal and can be advanced into the canal (4). *Used with permission from Brown DL. Spinal, epidural, and caudal anesthesia. In: Miller RD, ed, Miller's Anesthesia, 6th ed. Philadelphia, PA: Churchill Livingston, 2005, p. 1653.*

Caudal anesthesia requires identification of the sacral hiatus (Fig. 1-2 and Fig. 2-23). The sacrococcygeal ligament (i.e., extension of ligamentum flavum) overlying the sacral hiatus lies between sacral cornu. The sacral hiatus lies at the apex of an equilateral triangle whose base is a line connecting the posterior superior iliac crests. Alternatively, the sacral hiatus can be located by palpating the tip of the coccyx. The palpating finger is then moved cephalad approximately 4–5 cm until the tip overlies the sacral hiatus. The palpating finger(s) should remain in the sacral hiatus or on the cornu once it has been identified. It may be helpful to enter the skin toward the cephalad end of the hiatus since the caudal canal is deeper at this point. A skin wheal is raised by injecting local anesthetic through a 25-gauge needle. The caudal needle is introduced through the skin wheal at an angle of approximately 90–120 degrees to the skin (Fig. 2-23, inset). A distinct "pop" is perceived as the needle penetrates the sacrococcygeal ligament and enters the caudal canal.

Box 2-6

Indications of Correct Placement of a Needle in the Caudal Canal

Presence of bone surrounding tip of caudal needle

No CSF, blood, or air on aspiration

No tissue resistance to injection

No subcutaneous fluid or crepitus with rapid injection of 2–5 mL fluid or air

Positive "whoosh" test*

Ability of needle to pivot around point of penetration of sacrococcygeal ligament

No pain on injection of solution

Mild paresthesias or feeling of sacral "fullness" on injection

Grating of needle tip along anterior wall of canal when needle is advanced[†]

Free and easy advancement of epidural catheter through caudal needle

*A stethoscope is placed over the lumbar spine and 2–3 mL air is injected through the caudal needle. A "whoosh" sound should be heard through the stethoscope.

[†]This should not be intentionally elicited as the risk of vascular trauma is increased.

Source: Methods listed are from Willis RJ. Caudal epidural blockade. In: Cousins MJ, Bridenbaugh PO, eds, *Neural Blockade in Clinical Anesthesia and Management of Pain*, 3rd ed. Philadelphia, PA: Lippincott-Raven, 1998, p. 323.

bone and there should be no CSF or blood on aspiration. There should be no resistance to injection; the injection should feel similar to injection into the lumbar epidural space. The fingers or palm of the nondominant hand can be placed over the sacrum while 2–5 mL of anesthetic solution, saline, or air is injected rapidly through the needle. There should be no bulge or crepitus perceived by the hand during this procedure, or this indicates incorrect position of the needle outside and superficial to the sacral canal.

After ensuring correct needle position and before injecting the therapeutic dose of caudal anesthetic, aspiration should be performed and a test dose administered. The test dose should rule out both intrathecal and intravascular injection. The remaining dose of local anesthetic should be injected slowly. Concentrations of local anesthetic used for caudal epidural anesthesia mimic those for lumbar epidural anesthesia (Table 3-5). Twenty milliliters of local anesthetic solution is necessary to reliably block all the sacral nerves via the caudal approach.

If a continuous technique is planned, an epidural catheter is advanced through the caudal needle into the caudal canal. The depth of insertion may vary, depending on the anticipated site of surgery and the desired extent of anesthesia. Typically, the catheter is secured 2 cm or more in the caudal canal. In children, advancement of the catheter to the thoracic spine has been described (Chap. 15). The catheter should be secured in a manner that minimizes contamination from the perineum and avoids the surgical field. This is facilitated by application of a skin adhesive and sterile occlusive dressing.

Troubleshooting

The anatomy of the sacrum is such that identification of the sacral hiatus is inconsistent and often confusing, particularly in obese individuals. There is marked anatomic variation of the dorsum of the sacrum and sacral hiatus. The sacral hiatus may be absent in a small number of people, and the apex may extend cephalad to the lower half of S4. Total sacral spina bifida may also be present in 1% of the population.[94] The anatomy tends to be more consistent in children.

Needle penetration of a posterior sacral foramen may mimic the penetration of the sacrococcygeal ligament, since these are also openings in bone covered with ligament. The result is limited unilateral blockade. There are also bony depressions covered with ligament on the dorsal surface of the sacrum, although injection is difficult and should present resistance. One cornu may be less prominent than its twin. This may fool the anesthesiologist into identifying a tubercle of the lateral sacral crest as the second cornu. The needle tip may be positioned dorsal to the sacrum in the superficial tissue covering the sacrum, or may be ventral to the sacrum, in the rectum or even the fetal head.

Box 2-7

Indications for Cervical Epidural Anesthesia/Analgesia

Neck procedures

    Carotid endarterectomy

    Thyroidectomy

    Parathyroidectomy

Upper extremity procedures (bilateral)

    Cervical pain conditions

    Cervical radiculitis

    Postlaminectomy cervical syndrome

    Acute brachial plexitis

    Complex regional pain syndrome

    Chronic neck pain

Chest wall procedures

    Mammoplasty

    Mastectomy

CERVICAL EPIDURAL ANESTHESIA

Cervical epidural anesthesia is a technique used for surgical procedures of the neck, upper extremity (especially when the procedure is bilateral), chest wall, and in the conservative management of cervical pain conditions (Box 2-7). It has also been described in the treatment of refractory status asthmaticus during weaning from ventilatory support.[95]

▶ Equipment

The equipment necessary to perform cervical epidural injections mimics that of lumbar and thoracic epidural techniques. When using fluoroscopic guidance, additional equipment includes a fluoroscopy table, or an operating room table able to accommodate a C-arm fluoroscopy machine, along with sterile contrast dye. Contrast solution is commonly injected in 0.5–1 mL increments through the needle or epidural catheter. Lead gowns should be available for all those present in the room, including one for the patient to protect areas that do not need to be exposed to radiation.

▶ Patient Positioning

Several positions have been described for performing cervical epidural blockade. In the sitting position, the neck is anteflexed and the head is supported on a stable surface (Fig. 2-24). The patient can use his or her hand or folded

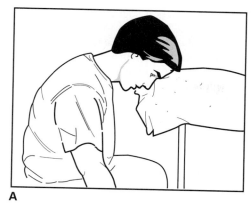

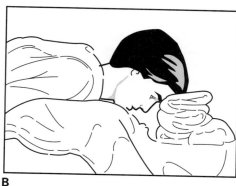

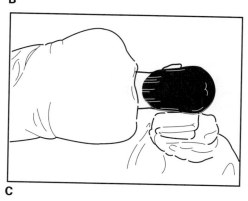

FIGURE 2-24. Positions for cervical epidural anesthesia: (A) sitting, (B) prone, and (C) lateral.

The prone position is also used for cervical epidural anesthesia. Specifically, this position is used when fluoroscopic guidance is used. The patient should lie prone with a roll under the clavicles and the neck flexed. The forehead is placed on the bed for support. A final alternative for cervical epidural blockade is the lateral decubitus position.

▶ Technique

The patient is prepared and monitored for cervical epidural anesthesia in a manner similar to that for thoracic or lumbar epidural anesthesia. The anesthesiologist may elect to omit intravascular venous access for single-shot cervical epidural steroid injections when sedation is not administered. If sedation is used, it should be carefully titrated to effect.

Midline Approach

The first description of the interlaminar cervical epidural technique using the LOR technique was described by Dogliotti in 1933. The hanging-drop technique was described by Gutierrez in the same year. Both techniques are currently used. The C7-T1 interspace is the widest and technically easiest interspace to access. The anteroposterior dimension measured from the anterior aspect of the ligamentum flavum to the dural sac on sagittal cut MRI images is largest at the C7-T1 and T1-T2 interspaces (mean distance 4 and 5 mm, respectively).[96] The mean distance from skin to the epidural space was 5.7 cm at C6-C7 and C7-T1 levels, but decreased to 5.4 cm at T1-T2 and 4.7 cm at T2-T3. Using human cadavers, Lirk et al. demonstrated that the ligamentum flavum fails to fuse in the midline in over 50% of specimens at cervical interlaminar spaces.[97] The authors hypothesized that this may make the LOR technique of identifying puncture of the epidural space less reliable at the cervical level compared to other vertebral levels.

In the sitting position with the neck flexed and the head supported, the spinous process of C7 (vertebra prominens) is the most prominent landmark. It is easily palpated in the majority of the patients. The patient's neck is widely prepped from the hairline to the upper thorax and draped in the usual sterile fashion. A clear plastic drape facilitates identification of surface landmarks. A skin wheal is raised using a local anesthetic with a 25- or 22-gauge needle in the C7-T1 interspace. The epidural needle is inserted through the skin wheal in a strict midsagittal plane to a depth of approximately 2 cm. The tip may be directed slightly cephalad, but with the head and neck in this position the needle is actually directed straight toward the floor. The stylet is removed once the needle is anchored in the interspinous ligament.

If the hanging-drop technique is chosen, a drop of saline is placed in the hub of the epidural needle. The needle is usually

arm to support the head on this surface. The acute flexion position increases the distance between the ligamentum flavum and the dura mater from 1.5–2 mm to 4–5 mm, thereby markedly increasing the safety of the technique. The sitting position also increases the negative pressure in the epidural space which assists in easier identification of the epidural space by the hanging-drop technique.

slowly advanced with a two-handed technique: the thumb and index finger of each hand grasp the wings of the epidural needle while the remaining fingers (tips or knuckles) are braced against either side of the neck to aid with needle control (Fig. 2-19). Some practitioners advocate needle advancement during inspiration as this increases the negative pressure in the epidural space. Entry into the epidural space is heralded by a sensation of "release" as the ligamentum flavum is pierced and inward displacement of the drop of fluid from the needle hub, at which point the advancement of the needle is immediately stopped. Confirmation of correct needle placement in the epidural space is by injection of a jet of saline into the hub of the epidural needle. The fluid should disappear into the epidural space.

If the LOR technique is used, needle advancement mimics that previously described. The ligamentum flavum is thinner at this level than at the lumbar or thoracic levels,[98] or it may be absent in the midline.[97] If the LOR to air technique is used, care should be taken to use a small volume of air (1–2 mL).

Paramedian (Paraspinous) Approach

The paramedian approach avoids both the spinous processes and their intervening ligaments and may facilitate advancement of an epidural catheter into the epidural space.

The skin is prepared and draped in the standard fashion. A skin wheal is raised with a 25-gauge needle 1.5 cm lateral to the spinous process of C7 or C6. A 22-gauge (38 mm) needle is inserted through the wheal at right angles to the skin, and the needle is advanced to the lamina. This allows the depth of the lamina to be determined. The needle is redirected while infiltrating the tissues with local anesthetic to assume a parasagittal angle of approximately 15 degrees. The 22-gauge needle is replaced with the epidural needle with the bevel facing cephalad. The epidural needle is introduced and advanced to the lamina. The stylet is removed and a syringe containing air or saline is attached. The needle is "walked" off the lamina in the cephalad and medial direction using the LOR technique previously described. Constant or intermittent pressure is applied to the plunger, and the complete unit is advanced until a LOR to the plunger advancement signals entry into the epidural space.

Injection into the cervical epidural space should be made slowly. If a catheter technique is planned, the catheter is advanced through the epidural needle as described previously. Two to three cm of catheter length is left in the epidural space. Longer lengths may increase the risk of migration through intervertebral foramina.

Fluoroscopically Assisted Technique

Even in experienced hands the blind technique may result in inaccurate needle placement.[99] Anesthesiologists are more likely to identify a cervical interspinous space that is more cranial than the one intended.[92] Fluoroscopic guidance for placement of epidural confirms the needle placement at the desired interspace. Epidural catheters can be accurately positioned at the site of the appropriate dermatome, in addition to the selective placement to the right or the left side of the spine. Unilateral catheter placement is easily obtained and is ideal for unilateral pain. Fluoroscopic guidance may provide greater safety, as using a lateral view gives clear indication of exactly where the needle is at all times, and may be used for epidural techniques at all vertebral levels.

Fluoroscopic-assisted identification of the cervical epidural space is performed with the patient in the prone or sitting position on a radiology table. After appropriate skin preparation the skin is anesthetized with 1% lidocaine. Under intermittent fluoroscopic guidance (lateral view), the Tuohy epidural needle is introduced at the C7-T1 interspace and advanced using LOR technique with normal saline until the posterior epidural space is located. An anteroposterior view is obtained to ensure the midline position, followed by the injection of contrast material (0.5–mL) to confirm epidural placement of the needle tip and to rule out intravascular, intrathecal, or soft tissue infiltration.

COMBINED SPINAL-EPIDURAL ANESTHESIA

Combined spinal-epidural anesthesia is a technique that combines the benefits and minimizes the disadvantages of continuous epidural and single-shot subarachnoid anesthesia. These include the ability to titrate the level of sensory blockade, a reduction in total drug dose, fewer failed blocks, and a continuous technique (Box 2-8). CSE anesthesia combines the rapid onset and dense blockade of spinal anesthesia with the flexibility afforded by an epidural catheter. Intrathecal surgical anesthesia can be followed by postoperative continuous epidural analgesia.

There are several techniques for combined spinal-epidural analgesia.[100] The most common technique is a *needle-through-needle* technique in which the epidural needle is sited in the epidural space and the spinal needle is passed through the epidural needle into the subarachnoid space. In essence, the epidural needle acts as an introducer for the spinal needle. This is the simplest technique, and is described in detail below. The disadvantage of this technique is that the correct placement of the epidural catheter cannot be tested until the spinal anesthetic wanes.

Alternatively, the epidural and spinal needles may be introduced through two different interspaces. If the epidural needle and catheter are sited first, the epidural catheter can be tested to ensure correct placement before the spinal anesthetic is initiated. A theoretical disadvantage of this technique

Advantages of CSE anesthesia

Advantages related to subarachnoid component

Rapid onset of profound motor and sensory block

Low local anesthetic dose

Advantages related to epidural component

Titratable levels of segmental anesthesia (minimizing the risk of high sympathetic blockade and attendant hemodynamic depression)

Extended surgical anesthesia and prolonged postoperative analgesia

Avoids/minimizes disadvantages related to single injection subarachnoid block

Limited and unpredictable duration

Unpredictable level

Hemodynamic depression associated with a high block level

Avoids/minimizes disadvantages inherent to epidural block

Slow onset of motor blockade and surgical anesthesia (20–30 min)

Incomplete motor blockade

Missed spinal segments—specifically L5 and S1 segments

Use of a large dose of local anesthetic with risks of:

Systemic toxicity (from intravascular injection or local anesthetic absorption)

Inadvertent subarachnoid or subdural injection resulting in total spinal anesthesia

---

is damage to the epidural catheter by the subsequently placed spinal needle. A large distance between the two interspaces decreases the probability of this occurrence (e.g., caudal or thoracic epidural catheter combined with lumbar spinal anesthesia). The disadvantage of placing the epidural needle and catheter after the intrathecal injection is the need to manipulate the epidural needle and catheter in a partially or completely anesthetized individual. Finally, the epidural needle and spinal needle can be introduced through two separate punctures in the same interspace with the disadvantages described earlier.

▶ **Equipment**

There are special epidural needle-spinal needle sets available for CSE (Fig. 2-25). These include epidural needles with a "back-eye" that allows the spinal needle to exit directly through the end of the epidural needle, and epidural-spinal needles that "lock" together at the hub. The technique, however, is easily performed using a standard epidural needle (3.5 in./8.9 cm) and long spinal needle (4 11/16–5 in./11.9–12.7 cm), usually 24- to 27-gauge. When used together, the spinal needle angles slightly as it exits the side-facing orifice of the epidural needle (Fig. 2-25).

It is critical that the spinal needle protrude an appropriate length from the tip of the epidural needle when fully inserted into the epidural needle. In a study of nonobstetric patients, the mean spinal needle protrusion from the tip of the epidural needle at dural puncture was 7.1 mm, with a range of 2.2–13.3 mm.[101] In obstetric patients, the incidence of failure to obtain CSF was 25% when the spinal needle protruded 9 mm, compared to 0% when the needle protruded 17 mm.[102] A 127-mm spinal needle is commonly used with a standard 9-cm epidural needle. Because of different epidural and spinal needle hub configurations, however, the two needle hubs do not always "fit" together and

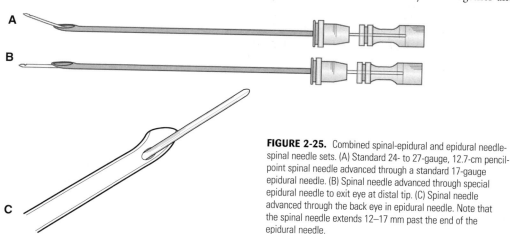

FIGURE 2-25. Combined spinal-epidural and epidural needle-spinal needle sets. (A) Standard 24- to 27-gauge, 12.7-cm pencil-point spinal needle advanced through a standard 17-gauge epidural needle. (B) Spinal needle advanced through special epidural needle to exit eye at distal tip. (C) Spinal needle advanced through the back eye in epidural needle. Note that the spinal needle extends 12–17 mm past the end of the epidural needle.

the length of protruding spinal needle may vary. In order to minimize the risk of failure, spinal needles should protrude 12–15 mm beyond the tip of the epidural needle when the spinal needle is seated in the epidural needle hub. Conversely, spinal needles that protrude more than 17 mm beyond the tip of the epidural needle may be associated with several problems, including difficulty stabilizing the spinal needle, increased risk of transient paresthesia,[103] and risk of puncturing the anterior dura.

A Luer-*slip* syringe is desirable for the spinal anesthetic medications, as a Luer-*lock* syringe requires more manipulation for secure attachment to the spinal needle, and therefore, risks needle movement during connection and injection. No other special equipment is necessary for the CSE procedure.

▶ Technique

Patient positioning and preparation are similar to those described for spinal and lumbar epidural anesthesia. Patient position should take into account the desired distribution of sensory blockade, spinal anesthetic baricity, and patient comfort. In addition, if the patient's position needs to be changed after the procedure to optimize intrathecal anesthetic distribution, the anesthesiologist should recall that it make take several minutes to insert and secure the epidural catheter, and this delay may influence the intrathecal distribution of drugs.

CSE anesthesia should be initiated in lumbar interspaces at or below the L2-L3 interspace as described for spinal anesthesia. The procedure mimics the initiation of lumbar epidural anesthesia up through the point when the epidural space is identified and the tip of the epidural needle resides in the epidural space. Some practitioners prefer using the LOR to air technique so that saline cannot be confused with CSF. However, there is no evidence that one method of LOR is superior to the other.

After identification of the epidural space, the syringe is removed from the epidural needle and the spinal needle is inserted through the epidural needle with the dominant hand (Fig. 2-27). A small amount of resistance is usually noted as the tip of the spinal needle exits the epidural needle orifice (because the shaft of the spinal needle impinges on the edge of the distal epidural needle orifice when using a standard epidural needle) (Fig. 2-25). The spinal needle is advanced until a "pop" is appreciated as the dura is punctured with the tip of the spinal needle. Further spinal needle advancement should be avoided. Similar to spinal anesthesia, the dura is tented with the tip of the spinal needle before it is actually punctured (Fig. 2-26). Therefore, immediately after dural puncture, the tip of the spinal needle is actually located inside the dura and the dura springs back to the neutral position. The orifice of the spinal needle will be located within the subarachnoid space and no further needle manipulation is necessary.

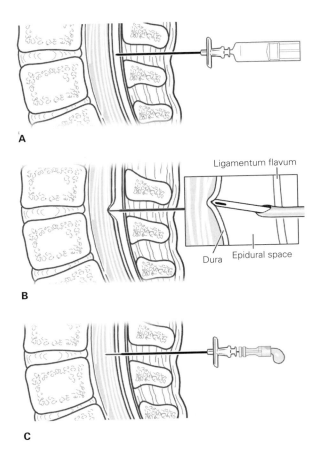

FIGURE 2-26. Combined spinal-epidural technique. (A) Insertion of the epidural needle using LOR into the epidural space. (B) Insertion of the spinal needle through the epidural needle. As the spinal needle exits the tip of the epidural needle the dura is tented. (C) The spinal needle "pops" through the dura into the subarachnoid space. CSF flows back through the spinal needle.

The hubs of the spinal and epidural needle should be stabilized by holding them together with the thumb and index finger of the nondominant hand. The back of the hand should be placed against the patient's back (Fig. 2-27). The spinal needle stylet is withdrawn with the dominant hand, and CSF return is noted through the spinal needle. Once CSF has reached the hub of the spinal needle, the spinal drug syringe is attached to the spinal needle with the dominant hand (during continued needle stabilization with the nondominant hand). Spinal needle stabilization during this maneuver is particularly important as the spinal needle is anchored only by the dura. Unlike traditional spinal anesthesia, in which the spinal needle exits the introducer well short

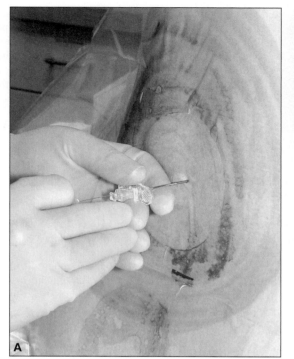

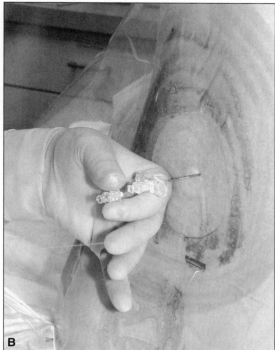

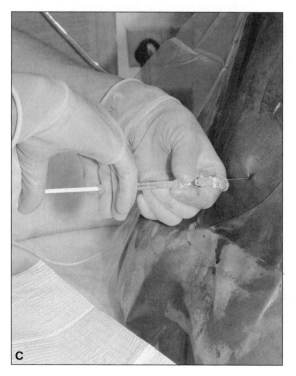

FIGURE 2-27. Needle-through-needle combined spinal-epidural technique. (A) Insertion of spinal needle through the epidural needle. (B) Stabilizing spinal needle while withdrawing spinal needle stylet. Note the thumb and index finger of the nondominant hand hold the hubs of the epidural and spinal needles so the spinal needle does not move within the epidural needle. (C) Syringe with intrathecal drug is attached to the spinal needle.

of the dura and is anchored along its shaft by surrounding tissue, the spinal needle during the CSE technique is surrounded by air in shaft of the much larger epidural needle.

Aspiration of CSF before injection of spinal drug is optional. Free aspiration of CSF is an indication that the spinal needle orifice is still correctly located after attachment of the syringe. In addition, any small air bubble at the syringe-CSF interface will be aspirated into the syringe and the inadvertent injection of air is less likely. However, it may not be feasible to freely aspirate CSF through long, small-gauge spinal needles, even if the orifice is correctly located in the subarachnoid space. The risk of inadvertently moving the tip of the needle during aspiration may be increased. Finally, the epidural catheter can be used to "rescue" failed spinal anesthesia should the spinal needle orifice be incorrectly placed.

After the spinal drugs are injected through the spinal needle, the spinal needle and attached syringe are removed as a unit. The epidural catheter is inserted and secured as described for continuous epidural anesthesia.

Spinal Drugs for CSE Anesthesia

Spinal drugs for CSE anesthesia can mimic those for single-shot spinal anesthesia (full-dose CSE anesthesia). Alternatively, a lower intrathecal dose can be chosen (sequential CSE anesthesia). This allows careful titration of the cephalad sensory level by slow, incremental injection through the epidural catheter and may be associated with less hemodynamic compromise than a single-shot spinal technique.[104]

The intrathecal distribution of anesthetic when injected as part of a CSE technique may be different than after the same injection as part of a single-shot spinal technique for several reasons. Firstly, once an epidural needle has been sited in the epidural space, and the LOR syringe has been removed, the epidural space pressure equilibrates with atmospheric pressure. Epidural pressure is usually less than atmospheric pressure. An increase in epidural pressure may alter the spinal CSF volume and dynamics. An increase in epidural pressure may cause an increase in spinal CSF pressure and the translocation of CSF out of the spinal canal, contributing to increased cephalad migration of drugs and a higher cephalad sensory level compared to single-shot spinal anesthesia. Indeed, the median effective dose of spinal bupivacaine was 20% less with a CSE compared to single-shot spinal technique.[105]

Secondly, if CSE anesthesia is initiated in the sitting position, there may be a delay in assuming the supine or lateral position compared to a single-shot spinal technique. Depending on the baricity of the injected spinal drugs, this may alter the subarachnoid distribution of drug. Finally, the epidural injection of fluid shortly after the intrathecal injection is associated with a higher cephalad sensory blockade.[106] This occurs whether the fluid is saline or local

anesthetic, although the cephalad sensory level is even higher when local anesthetic is injected compared to saline. The epidural volume injection increases cephalad migration of spinal anesthetics by compressing the dura and causing the translocation of CSF out of the spinal subarachnoid space. In addition, epidural local anesthetic may traverse the dural puncture site and contribute to increased CSF local anesthetic concentration.

Epidural Test Dose

A standard intrathecal test dose containing local anesthetic should not be injected through the epidural catheter immediately after the placement of the catheter after full-dose intrathecal injection. In the event of inadvertent intrathecal placement of the epidural catheter, high or total spinal anesthesia may result. Two options exist: a continuous epidural infusion (for maintenance of epidural anesthesia or analgesia) may be initiated through the epidural catheter. If inadvertent intrathecal or intravascular placement of the epidural catheter has occurred, epidural anesthesia will not result, but neither will total spinal anesthesia nor the intravascular injection of a toxic dose of local anesthetic. Alternatively, a traditional epidural test dose can be injected through the epidural catheter at the time the spinal anesthesia is expected to wane (e.g., 90 min after intrathecal bupivacaine injection).

Sequential CSE Anesthesia

Titration of epidural local anesthetic may be necessary to attain surgical anesthesia if sequential CSE anesthesia is planned. The spinal dose is intentionally chosen at the low end of the dose range, and therefore, some patients will require epidural supplementation. If the sensory block is inadequate 15 min after the intrathecal injection, small increments of local anesthetic (e.g., 2–3 mL) should be injected through the epidural catheter until a satisfactory block is obtained. Because the supplemental anesthesia is secondary to both an epidural volume effect and drug effect (see "Spinal Drugs for CSE Anesthesia," above), the amount of epidural local anesthetic necessary to obtain the desired block may be less than that necessary to supplement epidural anesthesia to the same degree. Care should be taken to wait for an appropriate amount of time before checking the new level of sensory blockade and injecting the next incremental epidural injection.

Maintenance of CSE Anesthesia

Epidural anesthesia as part of a CSE technique can be maintained with a continuous infusion (see Chap. 7) or intermittent bolus administration of local anesthetic. Intermittent bolus injection is similar to that following the initiation of neuraxial blockade with epidural local anesthetic. The epidural test dose should be injected at the time of expected regression of the spinal block (minus one standard deviation) (Table 3-4). Since the patient is already anesthetized, it may be difficult to recognize an inadvertent intrathecal injection. The authors recommend waiting 5–10 min after test dose administration before administering the remainder of the epidural bolus in 3 mL increments. The total bolus dose will approximate that necessary to maintain epidural anesthesia using a bolus technique (see "Anesthetic Bolus Dose," earlier).

Theoretical Issues Associated with CSE Anesthesia

Metallic Particle Contamination of CSF There is theoretical concern that the needle-through-needle technique could result in metallic particle contamination of the subarachnoid space. Two studies concluded that the technique does not produce metallic contaminants.[107,108]

Nervous Tissue Trauma There is a theoretical risk of masking nerve trauma with the CSE technique because the epidural catheter is threaded after the spinal dose has been injected, and therefore, the patient is partially anesthetized. However, the sensory blockade achieved within the first half minute after injection of intrathecal local anesthetic agents is not dense. In the authors' experience, patients still perceive paresthesias during epidural catheter insertion. As there is no further manipulation of the epidural needle at the time, the risk of tissue trauma is small.

Migration of the Epidural Catheter through the Dural Puncture Further concerns include a possible increased risk of the epidural catheter passing through the dural puncture site, either during insertion, or late migration. Using a cadaver model and epiduroscopy, several groups of investigators were unable to force an 18-gauge epidural catheter through a dural puncture made with a 25- or 27-gauge spinal needle.[107,109] In several large series of patients, there was a zero incidence of late migration of epidural catheters into the subarachnoid space.[110]

Troubleshooting CSE Anesthesia

Unable to Puncture the Dura with the Spinal Needle The failure rate for obtaining flow of CSF through the spinal needle is between 2 and 5%.[103,111] One reason for failure is that the epidural space depth is longer than the extension of the spinal needle beyond the end of the epidural needle (Fig. 2-28). This may be secondary to anatomic variation or the angle of the needle insertion. The distance will be longer

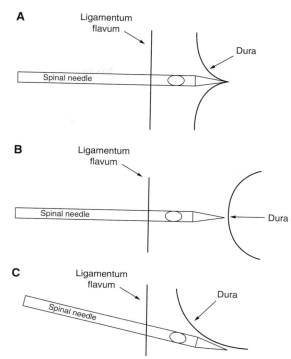

FIGURE 2-28. Reasons for failure of CSE technique. (A) The spinal needle tents the dura but does not penetrate it. (B) The spinal needle does not reach the dura. (C) The spinal needle passes to the side of the dural sac. *Used with permission from Riley ET, Hamilton CL, Ratner EF, et al. A comparison of the 24-gauge Sprotte and Gertie Marx spinal needles for combined spinal-epidural analgesia during labor. Anesthesiology 97:574, 2002.*

if the needle is angled more steeply in the midline, or during a paramedian approach. The risk may be increased if significant amounts of saline or air are injected into the epidural space during the LOR technique.

In addition, the pencil-point spinal needle may tent the dura, instead of puncturing it. Finally, if the spinal needle is angled off the midline, the needle may pass to the side of the dural sac. If the epidural and spinal needles enter the lateral epidural space perpendicular to the skin, but in a plane lateral and parallel to the midline, the spinal needle may not puncture the dura.

The anesthesiologist has several options at this point. If he or she is convinced that the epidural needle is in the epidural space, the CSE technique could be abandoned in favor of a pure epidural technique. Alternatively, the spinal and epidural needle can be withdrawn and the epidural needle repositioned in the same intervertebral space at a different angle, or in a different interspace. The authors do not recommend advancing the epidural needle as this may result in inadvertent dural puncture.

Paresthesias During Insertion of the Spinal Needle
Paresthesias during insertion of the spinal needle should be handled in a manner similar to that described for spinal anesthesia. Alternatively, the spinal needle can be withdrawn and the CSE technique abandoned in favor of epidural anesthesia.

CSF Dripping from Epidural Needle after Removal of the Spinal Needle Occasionally, following successful placement of the epidural and spinal needles, fluid appears slowly in the hub of the epidural needle after removal of the spinal needle. The fluid is CSF,[112] although in the authors' anecdotal experience, these patients do not seem to be at increased risk for PDPH. Presumably, CSF leaks through the dural puncture into the epidural needle.

DOCUMENTATION

Components of medical documentation of neuraxial blockade are listed in Box 2-9. Complete documentation of the procedure is useful as it allows for accurate review of the procedure in case of complications. In addition, complete documentation is useful for troubleshooting failed procedures

and for quality management purposes. Finally, complete documentation assists trainees in developing a consistent and organized approach to neuraxial blockade.

SUMMARY

Proper preparation, technique, and follow-up are important to the safe, successful, and efficient conduct of neuraxial anesthesia and analgesia. This requires knowledge of sterile technique, as well as an understanding of equipment options, and the risks and benefits of different neuraxial anesthesia techniques.

REFERENCES

1. Moen V. Meningitis is a rare complication of spinal anesthesia. Good hygiene and face masks are simple preventive measures [in Swedish]. *Lakartidningen* 95:628, 1998.
2. Browne IM, Birnbach DJ. Unmasked mischief. *Anesth Analg* 92:279, 2001.
3. Philips BJ, Fergusson S, Armstrong P, et al. Surgical face masks are effective in reducing bacterial contamination caused by dispersal from the upper airway. *Br J Anaesth* 69:407, 1992.
4. McLure HA, Mannam M, Talboys CA, et al. The effect of facial hair and sex on the dispersal of bacteria below a masked subject. *Anaesthesia* 55:173, 2000.
5. Panikkar KK, Yentis SM. Wearing of masks for obstetric regional anaesthesia. A postal survey. *Anaesthesia* 51:398, 1996.
6. Sleth JC. Evaluation of aseptic measures in the performance of epidural catheterization and perception of its risk of infection. Results of a survey in Languedoc-Roussillon [in French]. *Ann Fr Anesth Reanim* 17:408, 1998.
7. Tsen LC. The mask avenger. *Anesth Analg* 92:279; author reply 280, 2001.
8. Rotter MI. Hand washing and hand disinfection. In: Mayhall CG, ed, *Hospital Epidemiology and Infection Control*, 2nd ed. Philadelphia, PA: Lippincott Williams & Wilkins, 1999, p. 1339.
9. Boyce JM, Pittet D, Healthcare Infection Control Practices Advisory C, et al. Guideline for Hand Hygiene in Health-Care Settings. Recommendations of the Healthcare Infection Control Practices Advisory Committee and the HICPAC/SHEA/APIC/IDSA Hand Hygiene Task Force. Society for Healthcare Epidemiology of America/Association for Professionals in Infection Control/Infectious Diseases Society of America. *MMWR Recomm Rep* 51:1, 2002.
10. Hubble MJ, Weale AE, Perez JV, et al. Clothing in laminar-flow operating theatres. *J Hosp Infect* 32:1, 1996.
11. Anonymous. *Recommendations for Infection Control for the Practice of Anesthesiology*. Park Ridge, IL: American Society of Anesthesiologists, 1998.
12. Sato S, Sakuragi T, Dan K. Human skin flora as a potential source of epidural abscess. *Anesthesiology* 85:1276, 1996.
13. Simpson RS, Macintyre PE, Shaw D, et al. Epidural catheter tip cultures: Results of a 4-year audit and implications for clinical practice. *Reg Anesth Pain Med* 25:360, 2000.
14. Birnbach DJ, Meadows W, Stein DJ, et al. Comparison of povidone iodine and DuraPrep, an iodophor-in-isopropyl alcohol solution, for skin disinfection prior to epidural catheter insertion in parturients. *Anesthesiology* 98:164, 2003.

Box 2-9

Documentation of Neuraxial Anesthesia

Sterile technique, including skin preparation solution

Patient position

Equipment (size and type of needles)

Vertebral interspace

Description of technique

- Midline vs. paramedian
- LOR vs. hanging-drop

Drugs

- Local anesthetics and adjuvants
- Dose, concentration, volume

Placement of epidural catheter

- Depth of epidural space
- Length of catheter in space

Presence of paresthesias, blood, or CSF during procedure

Dermatome level of blockade

- Maximum
- End of procedure

Additional comments/notation of complications

15. Yentur EA, Luleci N, Topcu I, et al. Is skin disinfection with 10% povidone iodine sufficient to prevent epidural needle and catheter contamination? *Reg Anesth Pain Med* 28:389, 2003.

16. Sakuragi T, Yanagisawa K, Dan K. Bactericidal activity of skin disinfectants on methicillin-resistant Staphylococcus aureus. *Anesth Analg* 81:555, 1995.

17. Birnbach DJ, Stein DJ, Murray O, et al. Povidone iodine and skin disinfection before initiation of epidural anesthesia. *Anesthesiology* 88:668, 1998.

18. Hunt JR, Rigor BM Sr, Collins JR. The potential for contamination of continuous epidural catheters. *Anesth Analg* 56:222, 1977.

19. De Cicco M, Matovic M, Castellani GT, et al. Time-dependent efficacy of bacterial filters and infection risk in long-term epidural catheterization. *Anesthesiology* 82:765, 1995.

20. Zacher AN, Zornow MH, Evans G. Drug contamination from opening glass ampules. *Anesthesiology* 75:893, 1991.

21. Tunstall ME, MacLennan FM. Contamination of opioids during preparation for regional anaesthesia. *Anaesthesia* 52:290, 1997.

22. Holst D, Mollmann M, Ebel C, et al. In vitro investigation of cerebrospinal fluid leakage after dural puncture with various spinal needles. *Anesth Analg* 87:1331, 1998.

23. Vallejo MC, Mandell GL, Sabo DP, et al. Postdural puncture headache: A randomized comparison of five spinal needles in obstetric patients. *Anesth Analg* 91:916, 2000.

24. Santanen U, Rautoma P, Luurila H, et al. Comparison of 27-gauge (0.41-mm) Whitacre and Quincke spinal needles with respect to post-dural puncture headache and non-dural puncture headache. *Acta Anaesthesiol Scand* 48:474, 2004.

25. Flaatten H, Felthaus J, Kuwelker M, et al. Postural post-dural puncture headache. A prospective randomised study and a meta-analysis comparing two different 0.40 mm O.D. (27 g) spinal needles. *Acta Anaesthesiol Scand* 44:643, 2000.

26. Parker RK, White PF. A microscopic analysis of cut-bevel versus pencil-point spinal needles. *Anesth Analg* 85:1101, 1997.

27. Reina MA, de Leon-Casasola OA, Lopez A, et al. An in vitro study of dural lesions produced by 25-gauge Quincke and Whitacre needles evaluated by scanning electron microscopy. *Reg Anesth Pain Med* 25:393, 2000.

28. Smith EA, Thorburn J, Duckworth RA, et al. A comparison of 25 G and 27 G Whitacre needles for caesarean section. *Anaesthesia* 49:859, 1994.

29. Standl T, Stanek A, Burmeister MA, et al. Spinal anesthesia performance conditions and side effects are comparable between the newly designed Ballpen and the Sprotte needle: Results of a prospective comparative randomized multicenter study. *Anesth Analg* 98:512, 2004.

30. Dull RO, Peterfreund RA. Variations in the composition of spinal anesthetic solutions: The effects of drug addition order and preparation methods. *Anesth Analg* 87:1326, 1998.

31. Brooks RR, Oudekerk C, Olson RL, et al. The effect of spinal introducer needle use on postoperative back pain. *AANA J* 70:449, 2002.

32. Serpell MG, Gray WM. Flow dynamics through spinal needles. *Anaesthesia* 52:229, 1997.

33. Holman SJ, Robinson RA, Beardsley D, et al. Hyperbaric dye solution distribution characteristics after pencil-point needle injection in a spinal cord model. *Anesthesiology* 86:966, 1997.

34. Urmey WF, Stanton J, Bassin P, et al. The direction of the Whitacre needle aperture affects the extent and duration of isobaric spinal anesthesia. *Anesth Analg* 84:337, 1997.

35. Beardsley D, Holman S, Gantt R, et al. Transient neurologic deficit after spinal anesthesia: Local anesthetic maldistribution with pencil point needles? *Anesth Analg* 81:314, 1995.

36. Faure E, Moreno R, Thisted R. Incidence of postdural puncture headache in morbidly obese parturients [letter]. *Reg Anesth* 19:361, 1994.

37. Smith PS, Wilson RC, Robinson AP, et al. Regional blockade for delivery in women with scoliosis or previous spinal surgery. *Int J Obstet Anesth* 12:17, 2003.

38. de Filho GR, Gomes HP, da Fonseca MH, et al. Predictors of successful neuraxial block: A prospective study. *Eur J Anaesthesiol* 19:447, 2002.

39. Furness G, Reilly MP, Kuchi S. An evaluation of ultrasound imaging for identification of lumbar intervertebral level. *Anaesthesia* 57:277, 2002.

40. Grau T, Leipold RW, Fatehi S, et al. Real-time ultrasonic observation of combined spinal-epidural anaesthesia. *Eur J Anaesthesiol* 21:25, 2004.

41. Michael S, Richmond MN, Birks RJ. A comparison between open-end (single hole) and closed-end (three lateral holes) epidural catheters. Complications and quality of sensory blockade. *Anaesthesia* 44:578, 1989.

42. D'Angelo R, Foss ML, Livesay CH. A comparison of multiport and uniport epidural catheters in laboring patients. *Anesth Analg* 84:1276, 1997.

43. Collier CB, Gatt SP. Epidural catheters for obstetrics. Terminal hole or lateral eyes? *Reg Anesth* 19:378, 1994.

44. Norris MC, Ferrenbach D, Dalman H, et al. Does epinephrine improve the diagnostic accuracy of aspiration during labor epidural analgesia? *Anesth Analg* 88:1073, 1999.

45. Eckmann DM. Variations in epidural catheter manufacture: Implications for bending and stiffness. *Reg Anesth Pain Med* 28:37, 2003.

46. Banwell BR, Morley-Forster P, Krause R. Decreased incidence of complications in parturients with the Arrow (FlexTip Plus™) epidural catheter. *Can J Anaesth* 45:370, 1998.

47. Tyagi A, Kumar R, Bhattacharya A, et al. Filters in anaesthesia and intensive care. *Anaesth Intensive Care* 31:418, 2003.

48. Westphal M, Hohage H, Buerkle H, et al. Adsorption of sufentanil to epidural filters and catheters. *Eur J Anaesthesiol* 20:124, 2003.

49. Seow LT, Lips FJ, Cousins MJ. Effect of lateral posture on epidural blockade for surgery. *Anaesth Intensive Care* 11:97, 1983.

50. Huffnagle SL, Norris MC, Arkoosh VA, et al. The influence of epidural needle bevel orientation on spread of sensory blockade in the laboring parturient. *Anesth Analg* 87:326, 1998.

51. Richardson MG, Wissler RN. The effects of needle bevel orientation during epidural catheter insertion in laboring parturients. *Anesth Analg* 88:352, 1999.

52. Duffy BL. Don't turn the needle! *Anaesth Intensive Care* 21:328, 1993.

53. Borghi B, Agnoletti V, Ricci A, et al. A prospective, randomized evaluation of the effects of epidural needle rotation on the distribution of epidural block. *Anesth Analg* 98:1473, 2004.

54. Shenouda PE, Cunningham BJ. Assessing the superiority of saline versus air for use in the epidural loss-of-resistance technique: A literature review. *Reg Anesth Pain Med* 28:48, 2003.

55. Leiman BC, Katz J, Salzarulo H, et al. A comparison of different methods of lubrication of glass syringes used to identify the epidural space. *Anaesthesia* 43:397, 1988.

56. Rosenberg H, Keykhak MM. Distance to the epidural space in nonobstetric patients. *Anesth Analg* 63:539, 1984.

57. Palmer SK, Abram SE, Maitra AM, et al. Distance from the skin to the lumbar epidural space in an obstetric population. *Anesth Analg* 62:944, 1983.

58. Hamza J, Smida M, Benhamou D, et al. Parturient's posture during epidural puncture affects the distance from skin to epidural space. *J Clin Anesth* 7:1, 1995.

59. Rolbin SH, Halpern SH, Braude BM, et al. Fluid through the epidural needle does not reduce complications of epidural catheter insertion. *Can J Anaesth* 37:337, 1990.

60. D'Angelo R, Berkebile BL, Gerancher JC. Prospective examination of epidural catheter insertion. *Anesthesiology* 84:88, 1996.

61. Lim YJ, Bahk JH, Ahn WS, et al. Coiling of lumbar epidural catheters. *Acta Anaesthesiol Scand* 46:603, 2002.

62. Hamilton CL, Riley ET, Cohen SE. Changes in the position of epidural catheters associated with patient movement. *Anesthesiology* 86:778, 1997.

63. Mulroy MF, Norris MC, Liu SS. Safety steps for epidural injection of local anesthetics: Review of the literature and recommendations. *Anesth Analg* 85:1346, 1997.

64. Norris MC, Fogel ST, Dalman H, et al. Labor epidural analgesia without an intravascular "test dose." *Anesthesiology* 88:1495, 1998.

65. Colonna-Romano P, Padolina R, Lingaraju N, et al. Diagnostic accuracy of an intrathecal test dose in epidural analgesia. *Can J Anaesth* 41:572, 1994.

66. Ngan Kee WD, Khaw KS, Lee BB, et al. The limitations of ropivacaine with epinephrine as an epidural test dose in parturients. *Anesth Analg* 92:1529, 2001.

67. Moore DC, Batra MS. The components of an effective test dose prior to epidural block. *Anesthesiology* 55:693, 1981.

68. Guinard JP, Mulroy MF, Carpenter RL, et al. Test doses: Optimal epinephrine content with and without acute beta-adrenergic blockade. *Anesthesiology* 73:386, 1990.

69. Tanaka M, Sato M, Kimura T, et al. The efficacy of simulated intravascular test dose in sedated patients. *Anesth Analg* 93:1612, 2001.

70. Liu SS, Carpenter RL. Hemodynamic responses to intravascular injection of epinephrine-containing epidural test doses in adults during general anesthesia. *Anesthesiology* 84:81, 1996.

71. Liu SS. Hemodynamic responses to an epinephrine test dose in adults during epidural or combined epidural-general anesthesia. *Anesth Analg* 83:97, 1996.

72. Colonna-Romano P, Lingaraju N, Godfrey SD, et al. Epidural test dose and intravascular injection in obstetrics: Sensitivity, specificity, and lowest effective dose. *Anesth Analg* 75:372, 1992.

73. Colonna-Romano P, Lingaraju N, Braitman LE. Epidural test dose: Lidocaine 100 mg, not chloroprocaine, is a symptomatic marker of i.v. injection in labouring parturients. *Can J Anaesth* 40:714, 1993.

74. Mulroy MF, Neal JM, Mackey DC, et al. 2-Chloroprocaine and bupivacaine are unreliable indicators of intravascular injection in the premedicated patient. *Reg Anesth Pain Med* 23:9, 1998.

75. Leighton BL, Norris MC, DeSimone CA, et al. The air test as a clinically useful indicator of intravenously placed epidural catheters. *Anesthesiology* 73:610, 1990.

76. Leighton BL, Topkis WG, Gross JB, et al. Multiport epidural catheters. Does the air test work? *Anesthesiology* 92:1617, 2000.

77. Leighton BL, DeSimone CA, Norris MC, et al. Isoproterenol is an effective marker of intravenous injection in laboring women. *Anesthesiology* 71:206, 1989.

78. Yoshii WY, Miller M, Rottman RL, et al. Fentanyl for epidural intravascular test dose in obstetrics. *Reg Anesth* 18:296, 1993.

79. Morris GF, Gore-Hickman W, Lang SA, et al. Can parturients distinguish between intravenous and epidural fentanyl? *Can J Anaesth* 41:667, 1994.

80. Tsui BC, Gupta S, Finucane B. Confirmation of epidural catheter placement using nerve stimulation. *Can J Anaesth* 45:640, 1998.

81. Morris GN, Warren BB, Hanson EW, et al. Influence of patient position on withdrawal forces during removal of lumbar extradural catheters. *Br J Anaesth* 77:419, 1996.

82. Igarashi T, Hirabayashi Y, Shimizu R, et al. The epidural structure changes during deep breathing. *Can J Anaesth* 46:850, 1999.

83. Geernaert K, Hody JL, Adriaensen H, et al. Does epidural injection of physiological saline facilitate the advancement of catheters? *Eur J Anaesthesiol* 10:349, 1993.

84. Takeyama K, Yamazaki H, Maeda M, et al. Straight advancement of epidural catheter—comparative assessments by method and site of epidural needle puncture and angle of puncture. *Tokai J Exp Clin Med* 29:27, 2004.

85. Scott DA, Beilby DS. Epidural catheter insertion: The effect of saline prior to threading in non-obstetric patients. *Anaesth Intensive Care* 21:284, 1993.

86. Swenson JD, Wisniewski M, McJames S, et al. The effect of prior dural puncture on cisternal cerebrospinal fluid morphine concentrations in sheep after administration of lumbar epidural morphine. *Anesth Analg* 83:523, 1996.

87. Beilin Y, Zahn J, Bernstein HH, et al. Treatment of incomplete analgesia after placement of an epidural catheter and administration of local anesthetic for women in labor. *Anesthesiology* 88:1502, 1998.

88. Waters JH, Leivers D, Hullander M. Response to spinal anesthesia after inadequate epidural anesthesia. *Anesth Analg* 78:1033, 1994.

89. Furst SR, Reisner LS. Risk of high spinal anesthesia following failed epidural block for cesarean delivery. *J Clin Anesth* 7:71, 1995.

90. Langevin PB, Gravenstein N, Langevin SO, et al. Epidural catheter reconnection. Safe and unsafe practice. *Anesthesiology* 85:883, 1996.

91. Drasner K. Thoracic epidural anesthesia: Asleep at the wheal? *Anesth Analg* 99:578, 2004.

92. Lirk P, Messner H, Deibl M, et al. Accuracy in estimating the correct intervertebral space level during lumbar, thoracic and cervical epidural anaesthesia. *Acta Anaesthesiol Scand* 48:347, 2004.

93. Hsin ST, Chang FC, Tsou MY, et al. Inadvertent knotting of a thoracic epidural catheter. *Acta Anaesthesiol Scand* 45:255, 2001.

94. Willis RJ. Caudal epidural blockade. In: Cousin MJ, Bridenbaugh PO, eds, *Neural Blockade in Clinical Anesthesia and Management of Pain*, 3rd ed. Philadelphia, PA: Lippincott-Raven, 1998, p. 323.

95. Noda J, Ohama J, Suzuki S. The effectiveness of cervical epidural block for the treatment of status asthmaticus [Japanese]. *Masui* 43:1251, 1994.

96. Aldrete JA, Mushin AU, Zapata JC, et al. Skin to cervical epidural space distances as read from magnetic resonance imaging films: Consideration of the "hump pad." *J Clin Anesth* 10:309, 1998.

97. Lirk P, Kolbitsch C, Putz G, et al. Cervical and high thoracic ligamentum flavum frequently fails to fuse in the midline. *Anesthesiology* 99:1387, 2003.

98. Cousins MJ, Veering BT. Epidural neural blockade. In: Cousins MJ, Bridenbaugh PO, eds, *Neural Blockade in Clinical Anesthesia and Management of Pain*, 3rd ed. Philadelphia, PA: Lippincott-Raven, 1998, p. 243.

99. Stojanovic MP, Vu TN, Caneris O, et al. The role of fluoroscopy in cervical epidural steroid injections: An analysis of contrast dispersal patterns. *Spine* 27:509, 2002.

100. Cook TM. Combined spinal-epidural techniques. *Anaesthesia* 55:42, 2000.

101. Hoffmann VL, Vercauteren MP, Vreugde JP, et al. Posterior epidural space depth: Safety of the loss-of-resistance and hanging drop techniques. *Br J Anaesth* 83:807, 1999.

102. Riley ET, Hamilton CL, Ratner EF, et al. A comparison of the 24-gauge Sprotte and Gertie Marx spinal needles for combined spinal-epidural analgesia during labor. *Anesthesiology* 97:574, 2002.

103. Herbstman CH, Jaffee JB, Tuman KJ, et al. An in vivo evaluation of four spinal needles used for the combined spinal-epidural technique. *Anesth Analg* 86:520, 1998.

104. Choi DH, Ahn HJ, Kim JA. Combined low-dose spinal-epidural anesthesia versus single-shot spinal anesthesia for elective cesarean delivery. *Int J Obstet Anesth* 15:13, 2006.

105. Goy RW, Chee-Seng Y, Sia AT, et al. The median effective dose of intrathecal hyperbaric bupivacaine is larger in the single-shot spinal as compared with the combined spinal-epidural technique. *Anesth Analg* 100:1499, 2005.

106. Stienstra R, Dahan A, Alhadi BZ, et al. Mechanism of action of an epidural top-up in combined spinal epidural anesthesia. *Anesth Analg* 83:382, 1996.

107. Holst D, Mollmann M, Schymroszcyk B, et al. No risk of metal toxicity in combined spinal-epidural anesthesia. *Anesth Analg* 88:393, 1999.

108. Herman NL, Molin J, Knape KG. No additional metal particle formation using the needle-through-needle combined spinal-epidural technique. *Acta Anaesthesiol Scand* 40:227 1996.

109. Holmstrom B, Rawal N, Axelsson K, et al. Risk of catheter migration during combined spinal epidural block: Percutaneous epiduroscopy study. *Anesth Analg* 80:747, 1995.

110. Rawal N, Van Zundert A, Holmstrom B. Combined spinal-epidural technique. *Reg Anesth* 22:406, 1997.

111. Norris MC, Grieco WM, Borkowski M, et al. Complications of labor analgesia: Epidural versus combined spinal epidural techniques. *Anesth Analg* 79:529, 1994.

112. Haridas RP. Cerebrospinal fluid leak with combined spinal-epidural analgesia [abstract]. *Anesthesiology* 87:A785, 1997

Pharmacology of Drugs Used for Spinal and Epidural Anesthesia and Analgesia

Francis V. Salinas

INTRODUCTION

Successful spinal or epidural anesthesia requires an understanding of the pharmacology of local anesthetic agents and analgesic additives that are administered in the spinal (intrathecal) and epidural space. The following chapter will be divided into four basic sections. The first section will provide a clinically relevant review of the physiology of nerve conduction and mechanism of action of local anesthetics. The second section will provide an overview of the anatomy of the epidural and intrathecal structures that are clinically relevant to the pharmacokinetics and pharmacodynamics of neuraxial anesthetics, as well as other factors that influence variability in the response to the administration of local anesthetics in the spinal/epidural space. The third and fourth sections will provide a detailed discussion about the clinically useful local anesthetic agents and local anesthetic additives and their effects on the clinical efficacy of spinal and epidural anesthesia.

PHYSIOLOGY OF NEURAL CONDUCTION AND LOCAL ANESTHETIC ACTION

▶ Electrophysiologic Basis of the Resting Membrane Potential

Local anesthetics block neuronal conduction; thus an understanding of normal neuronal conduction is essential to the understanding of the mechanism of action of local anesthetics. The neuronal cell membrane is composed of a hydrophobic lipid bilayer embedded with transmembrane proteins. The lipid bilayer allows the passage of small nonpolar molecules, but is relatively impermeable to polar ions. Charged ions must traverse the cell membrane via ion-specific protein channels that permit the passage of certain ions across the cell membrane, while excluding others. Since the semipermeable nature of the lipid bilayer serves as a barrier to ion movement, it can electrically separate ionic charges between the intracellular and extracellular aqueous milieu. Ionic movement via the conductance pathways provided by the ion channels is based on two forces: (1) the relative concentration of the ions (concentration gradient) and (2) the relative charge (electrical potential gradient) on each side of the cell membrane. Thus, ions will tend to diffuse from areas of higher concentration to areas of lower concentration, as well as to areas of opposite polarity (electrical charge). The distribution of a specific ion across the neuronal cell membrane will reach equilibrium only when the electrical forces for that specific ion exactly balance the concentration forces.

The resting membrane potential of neuronal cells is usually about -60 to -70 mV, with the cell interior more negatively charged relative to the cell exterior. The resting membrane potential is a result of the dynamic balance between ionic concentration gradients created by a special transmembrane protein (the Na^+/K^+ ATPase ion pump) and the diffusion potential of ions. The Na^+/K^+ pump actively cotransports three Na^+ ions out of the cell and two K^+ ions into the cell powered by adenosine triphosphate (ATP) hydrolysis. The result is an intracellular to extracellular K^+ ratio of 120:4 mM (30:1) and an extracellular to intracellular Na^+ ratio 140:15 mM (10:1). The separation of the positive and negative charges carried by the net movement of these ions creates an electrical field across the cell membrane described as individual diffusion potentials (or transmembrane voltages) for Na^+ and K^+. The transmembrane voltage exerts a force on an ion toward the opposite polarity in a magnitude proportional to the voltage difference. The Nernst equation for a specific ion mathematically describes the magnitude of the transmembrane voltage (Nernst potential) that exerts a force that matches the diffusional force, thereby resulting in cessation of ion flow (equilibrium) through the channel.

At rest, the neuronal cell membrane predominantly demonstrates a selective permeability for K^+ ions. These K^+ channels are called nongated or "leak channels," indicating that they are always open, regardless of the membrane potential.[1] Thus, the resting cell membrane behaves primarily as a "K^+ electrode" with the Nernst equation predicting a resting membrane potential of −88 mV. The simplified Nernst equation can be described as follows:

$$E_K = (-58.1 \text{ mV}) \log ([K^+]_i/[K^+]_o)$$

where $[K^+]_i$ is the intracellular K^+ concentration and $[K^+]_o$ is the extracellular K^+ concentration. K^+ equilibrium, however, is not the only factor in determining the resting membrane potential. In addition to K^+ channels, neuronal cell membranes have additional voltage-independent channels that allow leak currents of Na^+, Cl^-, and other ions (each with their respective Nernst potentials) that also contribute to the final resting membrane potential of −60 to −70 mV.[2]

▶ Electrophysiologic Basis of the Action Potential

Generation of the Action Potential

The excitability of neurons (the ability to generate a large, rapid change of membrane voltage in response to a very small stimulus) is based on the action potential. It is the action potential that leads to the process of rapid depolarization (loss of the negative transmembrane potential due to inward current of positive charges), usually progressing to a positive transmembrane potential, and then rapidly repolarizing back to a negative transmembrane potential (Fig. 3-1a). In contrast to the dependence of the resting membrane potential on K^+ disequilibrium (and diffusion across nonvoltage-gated K^+ channels), the action potential depends on both Na^+ and K^+ disequilibrium that is maintained by the Na^+/K^+ pump, and ionic currents across voltage-gated Na^+ and K^+ channels.[2]

Voltage-gated Na^+ channels progress though several conformations based on temporal changes in the membrane potential. These channels are in a resting (closed) conformation at the resting membrane potential, but are suddenly

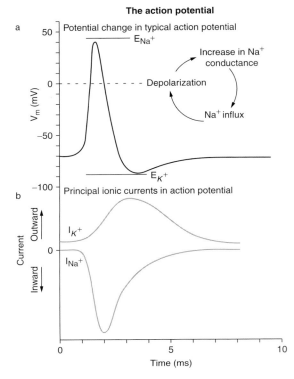

FIGURE 3-1. The action potential. (a) The membrane potential change of a typical action potential rapidly rises from a resting membrane potential of −70 mV, reaching a maximum near the Nernst potential for Na^+ (E_{Na^+}), then declines with a negative undershoot near the Nernst potential for K^+ (E_{K^+}). The action potential is triggered by a positive-feedback loop in which the initial depolarizing stimulus leads to opening of Na^+ channels, which leads to further depolarization. (b) Two principal ionic currents give rise to the action potential. Note that the outward K^+ current has a slower rate of rise in amplitude and is slightly delayed in onset compared to the rapidly rising initial inward Na^+ current. *Used with permission from Study RE. The structure and function of neurons. In: Hemmings H, Hopkins P, eds, Foundations of Anesthesia. Basic and Clinical Sciences. London: Mosby, 2000, p. 185.*

activated (opened) if membrane depolarization reaches a "threshold potential." Since the equilibrium potential for Na^+ is approximately +50 mV, activation of voltage-gated Na^+ channels (which now confers a relative selectively of the cell membrane for Na^+ ions) transforms the cell membrane into Na^+ electrode, and allows a large inward current of Na^+ ions due to the large electrochemical gradient generated by the Na^+/K^+ pump (Fig. 3-1b). The initial inward current of Na^+ through the voltage-gated channels leads to more depolarization and thus, more channel opening, initiating a positive-feedback loop until all the Na^+ channels that can be potentially activated are activated and the membrane potential reaches the equilibrium potential for Na^+ (Fig. 3-1a).

Following activation of Na^+ channels and initiation of the action potential, the process must be turned off in order for the membrane to return to its resting potential. After a few milliseconds of suddenly opening, the Na^+ channels spontaneously undergo another conformational change to an inactivated state. Almost simultaneously, the K^+-gated channels also become activated and open in response to depolarization produced by the action potential, but do so with a small delay and at a slower rate compared to the Na^+ channels. Since the equilibrium potential for K^+ is approximately –90 mV, when the K^+ channels open (during an action potential), the positive membrane potential creates a very strong electrochemical gradient for K^+ ions that leads to a positive outward ionic current that will tend to return the membrane potential back to its negative resting state (Fig. 3-1a). Because of the slight delay in the opening of the K^+ channels, the outward current of K^+ does not oppose the earlier inward current of Na^+ until after the action potential has been generated (Fig. 3-1b). The positive-feedback loop that generated the action potential continues until some of the Na^+ channels have become inactivated and enough of the K^+ channels have opened to change the balance of current to a net outward positive current that results in membrane repolarization. During the process of repolarization, inactivated Na^+ channels and open K^+ channels revert to resting (closed) conformations.

Thus, a three-state kinetic scheme conceptually describes the changes in Na^+ channel conformation that accounts for the changes in Na^+ conductance during depolarization and repolarization.[2] The resting (closed), activated (open), and inactivated conformations correspond to the state of the Na^+ channel during the resting membrane potential, during the action potential when the channel rapidly conducts an inward Na^+ current, and when the Na^+ channel stops conducting the inward Na^+ current immediately following the activated state, respectively. As a result of the voltage- and time-dependent conformational changes of the Na^+ and K^+ channels, the net movement of positive current is inward during the depolarizing phase of the action potential and outward during the phase of repolarization.

The initial change in membrane potential required to reach the activation threshold necessary to initiate the regenerative and self-sustaining process of the action potential is not an absolute value, but rather depends on the dynamic interactions between the voltage-gated Na^+ and K^+ channels. If the depolarizing stimulus is inadequate in duration, there will be insufficient time for Na^+ channels to become activated. If the rate of Na^+ channel activation is inadequate, then there will not be enough activated Na^+ channels at one time to reach the threshold potential. Furthermore, voltage-gated K^+ channels would begin to increase their outward current, thus, preventing the membrane from reaching the activation threshold. Thus, successful generation of an action potential requires a depolarizing stimulus of adequate speed, amplitude, and duration such that the depolarizing effect of the activated Na^+ channels becomes sufficiently self-sustaining to overcome the opposing influences of Na^+ channel inactivation and the hyperpolarizing effects of K^+ channel activation.

Propagation of the Action Potential

Once an action potential is generated, propagation of the electrical impulse along the axon is required for the information to be transmitted. Both the action potential and impulse propagation exhibit "all-or-none" behavior. This is particularly important in the case of impulse propagation, as either the locally generated action potential generates a threshold potential at adjacent membrane segments and causes propagation along the axon, or the local depolarization ceases. The action potential is propagated along the axon by continuous coupling between excited and nonexcited regions of the cell membrane.

The conduction velocity of the propagated impulse varies tremendously among neurons, and depending on their physiologic function, the velocity ranges from several meters per second (m/s) to as much as 75–120 m/s. The primary determinants of conduction velocity are axon diameter and myelination. The conduction velocity of an axon increases in proportion to the square root of the radius. Myelination can increase conduction velocity up to 10-fold over that achieved in nonmyelinated axons and all mammalian nerves with diameters greater than 1–2 μm are myelinated. Myelin is a tight, multilayered wrapping of the Schwann cell lipid bilayer membrane that encloses individual myelinated axons (Fig. 1-12). Although the myelin layer can account for over half the thickness of a neuron's diameter, it is not continuous along the length of the axon. Separating the myelinated regions, usually every 1–2 mm along the axon are very short distances where the neuronal cell membrane is exposed to the extracellular aqueous milieu. The Na^+ channels in the axon are concentrated in these areas, called *nodes of Ranvier*.[3]

An action potential generated from an adjacent node causes a depolarization that is sufficient to trigger the opening of enough Na^+ channels in the next node, resulting in an action potential that is then conducted to the next node. The process of an action potential propagated from node to node is called *saltatory conduction,* which allows very high conduction velocities along relatively small axons. The presence of myelin also accelerates conduction velocity due to increased electrical insulation of the axon. Thus, in contrast to nonmyelinated axons, which increase conduction velocity only with the square root of the diameter, conduction velocity increases directly with the axon diameter of myelinated axons. In summary, the action potential propagation along nonmyelinated axons requires achievement of the threshold potential at immediately adjacent membrane, whereas myelinated axons require generation of the threshold potential at a subsequent node of Ranvier.

Table 3-1

Classification of Afferent and Efferent Nerve Fibers Based on Axon Diameter and Conduction Velocity

Fiber Class	Diameter (μm)	Myelin	Conduction Velocity (m/s)	Innervation	Function
Aα	12–20	+++	75–120	Afferent from muscle spindle proprioceptors Efferents to skeletal muscle	Motor and reflex activity
Aβ	5–12	+++	30–75	Afferent from cutaneous mechanoreceptors	Touch and pressure
Aγ	3–6	++	12–35	Efferents to muscle spindles	Muscle tone
Aδ	1–5	++	5–30	Afferent pain and temperature Nociceptors	"Fast" pain, touch, and temperature
B	<3	+	3–15	Preganglionic sympathetic efferents	Autonomic function
C	0.2–1.5	−	0.5–2.0	Afferent pain and temperature	"Slow" pain, temperature

Data from Ref. 4.

The diameter and myelination of a neuron not only correlates with conduction velocity, but also with message-carrying function. Since different functions require different conduction velocities along axons, conduction velocity can be used to classify neurons. Most nerves (including the dorsal root ganglia) in the peripheral nervous system that transmit information between their axons and the central nervous system (CNS) contain a mixture of myelinated and nonmyelinated neurons that carry out both afferent and efferent functions. Neurons are categorized into three major classes, designated A, B, and C, corresponding to peaks in the temporal distribution of their conduction velocities (Table 3-1).[4] *Group A* includes large, myelinated somatic afferent and efferent axons, *group B* are smaller myelinated preganglionic autonomic efferents, and *group C* are the smallest and nonmyelinated afferents.

Group A axons are further subdivided based on decreasing conduction velocity and diameter (Table 3-1). $A\alpha$ fibers include both sensory afferents from proprioceptors of skeletal muscle and motor efferents to skeletal muscle responsible for motor function and reflex activity; $A\beta$ afferent fibers include cutaneous mechanoreceptors responsible for touch and pressure; $A\gamma$ efferent fibers include muscle spindles to control muscle tone; and $A\delta$ afferent fibers are responsible for temperature sensation and pain (typically described as sharp, intense, or lancinating). Group C fibers carry information about temperature, as well as pain, particularly pain that is perceived as dull, burning, or aching. Thus, afferent

sensory axons have two separate conduction pathways that carry pain-related information. The myelinated $A\delta$ fibers conduct signals (fast pain) rapidly and the nonmyelinated C fibers conduct signals (slow pain) relatively slower.

Refractory Period

An important characteristic of the action potential is the *refractory period:* the time after initiation of an action potential when it is impossible or more difficult to generate a second action potential. The *absolute refractory period* is the time from initial depolarization to when repolarization is almost complete. The basis for the absolute refractory period is Na^+ channel inactivation, when it is impossible to recruit a sufficient number of Na^+ channels to generate a second depolarizing stimulus until the previously activated Na^+ channels have recovered from inactivation, which takes several milliseconds.

The *relative refractory period*, when a stronger than predicted stimulus is required to generate a second action potential, follows the absolute refractory period. The basis for the relative refractory period is K^+ channel activation, when the repolarizing outward current of K^+ ions results in a brief period of hyperpolarization, such that a stronger depolarizing stimulus is required to activate the population of Na^+ channels that in the meantime have "reprimed" for activation. The refractory period limits the rate at which action potentials can be generated, an important

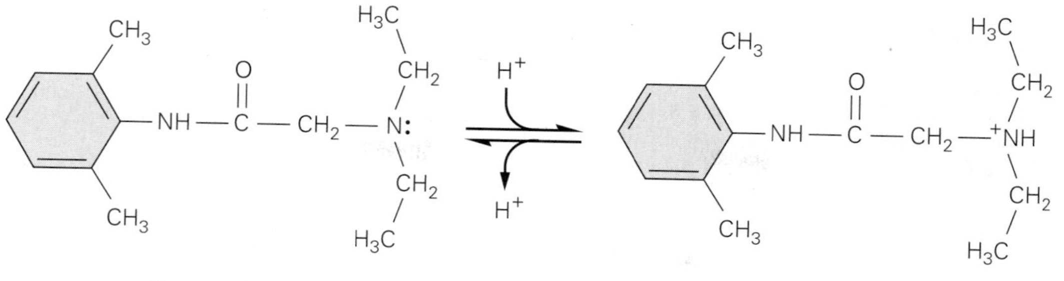

FIGURE 3-2. The basic (neutral) lipid-soluble and cationic (charged) hydrophilic forms of lidocaine. *Used with permission from Strichartz G. Neural physiology and local anesthetic action. In: Cousins MJ, Bridenbaugh PO, eds, Neural Blockade in Clinical Anesthesia and Pain Management. Philadelphia, PA: Lippincott-Raven, 1998, p. 41.*

aspect of neuronal signaling. Additionally, the refractory period facilitates unidirectional propagation of the action potential along the axon. Since the membrane on each side of the action potential is refractory, a second action potential approaching behind the first action potential will be terminated.

Molecular Mechanism of Action of Local Anesthetics

Local anesthetics render neurons less excitable by directly binding to and inhibiting the ability of voltage-gated Na^+ channels to conduct Na^+ currents.[5] They do so by inhibiting the conformational changes that form the basis of Na^+ channel activity. Therefore, local anesthetics fundamentally inhibit the generation and propagation of the action potential. Understanding the concepts of (1) local anesthetic ionization, (2) the three-state kinetic scheme of the Na^+ channel, and (3) tonic block versus phasic block provide the basis for understanding the mechanism of reversible local anesthetic-induced conduction blockade.

The most commonly used local anesthetics are tertiary amines that exist in a dynamic equilibrium between an electrically neutral base form and a positively charged protonated form. The relative concentrations of the two forms depend on the pK_a and the pH of the aqueous milieu where local anesthetics are deposited (Fig. 3-2). The ratio of the charged (ionized) form to the neutral form is described by the Henderson-Hasselbach equation:

$$[LAH^+]/[LA] = 10^{(pK_a - pH)}$$

Thus, the pK_a is the pH at which the concentration of the neutral form is equal to the concentration of the charged cation. Both ionized and nonionized drugs with local anesthetic

activity can inhibit Na^+ channels. Permanently neutral local anesthetics (such as the secondary amine benzocaine) freely permeate the hydrophobic neuronal membrane and inhibit Na^+ conductance and impulse conduction whether applied directly intracellular or deposited extracellular, demonstrating that ionization is not absolutely essential for local anesthetic activity.

In contrast, quaternary derivatives of local anesthetics (which are permanently charged) have very little membrane permeability, and exhibit potent inhibition of Na^+ conductance and conduction blockade only when they are directly infused into the neuronal cytoplasm.[6] Tertiary amines, which have pK_a values from about 7.7 to 8.9, exhibit more potent Na^+ channel inhibition when applied in an external alkaline pH, or when applied directly within neuronal cytoplasm at a neutral or slightly acidic pH. Thus, tertiary amine local anesthetics must first traverse the hydrophobic milieu of the neuronal membrane in the neutral form, and having reached the cytoplasm, become ionized to more avidly bind to the Na^+ channel.

The neutral local anesthetic benzocaine exhibits little change in Na^+ channel inhibition with an increased frequency of stimulation, whereas tertiary amine local anesthetics exhibit different degrees of Na^+ channel inhibition based on the frequency of neuronal stimulation. In the presence of local anesthetics, measures of Na^+ channel activity (either Na^+ currents or action potential amplitude) are decreased by 30–50% with low-frequency stimulation, which is known as "tonic block." If the stimulation is repeatedly applied at a higher frequency, Na^+ channel activation is decreased incrementally for each stimulus until a new steady-state level of Na^+ channel inhibition is reached. This is called frequency-dependent or "phasic block." The degree of Na^+ channel inhibition produced by the phasic block is quickly reversed to tonic levels when frequency of stimulation is decreased or stopped.

The differences in the degree of Na^+ channel inhibition exhibited by tertiary amine local anesthetics during tonic block compared to phasic block are best explained by the presence of a single local anesthetic receptor site within the Na^+ channel that demonstrates differing affinities (for local anesthetics) based on the specific Na^+ channel conformation.[5] Specifically, open and inactivated Na^+ channel conformations possess much higher affinities for local anesthetics as compared to the resting conformation. With each successive depolarization, the percentage of local anesthetic-bound Na^+ channels incrementally increase, and conversely, the percentage of resting Na^+ channels incrementally decrease. Local anesthetic binding to the Na^+ channels exhibits a dynamic equilibrium and dissociation occurs in the time interval between successive depolarizations. This is exemplified by an increase in Na^+ channel activity when the frequency of stimulation is decreased. However, the process of local anesthetic dissociation, which would allow the Na^+ channel to return to a resting conformation, occurs at a slower rate compared to the rapid voltage-regulated return to a resting Na^+ channel conformation that occurs during the physiologic process of repolarization.

FUNCTIONAL ANATOMY OF SPINAL AND EPIDURAL ANESTHESIA/ANALGESIA

▶ Structure and Functions of Neurons

Neurons are electrically excitable cells within the nervous system responsible for the processing and storage of information via electrical signaling. Neurons are able to generate and propagate electrical impulses (the action potential) that serve as the primary mechanism for communication in the nervous system. The typical neuron is composed of a *cell body,* multiple small processes close to the cell body called *dendrites,* and a single, long projection called an *axon.* The cell bodies of primary afferent sensory neurons are located in the dorsal root ganglia, adjacent to the respective spinal cord segment (Fig. 3-3). Each sensory neuron has only one axon, with the shorter branch projecting toward the dorsal root entry zone and a longer branch extending to the periphery as specialized sensory nerve endings (nociceptors) that form the somatosensory component of the sensory neuron.

Nociceptors innervate skin, subcutaneous and connective tissues, muscles, bones, joints, and visceral organs, and respond to noxious (painful) mechanical, thermal, and chemical stimuli. Intense mechanical and thermal stimuli (generally at temperatures exceeding 40–42°C trigger the process of *transduction,* which is the increased firing of

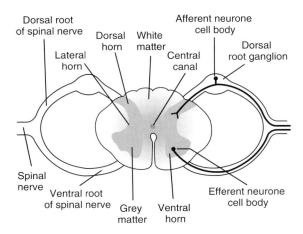

FIGURE 3-3. Transverse section through the spinal cord illustrating the location of the gray and white matter and the attachment of the dorsal and ventral spinal nerve roots. Note the afferent sensory neuron in the dorsal root ganglia, with the shorter branch projecting centrally toward the dorsal root entry zone. Note the efferent motor neuron with the cell body in the gray matter of the ventral horn. *Used with permission from Stranding S. Gray's Anatomy, 39th ed. Edinburgh: Churchill Livingstone, 2005, p. 229.*

impulses in the free sensory nerve endings.[7] Additionally, both nociceptor terminals and the surrounding damaged tissue release excitatory chemical substances (e.g., bradykinin, prostaglandins, substance P, H^+, histamine, and others) that directly excite the nociceptor terminals, and increase transduction of painful stimuli. The resulting series of impulses are then transmitted along the axon to the spinal cord.

Motor neurons have their cell bodies in the ventral (or anterior) gray horn of the spinal cord (Fig. 3-3). The cell body and dendrites receive and process information from other neurons and generate postsynaptic impulses. The postsynaptic impulses are then integrated into coordinated impulses that are transmitted along the efferent motor axon to the branched, distal terminal processes that form the proximal portion of the neuromuscular synaptic junction.[7] Each motor neuron and the set of muscle fibers that it innervates are collectively termed a *motor unit,* and a group of motor units responsible for controlling impulse output to a single muscle is known as a *motor-neuron pool.* Additionally, the cell bodies of the preganglionic sympathetic neurons are located within the intermediolateral gray horn (e.g., between the dorsal and ventral gray zones) of the T1 through L2 spinal cord segments. These sympathetic neurons also send efferent fibers via the ventral spinal roots to synapse with neurons located just outside the central neuraxial space in the sympathetic paravertebral ganglia.

▶ Functional Anatomy of the Vertebral Canal

Spinal Nerve Roots

An understanding of the functional anatomy of the structures within the spinal and epidural space provides a basis for understanding not only the clinical evaluation of central neuraxial blockade, but also provides a basis for understanding the pharmacokinetics and pharmacodynamics of local anesthetics administered in the intrathecal and epidural space.

The spinal cord is a cylindrical structure that gives rise to 31 pairs of spinal nerves, which arise from segments of the spinal cord specified by the intervertebral foramina through which the spinal nerves exit the vertebral canal (see Chap. 1). Each spinal cord segment gives rise to a ventral motor root and a dorsal sensory root, which cross the subarachnoid space and traverse the dura mater separately, uniting in or close to the intervertebral foramina to form the corresponding mixed spinal nerve (Fig. 3-4). Recent anatomic studies have demonstrated great interindividual variability in the size and cross-sectional area of human nerve roots.[8] The dorsal nerve roots are consistently larger compared with the ventral nerve roots. Based simply on a higher surface area to volume ratio, this should allow local anesthetics easier penetration and uptake into the smaller ventral nerve roots. However, detailed studies have demonstrated that dorsal nerve roots commonly divide into two to three separate bundles on exiting the spinal cord, while in the majority of cases, the ventral nerve root is formed as a single bundle. Moreover, as the dorsal nerve root bundles course laterally, they are observed to further subdivide into as many as 1–10 fascicles prior to the dorsal root expanding into the dorsal root ganglia.[8,9] Thus, the larger, but typically multistranded dorsal root offers a substantially larger surface area for local anesthetic uptake compared to the smaller, single ventral root. This anatomic finding may partially explain the relative ease of obtaining sensory blockade versus motor blockade.

Each dorsal root has an ovoid swelling, the dorsal root ganglia, just proximal to its junction with the corresponding ventral root in the intervertebral foramen (Fig. 3-3). After the dorsal and ventral nerve roots join to form a spinal nerve, the spinal nerve almost immediately divides into the dorsal primary ramus and the ventral primary ramus (Fig. 3-4). The dorsal rami innervate the skin and true muscles of the back while the ventral rami innervate the rest of the trunk and the limbs. Thus, the spinal nerves are united at ventral and dorsal roots, which are attached in series to the lateral aspect of the corresponding spinal cord segments. The term spinal nerve strictly applies only to the short segment between the union of the ventral and dorsal nerve roots within the intervertebral foramen up to the point at which the nerve splits into the rami. The spinal nerves (and rami) are mixed nerves in that they carry both afferent and efferent neural impulses. Since measuring local anesthetic concentrations within the spinal or

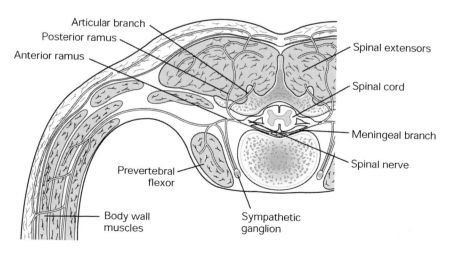

FIGURE 3-4. Illustration of the formation of the paired spinal nerves by the joining of the respective ventral and dorsal roots. Almost immediately after the paired spinal nerves are formed, they divide into ventral (anterior) and dorsal (posterior) primary rami. *Used with permission from Stranding S. Gray's Anatomy, 39th ed. Edinburgh: Churchill Livingstone, 2005, p. 780.*

epidural space is impractical, and dermatomes can be considered the sensory projections of the spinal cord segments, qualitative assessment of the loss of afferent sensory function (such as temperature, pinprick, and touch) provides an indirect, but clinically useful estimate of local anesthetic distribution within the spinal cord.

In adults, the spinal cord is shorter than the vertebral column, and typically ends at the conus medullaris at the lower third of the L1 vertebral body. The level of spinal cord termination, however, ranges between the upper third of the T12 vertebral body and the upper third of the L3 vertebral body, with a population distribution that is bell shaped (see Chap. 1 and Fig. 13-4).[10] Because the spinal cord is shorter than the vertebral column, there is progressive obliquity of the lower thoracic, lumbar, and sacral spinal nerve roots, which makes them travel increasingly longer distances within the subarachnoid space (from their spinal cord segments of origin) to the intervertebral foramina through which they exit as the spinal nerve (Fig. 1-7). The collection of spinal nerve roots in the subarachnoid space caudal to the conus medullaris is collectively termed the *cauda equina* due to its resemblance to a horse's tail. The enlargement of the subarachnoid space containing the cauda equina is termed the *lumbar cistern*. It is within the lumbar cistern that local anesthetics are injected during spinal anesthesia.

Meninges

Collectively, the spinal meninges consist of three membranes (*dura mater, arachnoid mater,* and *pia mater*) that along with the cerebrospinal fluid (CSF) in the subarachnoid space envelope, support and protect the spinal cord and spinal nerve roots. The spinal dura mater forms the dural sac, which is a long tubular sheath contained within the surrounding vertebral canal that extends from the foramen magnum to the lower border of the second sacral vertebra. The dura mater is the outermost and thickest meningeal membrane of the spinal cord. Thus, it incorrectly has been assumed to be the primary barrier to diffusion of epidurally administered drugs into the subarachnoid space. However, the dura mater is predominantly composed of collagen fibrils, interspersed with elastic fibers and ground substance in an anatomic arrangement that allows ready passage of drugs.[11] The inner surface of the dura mater is highly vascular and is composed of a rich capillary network.[12]

The arachnoid mater is closely applied to the inner surface of the dura mater, and is composed of overlapping layers of flattened epithelial-like cells that are connected by frequent tight junctions and occluding junctions.[12] Although much thinner than the dura mater, it is the anatomic arrangement of the arachnoid mater that accounts for greater than 90% of the resistance to drug diffusion through the spinal meninges.[13] The spinal pia mater closely invests the surface of the spinal cord and nerve roots. It is composed of three to six cell layers

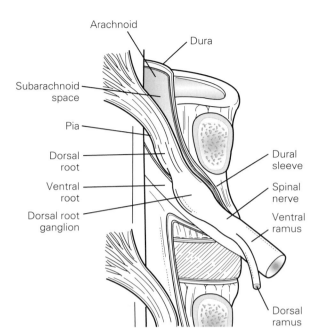

FIGURE 3-5. A spinal nerve, its roots, and meningeal coverings. *Used with permission from Stranding S. Gray's Anatomy, 39th ed. Edinburgh: Churchill Livingstone, 2005, p. 782.*

joined by desmosomes and other specialized junctions. There is underlying subpial tissue composed primarily of collagen that separates the pial cellular layer from the neural tissues. Scanning electron micrograph examination demonstrates fenestrations on the pial surface of the spinal cord and nerve roots that allows direct contact with the subarachnoid space.[14] Tubular extensions of the spinal dura mater, closely lined by the arachnoid, extend around the nerve roots and spinal nerves as they traverse through the lateral aspects of the vertebral canal and intervertebral foramina (Fig. 3-5). At the point where the nerve roots and nerves leave the subarachnoid space, the arachnoid mater is reflected onto their surfaces as they pass through the dura mater into the intervertebral foramina. The arachnoid mater becomes continuous with the perineurium and the dura mater becomes continuous with the epineurium.

Contents of the Epidural Space

The epidural space is the space that lies between the outer aspect of the dura mater and tissues that line the vertebral canal. The epidural space is not a closed space, but communicates freely with the paravertebral space via the intervertebral foramina. There is a rich venous plexus that courses primarily within the anterior and lateral portions of the epidural space with few if any veins in the posterior epidural space. The most widespread material within the epidural space is fat, primarily located in the posterior and lateral epidural space.[9] Epidural fat has a clinically important role in the pharmacokinetics of epidural drugs. Clinical studies have demonstrated that residence time for both local anesthetics and opioids administered in the epidural space is directly related to their lipid solubility, as is the amount of drug sequestered in the epidural fat.[15] Thus, sequestration in the epidural fat decreases the bioavailability of highly lipid-soluble drugs from their neural target sites of action.

CLINICAL PHARMACOLGY OF LOCAL ANESTHETIC AGENTS

The conduct of successful spinal and epidural anesthesia requires a block that is of sufficient sensory distribution to provide surgical anesthesia, and when required, motor blockade. Clinically successful spinal and epidural anesthesia also require a block of sufficiently fast onset to facilitate the timely start of surgery and adequate duration for the planned procedure, as well as prompt return of neurologic function (when needed) to facilitate a timely discharge. Conversely, central neuraxial blockade with unnecessary

cephalad spread may increase the risk for cardiovascular complications of hypotension and bradycardia.

Since there is considerable interpatient variability, it may be difficult to reliably predict the central neuraxial distribution and duration of a particular local anesthetic dose. Therefore, recommendations regarding specific local anesthetic choice and dose for an individual patient and specific surgical procedures (or for postoperative analgesia) must be made with a detailed knowledge of the determinants that govern the intrinsic activity and potency, as well as the distribution, uptake, and elimination of specific local anesthetics within the central neuraxial space.

▶ Physiochemical Properties of Local Anesthetics and Relationship to Activity and Potency

The clinically useful local anesthetics consist of a lipophilic, substituted benzene ring linked to a hydrophilic amine group via an intermediate alkyl chain consisting of either an ester or amide linkage (Fig. 3-6). The type of linkage separates local anesthetics into two chemically distinct groups based on their metabolism. The *aminoamides* are metabolized in

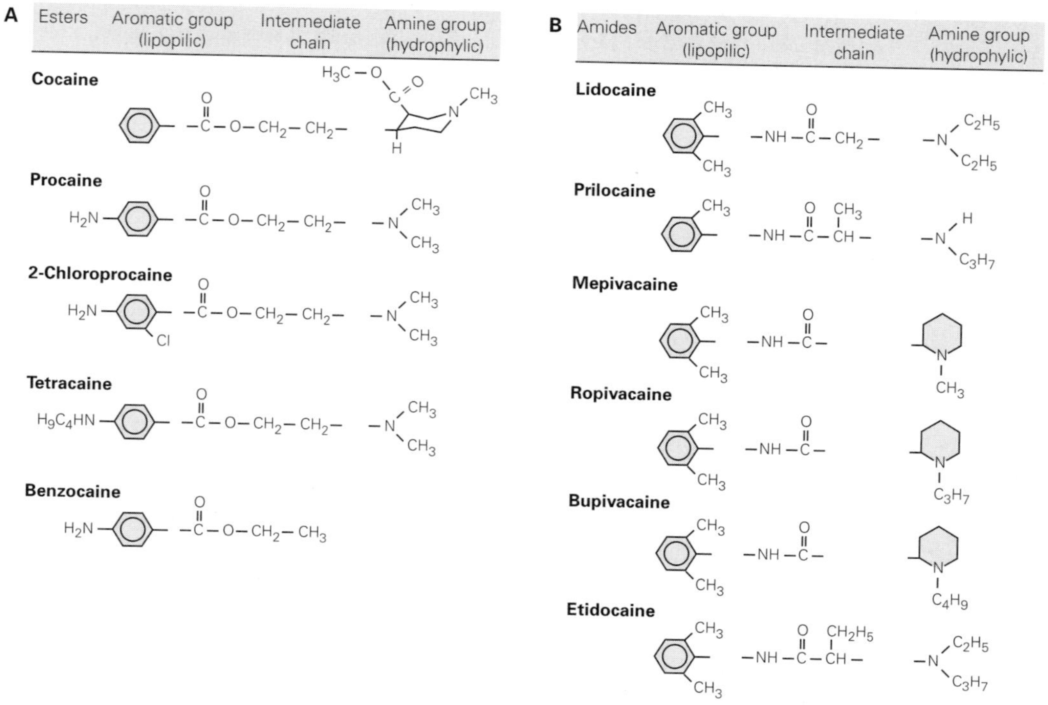

FIGURE 3-6. Local anesthetic structures. Clinically useful local anesthetics consist of a lipophilic, substituted benzene ring linked to a hydrophilic amine group via an intermediate chain consisting of either an ester (A) or amide (B) linkage. *Used with permission from Butterworth J. Mechanisms of local anesthetic action. In: Miller RA, Schwinn DA, eds, Atlas of Anesthesia. Scientific Principles of Anesthesia. Philadelphia, PA: Churchill Livingstone, Vol. 2, 1998, p. 162.*

Table 3-2

Physiochemical Properties of Clinically Useful Local Anesthetics for Spinal and Epidural Anesthesia

	pK_a	% Ionized (at pH 7.4)	Partition Coefficient (Lipid Solubility)	% Protein Building
Amides				
Lidocaine	7.9	76	366	64
Mepivacaine	7.6	61	130	77
Bupivacaine	8.1	83	3420	95
Levobupivacaine	8.1	83	3420	>97
Ropivacaine	8.1	83	775	94
Etidocaine	7.7	66	7317	94
Esters				
Chloroprocaine	8.7	95	810	NA
Procaine	8.9	97	100	6
Tetracaine	8.5	93	5822	94

Data from Ref. 16.

the liver by microsomal enzymes and the *aminoesters* are hydrolyzed by plasma cholinesterases. The clinical activity of local anesthetics is governed by several intrinsic physiochemical properties: ionization, lipid solubility, protein binding, and enantiomerism.

Ionization

The majority of clinically useful local anesthetics are weak bases that exist in a dynamic equilibrium either as a lipid-soluble neutral form or as a protonated (charged) hydrophilic form (Fig. 3-2). The pK_a, or dissociation constant, is the pH at which the two different forms exist at equivalent concentrations. The combination of local tissue pH where a local anesthetic is deposited and its pK_a determine the proportion of injected drug that exists in each form (Table 3-2).[16] For example, bupivacaine has a pK_a of 8.1, which means that 83% of the molecules exist in the charged ionized form and only 17% in the nonionized lipid-soluble form at a physiologic pH of 7.4. In contrast, etidocaine has a pK_a of 7.7, so that 66% exists in the ionized form and 34% exists in the unionized form at pH 7.4. Penetration of the hydrophobic lipid bilayer by the lipid-soluble form appears to be the primary mechanism by which local anesthetics gain access to the intracellular binding site of the Na^+ channel.[5] As previously discussed, the primary site of local anesthetic action is the intracellular side of the voltage-gated Na^+ channel, and the charged form appears to be the predominantly active species.[5] The percentage of local anesthetic found in the lipid-soluble neutral form is inversely

proportional to the pK_a of a specific agent. Thus, decreasing pK_a for a given local tissue pH will increase the percentage of lipid-soluble form, hastening the penetration of axonal membranes and onset of action (Fig. 3-7). Conversely, given that the pK_a of most local anesthetics is between 7.7 and 8.9 and that they are packaged in acidic solutions to maintain aqueous solubility, increasing the local tissue pH, for example, by addition of $NaHCO_3$, will also increase the percentage of the lipid-soluble form and hasten onset of action.

Lipid Solubility

Lipid solubility is another important determinant of intrinsic local anesthetic activity. Although increasing lipid solubility promotes penetration of neuronal membranes, it may also result in increased uptake and sequestration of local anesthetic in myelin and other lipid-soluble compartments. This creates a depot for the slow release of local anesthetics. Thus, increasing lipid solubility usually prolongs latency. Finally, increased lipid solubility parallels intrinsic local anesthetic potency. This observation may be explained by the correlation between lipid solubility and both Na^+ channel receptor affinity and the ability to alter Na^+ channel conformation by directly affecting the fluidity of the neuronal membrane.

Protein Binding

The degree of protein binding also affects local anesthetic activity as only the unbound form can diffuse across neural membranes and exert pharmacologic activity. In general,

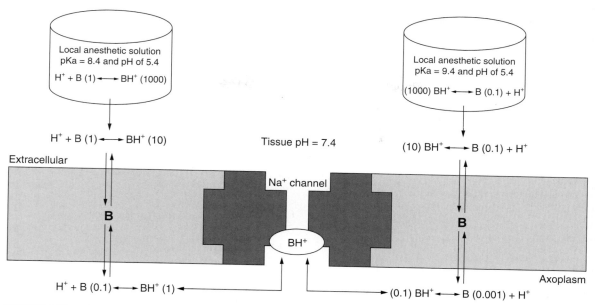

FIGURE 3-7. The ratio of a local anesthetic in the ionized (lipophobic) form to nonionized (lipophilic) base form is dependent on its pK_a and the pH of the surrounding solution. A local anesthetic with a pK_a of 8.4 is 3 pH units (10^3) away from its 50% equilibrium state when contained in a commercially prepared solution at a pH of 5.4, with an approximate unionized molecule to ionized molecule ratio of 1000:1. When the local anesthetic solution is injected into body tissues (physiologic pH of 7.4) and subsequently gains access to the axoplasm, the ratio decreases (by a factor of 10^2) to 10:1. For a local anesthetic with a pK_a of 9.4, the ratio of ionized to nonionized molecules in the commercially prepared solution is even higher (1000:0.1 or 10,000:1), with a ratio in body tissue of 100:1. The difference in the pK_a between the two local anesthetic solutions results in 10-fold difference in the amount of nonionized local anesthetic available to cross the lipid membrane, as well as 10-fold difference in the amount of the ionized active form of local anesthetic available to bind to the Na+ channel.

the more lipid-soluble and longer-acting local anesthetics also possess increased protein binding to tissue and plasma proteins. It has been erroneously assumed that increased protein binding correlates with increased duration of action. However, the degree of local anesthetic protein binding does not correlate with binding to the Na+ channel receptor. Studies suggest that binding and dissociation of local anesthetic molecules from the Na+ channel occurs in a matter of seconds regardless of the degree of protein binding. Thus, duration of action associated with an increased degree of protein binding must involve undefined interactions with extracellular or membranous proteins.

Chirality

Clinically useful local anesthetics, with the exception of lidocaine (achiral), ropivacaine (the S-enantiomer of a bupivacaine homolog with a propyl rather than a butyl chain at the tertiary amine), and levobupivacaine (S-bupivacaine), are packaged as racemic mixtures. Racemic drugs are 1:1 mixtures of two types of molecules (stereoisomers) bearing identical chemical composition and binding, but with a different spatial orientation around an asymmetric chiral carbon.[17] Local anesthetics exhibit a particular type of stereoisomerism known as

enantiomerism, where the pair of stereoisomers in three-dimensional projection cannot be superimposed on each other. Although enantiomers of local anesthetics have identical physiochemical properties, they exhibit potentially different pharmacodynamic, pharmacokinetic, and systemic toxic effects. For example, R-enantiomers appear to have increased in vitro potency for conduction blockade of both neuronal and cardiac Na+ channels and thus, may have increased therapeutic efficacy and potential for systemic toxicity.[17]

▶ Determinants of Clinical Efficacy of Spinal and Epidural Anesthesia

A basic definition of a few terms is essential for understanding the clinical pharmacology of spinal and epidural anesthesia. *Distribution* of local anesthetics within the subarachnoid or epidural space determines the spatial extent of sensory and motor block. *Uptake* of local anesthetics into neuronal tissues determines which neuronal functions are affected during spinal/epidural anesthesia. Uptake into neuronal tissue is a function of the CSF concentration and perineural tissue concentration in the epidural space, which is largely determined by the distribution, as the concentration of local anesthetic will decrease progressively from the area of initial highest concentration (injection site). *Elimination* of local anesthetics from the subarachnoid and epidural space determines the duration of action.

Since measuring local anesthetic concentrations within the spinal or epidural space is impractical, and dermatomes can be considered the sensory projections of the spinal cord segments, assessment of the loss of afferent sensory function provides an indirect, but clinically useful estimate of local anesthetic distribution. The most common methods are loss of temperature (most commonly cold), pinprick, and touch sensation, which correspond to inhibition of C, Aδ, and Aβ nerve fibers, respectively (Table 3-1). Thus, interpretation of studies of local anesthetic distribution and duration must be interpreted in the context of these clinically useful tests of afferent sensory blockade.

▶ Spinal Anesthesia and Determinants of Local Anesthetic Distribution

A number of factors have been proposed to influence the distribution of local anesthetic solutions within the subarachnoid space.[18] Many factors have been shown to have little if any clinical significance, while others clearly play a significant role. After injection within the subarachnoid space, the local anesthetic solution will initially spread simply by bulk flow created by displacement of CSF. Subsequently, the most important factor in determining intrathecal drug distribution is the baricity of the injected local anesthetic solution relative to the influence of gravity.

Baricity

Baricity is defined as the ratio of density of the local anesthetic solution relative to the density of CSF at 37°C. Density is the ratio of the mass of a substance to its volume (measured in weight/unit volume) and varies inversely with temperature. Thus, local anesthetic solutions that have the same density as CSF are classified as *isobaric*. Solutions that have a greater density than CSF are classified as *hyperbaric*, whereas solutions that have a lower density are classified as *hypobaric*. Baricity plays a key role in local anesthetic distribution because gravity causes hyperbaric solutions to distribute to the most dependent areas of the subarachnoid space, whereas hypobaric solutions rise upward toward the nondependent areas of the subarachnoid space. The effects of gravity are determined by choice of patient position (supine, prone, lateral, and sitting), and in the supine, horizontal position, by the curvatures of the vertebral canal (Fig. 1-3). Therefore, it is possible by choosing the appropriate baricity in combination with a specific patient position, to influence the distribution of the local anesthetic solution to

match the dermatomal segments that require surgical anesthesia. In contrast to hypobaric and hyperbaric solutions, patient position and the effects of gravity should exert little influence on intrathecal drug distribution for truly isobaric local anesthetic solutions.

The mean density of CSF varies significantly among specific patient population subgroups (Table 3-3).[19–24] The mean CSF density for males (1.00064 ± 0.00012 g/mL) and postmenopausal females (1.00070 ± 0.00018 g/mL) is very similar, while the density is only slightly lower for premenopausal females (1.00049 ± 0.00004 g/mL). Women at term pregnancy and immediately postpartum have a significantly lower mean CSF density (1.00030 ± 0.00004 g/mL). Because of the variability in CSF density, hyperbaric and hypobaric solutions must have densities three standard deviations above and below population mean CSF density, respectively, to predictably act in a hyperbaric or hypobaric manner. For clinically useful purposes, local anesthetic solutions with a baricity of greater than 1.0015 can be expected to predictably behave as a hyperbaric spinal anesthetic. Conversely, local anesthetic solutions with a baricity of less than 0.9990 can be expected to predictably function as a hypobaric spinal anesthetic. Table 3-3 lists the density range of commonly used local anesthetic solutions for spinal anesthesia.

Hyperbaric Spinal Anesthesia. Hyperbaric solutions are commonly prepared by mixing the local anesthetic solution with dextrose (glucose). There is a linear relationship between local anesthetic solution density and the concentration of dextrose.[19] A dextrose concentrations greater than 1.25%, there is no clinically significant difference in peak cephalad distribution of hyperbaric solutions. However, in nonpregnant patients, lower concentrations of dextrose have been shown to have a concentration-dependent effect on peak cephalad distribution of bupivacaine 0.5% injected with the patient in the right lateral position, followed by placement in the supine horizontal position: 0.33% produces mean sensory blockade to T10, 0.83% produces mean sensory blockade to T7, and 8.0% producing mean sensory blockade to T4.[25] In contrast, there is no clinically significant difference in the peak sensory blockade between bupivacaine 0.5% with 0.8% dextrose and bupivacaine 0.5% with 8% dextrose (T2 vs. T3) in term parturients undergoing cesarean delivery. This lack of difference in peak block height despite the 10-fold difference in dextrose concentration (0.8% vs. 8.0%) and marked difference in measured local anesthetic density (1.0016 g/mL vs. 1.0208 g/mL) is in part due to the decrease in density of CSF at term pregnancy (Table 3-3). Thus, the difference in density between CSF and the 0.8% dextrose local anesthetic solution is greater in pregnant patients than in nonpregnant patients, which will result in more extensive cephalad distribution, and demonstrates the importance of the relative density of local

Table 3-3

Density and Baricity of CSF in Different Patient Groups and Clinically Useful Local Anesthetics for Spinal Anesthesia

Population	Density at 37°C [Mean (SD)]	Range within 3 SD of mean
Men	1.00064 (0.00012)	1.00028–1.00100
Older women	1.00070 (0.00018)	1.00016–1.00124
Younger women	1.00049 (0.00004)	1.00037–1.00061
Pregnant/postpartum	1.00030 (0.00004)	1.00018–1.00042
Hyperbaric Solutions		
Lidocaine 5% in dextrose 7.5%	1.02650	
Tetracaine 0.5% in dextrose 5%	1.0136 (0.0002)	1.01300–1.0142
Bupivacaine 0.5% in dextrose 8%	1.02426 (0.00163)	1.01935–1.02913
Chloroprocaine 3%	1.00257 (0.00003)	1.00248–1.00266
Hypobaric Solutions		
Lidocaine 0.5% in water	0.99850	Hypobaric
Bupivacaine 0.35% in water	0.99730	Hypobaric
Tetracaine 0.2% in water	0.99250	Hypobaric
Isobaric or "Plain" Solutions		
Levobupivacaine 0.75%	1.00056 (0.00010)	1.00026–1.00086
Lidocaine 2%	1.00004 (0.00006)	0.99986–1.00022
Bupivacaine 0.5%	0.99944 (0.00012)	0.99908–0.99980
Ropivacaine 0.5%	0.99953 (0.00014)	0.99914–0.99992
Tetracaine (0.5%)*	1.0000 (0.0004)	0.99880–1.00120

*Tetracaine 1% diluted 1:1 with 0.9% saline.
Data from Refs. 19–24.

anesthetic solutions to CSF density in determining local anesthetic distribution.

When the patient is turned in the supine horizontal position after injection of hyperbaric local anesthetic solutions in the lumbar region, the curvatures of the vertebral canal will influence subsequent distribution. Hyperbaric solutions injected at the peak height of the normal lumbar lordosis (L4 to L5) will tend to distribute by the force of gravity toward the lowest points of the thoracic (T6 to T7) and sacral (S2) curvatures (Fig. 1-3).[26] Thus, pooling of hyperbaric local anesthetic solutions in the thoracic kyphosis has been postulated to explain the clinical observation that hyperbaric solutions tend to produce blocks with an average peak sensory block height in the midthoracic region.

Interestingly, hyperbaric solutions have been demonstrated to produce peak cephalad-sensory blockade with a bimodal distribution. One group of patients will have mean peak blockade located in the low thoracic region and a second group of patients with mean peak blockade located in the high thoracic region.[27] The presumed explanation for this clinical phenomenon is that injection at the apex of the lumbar lordosis splits the total dose into a fraction distributing cephalad toward the thoracic kyphosis and a fraction distributing caudal toward the sacrum. Thus, the peak cephalad distribution is determined by what percentage of the injected dose travels cephalad. Consistent with this hypothesis is the observation that decreasing the normal lumbar lordosis by maintaining the patient with the hips flexed for 5 min after injection of hyperbaric solution decreases the bimodal distribution of peak sensory block, without affecting peak sensory blockade.[27] Additionally, individual anatomic variations in the lowest point of the thoracic kyphosis, the maximum angle of decline of the lumbar spinal canal, and the maximum angle of incline of the upper thoracic spinal canal, may also explain the variability in peak sensory blockade of hyperbaric local anesthetic solutions.[26]

Injection of hyperbaric local anesthetic solution with the patient in the sitting position has been advocated as a means to restrict the distribution to the lumbosacral dermatomes, producing a "saddle block." However, this practice is based on the assumption that hyperbaric solutions will act in an isobaric manner at a point when they have become sufficiently diluted in the CSF, and are no longer influenced by gravity. Clinical studies, however, have demonstrated that a block initially restricted to the lumbosacral dermatomes (by maintaining the patient in the seated position) will eventually distribute to a peak thoracic sensory blockade height equivalent to that which would have been obtained had the patient been immediately placed in the horizontal supine position.[28] With the use of larger doses (15–20 mg) of a long-acting local anesthetic, such as bupivacaine, hyperbaric solutions may take as long as 60 min before the final peak sensory distribution is obtained.

Similar to the hypothesis of obtaining a saddle block with maintaining the patient in the sitting position, injection of hyperbaric local anesthetic solution with patients in the lateral position and maintaining the operative side in the dependent position has been advocated as a means to achieve "unilateral spinal anesthesia." One of the proposed advantages of unilateral spinal anesthesia is that limiting blockade of the sympathetic chain to one side decreases the degree of sympathetic blockade, with a lower incidence of hypotension. Unilateral spinal anesthesia with hyperbaric solutions has not been shown to eliminate significant changes in hemodynamic parameters as measured by decreases in blood pressure and cardiac index.[29] However, in comparison to conventional hyperbaric spinal anesthesia, unilateral spinal anesthesia has been shown to significantly reduce the incidence of clinically relevant decreases in blood pressure.[30] The major disadvantage of unilateral spinal anesthesia is that it requires a minimum of 15 min in the lateral position after injection to predictably obtain unilateral blockade.

Hypobaric Spinal Anesthesia. Hypobaric local anesthetic solutions are typically prepared by diluting commercially available local anesthetic preparations with sterile distilled water. For example, lidocaine 2% diluted with sterile water to 0.5% (baricity = 0.9985), as well bupivacaine 0.5% diluted with sterile water to 0.35% (baricity = 0.9973) will reliably result in "clinically hypobaric" spinal anesthesia.[31] The position of the patient during and after injection of hypobaric local anesthetic solutions determines distribution in the CSF. If the patient is maintained in the head-up position during and after injection, the local anesthetic solution will distribute primarily in the cephalad direction, and if head down, in a caudal direction.

Although less commonly used, hypobaric spinal anesthetics are ideally suited for perineal and rectal surgical procedures performed with the patient in the prone, jackknife position.

The advantages of this technique are twofold. First, local anesthetic is injected with the patient in the same position as that required for surgery, thus minimizing the need to change patient position. Second, the peak cephalad-sensory block height is restricted to the low thoracic dermatomes, while providing anesthesia of the lumbosacral dermatomes.[31] Hypo- and hyperbaric local anesthetics can redistribute for a significant period of time after intrathecal injection. For example, hyperbaric bupivacaine will distribute to the midthoracic dermatomes with position changes as long as 70 min after injection. Hypobaric lidocaine injected in the prone, jackknife position rose two to six dermatomes cephalad if an upright head-up position was allowed after surgery.

Hypobaric spinal anesthesia may also provide advantages for major hip surgery performed in the lateral position. Compared to isobaric spinal anesthetic solutions, hypobaric spinal anesthetic solutions demonstrated a significantly delayed onset of sensory regression on the nondependent operative side and more importantly, time till need for supplemental analgesia after hip surgery.[32] A hypobaric mixture of bupivacaine and fentanyl (or sufentanil) is used to initiate combined spinal-epidural (CSE) labor analgesia (see Chap. 7). Injection of hypobaric solutions with the patient maintained in the sitting position for several minutes after injection has been advocated as a way to achieve a predictable level of high thoracic sensory block distribution needed for abdominal operations, such as cesarean delivery.[33] However, this particular technique has two clinical disadvantages. First, maintaining the patient in the sitting position delays the progress of surgical preparation while the block distributes. Second, there is the possibility of significant hypotension due to venous pooling in the lower extremities as the local anesthetic uptake by the sympathetic fibers decreases sympathetic outflow.

Isobaric Spinal Anesthesia. An isobaric local anesthetic solution is most easily prepared by mixing equal volumes of tetracaine 1% solution with either CSF or sterile saline 0.9%. The density of tetracaine mixed with either CSF (0.9998) or saline 0.45% (1.0000) at 37°C allows it to predictably behave in a truly isobaric fashion. The only other commercially available plain local anesthetic solution that predictably behaves in an isobaric fashion is levobupivacaine 0.5–0.75% (Table 3-3). The densities of levobupivacaine 0.5% (1.00024 ± 0.00009 g/mL) and levobupivacaine 0.75% (1.00056 ± 0.00010 g/mL) at 37°C allow them to be truly isobaric (with a baricity greater than 0.9990) in all adult patient populations.[19] The major clinical advantage of truly isobaric solutions is that patient position during and after injection should have no effect on the distribution of the local anesthetic solution. Thus, isobaric solutions tend not to distribute as far from the site of injection (site of highest local anesthetic concentration). Isobaric spinal solutions are particularly useful when low thoracic dermatomal sensory blockade is desired, and when the degree of sympathetic blockade needs to be minimized. The most reliable method to produce low thoracic blockade is to mix 1 mL tetracaine 1% solution with 1 mL patient CSF. However, doses greater than 10 mg will produce peak sensory blockade in the mid to high thoracic dermatomes.

A major problem with interpreting previous studies of "isobaric spinal anesthetics" is that the densities of presumed isobaric local anesthetic solutions were reported at room temperature, which can vary considerably. It is important to keep in mind that local anesthetic solutions demonstrate a linear decrease in density with increasing temperature. The consequence of temperature is most evident with plain (diluted in saline) local anesthetic solutions. For example, one of the most commonly used plain local anesthetics for spinal anesthesia, bupivacaine 0.5%, is isobaric at 23°C (density 1.00376 ± 0.00002 g/mL, baricity of 1.0003 for nonpregnant females), but at 37°C (density 0.99944 ± 0.00012 g/mL) can be either "clinically isobaric" (baricity = 0.9992) or clinically hypobaric (baricity = 0.9985) within the normal distribution of densities for both the local anesthetic solution and individual patients' CSF (Table 3-3).[19] In fact, plain bupivacaine 0.5% has been considered an unpredictable spinal anesthetic agent. This is in part due to the fact that in many clinical situations, it is a hypobaric spinal anesthetic and thus, distribution in CSF will be affected by patient position during and after injection. This is clearly illustrated when directly comparing the median peak sensory blockade between equivalent doses of plain local anesthetic solutions versus hyperbaric local anesthetic solutions (Fig. 3-8). In this particular study, plain ropivacaine 0.5% resulted in median low thoracic peak sensory block, but with an extremely wide dermatomal distribution. In contrast, both hyperbaric ropivacaine solutions produced a median midthoracic peak sensory block with a much more predictable peak cephalad distribution.[34]

Dose, Volume, and Concentration

Clinical studies attempting to separate the individual effects of dose, volume, and concentration on local anesthetic distribution are difficult to interpret due to the fact that manipulating one of these variables affects either one or both of the other two variables. However, two well-done studies have addressed this issue.[35,36] In a study of plain bupivacaine, concentration, volume, and dose were systematically altered in six groups of patients. The peak sensory blockade levels were significantly higher in patients randomized to 15–20 mg (T2 to T4) compared to the level in patients given 10 mg (T5 to T8). Additionally, peak sensory blockade levels were similar in patients given 10 mg despite the differences in either concentration or volume. Lastly,

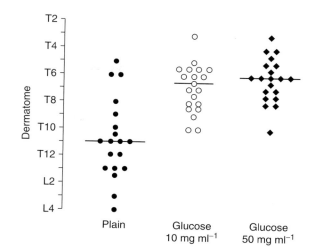

FIGURE 3-8. Illustration of upper levels of sensory blockade in individual patients after spinal anesthesia with ropivacaine plain, or combined with glucose 10 or 50 mg/mL. Horizontal bars represent the median values. Note the lower peak median blockade level and wider distribution for the plain compared to either of the hyperbaric (glucose-containing) solutions. *Used with permission from Whiteside JB, Burke D, Wildsmith JAW. Spinal anesthesia with ropivacaine 5 mg/mL in glucose 10 mg/mL or 50 mg/mL. Br J Anaesth 86:241, 2001.*

patients given the same volume (2 mL) had significantly higher peak sensory blockade levels with plain bupivacaine 0.75% (15 mg) compared to bupivacaine 0.5% (10 mg). The differences in concentration (0.5% vs. 0.75%), dose (10–20 mg), and volume (1.3–4.0 mL) may be criticized for being of relatively small magnitude. However, in a study of lidocaine 70 mg administered as 0.5, 1.0, 2.0, 5.0, and 10.0% solutions, the peak median sensory blockade (T4 to T5) did not differ among groups despite the 20-fold difference in concentration and range (injected volume 0.7–14 mL). Thus, for plain local anesthetic solutions, it appears that dose is more important than either volume or concentration in determining local anesthetic distribution.

Drug dose and volume appear to be relatively less important in determining the distribution of hyperbaric local anesthetic solutions in patients positioned supine after intrathecal injection. Increasing the dose of hyperbaric tetracaine from 7.5 to 15.0 mg, by increasing the volume and keeping the concentration constant, does not affect peak sensory block distribution.[37] Similarly, increasing the dose of hyperbaric bupivacaine 0.5% from 10 to 20 mg, simply by increasing the volume, does not increase peak sensory blockade height, but doses lower than 10 mg resulted in peak sensory block height approximately two to three dermatomes lower than those obtained with doses greater than 10 mg.[38] In a dose-response volunteer study of hyperbaric bupivacaine 0.75%, 3.75, 7.5, and 11.25 mg, the peak sensory blockade heights obtained were to T9, T7, and T4.[39] Conversely, in study of hyperbaric bupivacaine 0.75% for postpartum tubal ligation, doses ranging from 7.5 to 12.5 mg all resulted in peak sensory block distribution to T4.[40] The lack of difference in the dose-response in the postpartum patients may be explained in part by the lower CSF density in this patient population compared to nonpregnant patients, which makes baricity more important relative to the doses used in this study. Overall, it appears that bupivacaine dose is only important when doses less than 7.5 mg are used, and at higher doses, peak sensory distribution with hyperbaric solutions is primarily determined by baricity.

Intervertebral Space Injection Site

The location of the lumbar intervertebral injection site has been proposed to have a clinically significant effect on peak sensory cephalad distribution. In one study, mean peak cephalad-sensory block was decreased from T6 to T10 when plain bupivacaine 0.5% was injected initially at the L3-L4 intervertebral space, followed by repeat injection in the same patient at the L4-L5 interspace. In this study, plain bupivacaine 0.5% solutions at ambient room temperature were injected with the patient in the lateral position and then immediately placed in the horizontal supine position.[41] In contrast, when plain bupivacaine 0.5% solutions at either ambient room temperature or adjusted to 37°C are injected with the patient in the sitting position and maintained in the sitting position for 2 min prior to placing supine, there is no difference in peak sensory block height when injections at the L2-L3 versus L4-L5 intervertebral spaces are compared.[42] These seemingly conflicting data can be explained by the differences in baricity of the plain bupivacaine and patient position during and immediately after injection. Although often used as an "isobaric" spinal solution, plain bupivacaine 0.5% can clearly behave in a hypobaric manner. Thus, it appears that when nonisobaric solutions are injected in the sitting position, the effect of a higher or lower lumbar intervertebral space injection is outweighed by the effect of gravity on hypobaric solutions. Anesthesiologists frequently have difficulty in accurately identifying the actual vertebral level of injection and this may be an additional confounding factor.[43] In contrast to plain solutions, the level of lumbar intervertebral space injection has no clinically significant effect when clearly hyperbaric local anesthetic solutions are used, confirming that the effect of gravity has a dominant role during non-isobaric spinal anesthesia.[44,45]

Patient Characteristics

After injection of local anesthetic solutions, dilution within the CSF occurs before uptake by neuronal target sites. Therefore, the volume of lumbosacral CSF should have an effect on the distribution of spinal anesthesia. Two separate studies have demonstrated that lumbosacral CSF volume, as measured by MRI, is the primary determinant of both the extent and duration of sensory blockade, regardless of the baricity of the local anesthetic solutions.[46,47] These studies demonstrated a strong inverse correlation between lumbosacral CSF volume and peak sensory blockade level. Unfortunately, lumbosacral CSF volume correlates poorly with anthropomorphic physical measures, other than a weak correlation with patient weight. Therefore, CSF volume is difficult to accurately estimate from physical examination. Additionally, individual patient CSF density has been demonstrated to have a strong inverse correlation with peak sensory blockade level with the use of plain bupivacaine 0.5%.[48] Although these studies provide valuable mechanistic insight regarding the distribution of spinal anesthetic solutions, their application for guiding clinical practice is necessarily limited by the difficulty in determining an individual patient's CSF volume and CSF density.

During the administration of spinal or epidural anesthesia, pregnant women typically require lower doses of local anesthetics compared to nonpregnant women (see Chap. 13). Physiologic changes that contribute to increased local anesthetic distribution during pregnancy include decreases in CSF density, changes in the anatomic configuration of the spinal column and CSF volume, and hormonally mediated enhancement of neuronal sensitivity to local anesthetics.[49,50]

Although there is significant variation in the extent of local anesthetic distribution among patients using a standard technique, spinal anesthesia is very reproducible in the individual patient.[51] However, individual patient factors such as age, weight, height, body mass index, and gender have very little if any clinical significance in accurately predicting local anesthetic distribution differences from patient to patient.

▶ Spinal Anesthesia and Duration of Action

Clinically, spinal anesthetic blockade gradually recedes in a cephalad to caudal manner from peak block height. Depending on the criteria, duration of action can be defined as the time for two-dermatome regression from peak block height or as time to complete regression to sacral dermatomes. More importantly, duration of surgical anesthesia provided by the spinal anesthetic is dependent on peak block height, time-course of regression, and dermatomal location of the surgical procedure. For example, given an equivalent peak block height and time-course of regression, the duration of surgical anesthesia for an Achilles tendon repair would be considerably longer than that for an inguinal hernia repair. Time to complete regression of sensory and motor blocks are important considerations for proper selection of local anesthetic agents and dose, particularly in the ambulatory surgery setting (see Chap. 11).

Resolution of blockade after spinal anesthesia occurs when the neural tissue concentration of local anesthetic falls below the minimum blocking concentration (C_m). Thus, the rate at which a given dose of local anesthetic is removed from the neural tissues and CSF within the subarachnoid space determines the duration of spinal anesthesia. Elimination does not involve metabolism of local anesthetics within the subarachnoid space, but occurs completely by vascular absorption within the subarachnoid and epidural space. The blood supply (and surface area for absorption) in the subarachnoid space is significantly smaller compared to the epidural space. Therefore, as local anesthetics diffuse along a concentration gradient from the nerve roots and spinal cord into the CSF, they similarly diffuse along a concentration gradient across the spinal meninges from the CSF into the epidural space with subsequent rapid vascular absorption. Elimination of local anesthetics by diffusion from the neural tissues to the CSF and then to the epidural space occurs simultaneously, with vascular absorption within both the subarachnoid space and epidural space. Thus, duration of spinal anesthesia is primarily determined by the physiochemical properties of a specific local anesthetic agent that determine its availability for vascular absorption, the amount of local anesthetic administered in the subarachnoid space, and the degree of vascular absorption.

Local Anesthetic Choice

One of the primary determinants of the duration of spinal anesthesia is the choice of local anesthetic. Procaine is the shortest-acting local anesthetic for subarachnoid use. Procaine's short duration of action can be attributed to its very low lipid solubility and protein binding. Chloroprocaine is also a short-acting local anesthetic that has recently been evaluated in initial volunteer trials to determine its spinal anesthetic profile. Compared to an equivalent amount of plain lidocaine, plain chloroprocaine 40 mg demonstrated similar peak blockade height and duration of simulated surgical anesthesia in the low thoracic and lumbosacral dermatomes, but with a 20% faster time to complete recovery of sensory and motor function.[52] Lidocaine and mepivacaine are considered to have intermediate duration of action when used for spinal anesthesia, which are based on their intermediate degrees of lipid solubility and protein binding. Bupivacaine and tetracaine have the longest duration of action when used for spinal anesthesia. Although local anesthetic agents may be classified as having short, intermediate, and long durations of action, it is evident from the variability illustrated in Table 3-4 that there are other factors, which have significant effect on the duration of spinal anesthesia.[53–64] Additionally, in a study comparing the anesthetic profiles in 12 volunteers who underwent spinal anesthesia on three separate occasions with three hyperbaric local anesthetic solutions (lidocaine 100 mg, bupivacaine

15 mg, and tetracaine 15 mg) in random order and in a double-blind fashion, the time until complete resolution of sacral sensation to pinprick was highly variable within each local anesthetic group. For lidocaine, the average duration was 234 min (range 137–360 min); for bupivacaine, the average duration was 438 min (range 180–570 min); and for tetracaine, the average duration was 546 min (range 120–720 min).[53]

Local Anesthetic Dose

For any given local anesthetic agent, increasing the dose increases the duration of action. Within the clinically useful dose range of 30–60 mg of chloroprocaine, there was no significant difference in time to two-segment regression from peak blockade height. However, there was a 50% increase in the duration of surgical anesthesia at T10, and a 25% increase until complete recovery of sacral sensation with 60 mg compared to 30 mg.[54] In a study comparing the effects of escalating doses of hyperbaric bupivacaine (5, 7.5, 10, and 15 mg), the time until complete recovery of sensory block at S2 were 123, 144, 194, and 343 min, respectively.[65]

Block Distribution

For a given dose of local anesthetic, spinal blockade with higher peak cephalad distribution will completely regress faster compared to a lower peak cephalad distribution. In a study comparing equivalent doses of hyperbaric bupivacaine (15 mg), patients immediately placed in the horizontal position had higher peak block heights compared to patients placed with 30 degrees of torso elevation during the study period (T4 vs. T10). The patients with the lower peak blockade demonstrated significantly longer time until two-segment regression (159 min vs. 110 min) and regression to the L4 dermatome (337 min vs. 269 min) compared to patients with higher peak blockade.[55] In a study comparing equivalent doses of hyperbaric ropivacaine versus plain ropivacaine (15 mg) in patients immediately placed in the supine position, the peak blockade height was significantly higher (T4 vs. T9) in the hyperbaric group.[66] Although the total duration of sensory block to pinprick at the T10 dermatome was significantly longer (83 min vs. 33 min) in the hyperbaric group compared to the plain group, the time until complete sensory regression at the S2 dermatome was of significantly shorter duration in the hyperbaric ropivacaine group (210 min vs. 270 min). The pharmacokinetic basis for the shorter duration of action with higher peak cephalad blockade is based on a wider distribution within the CSF with resulting lower drug concentration throughout the CSF, as well as a larger surface area within the subarachnoid space for more rapid vascular absorption.[67] Consequently, it requires less time for the local anesthetic concentration within the subarachnoid space to fall below the minimum blocking concentration.

Table 3-4

Doses and Duration of Local Anesthetic Solutions for Spinal Anesthesia

Local Anesthetic Solution	Dose (mg)	Mean Peak Blockade Height	Duration of Sensory Block*		
			Onset of Two-dermatome Regression (min) (1 SD)	Regression to L1-L2 Dermatome (min) (1 SD)	Complete Regression (min) (1 SD)
Hyperbaric chloroprocaine	30[54]	T7	47 (8)	53 (30)	98 (20)
	40[54]	T7	45 (20)	64 (10)	114 (14)
	60[54]	T2	43 (50)	92 (13)	132 (23)
Plain lidocaine	40[57]	T12	44 (17)	60 (24)	142 (27)
	50[58]	T6	56 (5)	104 (5)	130 (18)
	60[57]	T8	40 (16)	67 (14)	157 (28)
	80[57]	T4	33 (16)	104 (23)	188 (27)
Hyperbaric lidocaine	50[59]	T4	50 (16)	80 (30)	123 (21)
	60[56]	T3	48 (12)	105 (20)	130 (25)
	100[53]	T2	59 (11)	NA[†]	234 (84)
Plain mepivacaine	45[60]	T6	76 (28)	140 (NA)[†]	203 (36)
	60[61]	T4	95 (21)	150 (32)	210 (18)
	80[61]	T4	100 (20)	160 (20)	225 (23)
Plain bupivacaine	10[62]	T7	33 (16)	127 (41)	178 (20)
	17.5[63]	T8	155 (50)	NA[†]	237 (88)
Hyperbaric bupivacaine	4[64]	T10	21 (4)	45 (12)	115 (42)
	8[64]	T5	59 (13)	135 (51)	198 (33)
	12[64]	T5	65 (32)	123 (44)	164 (30)
	15[53]	T3	60 (15)	NA[†]	438 (102)
	15[55]	T4[‡]	110 (30)	216 (46)	300 (NA)[†]
	15[55]	T10[§]	159 (49)	253 (64)	>360 (NA)[†]

*Duration of sensory block (to pinprick) dependent on baricity in relation to patient position, dose, and peak block height.
[†]NA: Data not available.
[‡]Hyperbaric bupivacaine 15 mg with patient in supine horizontal position.
[§]Hyperbaric bupivacaine 15 mg with patient supine with 30-degree torso elevation. Note the significant difference in onset of two-segment regression, duration of lumbar anesthesia, and complete regression.

▶ Epidural Anesthesia and Determinants of Local Anesthetic Distribution

Similar to spinal anesthesia, assessment of the onset, distribution, and duration of epidural anesthesia may be performed by standardized testing for the afferent sensory functions of temperature, pinprick, and touch. Although these measures of afferent sensory function are clinically useful, they are limited by the qualitative nature (presence or absence of sensation) of the response, and more importantly, may not accurately reflect surgical anesthetic requirements. Cutaneous current perception threshold (CPT) testing provides quantitative assessment of the depth of sensory blockade of different subpopulations of nerve fibers based on a specific sinusoidal frequency of low levels (less than 10 mA) of progressively increasing current delivered transcutaneously at different dermatomal levels. CPT selectively stimulates $A\beta$, $A\delta$, and C using 2000, 250, and 5 Hz, respectively. Higher intensity stimulation, such as that provided by tolerance to transcutaneous electrical nerve stimulation (TENS) with a 50-Hz square-wave stimulus at 60 mA provides a more accurate assessment of both the distribution and depth of surgical anesthesia. Thus, the differences in the method of assessment may explain some of the conflicting data regarding the extent of sensory blockade after local anesthetic injection in the epidural space.

Injection Site

Injection of local anesthetic in the epidural space produces sensory blockade with most rapid onset of action close to the site injection, with subsequent spread in a cephalad and caudad distribution to produce a segmental blockade. Consequently, the site of injection is a primary factor in determining local anesthetic distribution (and distribution of sensory/motor blockade) within the epidural space. Lumbar epidural injection volumes of less than 15 mL result in a slower onset and often, incomplete distribution caudal to the L5 spinal cord segments. The delayed onset of sensory anesthesia in the sacral segments is partially attributed to the fact that there is somewhat greater cranial than caudal distribution of local anesthetic. However, the primary reason is likely due to the larger size of the nerve roots below L5, resulting in a slower local anesthetic uptake.[8] Blockade of the lumbosacral segments is important when using epidural anesthesia for foot, ankle, and cystoscopic procedures of lower genitourinary tract.[68,69]

The cephalad distribution versus caudal distribution of local anesthetic injection in the thoracic region is dependent on site of injection in the thoracic region, as well as the total dose delivered. In general, the sensory block tends to spread quite evenly from the site of injection, but the number of blocked spinal segments cephalad to the injection site decreases significantly with ascending injection site.[70,71] Careful titration of local anesthetic dose in the thoracic region allows sparing of the lumbosacral nerve spinal segments and true segmental blockade. Avoiding lumbosacral sympathetic and motor blockade with a well-placed and titrated thoracic epidural catheter for postoperative analgesia facilitates maintenance of normal lower extremity and bladder function. Finally, caudal epidural blockade is largely restricted to the sacral and low lumbar spinal segments. As one may predict, the pattern of caudal epidural onset is cephalad from S5, with S1 and low lumbar segments the last to be blocked.

Dose, Volume, and Concentration

When using qualitative clinical measures of sensory blockade, and within the range typically used to provide surgical anesthesia, local anesthetic concentration is relatively unimportant in determining the spread of epidural block (Table 3-5).[72–78]

However, total local anesthetic dose (mg) and volume are important determinants of both spread and depth of epidural anesthesia. In a surgical population undergoing lumbar epidural anesthesia at the L1-L2 intervertebral space, there was no difference in upper level of sensory block to cold (T5 vs. T6), pinprick (T6 vs. T7), and touch (T12 in both groups) between lidocaine 2% 10 mL and lidocaine 1% 20 mL.[79] Additionally, in parturients undergoing lumbar epidural anesthesia at L1-L2 for elective cesarean delivery, there was no reported difference in the upper level of sensory block to pinprick (T4 in both groups) between lidocaine 1% 30 mL and lidocaine 2% 15 mL.[80] However, when the differences in concentration and volume are greater than twofold with the same total dose, the higher volume local anesthetic solutions result in a nonlinear increase of upper sensory blockade level. For example, tripling the injected volume of lidocaine from 10 to 30 mL while maintaining a constant dose (300 mg) increased the upper sensory blockade level by 4.3 dermatomes.[81] In a randomized, double-blind, crossover study of volunteers undergoing lumbar epidural anesthesia with 300 mg of 2-chloroprocaine as a 3% (10 mL) and a 1% (30 mL) solution, sensory blockade was assessed with pinprick, cold, touch, and TENS at 50 Hz (as a surrogate of surgical incision).[72] The number of dermatomes blocked to pinprick, cold, and touch was significantly higher with the 1% 2-chloroprocaine solution (on average two dermatomes higher). In contrast to the greater extent of sensory block to low intensity stimuli with high volume of low concentration, sensory block to TENS was similar with either the 1% or 3% solution at the T12 and L2 dermatomes, suggesting that surgical epidural anesthesia (and intensity of blockade) is primarily dependent on total dose of local anesthetic. A popular theory for the mechanism of epidural anesthesia focuses on the finding that a critical length of nerve fiber needs to be blocked by local anesthetic for sensory function to terminate.[82,83] The greater length of spinal nerve exposed to higher volumes of local anesthetic at a lower concentration, or in the case of epidural anesthesia, a higher cephalad spread in the epidural space, would explain the greater extent of sensory block to low intensity stimuli.

Age

When a given dose of local anesthetic (fixed volume and concentration) is administered to patients of different age groups, increasing age has been demonstrated to increase the longitudinal spread within the epidural space (Table 3-5).[73–75] The magnitude of the effect of age is greatest when comparing age groups with more than 30 years difference, and even then the difference in peak sensory levels after lumbar epidural injection is only two to four dermatomes. However, even within the same age groups, there is moderate interindividual variability. Older patients exhibit physiologic and anatomic changes that influence the

Table 3-5

Local Anesthetic Agents for Epidural Anesthesia: Approximate Two-Segment Regression Time and Redosing (Top-up) Intervals for Lumbar (L2 to L4) Epidural Anesthesia

Local Anesthetic	Dose (mg)	Peak Cephalad Block Height	Time to Two-segment Regression (1 SD or Range) (min)*	Recommended Time Interval for Top-up Dose (min)[†]
Chloroprocaine 2–3% plus 1:200,000 epinephrine[72,76.]	600	T5	80 (15)	45
Lidocaine 1.5–2% plus 1:200,000 epinephrine[76,77]	300–400	T4	100 (50–60)	60
Mepivacaine 1.5–20% plus 1:200,000 epinephrine[76,77]	300–400	T4	110–120 (40–50)	60
Bupivacaine 0.5–0.75% (plain)[73,78]	100–150	T5	150–190 (60–80)	120
Ropivacaine 1% (plain)[74] Age 30 (18–40)[‡]	150	T8[§]	143 (45–298)	120
Ropivacaine 1% (plain)[74] Age 51 (41–59)[‡]	150	T6	190 (100–340)	120
Ropivacaine 1% (plain)[74] Age 71 (61–82)[‡]	150	T4[§]	203 (105–378)	120
Levobupivacaine 0.75% (plain)[75] Age 32 (18–44)[‡]	125	T8[§]	166 (51)	120
Levobupivacaine 0.75% (plain)[75] Age 57 (47–69)[‡]	125	T5	158 (59)	120
Levobupivacaine 0.75% (plain)[75] Age 78 (72–85)[‡]	125	T5[§]	174 (61)	120

*Mean (1 SD or range).
[†]Dosing intervals are approximate guidelines. In awake and cooperative patients, clinical monitoring for signs and symptoms (increase in blood pressure and heart rate or objective evaluation of dermatomal level of block) of dermatomal regression will indicate the need for a top-up dose.
[‡]Ages expressed as mean (range).
[§]Note for ropivacaine and levobupivacaine the significant difference in peak block height between the youngest and oldest age groups.

pharmacokinetic profile during epidural anesthesia. Normally, local anesthetic solution flows outward through the intervertebral foramina in clefts between lobules of fat and between nerves and the foraminal walls.[84] In older patients, lateral escape of local anesthetic solution is decreased due to sclerosis and calcification of the interverte-bral foramina.[85] Additionally, epidural fat content decreases with increasing age, which leads to a more compliant and

less resistant epidural space.[86] Together, these age-related changes may contribute to the increased longitudinal spread of local anesthetic solutions within the epidural space.

Pregnancy

Studies evaluating the influence of pregnancy on longitudi-nal spread of local anesthetic solutions within the epidural space are conflicting. Some studies have not reported a significant difference in the spread of epidural blockade between pregnant and nonpregnant women.[87,88] However, studies have demonstrated increased cephalad spread in pregnant patients compared to nonpregnant when using low-level stimulus to assess for the upper level of sensory blockade, but no difference in latency or density of sensory blockade when quantitative measures of higher intensity pain stimuli were used.[89]

Injection Technique

Although rapid injection of local anesthetic solution has been demonstrated to increase the spread of sensory block initially, there is no difference in the final extent of sensory block.[90,91] Given the potential for increased systemic toxicity with rapid injection of a large dose of local anesthetic, injections should be made slowly and preferentially in incremental doses.

Injection of local anesthetic solution via the catheter probably does not increase the cephalad extent of sensory blockade, although this is often assumed to be the case. The higher velocity injection of local anesthetic via the longer and smaller diameter epidural catheter might be assumed to result in increased bulk flow. However, rapidity of injection has not been shown to increase the final extent of sensory blockade. It is often assumed that epidural catheters ascend rostrally in the posterior midline epidural space when the bevel of the epidural needle is oriented cephalad. Thus, local anesthetics would emerge from the catheter tip cephalad to the needle tip based on the length of catheter inserted into the epidural space. Contrary to this popular assumption, however, many catheters actually travel lateral in the epidural space toward the intervertebral foramina, and at times may even travel caudal to the needle insertion point.[92,93] It should not be surprising that catheters do not usually ascend rostrally when a lumbar midline approach is used, as the catheter approaches the cylindrical dural sac at approximately a right angle, whereupon it is deflected laterally by the convex posterior dura mater into the lateral aspects of the epidural space. A recent study demonstrated that there is no difference in either the upper level of sensory blockade or radiographic spread of contrast medium when injected via either a Tuohy needle or a catheter inserted 3 cm into the epidural space.[93]

Epidural "Top-Up" of an Established Block

After the initial dose of local anesthetic solution is given to establish surgical anesthesia, repeat injections may be delivered via the epidural catheter. A single repeat dose (20% of the initial induction dose) given 20 min after the induction dose has been proposed to consolidate an epidural block within the distribution of the established block (*repainting*

the fence). Thus, an incomplete or "patchy" epidural block may be reinforced without extending the sensory distribution of the initial block. This technique is especially useful for pelvic or abdominal surgical procedures when noxious stimulation of the viscera may not be totally blocked by the initial epidural dose, despite adequate dermatomal extent of blockade. Alternatively, an epidural top-up (repeated doses of approximately 50% of the initial induction dose) will maintain the initial segmental distribution of sensory block if given when the upper level of sensory block begins to recede by one to two dermatomal segments or at the time of predicted duration of a given dose of local anesthetic solution (Table 3-5). Delivery of the epidural top-up dose greater than 10 min after the onset of regression of sensory block (the interanalgesic interval) may require an increased dose to maintain the distribution of sensory block.[94]

Epidural top-ups are most commonly used to maintain continuous epidural anesthesia. In addition, they are employed in CSE anesthesia to either increase the level of sensory block shortly after the subarachnoid injection or to extend the duration of central neuraxial anesthesia beyond the expected duration of the initial subarachnoid injection. The extension of the sensory blockade induced by an epidural top-up with local anesthetic in CSE anesthesia appears to be due to two primary mechanisms. There is an initial rapid increase in sensory blockade caused by compression of the dural sac by an epidural volume effect. This results in the cranial shift of CSF already containing local anesthetic. This effect is augmented by a local anesthetic effect that occurs independent of the volume effect.[95,96] In contrast, the mechanism of action of increased sensory blockade with an epidural top-up during epidural anesthesia is primarily due to local anesthetic effect and not via compression of the dural sac.[97,98] Although clinically relevant concentrations of local anesthetic appear in the CSF after epidural injection of local anesthetic, the combination of the uptake of local anesthetics from the epidural space and the elimination of local anesthetics from the CSF prevents accumulation of a sufficient amount of local anesthetic to allow the volume effect seen with CSE anesthesia.

▶ Epidural Anesthesia and Duration of Action

Local Anesthetic Choice

Similar to spinal anesthesia, the choice of local anesthetic is the primary determinant of epidural anesthesia duration. 2-Chloroprocaine has the shortest duration of action due to its rapid hydrolysis by plasma cholinesterases.[99] Lidocaine and mepivacaine have essentially the same pharmacokinetic profile and are considered to have an intermediate duration of action. Lidocaine 400 mg (20 mL 2%) compared to bupivacaine 100 mg (20 mL 0.5%) produces the same peak block distribution, but bupivacaine results in an approximately 30% longer time until two- and four-segment dermatome regression.[100] Etidocaine has the same duration of sensory blockade as bupivacaine, but has a significantly longer duration of motor blockade. Etidocaine is unique among clinically useful local anesthetics in that its motor blockade may be significantly longer than its sensory blockade. This property of etidocaine is most likely due to the fact that it is the most lipid soluble of the local anesthetics (Table 3-2), which allows it to rapidly partition and then become sequestered within the heavily myelinated Aα efferent motor fibers within the central neuraxial space.

Dose, Alkalinization, and Age

Increasing the dose of epidurally administered local anesthetic results in dose-related prolongation of sensory and motor blockade.[101] Interestingly, alkalinization of ropivacaine has been shown to also increase the duration of sensory blockade.[102] Alkalinization has been used to decrease the latency of local anesthetics by increasing the pH of the local anesthetic solution, which increases the fraction of nonionized local anesthetic molecules available to penetrate and cross the lipid membrane. Alkalinization also increases the PCO_2 of the local anesthetic solution. PCO_2 is highly diffusible into the cell. In turn, this increases the intracellular fraction of the ionized (active) form of the local anesthetic and not only increases block intensity, but also duration. The effects of age on the duration of epidural anesthesia are conflicting. The duration of lumbar lidocaine epidural anesthesia is only slightly prolonged (10–12%) in older men.[103] In contrast, increasing age does not significantly increase the duration of epidural anesthesia with bupivacaine, levobupivacaine, or ropivacaine.[73–75]

▶ Clinical Pharmacokinetics of Spinal and Epidural Anesthesia

Absorption

Local anesthetics are not metabolized in the intrathecal or epidural space. Rather, they are eliminated from the intrathecal and epidural space almost completely via vascular absorption into the systemic circulation. Thus, the duration of anesthesia is primarily determined by the rate of systemic absorption, which is influenced by the physiochemical properties of the individual local anesthetics, as well as the site of administration, which in the case of intrathecal and epidural anesthesia also determines the administered dose.

Pharmacokinetic evaluation of local anesthetics allows prediction of the time course (T_{max}) of maximal plasma concentrations (C_{max}), which is clinically relevant based on the fact that systemic toxicity is primarily dependent on both the rate of rise and absolute plasma concentrations of unbound local anesthetics (see Chap. 6). Peak plasma levels of local anesthetics after spinal anesthesia are well below the threshold for systemic toxicity and are thus, not clinically relevant. Conversely, clinical doses of local anesthetics for epidural anesthesia are typically 5–10 times greater than for spinal anesthesia and have the potential for systemic toxicity. The typical C_{max} and T_{max} after common clinical epidural doses of local anesthetics are listed in Table 3-6,[104–107] along with effect of added epinephrine. Typical doses used for epidural anesthesia produce local anesthetic plasma concentrations that are well below the threshold for the early signs of systemic toxicity.

Continuous epidural infusions of dilute long-acting amide local anesthetics are commonly used to provide postoperative analgesia. Over the time course of the continuous epidural infusion, local anesthetic plasma concentrations may progressively increase, raising the concern of systemic

Table 3-6					
Typical C_{max} after Epidural Anesthesia with Commonly Used Local Anesthetics					
Local Anesthetic	Toxic Plasma Concentration (µg/mL)	Dose (mg)	C_{max} (µg/mL)*	T_{max} (min)†	Effect of Epinephrine (C_{max}/T_{max})
Lidocaine[104]	5–7	400	2.2	27	1.7/32
Bupivacaine[104]	3	100	0.73	19	0.53/21
Mepivacaine[105]	5–7	460	3.1	18	–
Ropivacaine[106]	4	85	1.31	12	0.82/23
Levobupivacaine[107]	3	112.5	0.81	24	–

*C_{max} is peak venous plasma level.
†T_{max} is the time from injection until peak plasma level.

toxicity. Recent pharmacokinetic data have demonstrated that total local anesthetic plasma concentrations increase steadily during 48–72 h of continuous administration.[108,109] However, despite the progressive increase in total plasma concentration, unbound concentration reached peak steady-state levels well below the thresholds for systemic toxicity. During continuous epidural infusions, postoperative increases in plasma proteins (predominantly α_1-acid glycoprotein) enhance the protein binding of local anesthetics, causing divergence of the total and unbound concentrations.[108,109] Thus, the pharmacokinetic data confirm the clinical experience of the safety of continuous epidural infusions of dilute local anesthetic solutions.

Distribution, Elimination, and Excretion

After systemic absorption, local anesthetics are rapidly distributed throughout all body tissues, with the relative concentrations in different tissue compartments based on tissue perfusion, lipid solubility, and plasma protein binding. For a detailed discussion of the pharmacokinetics of epidural anesthesia, the reader is referred to two extensive reviews.[110,111] The clearance of aminoesters is primarily dependent on hydrolysis of the ester bond by plasma cholinesterases. The rate of enzymatic degradation varies, with chloroprocaine undergoing the most rapid hydrolysis, tetracaine the slowest, and procaine intermediate between the two. The aminoamides undergo enzymatic degradation, primarily in the liver. Thus, hepatic extraction, perfusion, and metabolism determine the rate of clearance of aminoamides. Excretion of aminoamides occurs via the kidneys, with less than 5% of the unchanged drug excreted in the urine.

PHARMACOLOGY OF INTRATHECAL AND EPIDURAL OPIOIDS

Administration of central neuraxial opioids in either the intrathecal or epidural space is a widespread clinical practice. Lipophilic opioids (most commonly fentanyl) are adminis-

tered as additives to local anesthetics to augment the efficacy of spinal anesthesia, while hydrophilic opioids (most commonly morphine) are administered in the intrathecal or epidural space to provide postoperative analgesia. Additionally, opioids are commonly administered in the epidural space as the sole agent for postoperative analgesia or to augment the efficacy of continuous epidural local anesthetic infusions in an effort to decrease local anesthetic requirements and side effects. The rational for administering opioids in either the intrathecal or epidural space is to produce selective spinally mediated analgesia by interacting with opioid receptors in the dorsal horn of the spinal cord, and thereby minimize the dose-limiting supraspinal effects (e.g., respiratory depression, sedation, and nausea) that occur when systemically administered opioids reach the brainstem opioid receptor sites.

Despite widespread use of intrathecal and epidural opioids, and widespread belief that their analgesic effects are predominantly spinally mediated, accumulating evidence indicates that there are significant differences in the mechanism of action of different opioids based on their individual physiochemical properties (Table 3-7),[112] site of delivery (intrathecal vs. epidural), and method of administration (bolus infusion vs. continuous infusion). The result is that opioid administration in either the intrathecal or epidural space can result in systemically mediated analgesia (and side effects) because of distribution to supraspinal sites. This occurs due to cephalad migration in the CSF or because of systemic absorption and subsequent redistribution to the brainstem. The following sections will review recent pharmacokinetic data that illustrate the interaction between key anatomic structures within the epidural space, spinal meninges, and spinal cord and the physiochemical properties of the clinically useful opioids that govern their ability to produce spinally mediated effects.

▶ Mechanism and Site of Action

The site of action of opioids administered either in the intrathecal or epidural space is located in the dorsal horn of the spinal cord. More specifically, opioid receptors are

---

Table 3-7

Physiochemical Properties of Opioids for Spinal and Epidural Anesthesia

	% Protein Binding	pK_a	% Ionized (at pH 7.4)	Partition Coefficient (Lipid Solubility)
Morphine	35	7.9	76	1.4
Alfentanil	92	6.5	11	128
Fentanyl	84	8.4	91	860
Sufentanil	93	8.0	80	1778

Data from Ref. 112.

located primarily within the gray matter of the substantia gelatinosa. This provides the anatomic basis for selective spinal analgesia after direct neuraxial administration of opioids. Intrathecal opioids selectively block transmission of afferent nociceptive stimuli from Aδ and C fibers by binding at presynaptic and postsynaptic opioid receptors. Postsynaptically, opioids increase K^+ conductance, hyperpolarizing ascending second-order projecting neurons without any effect on somatosensory or motor evoked potentials.[113,114] Presynaptic effects include the release of spinal adenosine, which seems to be an important mediator specific for spinally mediated analgesia,[115] as well as inhibiting Ca^{2+} influx and the subsequent release of glutamate and neuropeptides (such as substance P) from primary afferent terminals.[116,117]

▶ Pharmacokinetics of Opioids Relevant to Spinal Bioavailability

Epidural Administration

In order for epidurally administered opioids to exert spinal analgesia, they must redistribute out of the epidural space to ultimately reach their intended site of action in the spinal cord dorsal horn. Opioids will diffuse down a concentration gradient into surrounding tissues at a rate and extent governed by the volume and physiochemical properties of the tissues relative to the physiochemical properties of a particular opioid. Two important structures that govern redistribution from the epidural to the intrathecal spaces are epidural fat and the epidural venous plexus. Highly lipophilic opioids (fentanyl and sufentanil) preferentially distribute into epidural fat, which subsequently makes them unavailable for diffusion into the intrathecal space. The inner surface of the dura mater contains a rich capillary network, which eventually drains into the epidural venous plexus. Thus, drugs diffusing into the epidural tissues (e.g., epidural fat and dura mater) have the potential to be absorbed and cleared from the epidural space via capillaries into the epidural venous plexus.

In an elegantly designed animal study employing microdialysis catheter techniques to allow continuous sampling of opioid concentrations in the intrathecal and epidural spaces, the redistribution of bolus doses of morphine, alfentanil, fentanyl, and sufentanil out of the epidural space were quantified.[15] The study clearly demonstrated a strong linear relationship between increasing lipid solubility and both mean residence time in the epidural space (Fig. 3-9a) and terminal elimination half-life (Fig. 3-9b). The lipid-solubility-dependent differences in pharmacokinetics among the opioids were primarily determined by the

differences in the extent to which they partitioned into the epidural fat. At the end of the study period, the epidural fat was sampled and later analyzed for opioid concentration. The concentration of opioid in the epidural fat demonstrated a linear relationship with lipid solubility (Fig. 3-9c). As a whole, these findings indicate that the relatively longer persistence of lipid-soluble opioids (fentanyl and sufentanil) in the epidural space is due to their increased sequestration into epidural fat, with subsequent slow continuous redistribution back into the epidural space. As a result of the increase in the mean residence in the epidural space, lipophilic opioids should have a lower concentration in the CSF. This is illustrated by the dose-normalized area under the spinal CSF concentration time curve (AUC) of morphine, alfentanil, fentanyl, and sufentanil in the intrathecal space adjacent to the site of epidural administration, wherein morphine has the highest AUC.[118] Conversely, the lower AUC for fentanyl and sufentanil indicate that a significantly smaller proportion of the epidural dose reaches the CSF compared to morphine.

The CSF concentration of alfentanil can be explained by its physiochemical properties. The increased mean residence time, terminal elimination half-life, and dose-normalized concentration within the epidural space of alfentanil compared to morphine are due to the increased lipid solubility of alfentanil in relation to morphine. Additionally, the plasma concentration of alfentanil after epidural administration was significantly higher than that of morphine, fentanyl, and sufentanil at all time points. Thus, alfentanil's lower CSF bioavailability, relative to morphine, is due to a combination of greater partitioning into epidural fat, and to a greater degree of systemic absorption from the epidural fat and dural capillary network because of its lower lipid solubility (and subsequent faster release from the epidural fat) relative to fentanyl and sufentanil.

Intrathecal Administration

Once opioids reach the CSF, either by intrathecal or epidural administration, they must partition into the spinal cord to reach the opioid target sites in the dorsal horn. The extent of uptake of intrathecal opioids from the CSF into the neural tissues of the spinal cord, as well as the brainstem, is also governed predominantly by lipid solubility. The spinal cord consists of gray matter surrounded by white matter. White matter consists primarily of axonal membranes, which are wrapped in multiple layers of lipid-rich myelin. Thus, one would expect that lipophilic opioids would preferentially distribute into the white matter. In a classic animal study, radiolabeled morphine, dihydromorphine, and fentanyl were administered into the CSF of the lateral ventricle of rabbits, followed by autoradiography to measure the depth that the

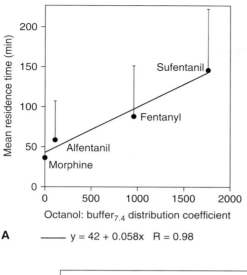

A ——— y = 42 + 0.058x   R = 0.98

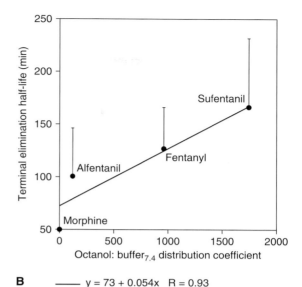

B ——— y = 73 + 0.054x   R = 0.93

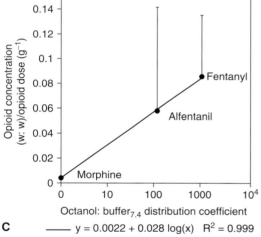

C ——— y = 0.0022 + 0.028 log(x)   R^2 = 0.999

FIGURE 3-9. (A) Relationship between opioid mean residence time in the epidural space and opioid lipid solubility (octanol:buffer distribution coefficient). (B) Relationship between opioid lipid solubility (octanol:buffer distribution coefficient) and terminal elimination half-life in the epidural space. (C) Relationship between opioid lipid solubility (octanol:buffer distribution coefficient) and the dose-normalized concentration (w:w) in fat taken from the lumbar epidural space. *Used with permission from Bernards CM. Recent insights into the pharmacokinetics of spinal opioids and the relevance to opioid selection. Curr Opin Anaesthesiol 17:441, 2004.*

three opioids penetrated into the substance of the adjacent CNS tissue.[119] Over time, both morphine and dihydromorphone penetrated the CNS tissue more deeply than fentanyl. More importantly, morphine and dihydromorphone preferentially distributed into gray matter, while fentanyl demonstrated a marked preferential accumulation in white matter.

Because the target sites for opioids reside within the substantia gelatinosa of the spinal gray matter, which is surrounded by white matter, the physiochemical properties of the different opioids are important in determining their ability (bioavailability) to reach opioid receptors. Therefore, hydrophilic opioids that are not sequestered within the lipid-rich myelin of the more peripherally located white matter should be available in the extracellular environment

of the spinal cord to diffuse into the more centrally located dorsal horn which is comprised primarily of gray matter. This has been substantiated in another microdialysis probe study, where equal doses of morphine, alfentanil, fentanyl, and sufentanil were administered in the L3 intrathecal space, followed by CSF sampling at multiple cephalad levels over time, as well as sampling spinal cord tissue at the same levels as the CSF sampling.[120] The analysis of the cephalad CSF sampling sites demonstrated that morphine was found in significantly higher concentrations compared to either fentanyl or sufentanil. Additionally, the morphine concentration over time in the spinal cord tissue (measure of its bioavailability) was significantly greater compared to the other opioids at both the lumbar and the more cephalad spinal cord segments. The apparent volume of distribution in the spinal cord (V_{cord}) represents the unbound (to target sites), freely diffusible, and therefore pharmacologically relevant, opioid in the extracellular space. V_{cord} is expected to increase as more opioid is nonspecifically bound to tissue compartments (myelin) because opioid so bound is not available to opioid receptors. Because lipid solubility is a determinant of the extent of this nonspecific binding, it makes sense that V_{cord} parallels a particular opioid's partition coefficient (Table 3-7), with morphine having the smallest median Vcord, and sufentanil having the largest median V_{cord}.

Taken together, these animal studies provide a mechanistic explanation for the pharmacokinetic and pharmacodynamic behavior of the different opioids administered in the epidural and intrathecal space. The preferential partitioning of lipophilic opioids into lipid-rich tissues (epidural fat and myelin) decreases their spinal bioavailability relative to morphine. The intermediate lipid solubility of alfentanil not only increases its sequestration in lipid-rich tissues, but also significantly increases its systemic absorption relative to both the lipophilic and hydrophilic opioids, which together decreases its spinal bioavailability. These observations should provide a rational basis for interpreting the clinical studies that illustrate the limited selective spinal action of lipophilic opioids administered in the epidural and intrathecal space.

▶ Clinical Pharmacology of Intrathecal and Epidural Opioids

Intrathecal Administration

The physiochemical properties of the different opioids not only determine their primary mechanism (spinal vs. supraspinal), but also their relative potencies, onset and duration of action, and side effects when administered within the intrathecal space. All opioids administered into the intrathecal space can be expected to initially result in spinally mediated analgesia. The principal differences that affect their relative potency, time course of analgesia, and side effects will be determined by their speed of redistribution to brainstem opioid sites and the mechanism by which a particular opioid reaches brainstem sites.

A hydrophilic opioid such as morphine provides long-lasting (up to 24 h) selective spinal analgesia, because of its small V_{cord} and slow clearance from the spinal cord. The relatively slower spinal cord uptake and prolonged residence time in the CSF due to its hydrophilic nature results in a slow onset of action (greater than 30 min), but also a prolonged duration of action, which makes it well suited for extended postoperative analgesia. The prolonged residence time in the CSF is the mechanism for the cephalad spread to the brainstem via CSF migration and the risk for delayed respiratory depression. Morphine does not inherently have greater availability to distribute cephalad in the CSF compared to more lipid-soluble opioids. Independent of density-related differences between the CSF and intrathecally administered anesthetic/analgesic solutions; the primary determinant of drug spread in the CSF is the movement of CSF itself. The spinal cord moves caudally within the vertebral canal early in the cardiac cycle in conjunction with the pulsatile flow of blood into the CNS. This is accompanied by the rapid movement of CSF in the caudal direction down the dorsal surface of the spinal cord. Later in the cardiac cycle, CSF moves along the ventral surface of the spinal cord, with a net flow in the cephalad direction.[121] Thus, morphine is able to reach brainstem sites due to its lower clearance from the CSF, with more drug available to be carried by the cephalad flow of CSF.

The risk of respiratory depression with neuraxial morphine is dose-related, with few instances of clinically significant respiratory depression reported with intrathecal doses less than 0.4 mg. Based on human studies, the terminal elimination half-life of intrathecally administered morphine is reported to be 90 min, with a range of 60–140 min. This would result in morphine being completely eliminated from the lumbar CSF in approximately 6–12 h. However, the duration of analgesia, as well as inhibition of the ventilatory response to hypoxia clearly persists well after morphine's CSF concentrations and plasma concentrations are expected to be negligible.[122] This can be partially explained by large interindividual differences in CSF pharmacokinetics. Additionally, it is likely that morphine persists at spinal cord and brainstem opioid receptors much longer than in the CSF, reflecting a difference between CSF pharmacokinetics and effect-site pharmacokinetics.

Fentanyl and sufentanil are the most commonly administered intrathecal lipophilic opioids. Clinical studies suggest that sufentanil may produce selective spinal analgesia, but pharmacokinetic studies suggest that rapid systemic uptake followed by supraspinal-mediated analgesia may be the dominant mechanism of action. In a dose-response volunteer study of intrathecal sufentanil (12.5, 25, or 50 μg), all three doses resulted in equivalent analgesic thresholds.[123] Plasma sufentanil concentrations from all three doses exceeded the minimum effective concentration demonstrated to produce effective systemic analgesia in patients.[124] Additionally, all three doses resulted in significant depression of ventilation peaking at 90–120 min, paralleling the time course of peak analgesic effect and maximal plasma sufentanil concentrations. Since respiratory depression is a supraspinal effect, it is likely that some part of the analgesia was in fact supraspinally mediated. The large V_{cord} for sufentanil and the rapid clearance into the systemic circulation, with peak plasma levels occurring within 30–60 min, provides a pharmacokinetic basis for the numerous case reports of significant early respiratory depression after the administration of clinically relevant doses of intrathecal sufentanil.[125,126]

Fentanyl is by far the most commonly used intrathecal lipophilic opioid. It is less lipid soluble than sufentanil and will maintain a modest spinally mediated analgesic effect when administered intrathecally, although there is a paucity of pharmacokinetic data to determine the extent of its spinal selectivity. Dose-response data indicate that intrathecal fentanyl alone provides analgesia with a minimal effective dose of 10 μg in adults.[127] Fentanyl has a rapid onset (5–10 min) and intermediate duration of action (60–120 min), which makes it an ideal agent as an additive to local anesthetics to augment the efficacy of spinal anesthesia. Addition of fentanyl 10–25 μg to local anesthetic solutions permits the use of smaller doses of local anesthetic, which increases the success of spinal anesthesia and prolongs the duration without significantly prolonging complete sensory resolution of the block.[128] The ability to use lower doses of local anesthetic with the addition of intrathecal fentanyl also results in a significantly lower incidence of hypotension compared to a higher dose of local anesthetic alone.[129]

Epidural Administration

Opioids injected in the epidural space produce analgesia by one of two mechanisms. As previously discussed, to produce selective spinally mediated analgesia, epidural opioids must diffuse though the spinal meninges to reach the CSF, and then diffuse into the dorsal horn of the spinal cord. Supraspinally mediated analgesia from epidural opioids is either due to cephalad redistribution within the CSF to interact with brainstem opioid receptors or via systemic absorption into plasma and redistribution to the brainstem via the bloodstream or both.

Hydrophilic Opioids. The predominant mechanism of analgesia for epidural hydrophilic opioids (morphine and hydromorphone) is spinally mediated. This was well illustrated in a prospective, although nonrandomized, study comparing epidural morphine to intravenous patient-controlled morphine analgesia (IV-PCA) after major knee ligament surgery.[130] Over a 24-h period, the patients in the IV-PCA group required a mean morphine dose of 64 mg compared to the epidural morphine group, which required a mean dose of only 12 mg. Despite requiring less than 20% as much morphine, the patients in the epidural morphine group reported significantly lower rest and dynamic pain scores. In a prospective randomized trial, patients undergoing major intra-abdominal surgery under general anesthesia

were randomized to receive preoperative epidural saline or epidural morphine 5 mg.[131] Postoperative analgesia was provided by IV-PCA morphine to both groups. The patients who received epidural morphine preoperatively had significantly lower intraoperative fentanyl requirements (465 μg vs. 983 μg), cumulative postoperative IV-PCA morphine consumption (37 mg vs. 86 mg), and significantly better analgesia compared to the patients who did not receive epidural morphine. In another prospective trial, women undergoing elective cesarean delivery under bupivacaine epidural anesthesia were randomized postoperatively to either patient-controlled epidural analgesia (PCEA) or IV-PCA hydromorphone.[132] There was no difference in analgesia during the 48-h study period, but patients randomized to the epidural hydromorphone group required four times less hydromorphone and significantly fewer PCA demands (33 vs. 105). Taken together, these studies demonstrating improved, or at a minimum equivalent, analgesia with much less systemic opioid requirement provide evidence of a spinal site of action for these two hydrophilic opioids.

Lipophilic Opioids. Fentanyl is by far the most commonly used lipophilic opioid for epidural analgesia. However, a number of studies bring into question the mechanism of epidurally administered fentanyl, particularly as a continuous infusion. In a prospective double-blind study, patients undergoing major knee ligament reconstruction were randomized to either epidural or IV fentanyl.[133] There were no differences in the quality of postoperative analgesia, fentanyl requirements, or frequency of opioid-related side effects between the two groups. Additionally, there was no difference in the plasma fentanyl concentrations between the epidural and IV infusions. In a different surgical population (postthoracotomy), patients were randomized in a double-blind fashion to either lumbar epidural or IV infusions of fentanyl.[134] There were no differences in the quality of analgesia, respiratory depression, other opioid-related side effects (nausea, vomiting, or pruritus), and plasma fentanyl concentrations between the epidural and IV infusions of fentanyl. It is possible that administration of epidural fentanyl via a catheter in the lumbar epidural space for postthoracotomy pain precludes its ability to provide selective spinal analgesia because its limited cephalad distribution prevents it from acting at the segmental level of painful afferent stimuli. However, this was addressed in a study where postthoracotomy patients were randomized to receive IV-PCA fentanyl, lumbar (L4 to L5) PCEA fentanyl, or thoracic (T4 to T5) PCEA fentanyl infusions.[135] There were no differences among the three groups in overall quality of resting or dynamic analgesia, mean fentanyl requirements, and opioid-related side effects. Thus, even when fentanyl is administered in the epidural space close to the spinal cord segment receiving the painful afferent stimuli, there is no evidence to support a clinically important spinally mediated analgesic effect.

There are data, however, that suggest that the method of delivery influences the primary anatomic site of action of epidurally administered fentanyl. In a recent randomized, double-blind study, the analgesic effects of both epidural fentanyl infusion and epidural fentanyl bolus were evaluated using a crossover design.[136] Volunteers received both infusions and bolus doses of fentanyl in random order and were then subjected to painful stimuli at the lumbar (thigh) and cranial (cheek and ear) dermatomes. Epidural bolus administration of fentanyl resulted in segmental analgesia (lumbar dermatome analgesia greater than cranial dermatome analgesia), whereas epidural infusion produced nonsegmental analgesia (lumbar = cranial). Nonsegmental analgesia (suggesting relevant opioid binding in the brain) during the continuous epidural infusion of fentanyl and segmental analgesia (suggesting relevant opioid binding in the spinal cord) after bolus administration is likely explained by the fact that an epidural fentanyl bolus results in a significantly larger amount of fentanyl in the epidural space compared to that which occurs at any single time point during a fentanyl infusion. Thus, even though only a small fraction of the administered fentanyl is able to distribute to the spinal cord opioid receptors, in the case of bolus administration, the fraction is sufficient to produce a spinally mediated analgesic effect.

The physiochemical properties and animal data would indicate that epidurally administered sufentanil produces supraspinally mediated analgesia due to its systemic absorption and redistribution to brainstem opioid receptors. This has been demonstrated in a prospective randomized double-blind study comparing continuous IV sufentanil to low thoracic continuous epidural sufentanil infusion after major abdominal surgery.[137] Similar to the fentanyl infusion studies, there were no differences in analgesic efficacy at rest or with movement, opioid-related side effects, and plasma sufentanil concentrations between the two methods of administration.

PHARMACOLOGY OF ADRENERGIC RECEPTOR AGONISTS

Epinephrine has long been administered into the intrathecal and epidural spaces with the intent of prolonging block duration, intensifying the analgesic effects of local anesthetics and opioids, and reducing plasma concentrations (and undesired systemic side effects) of local anesthetics and opioids. The mechanism by which epinephrine exerts these actions is complex and is dependent on the anatomic site of injection and the physiochemical properties of the particular local anesthetic.

▶ Intrathecal Epinephrine

Spinal Cord and Dural Blood Flow

The mechanism by which intrathecal administration of epinephrine (and phenylephrine, which is used infrequently) prolongs the duration of spinal anesthesia is believed to be due to α-adrenergic-mediated vasoconstriction, thereby leading to decreased vascular absorption and subsequent increased neural tissue uptake of local anesthetics. The intrathecal administration of epinephrine by itself has not been demonstrated to significantly decrease spinal cord blood flow, but does result in a significant decrease in dural blood flow.[138] However, the vasoactive effects of intrathecal epinephrine are more complex when it is administered with local anesthetics. Local anesthetics have different effects on spinal cord and dural blood flow, which are modified by the addition of epinephrine (Fig. 3-10). In a canine model, intrathecal lidocaine and tetracaine have been demonstrated to significantly increase spinal cord and dural blood flow, which is prevented by the addition of 0.2 mg of epinephrine.[139,140] In the same canine model, intrathecal bupivacaine produced an approximately 25% reduction in both spinal cord and dura mater blood flow and addition of 0.2 mg of epinephrine resulted in a 25–50% further reduction in spinal cord and dural blood flow.[141]

Epinephrine Interaction with Local Anesthetics

Clinically, the effectiveness of intrathecal epinephrine is dependent on the local anesthetic with which it is combined, which may be partly explained by the previously discussed animal studies. Epinephrine is typically administered at a dose of 0.2–0.3 mg and at these doses is effective at prolonging the block duration in only the lumbosacral dermatomes.[56] Previous studies that showed no benefit with the addition of epinephrine to lidocaine spinal anesthesia were based on the lack of prolongation of two-dermatome regression from peak block height.[142] However, closer inspection of these studies and more recent investigations clearly demonstrates that epinephrine significantly prolongs the duration of lumbosacral anesthesia, which would be clinically relevant for lower extremity and perineal surgery.[143] Thus, conclusions regarding the effectiveness of the addition of epinephrine to lidocaine spinal anesthesia are dependent on the criteria used to define the duration of anesthesia (two dermatome regression vs. complete regression) in clinical studies.

The duration of bupivacaine spinal anesthesia is also prolonged with the addition of epinephrine. Epinephrine 0.2 mg added to plain bupivacaine 15 mg did not significantly

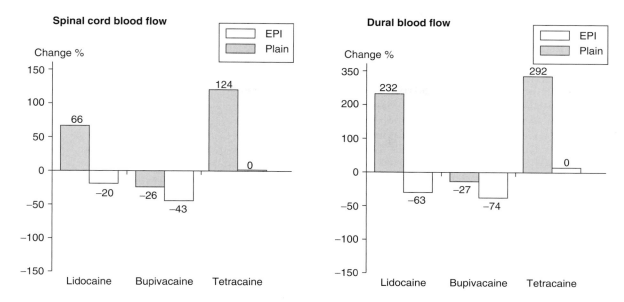

FIGURE 3-10. Effect of epinephrine on spinal cord and dural blood flow during spinal anesthesia with lidocaine, bupivacaine, and tetracaine. *Used with permission from Covino BG, Scott DB, Lambert DH. Handbook of Spinal Anesthesia. Philadelphia, PA: W.B. Saunders, 1994, p. 89.*

prolong the time until two-segment regression from a peak block height of T9 to T10, but increased duration until regression to L2 by 20%.[144] When the dose of epinephrine is increased to 0.3–0.5 mg, there is significant prolongation until time regression from a peak block height (30–35%) and time until regression to L2 (25–30%). Thus, higher epinephrine doses appear to increase the duration of anesthesia in both lower thoracic and lumbosacral dermatomes.[145] In contrast, the addition of 0.2 mg of epinephrine to hyperbaric bupivacaine 15 mg has not been shown to prolong the duration until two-segment regression from peak block height, or the duration of thoracic anesthesia, but again, this study failed to evaluate regression to the lumbosacral dermatomes.[146] In a volunteer crossover study, the addition of 0.2 mg of epinephrine to low-dose (7.5 mg) hyperbaric bupivacaine spinal anesthesia did not prolong the duration of simulated surgical stimulus anesthesia in the thoracic dermatomes, but clearly prolonged the duration to simulated surgical stimulus anesthesia in the lumbosacral dermatomes by 30%.[147]

The effects of epinephrine in combination with lidocaine or bupivacaine on spinal cord and dural blood flow are reflected in the observed peak plasma concentrations of these drugs. Addition of epinephrine 0.15 mg to intrathecal hyperbaric lidocaine has been demonstrated to significantly decrease peak plasma concentrations of lidocaine, but did not decrease peak plasma concentrations when added to

intrathecal hyperbaric bupivacaine.[148] Epinephrine 0.2–0.3 mg significantly prolongs the duration of both plain and hyperbaric tetracaine spinal anesthesia by 30–50% at all dermatomal levels, with a slightly greater effect in the lumbosacral dermatomes.[149,150]

Phenylephrine

Phenylephrine has effects similar to epinephrine on spinal cord and dural blood flow.[138] Clinically, phenylephrine 5 mg also prolongs the duration of spinal anesthesia, but its use with spinal tetracaine has been implicated as a significant risk factor for transient neurologic symptoms (10-fold increase), and this has significantly reduced its clinical use.[151]

▶ Epidural Epinephrine

Epinephrine is added most often to epidural local anesthetics in a concentration of 5 µg/mL (1:200,000). Although epinephrine has been shown to significantly increase the duration of epidural anesthesia with the shorter-acting amide local anesthetics (e.g., lidocaine), it has not been shown to affect anesthesia duration with the longer-acting agents (e.g., bupivacaine).[152,153] The mechanism by which epidural epinephrine prolongs the duration of epidural anesthesia is also assumed to be due to regional vasoconstriction resulting in decreased vascular absorption of local anesthetics from the epidural space. Consistent with the mechanism of decreased systemic absorption, epinephrine administered in the epidural space has been demonstrated to decrease the peak plasma concentrations of epidurally administered local anesthetics.[104,153] However, IV infusions of low-dose epinephrine have also been shown to decrease peak plasma concentrations of local anesthetics.[154] Thus, it is possible that systemic absorption of epinephrine from the epidural space can lead to β-adrenergic-mediated increases in cardiac output (promoting hepatic uptake and renal excretion) and an increased volume of distribution (due to increased vascular capacitance), either of which can account for decreased plasma concentrations.

Although it appears that epinephrine does not significantly prolong the duration of epidural anesthesia when added to concentrated long-acting local anesthetics administered for surgical anesthesia, epinephrine has been demonstrated to significantly improve the quality of postoperative thoracic epidural analgesia provided by dilute concentrations of local anesthetic-opioid solutions. In a series of randomized double-blind crossover studies in patients undergoing major thoracic or abdominal procedures, effective thoracic epidural analgesia was provided by a combination of low-dose epinephrine (2 μg/mL), fentanyl (2 μg/mL), and dilute concentrations (0.1%) of either bupivacaine or ropivacaine.[155,156] Additionally, plasma fentanyl concentrations in all patients whose infusions contained epinephrine were well below the minimum mean effective fentanyl concentration (0.63 ng/mL) necessary for effective analgesia during IV administration.[157] Conversely, when epinephrine was omitted from the bupivacaine/fentanyl epidural infusion, dynamic pain and need for IV rescue analgesia significantly increased, hypoesthetic dermatomal segments decreased, and plasma fentanyl concentrations doubled with 25% of the patients achieving plasma concentrations well above 0.63 ng/mL.[155] The increase in the plasma fentanyl concentrations, along with significant increase in pain, provide indirect evidence that epinephrine-induced vasoconstriction leads to accumulation of fentanyl at spinal opioid receptor sites.

The possible benefits of the addition of epinephrine to fentanyl local anesthetic solutions may go beyond a simple pharmacokinetic effect. Epidural administration of epinephrine by itself has been observed to possess segmental hypoalgesic effects, which is most likely explained by absorption into the CSF and binding to spinal α₂-adrenergic receptors and subsequent hyperpolarization of afferent neurons in the spinal cord dorsal horn.[158] As local anesthetics, opioids and epinephrine have different pharmacodynamic effects on modulating afferent nociceptive transmission; together they may produce a supra-additive analgesic interaction.

▶ Pharmacology of Intrathecal and Epidural Clonidine

Mechanism of Action

Clonidine is a α₂-adrenergic receptor agonist that produces dose-dependent analgesia, sedation, and hypotension. There are three primary subtypes of α₂ receptors (designated α₂A, α₂B, and α₂C), with each subtype distributed widely throughout the body. The α₂A receptor subtype has been positively identified as mediating the primary clinical effects of analgesia, sedation, and sympatholysis. Pain and systemic opioids trigger the release of endogenous norepinephrine from descending inhibitory neurons in the CNS, which decreases the activity of second-order neurons in the dorsal horn of the spinal cord by attenuating input from Aδ and C peripheral nociceptive fibers.[117] At the level of the spinal cord, intrathecal or epidural administration of clonidine mimics the effect of norepinephrine and produces analgesia in humans.

Oral clonidine has virtually 100% bioavailability and peak plasma concentration occurs 1–3 h after administration. Clinical studies have demonstrated that oral clonidine 0.2 mg 1–2 h prior to lidocaine spinal anesthesia prolongs sensory and motor block.[159] Clonidine is moderately lipid soluble and easily crosses the blood-brain barrier, and therefore systemic administration may lead to clonidine binding with supraspinal and spinal receptors. Although IV and epidurally administered clonidine can provide postoperative analgesia, the spinal cord appears to be the primary site for the analgesic effect of clonidine.[160] The analgesic effects of intrathecal and epidural administration of clonidine appear to be more effective than after IV administration.[161,162] Furthermore, epidural clonidine has been demonstrated to produce segmental hypoalgesia to different experimentally applied painful stimuli.[158]

Clinical Applications

Clinically, intrathecal clonidine is primarily administered in conjunction with lower doses of local anesthetics to augment the success and duration of spinal anesthesia. Intrathecal clonidine doses as low as 15 μg have been shown to decrease local anesthetic dose requirements and prolong the duration of postoperative analgesia for ambulatory spinal anesthesia.[163,164] When added to local anesthetics, intrathecally administered clonidine up to 150 μg provides dose-related prolongation of postoperative analgesia with minimal side effects of sedation or hypotension.[165] Epidural clonidine at 2 μg/kg/h as the sole analgesic agent has been shown to provide complete postoperative analgesia for up to 6 h without major side effects.[166] Low-dose epidural clonidine (2 μg/mL) added to low-dose epidural ropivacaine-fentanyl infusions significantly reduced the need for systemic opioid analgesia after total knee arthroplasty.[167] Thus, there is accumulating evidence that intrathecal and epidural clonidine produce predominantly spinally mediated analgesia. Further investigation is warranted to define its place in intrathecal and epidural anesthesia/analgesia.

REFERENCES

1. Wann KT. Neuronal sodium and potassium channels: Structure and function. *Br J Anaesth* 71:2, 1993.
2. Caterall WA: The molecular basis of neuronal excitability. *Science* 223:653, 1984.
3. Landon N, Williams PL. Ultrastructure of the node of Ranvier. *Nature* 199:575, 1963.
4. Stranding S. Peripheral nerves. In: Stranding S, Ellis H, Healy JC, et al., eds, *Grays' Anatomy,* 39th ed. Edinburgh: Churchill Livingstone, 2005, p. 55.
5. Butterworth JF, Strichartz GR. Molecular mechanisms of local anesthetics: A review. *Anesthesiology* 72:711, 1990.
6. Strichartz GR. The inhibition of sodium currents in myelinated nerve by quaternary derivatives of lidocaine. *J Gen Physiol* 62:37, 1973.
7. Kelly DJ, Ahmad M, Brull SJ. Preemptive analgesia I: Physiological pathways and pharmacological modalities. *Can J Anaesth* 48:1000, 2001.
8. Hogan QH. Size of human lower thoracic and lumbosacral nerve roots. *Anesthesiology* 85:37, 1996.
9. Hogan QH, Toth J. Anatomy of soft tissues of the spinal canal. *Reg Anesth Pain Med* 24:303, 1999.
10. Kim JT, Bahk JH, Sung J. Influence of age and sex on the position of the conus medullaris and Tuffier's line in adults. *Anesthesiology* 99:1359, 2003.
11. Fink BR, Walker S. Orientation of fibers in the human dorsal lumbar dura mater in relation to lumbar puncture. *Anesth Analg* 69:768, 1989.
12. Vandenabeele F, Creemers J, Lambrichts I. Ultrastructure of the human spinal and dura mater. *J Anat* 189:417, 1996.
13. Bernards CM, Hill HF. Morphine and alfentanil permeability through the spinal dura, arachnoid, and pia mater of dogs and monkeys. *Anesthesiology* 73:1214, 1990.
14. Reina MA, Casasola OD, Villaneuva MC, et al. Ultrastructural findings in human spinal pia mater in relation to subarachnoid anesthesia. *Anesth Analg* 98:1479, 2004.
15. Bernards CM, Shen DD, Sterling ES, et al. Epidural, cerebrospinal fluid, and plasma pharmacokinetics of epidural opioids (part 1): Differences among opioids. *Anesthesiology* 99:455, 2002.
16. Salinas FV. Analgesic: Ion channel ligands/sodium channel blockers/local anesthetics. In: Evers AS, Maze M, eds, *Anesthetic Pharmacology: Physiologic Principles and Clinical Practice.* The Netherlands: Elsevier, 2003, p. 507.
17. Nau C, Strichartz GR. Drug chirality in anesthesia. *Anesthesiology* 97:497, 2002.
18. Green NM. Distribution of local anesthetic solutions within the subarachnoid space. *Anesth Analg* 64:715, 1985.
19. McLeod GA. Densities of spinal anesthetic solutions of bupivacaine, levobupivacaine, and ropivacaine with and without dextrose. *Br J Anaesth* 92:547, 2004.
20. Greene NM. Distribution of local anesthetic solution within the subarachnoid space. *Anesth Analg* 64:715, 1985.
21. Richardson MG, Wissler RN. Density of cerebrospinal fluid in pregnant and nonpregnant humans. *Anesthesiology* 85:326, 1996.
22. Schiffer E, Van Gessel E, Gamulin Z. Influence of sex on cerebrospinal fluid density in adults. *Br J Anaesth* 83:943, 1999.
23. Richardson MG, Wissler RN. Densities of dextrose-free intrathecal local anesthetics, opioids, and combinations measured at 37°C. *Anesth Analg* 84:95, 1997.
24. Na KB, Kopacz DJ. Spinal chloroprocaine solutions: density at 37°C and pH titration. *Anesth Analg* 98:70, 2003.
25. Bannister J, McClure JH, Wildsmith JA. Effect of glucose concentration on the intrathecal spread of 0.5% bupivacaine. *Br J Anaesth* 64:232, 1990.
26. Hirabayashi Y, Shimizu R, Saitoh K, et al. Anatomical configuration of the spinal column in the supine position. I. A study using magnetic resonance imaging. *Br J Anaesth* 75:3, 1995.
27. Logan MR, Drummond GB. Spinal anesthesia and lumbar lordosis. *Anesth Analg* 67:338, 1988.
28. Veering BT, Immink-Speet TT, Burm AG, et al. Spinal anaesthesia with 0.5% hyperbaric bupivacaine in elderly patients: Effects of duration spent in the sitting position. *Br J Anaesth* 87:738, 2001.
29. Donati A, Mercuri G, Iuorio S, et al. Haemodynamic modifications after unilateral subarachnoid anaesthesia evaluated with transthoracic echocardiography. *Minerva Anestesiol* 71:75, 2005.
30. Casati A, Fanelli G, Aldegheri G, et al. Frequency of hypotension during conventional or asymmetric hyperbaric spinal block. *Reg Anesth Pain Med* 24:214, 1999.
31. Bodily MN, Carpenter RL, Owens BD. Lidocaine 0.5% spinal anaesthesia: A hypobaric solution for short-stay perirectal surgery. *Can J Anaesth* 39:770, 1992.
32. Faust A, Fournier, Van Gessel E, et al. Isobaric versus hypobaric spinal bupivacaine for total hip arthroplasty in the lateral position. *Anesth Analg* 97:589, 2003.
33. Stienstra R, Veering BT. Intrathecal drug spread: Is it controllable? *Reg Anesth Pain Med* 23:347, 1998.
34. Whiteside JB, Burke D, Wildsmith JAW. Spinal anesthesia with ropivacaine 5 mg/mL in glucose 10 mg/mL or 50 mg/mL. *Br J Anaesth* 86:241, 2001.
35. Shesky MC, Rocco AG, Bizzarri-Schmid M, et al. A dose-response study of bupivacaine for spinal anesthesia. *Anesth Analg* 62:931, 1983.
36. Van Zundert AA, Grouls RJ, Korsten HH, et al. Spinal anesthesia. Volume or concentration: What matters? *Reg Anesth* 21:112, 1996.
37. Brown DT, Wildsmith JAW, Covino BG, et al. Effect of baricity on spinal anesthesia with amethocaine. *Br J Anaesth* 52:589, 1980.
38. Wildsmith JAW, McClure J, Brown D, et al. Effects of posture on spread of isobaric and hyperbaric amethocaine. *Br J Anaesth* 53:273, 1981.
39. Liu SS, Ware PD, Allen HW, et al. Dose-response characteristics of spinal bupivacaine in volunteers: Clinical implications for ambulatory anesthesia. *Anesthesiology* 85:729, 1996.
40. Huffnagle SL, Norris MC, Huffnagle J, et al. Intrathecal hyperbaric bupivacaine dose response in postpartum tubal ligation patients. *Reg Anesth Pain Med* 27:284, 2002.
41. Tuominen M, Pitkanen M, Taivainen T, et al. Prediction of the spread of repeated spinal anaesthesia with bupivacaine. *Br J Anaesth* 68:136, 1992.

42. Olson KH, Nielsen TH, Kristofferson E, et al. Spinal analgesia with plain 0.5% bupivacaine administered at spinal interspace L2/L3 or L4/L5. *Br J Anaesth* 64:170, 1990.

43. Broadbent CR, Maxwell WB, Ferrie R, et al. Ability of anaesthetists to identify a marked lumbar interspace. *Anaesthesia* 55:1122, 2000.

44. Veering BT, Ter Reit PM, Burm AG, et al. Spinal anaesthesia with 0.5% hyperbaric bupivacaine in elderly patients: Effect of site of injection on spread of analgesia. *Br J Anaesth* 77:343, 1996.

45. Sakura S, Sumi M, Morimoto N, et al. Spinal anesthesia with tetracaine in 0.75% glucose: Influence of vertebral interspace for injection. *Reg Anesth Pain Med* 23:170, 1998.

46. Carpenter RL, Hogan QH, Liu SS, et al. Lumbosacral cerebrospinal fluid volume is the primary determinant of sensory block extent and duration during spinal anesthesia. *Anesthesiology* 89:24, 1998.

47. Higuchi H, Hirata J, Adachi Y, et al. Influence of lumbosacral cerebrospinal fluid density, velocity, and volume on extent and duration of plain bupivacaine spinal anesthesia. *Anesthesiology* 100:106, 2004.

48. Schiffer E, Van Gessel E, Fournier R, et al. Cerebrospinal fluid density influences extent of plain bupivacaine spinal anesthesia. *Anesthesiology* 96:1325, 2002.

49. Hirabayashi Y, Shimizu R, Fukuda H, et al. Anatomical configuration of the spinal column in the supine position. II. Comparison of pregnant and non-pregnant women. *Br J Anaesth* 75:6, 1995.

50. Butterworth JF, Walker FO, Lysak SZ. Pregnancy increases median nerve susceptibility to lidocaine. *Anesthesiology* 72:962, 1990.

51. Taivainen TR, Tuominen MK, Kuulasmaa KA, et al. A prospective study on reproducibility of the spread of spinal anesthesia using plain 0.5% bupivacaine. *Reg Anesth* 15:12, 1990.

52. Kouri ME, Kopacz DJ. Spinal 2-chloroprocaine: A comparison with lidocaine in volunteers. *Anesth Analg* 98:75, 2004.

53. Frey K, Holman S, Mikat-Stevens M, et al. The recovery profile of hyperbaric spinal anesthesia with lidocaine, tetracaine, and bupivacaine. *Reg Anesth Pain Med* 23:159, 1998.

54. Smith KN, Kopacz DJ, McDonald SB. Spinal 2-chloroprocaine: A dose-ranging study and the effect of added epinephrine. *Anesth Analg* 98:81, 2004.

55. Kooger Infante NE, Van Gessel E, Forster A, et al. Extent of hyperbaric spinal anesthesia influences the duration of block. *Anesthesiology* 92:1319, 2000.

56. Kito K, Kato H, Shibata M, et al. The effect of varied doses of epinephrine on duration of lidocaine spinal anesthesia in the thoracic and lumbosacral dermatomes. *Anesth Analg* 86:1018, 1998.

57. Liam BL, Yim CF, Chong JL. Dose response study of 1% lidocaine for spinal anesthesia for lower limb and perineal surgery. *Can J Anaesth* 45:645, 1998.

58. Liu SS, Pollock JE, Mulroy MF, et al. Comparison of 5% with dextrose, 1.5% with dextrose, and 1.5% dextrose-free lidocaine solutions for spinal anesthesia in human volunteers. *Anesth Analg* 81:697, 1995.

59. Liu SS, Chiu AA, Carpenter RL, et al. Fentanyl prolongs lidocaine spinal anesthesia without prolonging recovery. *Anesth Analg* 80:730, 1995.

60. Zayas VM, Liguori GA, Chisolm MF, et al. Dose response relationships for isobaric spinal mepivacaine using the combined spinal epidural technique. *Anesth Analg* 89:1167, 1999.

61. Pawlowski J, Sukhani R, Pappas A, et al. The anesthetic and recovery profile of two doses (60 and 80 mg) of plain mepivacaine for ambulatory anesthesia. *Anesth Analg* 91:580, 2000.

62. Malinovsky JM, Charles F, Kick O, et al. Intrathecal anesthesia: Ropivacaine vs. bupivacaine. *Anesth Analg* 91:1457, 2001.

63. Glaser C, Marhofer P, Zimpfer G, et al. Levobupivacaine versus racemic bupivacaine for spinal anesthesia. *Anesth Analg* 94:194, 2002.

64. Alley EA, Kopacz DJ, McDonald SB, et al. Hyperbaric spinal levobupivacaine: A comparison to racemic bupivacaine in volunteers. *Anesth Analg* 94:188, 2002.

65. Ben-David B, Levin H, Solomon E, et al. Spinal bupivacaine in ambulatory surgery: The effects of saline dilution. *Anesth Analg* 83:716, 1996.

66. Kallio H, Snall EVT, Tuomas CA, et al. Comparison of hyperbaric and plain ropivacaine 15 mg in spinal anesthesia for lower limb surgery. *Br J Anaesth* 93:664, 2004.

67. Burm AG, van Kleef JW, Gladines MP, et al. Plasma concentrations of lidocaine and bupivacaine after subarachnoid administration. *Anesthesiology* 59:191, 1983.

68. Gosteli P, Van Gessel E, Gamulin Z. Effects of pH adjustment and carbonation of lidocaine during epidural anesthesia for foot and ankle surgery. *Anesth Analg* 81:104, 1995.

69. Asato F, Kanai A. Sensory block of S3 dermatome prevents pain during bladder catheterization. *Can J Anaesth* 48:379, 2001.

70. Visser WA, Liem TH, Egmond J, et al. Extension of sensory block after thoracic administration of a test dose of lidocaine at three different levels. *Anesth Analg* 86:332, 1998.

71. Yokoyama M, Hanazaki M, Fujii H, et al. Correlation between the distribution of contrast medium and the extent of blockade during epidural anesthesia. *Anesthesiology* 100:1504, 2004.

72. Liu SS, Ware PD, Rajendran S. Effects of concentration and volume of 2-chloroprocaine on epidural anesthesia in volunteers. *Anesthesiology* 86:1288, 1997.

73. Veering BT, Burm AGL, Van Kleef JW, et al. Epidural anesthesia with bupivacaine: Effects of age on neural blockade and pharmacokinetics. *Anesth Analg* 66:589, 1987.

74. Simon MJG, Veering BT, Stienstra R, et al. The effects of age on neural blockade and hemodynamic changes after epidural anesthesia with ropivacaine. *Anesth Analg* 94:1325, 2002.

75. Simon MJG, Veering BT, Stienstra R, et al. Effect of age on the clinical profile and systemic absorption and disposition of levobupivacaine after epidural administration. *Br J Anaesth* 93:512, 2004.

76. Kopacz DJ, Mulroy MF. Chloroprocaine and lidocaine decrease hospital stay and admission rate after outpatient epidural anesthesia. *Reg Anesth* 15:19, 1990.

77. Terai T, Yukioka H, Fujimori M. A double-blind comparison of lidocaine and mepivacaine during epidural anaesthesia. *Acta Anaesthesiol* 37:607, 1993.

78. Kopacz DJ, Allen HW, Thompson GT. A comparison of epidural levobupivacaine 0.75% with racemic bupivacaine for lower abdominal surgery. *Anesth Analg* 90:642, 2000.

79. Sakura S, Sumi M, Kushizaki H, et al. Concentration of lidocaine affects intensity of sensory block during lumbar epidural anesthesia. *Anesth Analg* 88:123, 1999.

80. Nakayama M, Yamamoto J, Ichinose H, et al. Effects of volume and concentration of lidocaine on epidural anaesthesia in pregnant females. *Eur J Anaesthesiol* 19:808, 2002.

81. Erdemir HA, Soper LE, Sweet RB. Studies of factors affecting peridural anesthesia. *Anesth Analg* 44:400, 1965.

82. Fink BR. Mechanisms of differential axial block in epidural and spinal anesthesia. *Anesthesiology* 70:851, 1989.

83. Raymond SA, Steffensen SC, Gigion LD, et al. The role of length of nerve exposed to local anesthetic in impulse blocking action. *Anesth Analg* 68:563, 1989.

84. Hogan QH. Distribution of solution in the epidural space: Examination by cryomicrotome section. *Reg Anesth Pain Med* 27:150, 2002.

85. Hogan QH. Epidural anatomy examined by cryomicrotome section: Influence of age, vertebral level, and disease. *Reg Anesth* 21:395, 1996.

86. Igarashi T, Hirabayshi Y, Shimuzu R, et al. The lumbar extradural changes with increasing age. *Br J Anaesth* 78:149, 1997.

87. Grundy EM, Zamora AM, Winnie AP. Comparison of spread of epidural anesthesia in pregnant and nonpregnant women. *Anesth Analg* 57:544, 1978.

88. Kalas DB, Senfeld RM, Hehre FW. Continuous lumbar peridural anesthesia in obstetrics, IV: Comparison of the number of segments blocked in pregnant and nonpregnant subjects. *Anesth Analg* 45:848, 1966.

89. Arakawa M. Does pregnancy increase the efficacy of lumbar epidural anesthesia? *Int J Obstet Anesth* 13:86, 2004.

90. Kanai A, Suzuki A, Hoka S. Rapid injection of epidural mepivacaine speeds onset of nerve blockade. *Can J Anaesth* 52:281, 2005.

91. Griffiths RB, Horton WA, Jones IG, et al. Speed of injection and spread of bupivacaine in the epidural space. *Anesthesia* 42:160, 1987.

92. Hogan QH. Epidural catheter tip position and distribution of injectate evaluated by computed tomography. *Anesthesiology* 90:964, 1999.

93. Yun MJ, Kim YC, Lim YJ, et al. The differential flow of epidural local anesthetic via needle or catheter: A prospective randomized double-blind study. *Anaesth Intensive Care* 32:377, 2004.

94. Bromage PR, Pettigrew RT, Crowell DE. Tachyphylaxis in epidural analgesia. I. Augmentation and decay of local anesthesia. *J Clin Pharmacol* 9:30, 1969.

95. Stienstra R, Dahan A, Alhadi BZ, et al. Mechanism of action of epidural top-up in combined spinal epidural anesthesia. *Anesth Analg* 83:382, 1996.

96. Stienstra R, Dilrosun-Alhadi BZ, Dahan A, et al. The epidural "top-up" in combined spinal-epidural anesthesia: The effect of volume versus dose. *Anesth Analg* 88:810, 1999.

97. Takiguchi T, Okano T, Egawa H, et al. The effect of epidural saline injection on analgesic level during combined spinal and epidural anesthesia assessed clinically and myelographically. *Anesth Analg* 85:1097, 1997.

98. Leeda M, Stienstra R, Arbous S, et al. The epidural "top-up." Predictors of increased sensory blockade. *Anesthesiology* 96:1310, 2002.

99. Neal JM, Deck JJ, Kopacz DJ, et al. Hospital discharge after ambulatory knee arthroscopy: A comparison of epidural 2-chloroprocaine versus lidocaine. *Reg Anesth Pain Med* 26:35, 2001.

100. Seoew LT, Lips FJ, Cousins MJ. Lidocaine and bupivacaine mixtures for epidural block. *Anesthesiology* 56:177, 1982.

101. Finucane BT, Sandler AN, McKenna J, et al. A double-blind comparison of ropivacaine 0.5%, 0.75%, 1.0%, and bupivacaine 0.5% injected epidurally, in patients undergoing abdominal hysterectomy. *Can J Anaesth* 43:442, 1996.

102. Ramos G, Pereira E, Simonetti MP. Does alkalinization of 0.75% ropivacaine promote a lumbar peridural block of higher quality? *Reg Anesth Pain Med* 26:357, 2001.

103. Park WY, Massengale M, Kin SI, et al. Age and the spread of local anesthetic solutions in the epidural space. *Anesth Analg* 59:867, 1980.

104. Burm AG, van Kleef JW, Gladines MP, et al. Epidural anesthesia with lidocaine and bupivacaine. Effects of epinephrine on the plasma concentration profiles. *Anesth Analg* 65:1281, 1986.

105. Lee BB, Ngan Kee WD, Plummer JL, et al. The effect of the addition of epinephrine on the early systemic absorption of epidural ropivacaine in humans. *Anesth Analg* 95:1402, 2002.

106. Groen K, Mantel M, Zeijlmans, et al. Pharmacokinetics of the enantiomers of bupivacaine and mepivacaine after epidural administration of the racemates. *Anesth Analg* 86:361, 1998.

107. Foster RH, Markham A. Levobupivacaine: A review of its pharmacology and use as a local anesthetic. *Drugs* 59:551, 2000.

108. Burm AG, Stienstra R, Brouwer RP, et al. Epidural infusion of ropivacaine for postoperative analgesia after major orthopedic surgery. *Anesthesiology* 93:395, 2000.

109. Veering BT, Burm AG, Feyen HM, et al. Pharmacokinetics of bupivacaine during postoperative epidural infusion. *Anesthesiology* 96:1062, 2002.

110. Burm AG. Clinical pharmacokinetics of epidural and spinal anaesthesia. *Clin Pharmacokinet* 16:283, 1989.

111. Thomas JM, Schug SA. Recent advances in the pharmacokinetics of local anesthetics. *Clin Pharmacokinet* 36:67, 1999.

112. Stein C. Analgesic: Receptor ligands and opiate narcotics. In: Evers AS, Maze M, eds, *Anesthetic Pharmacology: Physiologic Principles and Clinical Practice.* The Netherlands: Elsevier, 2003, p. 457.

113. Schubert A, Licina MG, Lineberry PJ, et al. The effects of intrathecal morphine on somatosensory evoked potentials in awake volunteers. *Anesthesiology* 75:401, 1991.

114. Fernandez-Galinski SM, Monells J, Espadaler JM, et al. Effects of subarachnoid lidocaine, meperidine, and fentanyl on somatosensory and motor evoked responses in awake humans. *Acta Anaesthesiol Scand* 40:39, 1996.

115. Eisenach JC, Hood DD, Curry R, et al. Intrathecal but not intravenous opioids release adenosine from the spinal cord. *J Pain* 5:64, 2004.

116. Dickenson AH. Spinal cord pharmacology of pain. *Br J Anaesth* 75:193, 1995.

117. Chiari A, Eisenach JC. Spinal anesthesia: Mechanisms, agents, methods, and safety. *Reg Anesth Pain Med* 23:357, 1998.

118. Bernards CM. Pharmacokinetics of spinal opioids. *Curr Opin Anaesthesiol* 17:441, 2004.

119. Herz A, Teschemacher H. Activities and sites of antinociceptive action of morphine-like analgesics and kinetics of distribution following intravenous, intracerebral, and intraventricular application. In: Simmonds A, ed, *Advances in Drug Research.* London: Academic Press, 1971, p. 79.

120. Ummenhofer WC, Arends RH, Shen DD, et al. Comparative spinal distribution and clearance kinetics of intrathecally administered morphine, fentanyl, alfentanil, and sufentanil. *Anesthesiology* 92:729, 2000.

121. Bhadelia RA, Bogdan AR, Kaplan RF, et al. Cerebrospinal fluid pulsation amplitude and its quantitative relationship to cerebral blood flow pulsations: A phase contrast MR flow imaging study. *Neuroradiology* 39:258, 1997.

122. Bailey PL, Lu JK, Pace NL, et al. Effects of intrathecal morphine on the ventilatory response to hypoxia. *N Engl J Med* 343:1228, 2000.

123. Lu JK, Schafer PG, Gardner TL, et al. The dose-response pharmacology of intrathecal sufentanil in female volunteers. *Anesth Analg* 85:372, 1997.
124. Lehmann KA, Gerhard A, Horrichs-Haermeyer G, et al. Postoperative patient-controlled analgesia with sufentanil: Analgesic efficacy and minimum effective concentration. *Acta Anaesthesiol Scand* 35:221, 1991.
125. Ferouz F, Norris MC, Leighton BL. Risk of respiratory arrest after intrathecal sufentanil. *Anesth Analg* 85:1088, 1997.
126. Fournier R, Gamulin Z, Van Gessel E. Respiratory depression after 5 µg of intrathecal sufentanil. *Anesth Analg* 87:1377, 1998.
127. Reuben SS, Dunn SM, Duprat KM, et al. An intrathecal dose-response study in lower extremity revascularization procedures. *Anesthesiology* 81:1371, 1994.
128. Salinas FV, Liu SS. Spinal anaesthesia: Local anesthetics and adjuncts in the ambulatory setting. *Best Pract Res Clin Anaesthesiol* 16:195, 2002.
129. Ben-David B, Frankel R, Arzumonov T, et al. Minidose bupivacaine-fentanyl spinal anesthesia for surgical repair of hip fracture in the aged. *Anesthesiology* 92:6, 2000.
130. Loper KA, Ready LB. Epidural morphine after anterior cruciate ligament repair: A comparison with patient-controlled intravenous analgesia. *Anesth Analg* 68:350, 1989.
131. Negre I, Gueneron JP, Jamali SJ, et al. Preoperative analgesia with epidural morphine. *Anesth Analg* 79:298, 1994.
132. Parker RK, White PF. Epidural patient-controlled analgesia: An alternative to intravenous patient-controlled analgesia for pain relief after cesarean delivery. *Anesth Analg* 75:245, 1992.
133. Loper KA, Ready LB, Downey M, et al. Epidural and intravenous fentanyl are clinically equivalent after knee surgery. *Anesth Analg* 70:72, 1990.
134. Sandler AN, Stringer D, Panos L, et al. A randomized, double blind comparison of lumbar epidural and intravenous fentanyl infusions for postthoracotomy pain relief. *Anesthesiology* 77:626, 1992.
135. Guinard JP, Mavrocodatos P, Chiolero R, et al. A randomized comparison of intravenous versus lumbar and thoracic epidural fentanyl for analgesia after thoracotomy. *Anesthesiology* 77:1108, 1992.
136. Ginosar Y, Riley ET, Angst MS. The site of action of epidural fentanyl in humans: The difference between infusion and bolus administration. *Anesth Analg* 97:1428, 2003.
137. Miguel R, Morrell M, Scharf J, et al. A prospective, randomized, double blind comparison of epidural and intravenous sufentanil infusions. *Anesthesiology* 81:346, 1994.
138. Kozody R, Palahniuk RJ, Wade JG, et al. The effect of subarachnoid epinephrine and phenylephrine on spinal cord blood flow. *Can Anaesth Soc J* 31:503, 1984.
139. Kozody R, Swartz J, Palahniuk RJ, et al. Spinal cord blood flow following subarachnoid lidocaine. *Can Anaesth Soc J* 32:472, 1985.
140. Kozody R, Palahniuk RJ, Cumming MO. Spinal cord blood flow following subarachnoid tetracaine. *Can Anaesth Soc J* 32:23, 1985.
141. Kozody R, Ong B, Palahniuk RJ, et al. Subarachnoid bupivacaine decreases spinal cord blood flow in dogs. *Can Anaesth Soc J* 32:216, 1985.
142. Chambers WA, Littlewood DG, Logan MR, et al. Effect of added epinephrine on spinal anesthesia with lidocaine. *Anesth Analg* 60:417, 1981.
143. Chiu AA, Liu SS, Carpenter RL, et al. The effects of epinephrine on lidocaine spinal anesthesia: A crossover study. *Anesth Analg* 80:735, 1995.
144. Racle JP, Benkhadra A, Poy JY, et al. Prolongation of isobaric spinal anesthesia with epinephrine and clonidine for hip surgery in the elderly. *Anesth Analg* 66:442, 1987.
145. Racle JP, Benkhadra A, Poy JY, et al. Effect of increasing amounts of epinephrine during isobaric bupivacaine spinal anesthesia in elderly patients. *Anesth Analg* 66:882, 1987.
146. Chambers WA, Littlewood DG, Scott DB. Spinal anesthesia with hyperbaric bupivacaine: Effect of added vasoconstrictors. *Anesth Analg* 61:49, 1982.
147. Moore JM, Liu SS, Pollock JE, et al. The effect of epinephrine on small dose hyperbaric bupivacaine spinal anesthesia: Clinical implications for ambulatory surgery. *Anesth Analg* 86:973, 1998.
148. Burm AG, van Kleef JW, Gladines MP, et al. Spinal anesthesia with hyperbaric lidocaine and bupivacaine: Effects of epinephrine on plasma concentration profiles. *Anesth Analg* 66:1104, 1987.
149. Armstrong IR, Littlewood DG, Chambers WA. Spinal anesthesia with tetracaine-effect of added vasoconstrictors. *Anesth Analg* 62:793, 1983.
150. Concepcion M, Maddi R, Francis D, et al. Vasoconstrictors in spinal anesthesia with tetracaine-comparison of epinephrine and phenylephrine. *Anesth Analg* 63:134, 1984.
151. Sakura S, Sumi M, Sakaguchi Y, et al. The addition of epinephrine contributes to the development of transient neurologic symptoms after spinal anesthesia with 0.5% tetracaine. *Anesthesiology* 87:771, 1997.
152. Tucker G. Pharmacokinetics of local anesthetics. *Br J Anaesth* 58:717, 1986.
153. Kopacz DJ, Helman JD, Nussbaum CE, et al. A comparison of epidural levobupivacaine 0.5% with or without epinephrine for lumbar spine surgery. *Anesth Analg* 93:755, 2001.
154. Sharrock N, Go G, Mineo R. Effect of i.v. low-dose adrenaline and phenylephrine infusions on plasma concentrations of bupivacaine after epidural anesthesia in elderly patients. *Br J Anaesth* 67:694, 1991.
155. Niemi G, Breivik H. Adrenaline markedly improves thoracic epidural analgesia produced by low-dose infusion of bupivacaine, fentanyl and adrenaline after major surgery. *Acta Anaesthesiol Scand* 42:897, 1998.
156. Niemi G, Breivik H. Epinephrine markedly improves thoracic epidural analgesia produced by small-dose infusion of ropivacaine, fentanyl, and epinephrine after major thoracic or abdominal surgery: A randomized, double-blinded crossover study with and without epinephrine. *Anesth Analg* 94:1598, 2002.
157. Gourlay GK, Kowalski SR, Plummer JL, et al. Fentanyl blood concentration-analgesic response relationship in the treatment of postoperative pain. *Anesth Analg* 67:329, 1988.
158. Curatolo M, Petersen-Felix S, Arendt-Nielsen L, et al. Epidural epinephrine and clonidine: Segmental analgesia and effects on different pain modalities. *Anesthesiology* 87:785, 1997.
159. Liu SS, Chiu AA, Neal JM, et al. Oral clonidine prolongs lidocaine spinal anesthesia in human volunteers. *Anesthesiology* 82:1353, 1995.
160. Eisenach JC, Detweiler D, Hood DH. Hemodynamic and analgesic actions of epidurally administered clonidine. *Anesthesiology* 78:277, 1993.

161. Eisenach JC, Hood DH, Curry R. Intrathecal, but not intravenous, clonidine reduces experimental thermal or capsaicin-induced pain and hyperalgesia in normal volunteers. *Anesth Analg* 87:591, 1998.

162. Bernard JM, Kick O, Bonnet F. Comparison of intravenous and epidural clonidine for postoperative patient-controlled analgesia. *Anesth Analg* 81:706, 1995.

163. De Kock M, Gautier P, Fanard L, et al. Intrathecal ropivacaine and clonidine for ambulatory knee arthroscopy. *Anesthesiology* 94:574, 2001.

164. Dobrydnjov I, Axelsson K, Thorn E, et al. Clonidine combined with small-dose bupivacaine during spinal anesthesia for inguinal herniorrhaphy: A randomized double-blinded study. *Anesth Analg* 96:1496, 2003.

165. Strebel S, Gurzeler JA, Schneider MC, et al. Small-dose intrathecal clonidine and isobaric bupivacaine for orthopedic surgery: A dose-response study. *Anesth Analg* 99:1231, 2004.

166. De Kock M, Weiderkher P, Laghmiche A, et al. Epidural clonidine used as the sole analgesic agent during and after abdominal surgery: A dose-response study. *Anesthesiology* 86:285, 1997.

167. Forster JG, Rosenberg PH. Small dose of clonidine mixed with low-dose ropivacaine and fentanyl for epidural analgesia after total knee arthroplasty. *Br J Anaesth* 93:670, 2004.

Physiologic Effects of Neuraxial Anesthesia

CHAPTER 4

Barbara M. Scavone
John Ratliff
Cynthia A. Wong

INTRODUCTION

Induction of spinal and epidural anesthesia has widespread direct and indirect effects on a number of physiologic systems, including the cardiovascular, respiratory, gastrointestinal, renal, endocrine, and coagulation systems. Understanding these effects and the ability to manage physiologic side effects is important to the safe conduct of neuraxial anesthesia. This chapter will review the mechanisms of physiologic effects of neuraxial analgesia. Treatment of adverse effects is discussed in detail in Chap. 6.

DIFFERENTIAL NEURAXIAL BLOCKADE

The ability to obtund sensory, motor, and sympathetic nerve functions to different degrees is called "differential" blockade. Neural blockade is not complete or absolute. For example, blockade to temperature occurs earlier and to a greater extent than motor blockade after intrathecal injection of local anesthetic. The mechanism of differential blockade has not been completely elucidated and may result from several mechanisms.[1,2] Nerves may be blocked at different rates, and blockade may resolve at different rates, so that differential blockade may be observed during block onset and resolution, but not at equilibrium. Anatomic features of different nerves, including the presence or absence of myelin, and nerve diameter, may affect the concentration of local anesthetic necessary to block conduction (see Chap. 3). The length of blocked nerve affects conduction blockade since it is necessary to block a certain length of nerve to prevent the action potential from "jumping" to an unblocked segment. In the neuraxial canal the length of spinal nerve exposed to local anesthetic may differ, depending on where the drug is injected. For example, the length of nerve exposed to local anesthetic injected into the epidural space may differ from the length of nerve exposed after injection into the subarachnoid space.[2] The length of exposed spinal nerve differs in the lumbar subarachnoid space, around the cauda equina, compared to the thoracic subarachnoid space. Ion channels and lipid membranes of nerves differ, and this may also affect the concentration of local anesthetic required to block conduction. In addition, blockade of nerve sodium channels depends on the frequency of axon firing. Therefore, ongoing nerve activity at the time of blockade may contribute to the degree of differential blockade. During neuraxial blockade, the concentration of local anesthesia decreases as a function of distance from the injection site. Finally, differential blockade may be explained by the use of specific local anesthetics, as individual agents have different abilities to penetrate lipid membranes.

The classical teaching is that the sympathetic blockade extends two dermatomes higher than sensory blockade during spinal anesthesia. This conclusion was based on measurement of sympathetic activity using skin temperature or loss of cold sensation. Other methods of measuring sympathetic nervous system activity, however, have demonstrated that the differential may be as great as 6 dermatomes, and sympathetic blockade may not be complete.[3]

In general, during neuraxial anesthesia, sensory function is blocked with a lower concentration/mass of local anesthetic compared to motor function, and is also blocked at a faster rate. Sensory blockade to temperature (warm and cold) is blocked first, followed by prick and finally touch. The clinical manifestations of differential blockade are important to appreciate when assessing the adequacy of sensory and motor blockade before the start of a surgical procedure (see Chap. 2).

CARDIOVASCULAR EFFECTS

Spinal and epidural analgesia/anesthesia have primarily indirect effects on the cardiovascular system (Table 4-1). In contrast to spinal anesthesia, drugs absorbed into the systemic

Table 4-1

Hemodynamic Effects of Neuraxial Anesthesia[a]

Parameter	Effect[b]
Blood pressure	↓
Central venous pressure	↓
Heart rate	↓, →, ↑
Cardiac output	↓
Stroke volume	↓
SVR	↓

[a]Extent of hemodynamic changes largely depend on extent of neural blockade and baseline hemodynamic status of patient.
[b]↓ = decrease, → = no change, ↑ = increase.

Box 4-1

Risk Factors for Neuraxial Anesthesia-Associated Hypotension

- Block height higher than T5
- Older age
- Baseline systolic blood pressure < 120 mmHg
- Combined neuraxial-general anesthesia
- Dural puncture higher than L3-L4 interspace

circulation from the epidural space may have direct effects on organ systems. The indirect effects are mediated primarily through blockade of the sympathetic nervous system and include reflex responses to the primary cardiovascular effect. The extent of the effect of neuraxial blockade on the cardiovascular system depends on the number and position of blocked spinal segments.

The cell bodies of preganglionic sympathetic nerve fibers reside in the thoracic and high lumbar spinal cord (T1 through L1 to L2), and are blocked to a variable degree during spinal anesthesia. The rostral extent of sympathetic blockade exceeds that of sensory blockade by as many as six dermatomes, although sympathetic blockade is often incomplete.[4–7] Because spinal anesthesia is always initiated at the lumbar level, it is almost always associated with some degree of sympathetic blockade. Caudal epidural anesthesia that blocks only sacral dermatomes may avoid sympathetic blockade. Hemodynamic derangements during spinal/epidural anesthesia are related to the extent of sympathetic blockade, with increasing levels of sympathectomy associated with increasing degrees of systemic arterial hypotension and bradycardia.[8–10] In addition, the degree of cardiovascular compromise is influenced by patient position and intravascular volume, the presence of other drugs administered chronically or acutely, and underlying patient disease states.

▶ Hypotension

The most notable effect of spinal anesthesia is *systemic hypotension*, which is estimated to occur at a rate of 16–33%. Risk factors for developing hypotension include block height higher than T5, increasing age, baseline systolic

pressure less than 120 mmHg, combination general-neuraxial anesthesia, and spinal puncture at or above the L2-L3 interspace (Box 4-1).[8,10] Maximum decreases in mean arterial pressure occur at a mean of 28 min after administration of spinal anesthesia, and can occur in patients who were previously stable for an hour or more.[8,10,11]

Mean arterial blood pressure is the product of cardiac output and total peripheral resistance, and both are affected during neuraxial anesthesia. In a canine model, Butterworth et al. used cardiopulmonary bypass to isolate the effects of spinal anesthesia to the venous or arterial circulations.[12,13] Decreases in venous reservoir blood volume indicated increases in venous capacitance and, in the setting of constant pump flow and central venous pressure, decreases in mean arterial pressure indicated decreases in systemic vascular resistance (SVR). Spinal anesthesia both increased venous capacitance and decreased SVR.

Rooke et al. investigated the effects of spinal anesthesia on central hemodynamic parameters using a pulmonary artery catheter, and the effect on regional blood flow using radiolabeled red cell scans.[14] Fifteen elderly male patients with known cardiac disease received hyperbaric lidocaine spinal anesthesia (median block height T4, range T1 to T10). Mean arterial pressure decreased by an average of 33% as a consequence of an average 10% decrease in cardiac output and 26% decrease in SVR. The decrease in cardiac output primarily resulted from a 10% reduction in stroke volume, not a reduction in heart rate (Fig. 4-1A). The decrease in stroke volume was due to a 19% decrease in left ventricular end-diastolic volume, without any change in ejection fraction. There was a redistribution of blood away from the heart to the periphery, where pooling occurred (Fig. 4-1B).

Sympathetic blockade results in arterial and venous vasodilation via two mechanisms: direct inhibition of sympathetic outflow to nerves innervating blood vessels, and a decrease in circulating catecholamines via inhibition of

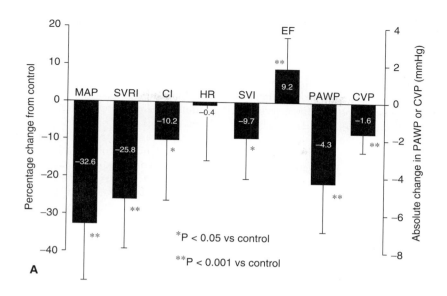

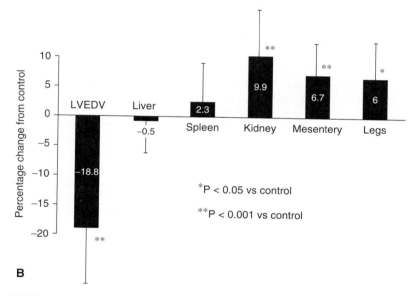

FIGURE 4-1. The percentage of change or absolute change from baseline (± SD) in response to spinal anesthesia in 15 elderly men with cardiac disease. (A) MAP = mean arterial pressure, SVRI = systemic vascular resistance index, CI = cardiac index, HR = heart rate, SVI = stroke volume index, EF = left ventricular ejection fraction, PAWP = pulmonary artery wedge pressure, CVP = central venous pressure. The major cause of the decrease in MAP was a decrease in SVR, not a decrease in CI. The major cause of the decrease in CI was SVI, not HR. (B) Changes in organ blood volume. LVEDV = left ventricular end-diastolic volume. Blood shifted from the heart to the abdomen and legs, but not into the liver or spleen. *(Modified with permission from Rooke GA, Freund PR, Jacobson AF. Hemodynamic response and change in organ blood volume during spinal anesthesia in elderly men with cardiac disease. Anesth Analg 85:99, 1997.)*

nerves innervating the adrenal gland. Arteriolar smooth muscle maintains autonomous tone even after complete sympathectomy, so that although total peripheral resistance decreases, blood pressure will be maintained close to baseline as long as cardiac output is maintained. In contrast, veins and venules have very little smooth muscle. Therefore, they may dilate maximally after sympathectomy, depending on intraluminal hydrostatic pressure. This is largely a function of gravity and the position of the vessel relative to the right atrium.

The extent of blockade is loosely correlated with the severity of hemodynamic perturbations. The incidence of systemic hypotension and bradycardia increases as blockade height increases, especially to T5 or above (Fig. 4-2).[8,10] Blockade of sympathetic outflow to the splanchnic bed (T6 to L1) results in dilated splanchnic veins and a markedly increased venous capacitance. In contrast, muscle veins have no sympathetic innervation so neuraxial blockade limited to the lumbar and caudal regions results in minimal vasodilation and change in venous capacitance. Compensatory vasoconstriction can occur above the level of the block, but as block height increases, compensatory vasoconstriction diminishes, and eventually it is no longer sufficient to offset the sympatholytic effects in the lower body.

As noted above, hypotension is accompanied by arteriolar dilation, which serves to increase blood flow through the capillary beds at any given arterial pressure. Blood flow is not expected to increase, however, in patients with atherosclerotic disease that prevents vasodilation, or in patients with mean arterial pressures so low that insufficient hydrostatic pressure is maintained to keep the capillaries open. Also, compensatory vasoconstriction may occur in areas of the body above the level of the block, and regional capillary blood flow may decrease in the setting of systemic hypotension. Hemodynamic effects become more marked during hypovolemia and the clinician is cautioned against the use of central neuraxial techniques in this setting.

Arginine vasopressin (AVP) and the renin-angiotensin system may play a role in maintaining blood pressure during neuraxial anesthesia. Plasma renin concentration, but not AVP increased after sodium nitroprusside-induced hypotension.[15] In the presence of T11-T1 sympathetic blockade, plasma renin levels did not increase, but AVP levels did. In a volunteer study, blood pressure dropped significantly after induction of epidural anesthesia to a T2 sensory level when both enalapril (an angiotensin-converting enzyme [ACE] inhibitor) and an AVP V1 receptor antagonist were infused, but did not change after either antagonist drug administered alone or after saline control infusion.[16] Finally, the blood pressure decrease in patients with long-term ACE inhibitor therapy did not differ from control patients.[17] Plasma AVP concentration, however, was increased in the ACE inhibitor therapy group compared to control. Taken together, these results suggest that these two systems complement one another to maintain blood pressure during neuraxial anesthesia.

In summary, both venous pooling (which serves to decrease preload and therefore, cardiac output) and arterial dilation (which serves to decrease SVR) combine to cause a decrease in mean arterial pressure. Additional vascular dilation, resulting from hypoxemia, hypercarbia, acidemia, lactate accumulation, or systemic drugs, could serve to further decrease systemic blood pressure. The incidence and treatment of hypotension are discussed in detail in Chap. 6.

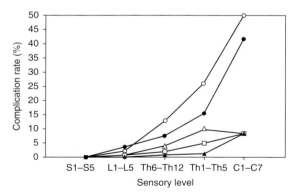

FIGURE 4-2. Correlation between extend of blockade and incidence of side effects. The incidence of hypotension, bradycardia, nausea (*P* < 0.0001), and shivering (*P* < 0.005) were significantly higher with higher sensory levels. ○ = hypotension, ● = bradycardia, △ = nausea, □ = shivering, ▲ = vomiting. (*Used with permission from Tarkkila PJ, Kaukinen S. Complications during spinal anesthesia: A prospective study. Reg Anesth 16:101, 1991.*)

Box 4-2

Risk Factor for Neuraxial Anesthesia-Associated Bradycardia

▷ Block height higher than T5

▷ Younger age

▷ ASA PS I

▷ Baseline heart rate < 60 bpm

▷ Prolonged PR interval

▷ β-blocker therapy

Heart Rate

Although decreases in preload are the primary cause of diminished cardiac output, heart rate also plays a role. In general, as blockade level increases, heart rate decreases. Bradycardia to rates less than 50 bpm is estimated to occur in 9–13% of spinal anesthetics. Risk factors for bradycardia include block height higher than T5, decreasing age, American Society of Anesthesiologists Physical Status I (ASA PS I), baseline heart rate less than 60 bpm, prolonged PR interval, and therapy with β-adrenergic blocking medications (Box 4-2).[8,10,18]

Heart rate is a complex function of the balance between sympathetic and parasympathetic tone, as well as cardiac filling, and reflex responses to decreased preload.

During spinal anesthesia restricted to low thoracic dermatomes or below, reflex increases in sympathetic activity above the level of blockade, as well as decreases in vagal activity tend to increase heart rate, helping to preserve cardiac output. High thoracic spinal anesthesia decreases sympathetic output to the heart. However, uninterrupted central sympathetic outflow may cause reflex vagal inhibition, so that sympathetic-parasympathetic nervous system balance, as assessed by heart rate variability[19] and spontaneous cardiac baroreflex activity[20] appears to be maintained in most patients during high thoracic spinal anesthesia. Both sympathetic and parasympathetic outflow decrease (Fig. 4-3).[19]

In a few patients, however, severe bradycardia associated with hypotension occurs following spinal anesthesia and

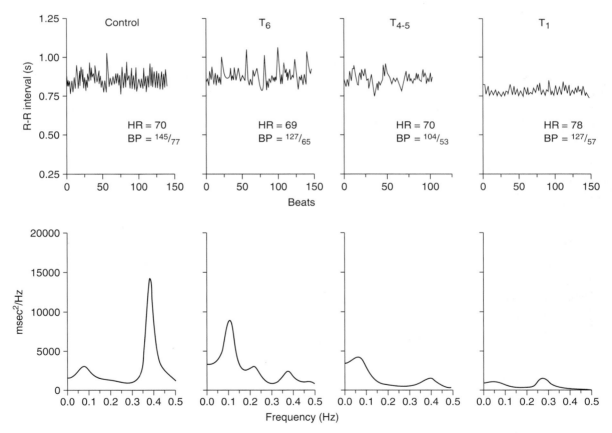

FIGURE 4-3. The sympathovagal effects of spinal anesthesia assessed by heart rate variability analysis. Tachygrams (upper panels) and the corresponding power spectra of the tachygrams (lower panels) obtained from an individual patient as spinal blockade progressed to the T1 dermatome. Total power (area under the curve) changes little between control and T6, but progressively decreases as the block level climbs to T1. The power spectral component between 0.05 and 0.1 Hz primarily reflects sympathetic activity and the component between 0.3 and 0.4 Hz reflects parasympathetic activity. HR = heart rate, BP = blood pressure. (*Used with permission from Introna R, Yodlowski E, Pruett J, et al. Sympathovagal effects of spinal anesthesia assessed by heart rate variability analysis. Anesth Analg 80:315, 1995.*)

this may be a result of an increase in parasympathetic activity relative to sympathetic activity. Patients who developed bradycardia and hypotension during spinal anesthesia had increased vagal activity as assessed by the slope of the spontaneous cardiac baroreflex, whereas patients who remained hemodynamically stable did not demonstrate this increased vagal activity.[20] Similarly, during recovery from total spinal anesthesia, bradycardia and hypotension were associated with increases in the high frequency component of heart rate variability, which is mediated by the parasympathetic nervous system.[21] Finally, in support of autonomic imbalance as an explanation of severe bradycardia, the aforementioned risk factors for bradycardia (e.g., decreasing age, slow resting heart rate, and prolonged PR interval) indicate a high degree of resting parasympathetic tone.

Several reflex responses to decreased preload may also play a role in severe bradycardia.[22] Intrinsic cardiac pacemaker activity slows with decreased stretch of myocardial cells. Also, cardiac and vena cava mechanoreceptors show increased activity during periods of decreased cardiac filling, and a vagal-mediated reflex bradycardia ensues. It is postulated that these reflex mechanisms serve a protective function, allowing for increased venous filling in cases of critical reductions in preload.[23,24] The decrease in venous return that occurs during lumbar epidural anesthesia enhances cardiac vagal tone, as decreased ventricular diameter on echocardiogram heralds the onset of bradycardia.[25,26] In sympathetically intact individuals, decreased preload and resulting hypotension would be expected to stimulate the cardiac baroreceptor reflex, which increases heart rate. The efferent limb of the baroreceptor reflex, however, is mediated through the sympathetic nervous system and therefore may not be functional in the presence of decreased sympathetic tone.

The incidence and treatment of severe bradycardia and cardiac arrest are discussed in Chap. 6. Closed claim analysis of cases of cardiac arrest following spinal anesthesia identified the administration of sedatives and a lack of appreciation of respiratory insufficiency and quick resuscitation as contributing factors.[27] Most of these cases, however, occurred before the widespread use of pulse oximetry and more recent data and case reports suggest that respiratory insufficiency does not play a role in these events.[22] In a review of spinal anesthesia-associated cardiac arrest, Pollard makes a convincing argument in favor of a circulatory etiology, arguing that asystole represents the far end of a spectrum that begins with bradycardia. If this is true, the risk factors for bradycardia noted above are also risk factors for cardiac arrest. Maintenance of adequate preload may be key in decreasing the incidence of bradycardia and asystole.[22]

Organ Blood Flow

Cerebral blood flow is maintained during high thoracic spinal anesthesia within the range of cerebral autoregulation. Coronary blood flow likewise appears minimally affected.[28] Any decrease in coronary blood flow that accompanies systemic hypotension appears to be offset by favorable effects on cardiac work, presumably due to decreases in preload, afterload, and heart rate. Coronary blood flow may increase in patients with severe coronary artery disease during thoracic epidural anesthesia, and, indeed, thoracic epidural anesthesia is associated with decreased infarct size during cardiac ischemia.[29,30] Also, motor and sympathetic blockade are associated with decreases in oxygen consumption, and thus would be expected to have a favorable effect on total body oxygen supply and demand.[31] Hepatic blood flow decreases in proportion to decreases in mean arterial pressure while renal blood flow, and consequently urine output, is well maintained within the range of autoregulation of the kidneys.[32]

Spinal Blockade Compared to Epidural Blockade

Differences exist between the cardiovascular effects of spinal and epidural blockade. Hypotension occurs less often during cesarean delivery performed under epidural compared to spinal anesthesia.[33] The reason(s) for this is not clear. The degree of sympathetic blockade which occurs during epidural anesthesia is equivalent to that which occurs during spinal anesthesia. In both cases, sympathetic blockade is probably not complete even after high thoracic blockade.[3–5,7] It has been postulated that sympathetic blockade occurs more slowly during epidural blockade than subarachnoid blockade, allowing time for the body's various compensatory mechanisms to offset negative hemodynamic consequences.

The absorption of local anesthetic and epinephrine from the epidural space may have direct cardiovascular effects. Moderate circulating levels of lidocaine, such as that occur during epidural anesthesia, appear to have a cardiac-stimulating effect. Heart rate and cardiac output increase, thereby partially offsetting some of the negative effects of sympathetic blockade.[34] Subconvulsant doses of mepivacaine result in a mild increase in cardiac output via increases in both heart rate and stroke volume.[35] Systemic absorption of epidural epinephrine (80–120 µg) results in predominantly β-adrenergic agonist effects: increasing heart rate, stroke volume and cardiac output, and lowering SVR. Compared to plain epidural lidocaine anesthesia or spinal anesthesia, the mean arterial pressure decreases to a greater extent when epinephrine is added to epidural lidocaine because the decrease in SVR outweighs the increase in cardiac output.[36,37]

PULMONARY EFFECTS

Lumbar and thoracic neuraxial anesthesia and analgesia have minor effects on respiratory physiology (Table 4-2; Fig. 4-4); these changes have minimal clinical consequences in otherwise healthy patients. During high thoracic epidural anesthesia, vital capacity (VC) decreased by 6%, total lung capacity (TLC) decreased by 3.5%, and the absolute value of forced expiratory volume in 1 s (FEV1) decreased by 5%.[38] The FEV1/FVC ratio remained unchanged. Tidal volume (TV) remains unchanged during high spinal and epidural anesthesia. However, peak expiratory flow rate (PEFR) decreased after spinal anesthesia in term pregnant patients[39] and peak expiratory pressure (PEP) was significantly reduced after epidural anesthesia with 2% lidocaine with epinephrine.[40] In contrast, PEP was only mildly reduced in patients randomized to receive epidural bupivacaine 0.5%. The negative change in peak expiratory flow increased as block height increased. These results are probably due to denser abdominal and thoracic motor blockade after epidural lidocaine with epinephrine compared to bupivacaine, and as sensory blockade height increases. Therefore, although high spinal and dense epidural anesthesia does not affect normal, at-rest respiratory function, the ability to cough and clear secretions may be adversely affected.

Gas exchange and ventilation/perfusion matching remained constant in elderly patients after lumbar epidural anesthesia.[41] Neither lumbar nor thoracic epidural anesthesia impaired the ventilatory response to hypercarbia or hypoxia in elderly patients.[42]

Bronchial tone at rest is predominantly vagal. Tone is also modulated by the sympathetic nervous system via β1- and β2-adrenergic receptors. There is theoretical concern that blockade of the sympathetic nervous system will result in increased airway resistance, particularly in individuals with baseline airway hyperreactivity. Groeben et al. administered high thoracic anesthesia (sensory blockade T8 to C5) to patients with chronic obstructive pulmonary disease.[43] Airway resistance was unchanged (Fig. 4-5), as were FEV1/FVC and functional residual capacity, and arterial blood gases (ABG). The authors concluded that high thoracic anesthesia is safe for patients with bronchospastic disease.

In the event of an inadvertent high or total spinal anesthetic, a patient may experience respiratory arrest and even lose consciousness. This is usually not secondary to phrenic nerve paralysis, or direct depression of the brain by local anesthetic. Instead, profound hypoperfusion of the brain and respiratory centers in the brainstem causes apnea and loss of consciousness. As soon as blood pressure is corrected the apnea usually resolves.

Table 4-2

Pulmonary Effects of High Thoracic Blockade

Parameter	Effect[a]
Lung volumes and spirometry	
VC, TLC, FEV1	↓ ≈ 5%
FEV1/FVC	→
TV	→
PEFR, PEP	↓[b]
Gas exchange, ABG	→
Ventilatory response to hypoxemia, hypercarbia	→
Bronchial tone	→

Abbreviation: FVC = forced vital capacity.
[a]↓ = decrease, → = no change, ↑ = increase.
[b]Depends on density of thoracic motor block.

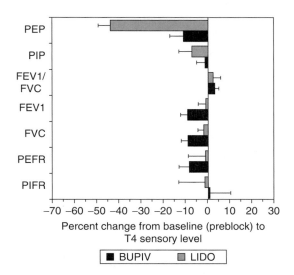

FIGURE 4-4. Percentage change in pulmonary function tests from baseline (preblock) to T4 sensory level during epidural anesthesia with lidocaine 2% with epinephrine 1:200,000 or bupivacaine 0.5%. Error bars indicated standard error of the mean (SEM). PEP = peak expiratory pressure, PIP = peak inspiratory pressure, FEV1 = forced expiratory volume in 1 s, FVC = forced vital capacity, PEFR = peak expiratory flow rate, PIFR = peak inspiratory flow rate, BUPIV = bupivacaine, LIDO = lidocaine. The top bar in each pair is lidocaine. (*Used with permission from Yun E, Topulos GP, Body SC, et al. Pulmonary function changes during epidural anesthesia for cesarean delivery. Anesth Analg 82:750, 1996.*)

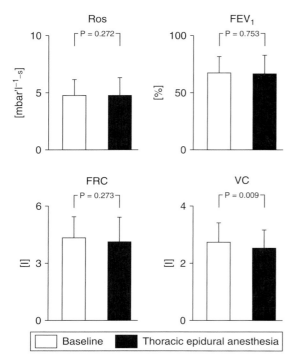

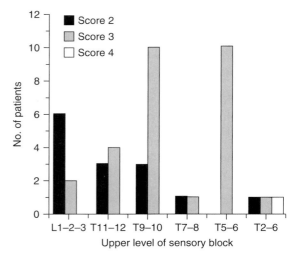

FIGURE 4-6. Maximum Ramsey scale sedation scores (5–45 min after intrathecal injection) corresponding to level of sensory blockade following bupivacaine spinal anesthesia (1 = anxious and agitated, 2 = cooperative and tranquil, 3 = drowsy but responsive to command, 4 = asleep but responsive to a glabellar tap, 5 = asleep with a sluggish response to tactile stimulation, 6 = asleep with no response). There was a significant correlation with maximum cephalad level of sensory blockade and level of sedation ($P < 0.05$). (*Used with permission from Gentili M, Huu PC, Enel D, et al. Sedation depends on the level of sensory block induced by spinal anaesthesia. Br J Anaesth 81:970, 1998.*)

FIGURE 4-5. Lung function at baseline and after high thoracic epidural anesthesia with bupivacaine 0.75% measured in the supine position. Data are mean ± SD. Ros = airway resistance, FRC = forced vital capacity, FEV1 = forced expiratory volume in 1 s, VC = vital capacity. Ros, FEV1/VC, and FRC were unchanged, while VC and FEV1 decreased by 7–9%. (*Used with permission from Groeben H. Effects of high thoracic epidural anesthesia and local anesthetics on bronchial hyperreactivity. J Clin Monit Comput 16:457, 2000.*)

The effects of neuraxial anesthesia/analgesia on postoperative pulmonary morbidity are discussed in detail in Chap. 16. Current evidence suggests that neuraxial anesthesia/analgesia is associated with improved pulmonary morbidity[44]; however, this remains controversial.

CENTRAL NERVOUS SYSTEM EFFECTS

Cerebral blood flow is autoregulated; thus blood flow to the central nervous system remains constant during neuraxial anesthesia unless there is profound hypotension (mean arterial pressure less than 55 mmHg in a normotensive individual).

Both animal and human studies support the notion that neuraxial blockade may have direct effects on level of consciousness. It is unlikely that sedation during neuraxial anesthesia is a result of clinical levels of local anesthetic in the brain, as rat studies found a decrease in the hyponotic dose of thiopental necessary to obtund certain reflex responses during bupivacaine spinal anesthesia despite undetectable levels of bupivacaine in the brain.[45] In humans, minimum alveolar concentration of sevoflurane (MAC) was decreased approximately 50% during high thoracic lidocaine epidural anesthesia.[46] Similarly, the median effective dose (ED_{50}) of propofol was reduced by 39% during bupivacaine spinal anesthesia to the midthoracic level.[47] Sedation scores were directly related to the extent of spinal blockade with high thoracic blockade producing more sedation than blockade limited to lumbar dermatomes (Fig. 4-6).[48] Taken together, these data suggest a decrease in afferent input to the reticular-activating system results in sedation during neuraxial anesthesia, and decreased requirements for supplemental systemic central nervous system depressants during neuraxial anesthesia.

The effects of neuraxial anesthesia on postoperative cognitive dysfunction are discussed in detail in Chap. 7. Neuraxial anesthesia may be associated with a decreased incidence of early postoperative cognitive dysfunction; however, the long-term outcome does not appear to be different compared to general anesthesia.

NEUROENDOCRINE EFFECTS

Surgical trauma induces local and systemic endocrine-metabolic and immune responses, often called the *stress response*.[49] The neuroendocrine system plays an important role in this response. The stress response may be influenced by the type of surgical anesthesia and postoperative analgesia. From a teleologic standpoint the stress response probably contributed to survival. In the modern era, however, these responses may be detrimental. Examples of undesirable effects of the stress response include postoperative ileus, hypercoagulability, and hyperglycemia. Therefore, the ability to influence the stress response by modulating anesthesia care or other aspects of perioperative care may affect outcome (see Chap. 16).

The stress response involves increases in plasma concentrations of catabolic hormones (e.g., adrenocorticotropic hormone [ACTH], cortisol, catecholamines, renin, angiotensin-II, aldosterone, glucagons, and interleukin-6 [IL-6]), as well as decreased concentrations of anabolic hormones (e.g., insulin and testosterone). These changes, in turn, influence metabolic pathways, and changes in fluid and electrolyte balance. The intensity and duration of the stress response is directly related to the degree and duration of surgical trauma. Afferent stimuli conducted through the somatosensory and sympathetic nervous systems play a major role in eliciting the neuroendocrine response to trauma. Humoral factors, released at the site of trauma, also play a role, both systemically and through stimulation of the afferent nervous system. Other factors, such as hemorrhage, acidosis, or hypoxemia, may also contribute to eliciting the stress response. Responses may occur over minutes to hours.

The mechanism(s) by which neuraxial anesthesia influence(s) these responses has not been thoroughly elucidated. Neuraxial blockade may contribute to a mitigated stress response by direct blockade of both efferent and afferent signals. There is evidence that local anesthetics directly block certain aspects of the stress response[49] and this may be an additional mechanism of epidural blockade-related alterations in the stress response. The effects on the stress response of spinal compared to epidural blockade, extent and duration of blockade, and specific local anesthetics require further study. Preliminary data suggest that suppression of the stress response is directly related to the extent and duration of neuraxial blockade. In contrast to neuraxial anesthesia, inhalational, intravenous, or balanced general anesthesia has minimal effects on the stress response, either alone or combined with neuraxial anesthesia. Epidural morphine compared to local anesthetics is less effective at blunting the stress response, even when pain control is similar.[50]

The initiation of the stress response during and after surgical procedures is evidenced by increases in serum levels of

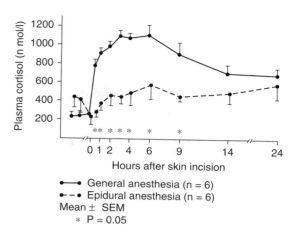

FIGURE 4-7. Intra- and postoperative plasma cortisol levels in patients undergoing abdominal hysterectomy under general (inhalational) or epidural (bupivacaine) anesthesia (followed by epidural postoperative analgesia). Plasma cortisol levels were increased at all times after the start of surgery in patients who received general, but not epidural anesthesia. (*Used with permission from Brandt MR, Fernandes A, Mordhorst R, et al. Epidural analgesia improves postoperative nitrogen balance. Br Med J 1:1106, 1978.*)

various stress hormones and an altered metabolic response. Spinal and epidural anesthesia attenuated, but did not inhibit, intraoperative increases in stress hormones such as glucose, cortisol, catecholamine, and ACTH (Fig. 4-7; Tables 4-3 and 4-4).[51–53] Epidural compared to general anesthesia resulted in an increase in tissue oxygenation.[54,55]

Neuraxial blockade may influence neuroendocrine function. Neuraxial blockade higher than T9-T10 is associated with decreased plasma epinephrine and norepinephrine concentrations. Catecholamine concentrations decrease in a direct relationship to extent of cephalad sensory blockade during tetracaine spinal anesthesia.[56] Plasma renin and vasopressin responses may be altered (see "Hypotension," earlier). High thoracic blockade may inhibit the normal response to acute hyperglycemia.[57] Aside from the direct and indirect effects of inhibition of the sympathetic nervous system, neuraxial blockade per se does not appear to have major effects on endocrine and metabolic function in general.

▶ Oxygen Consumption

Decreased oxygen consumption (VO_2) and extraction (VO_2/DO_2) accompany spinal anesthesia.[31] This decrease is likely a response to the reduction in metabolic demand due to reduced cardiac workload, muscle paralysis, and an overall decrease in metabolism. The overall effect of neuraxial

Table 4-3

Influence of Neuraxial Blockade on the Endocrine Response to Lower Abdominal or Lower Extremity Surgery

Plasma Hormone	Intraoperative Response[a]
Growth hormone	↓
ACTH	↓
ADH	↓
TSH	↓
β-Endorphin	↓
Cortisol	↓
Aldosterone	↓
Renin	↓
Epinephrine	↓
Norepinephrine	↓
Insulin	↘
Glucagon	→
T3 and T4	→

Abbreviation: ADH = antidiuretic hormone.
[a]↓ = decreased plasma concentration, → = no change in plasma concentration, ↘ = slight decrease in plasma concentration.
Modified with permission from Kehlet H. Modifications of responses to surgery by neural blockade. In: Cousins MJ, Bridenbaugh PO, eds, Neural Blockade in Clinical Anesthesia and Management of Pain, 3rd ed. Philadelphia, PA: Lippincott-Raven, 1998, p 129.

Table 4-4

Influence of Neuraxial Blockade on the Metabolic Response to Lower Abdominal or Lower Extremity Surgery

Metabolic Parameter	Response[a]
Plasma glucose	↓
Glucose tolerance	↑
Insulin clearance	↓
FFA and glycerol	↓
Plasma ketones	↓
Plasma lactate	↓
Liver glycogen	↓
Muscle amino acids	?
Nitrogen balance	?
Plasma acute phase proteins	→
IL-6	→
Oxygen consumption	?

Abbreviation: FFA = free fatty acids.
[a] ↑ = increased plasma concentration, ↓ = decreased plasma concentration, → = no change in plasma concentration, ↘ = slight decrease in plasma concentration, ? = no data.
Modified with permission from Kehlet H. Modifications of responses to surgery by neural blockade. In: Cousins MJ, Bridenbaugh PO, eds, Neural Blockade in Clinical Anesthesia and Management of Pain, 3rd ed. Philadelphia, PA: Lippincott-Raven, 1998, p 129.

anesthesia on oxygen consumption, however, may be influenced by altered thermoregulation and shivering, as these may increase oxygen consumption.

THERMOREGULATION

Hypothermia is associated with an increased incidence of myocardial ischemia and other cardiac morbidity, wound infection, impairment of coagulation, and blood loss.[58] Hypothermia appears to occur at a similar rate and with similar severity during major neuraxial anesthesia (spinal and epidural anesthesia) as compared to general anesthesia (Fig. 4-8).[59,60] Unfortunately, a recent survey revealed that a majority of practitioners do not routinely monitor temperature during spinal and epidural anesthesia.[61] When they do undertake temperature monitoring, practitioners most commonly monitor forehead skin temperature, which is an inaccurate estimate of core temperature, especially during spinal anesthesia.[61,62]

Perioperative heat balance results from a complex interplay of heat production, heat loss to the environment, distribution of heat from the core to the periphery, and thermoregulatory responses by the body to increase heat production and decrease loss during hypothermia.[63] The predominant cause of decreased core temperature during neuraxial anesthesia is redistribution of heat from the core to the periphery due to peripheral vasodilatation. During the first hour of anesthesia, redistribution accounts for 89% of core heat loss, and during the second and third hours, it accounts for 62% of core heat loss. Even after 3 h of anesthesia, redistribution remains the predominant cause of core hypothermia (Fig. 4-9).[64]

In addition to heat redistribution, a state of slight negative heat balance (heat loss exceeds heat production) exists (Fig. 4-9). Several factors contribute to the net negative heat balance. The metabolic rate is decreased below the level of blockade. Concurrently, heat loss to the environment (through radiation, conduction, convection, and evaporation) occurs.[63]

In addition, central thermoregulatory control is impaired during neuraxial anesthesia. Sympathetic and motor blockade

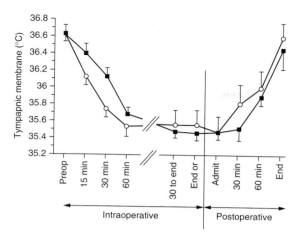

FIGURE 4-8. Tympanic temperature during epidural compared to general anesthesia. There were no differences between the two techniques at any time. ○ = general anesthesia, ■ = epidural anesthesia. (*Used with permission from Frank SM, Shir Y, Raja SN, et al. Core hypothermia and skin-surface temperature gradients. Epidural versus general anesthesia and the effects of age. Anesthesiology 80:502, 1994.*)

preclude vasoconstriction and shivering in the lower half of the body, but even in the upper half of the body, spinal and epidural anesthesia lower thermoregulatory vasoconstriction and shivering thresholds. Similar to general anesthesia, vasoconstriction and shivering, which counteract hypothermia, are triggered at lower core temperatures during spinal and epidural anesthesia.[65,66] This central thermoregulatory

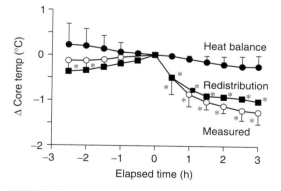

FIGURE 4-9. Contribution of decreased overall heat balance and internal redistribution of body heat to decrease the core temperature associated with epidural anesthesia. Induction of epidural anesthesia is identified as elapsed time 0. Redistribution contributed 80% to the entire 1.2 ± 0.3°C decrease in core temperature during the 3 h of anesthesia. *Values differing significantly from time 0. (*Used with permission from Matsukawa T, Sessler DI, Christensen R, et al. Heat flow and distribution during epidural anesthesia. Anesthesiology 83:961, 1995.*)

impairment is secondary to decreases in afferent input from the lower body. Epidural anesthesia also decreases the gain (incremental intensity increase) and maximum intensity of shivering because only the upper part of the body, above the blocked area, is participating in the shivering response.[67]

Patients randomized to spinal anesthesia versus epidural anesthesia for cesarean delivery cooled more rapidly during the first 30 min if they received spinal anesthesia.[68] After the first 30 min both groups cooled at the same rate. Overall, this resulted in lower core temperatures in patients in the spinal group. The incidence of shivering was similar in both groups, but shivering threshold was decreased to a greater extent, and shivering intensity was reduced in the spinal as compared to the epidural group. The authors concluded that thermoregulation was impaired more by spinal than epidural anesthesia. Other predictors of hypothermia include age and extent of blockade.[69] The decrease in shivering threshold that occurs after spinal blockade is proportional to the number of dermatomes blocked.[70]

Finally, when forced air rewarming is applied postoperatively, patients given spinal anesthesia rewarm to 36.5°C more quickly than patients given general anesthesia, presumably because vasodilation augments peripheral to core heat transfer.[71]

COAGULATION SYSTEM EFFECTS

Postoperative hypercoagulability is a known complication of major surgery. Alterations in both coagulation and fibrinolysis contribute to an overall increase in coagulability. Immobility and a decrease in lower extremity blood flow also contribute to an increased incidence of thrombotic events in the postoperative period. Neuraxial compared to general anesthesia is associated with a decreased risk of deep venous thrombosis and pulmonary embolism[72] and a decreased risk of venous and arterial thrombosis after vascular procedures.[73] The mechanism(s) by which neuraxial anesthesia modifies the risk of thromboembolic events may be due to efferent and afferent blockade or direct effects of local anesthetics. Neuraxial anesthesia may modify Virchow's triad (i.e., blood flow, vessel wall, and chemical composition of blood coagulation components) by influencing blood flow and the concentration and activity of coagulation components. Although there is clearly a salutary effect of neuraxial anesthesia on the incidence of postoperative thromboembolic complications, it is not clear whether this effect is dependent on the type and extent of anesthesia (epidural vs. spinal), the duration of neuraxial blockade (intraoperative only vs. intraoperative and postoperative), and specific neuraxial drugs (local anesthetics vs. opioids).

Data are conflicting as to the effects of neuraxial anesthesia on individual coagulation and fibrinolytic factors. For example, studies have shown both an increase in von Willebrand factor antigen[74] and no change.[75] Neuraxial blockade had no effect on postoperative platelet count,[74] but inhibited platelet aggregation.[76] Postoperative hypercoagulation as assessed by thromboelastography (TEG) was inhibited by combined epidural-general anesthesia compared to general anesthesia in vascular surgery patients (smaller α-angle and maximum amplitude [MA]).[73]

Estimated blood loss was decreased about 30% in studies comparing neuraxial to general anesthesia for hip replacement surgery (see Chap. 7) and prostatectomy. The mechanism is unclear, but may be related to a reduction in both arterial and venous pressure, leading to decreased venous oozing.[77]

GENITOURINARY EFFECTS

▶ Renal Effects

Innervation to the kidney originates from T10 to L1 (Fig. 1-20). Central neuraxial blockade may alter renal function by several mechanisms. These include indirect effects, via neuraxial anesthesia-induced changes in cardiac output and blood pressure or the endocrine system; or direct effects due to blockade of efferent nerves to the kidney, or altered reflex responses due to afferent nerve blockade.[78] In addition, the renal response to neuraxial blockade is probably dependent on the type and duration of surgical procedure, the type, duration, and extent of neuraxial blockade, and intra- and postoperative fluid management.

The alterations in renal function accompanying central neuraxial blockade are of little physiologic importance in the healthy individual due to a large reserve. As a result of autoregulation, renal blood flow, and subsequently, glomerular filtration rate, remain constant over a wide range of mean arterial pressures (50–150 mmHg). The kidney primarily achieves this homeostasis through afferent arteriolar dilation secondary to over-reabsorption of chloride ion and efferent arteriolar vasoconstriction through activation of the renin-angiotensin cascade. These two feedback mechanisms, which occur within minutes of alterations in mean arterial pressure, allow the healthy kidney to maintain a constant renal blood flow. Therefore, adequate preoperative hydration and maintenance of systemic blood pressure within the range of autoregulation act to preserve renal function in the presence of the hemodynamic response to neuraxial blockade. In the presence of hypotension (mean arterial pressure less than 50 mmHg), renal blood flow is deceased, but oxygen delivery is usually sufficient so that renal function returns to normal once blood pressure normalizes.

The renal effects of neuraxial anesthesia in patients with significant preexisting renal disease are not well studied. In a retrospective review of patients undergoing total hip replacement with hypotensive epidural anesthesia, 54 patients with chronic renal dysfunction were matched to patients with normal renal function with and without hypertension.[79] No patients developed acute renal dysfunction, although three patients with chronic renal dysfunction had worsening renal function 2–3 days after surgery associated with acute blood loss and ileus. The authors suggested that this anesthetic technique is appropriate for a patient with chronic renal dysfunction as long as intravascular volume is maintained.

▶ Bladder Effects

Urinary retention is a complication of both neuraxial and general anesthesia and is discussed in detail in Chaps. 6 and 11. The bladder is innervated by nerves traveling with the S2 through S4 nerve roots (Figs. 1-19 and 1-20). Sympathetic nerves to the bladder originate at the low thoracic/high lumbar level and parasympathetic innervation originates at the sacral level. Blockade of these nerve roots can directly affect detrusor muscle and urinary sphincter function (Box 4-3). The etiology of urinary retention is multifactorial; however, appropriate choice of local anesthetic and extent of blockade, choice of adjunct agents (e.g., short-acting opioids vs. long-acting opioids and

---

Box 4-3

Neuraxial Anesthesia Effects on Bladder Function

Local anesthetics

▶ Block efferent and afferent signals to/from the detrusor muscle

  ▶ Decrease sensation/urge to void

  ▶ Decrease detrusor contractility

▶ Block efferent and afferent signals to/from the internal uretheral sphincter[a]

▶ Block efferent and afferent signals to/from the external urethral sphincter

Opioids

▶ Decrease detrusor contractility

▶ Decrease sensation, urge to void

Epinephrine

▶ Potentiate actions of local anesthetics

[a]The male bladder neck has a more developed middle muscle layer compared to the female and this layer is richly innervated with adrenergic nerve fibers.

epinephrine), and intraoperative fluid administration may influence the incidence of urinary retention. The incidence also depends on patient age, type of surgical procedure, anxiety, and pain.[80] Recent evidence suggests that intrathecal opioids alter lower urinary tract function by decreasing detrusor contractility and decreasing the sensation, or urge to void.[81]

GASTROINTESTINAL EFFECTS

The sympathetic supply to the abdominal viscera originates from T6 to T12-L1 (Fig. 1-20), while the parasympathetic supply to the gut is via the vagus nerve (Fig. 1-19). Therefore, neuraxial blockade at the mid to low thoracic levels results in sympathetic denervation of the gut and parasympathetic dominance. The result is a contracted gut, relaxed sphincters, and normal peristalsis (Box 4-4).[82]

Results of human and animal studies of neuraxial anesthesia and intestinal blood flow are conflicting. For example, a study of bupivacaine thoracic epidural anesthesia in humans found decreased colonic serosal red cell flux and inferior mesenteric artery blood flow associated with epidural anesthesia-induced hypotension.[83] Another human study found an increase in intestinal blood flow associated with epidural anesthesia[84] and yet another study found no change.[85] These conflicting results may be a result of different levels of neuraxial blockade and dose of bupivacaine, blood pressure and fluid management differences between study groups, and technique of blood flow measurement (e.g., tonometry and Doppler flowmetry). In general, animal studies have found a favorable effect of epidural anesthesia on intestinal blood flow.[86,87]

There is theoretical concern that parasympathetic dominance and the enhanced gastrointestinal motility associated with neuraxial blockade could increase the risk of breakdown of surgical anastomosis. A retrospective study of factors associated with anastomotic leakage after esophagectomy found that thoracic epidural anesthesia was independently associated with a *decreased* risk of leakage (odds ratio 0.13, 95% confidence interval 0.02–0.71).[88] Recent systemic reviews suggest that epidural blockade is not associated with an increased risk of anastomotic breakdown.[89,90] The risk of a false negative result, however, was 67% and larger studies are needed to address this question.[89]

The overall effects of these changes on postoperative outcome, including the duration of postoperative ileus, are discussed in detail in Chaps. 9 and 16. A meta-analysis of studies comparing epidural to systemic analgesia and epidural local anesthetic to epidural opioid analgesia found that thoracic (not lumbar) epidural analgesia with local anesthetics has a beneficial effect on postoperative pain and recovery of bowel function after major abdominal surgery.[82] Further studies are required to determine the optimal extent of neuraxial blockade, drug combination (with and without opioids), and timing (start and end time) in order to most effectively influence gastrointestinal outcome.

▶ Liver Function

The effects of neuraxial anesthesia on hepatic function per se, or its effects on surgically induced alterations in hepatic function are not well studied. Midthoracic spinal anesthesia did not alter propranolol clearance or elimination half-life in a dog model.[91] Plasma glutathione S-transferase, a marker of hepatocellular injury, was not increased after spinal anesthesia, as long as profound hypotension was avoided.[92]

SUMMARY

Neuraxial blockade results in physiologic alternations of many organ systems. These changes are largely a result of the autonomic nervous system effects of neuraxial blockade and are dependent on the extent of sympathetic blockade. In general, lumbar blockade results in less physiologic perturbation than thoracic blockade. Additionally, there may be direct effects of local anesthetics and adjuvant drugs associated with epidural anesthesia. Direct effects after spinal anesthesia are unlikely because of the low drug doses necessary for spinal blockade. Physiologic alternations associated with neuraxial blockade may be beneficial to the patient and surgical outcome, or may represent a hazard to the patient unless carefully monitored and treated by the anesthetist. An understanding of these alterations is important to the safe practice and outcome of neuraxial anesthesia.

Box 4-4

Mechanisms by which Thoracic Epidural Anesthesia may Promote Gastrointestinal Motility

▶ Blockade of nociceptive afferent nerves

▶ Blockade of thoracolumbar sympathetic efferent nerves

▶ Unopposed parasympathetic efferent nerves

▶ Reduced need for postoperative opioids

▶ Increased gastrointestinal blood flow

▶ Systemic absorption of local anesthetics

Source: Used with permission from Steinbrook RA. Epidural anesthesia and gastrointestinal motility. Anesth Analg 86:837, 1998.

REFERENCES

1. Raymond SA, Glisson AJ. *Mechanisms of differential blockade.* Berlin, Heidelberg: Springer-Verlag, 1987.
2. Fink BR. Mechanisms of differential axial blockade in epidural and subarachnoid anesthesia. *Anesthesiology* 70:851, 1989.
3. Stevens RA, Beardsley D, White JL, et al. Does spinal anesthesia result in a more complete sympathetic block than that from epidural anesthesia? *Anesthesiology* 82:877, 1995.
4. Chamberlain DP, Chamberlain BD. Changes in the skin temperature of the trunk and their relationship to sympathetic blockade during spinal anesthesia. *Anesthesiology* 65:139, 1986.
5. Malmqvist LA, Bengtsson M, Bjornsson G, et al. Sympathetic activity and haemodynamic variables during spinal analgesia in man. *Acta Anaesthesiol Scand* 31:467, 1987.
6. Brull SJ, Greene NM. Time-courses of zones of differential sensory blockade during spinal anesthesia with hyperbaric tetracaine or bupivacaine. *Anesth Analg* 69:342, 1989.
7. Cook PR, Malmqvist LA, Bengtsson M, et al. Vagal and sympathetic activity during spinal analgesia. *Acta Anaesthesiol Scand* 34:271, 1990.
8. Carpenter RL, Caplan RA, Brown DL, et al. Incidence and risk factors for side effects of spinal anesthesia. *Anesthesiology* 76:906, 1992.
9. Hartmann B, Junger A, Klasen J, et al. The incidence and risk factors for hypotension after spinal anesthesia induction: An analysis with automated data collection. *Anesth Analg* 94:1521, 2002.
10. Tarkkila PJ, Kaukinen S. Complications during spinal anesthesia: A prospective study. *Reg Anesth* 16:101, 1991.
11. Arndt JO, Bomer W, Krauth J, et al. Incidence and time course of cardiovascular side effects during spinal anesthesia after prophylactic administration of intravenous fluids or vasoconstrictors. *Anesth Analg* 87:347, 1998.
12. Butterworth JFT, Austin JC, Johnson MD, et al. Effect of total spinal anesthesia on arterial and venous responses to dopamine and dobutamine. *Anesth Analg* 66:209, 1987.
13. Butterworth JFT, Piccione W Jr, Berrizbeitia LD, et al. Augmentation of venous return by adrenergic agonists during spinal anesthesia. *Anesth Analg* 65:612, 1986.
14. Rooke GA, Freund PR, Jacobson AF. Hemodynamic response and change in organ blood volume during spinal anesthesia in elderly men with cardiac disease. *Anesth Analg* 85:99, 1997.
15. Hopf HB, Schlaghecke R, Peters J. Sympathetic neural blockade by thoracic epidural anesthesia suppresses renin release in response to arterial hypotension. *Anesthesiology* 80:992, 1994.
16. Carp H, Vadhera R, Jayaram A, et al. Endogenous vasopressin and renin-angiotensin systems support blood pressure after epidural block in humans. *Anesthesiology* 80:1000, 1994.
17. Hohne C, Meier L, Boemke W, et al. ACE inhibition does not exaggerate the blood pressure decrease in the early phase of spinal anaesthesia. *Acta Anaesthesiol Scand* 47:891, 2003.
18. Liu S, Paul GE, Carpenter RL, et al. Prolonged PR interval is a risk factor for bradycardia during spinal anesthesia. *Reg Anesth* 20:41, 1995.
19. Introna R, Yodlowski E, Pruett J, et al. Sympathovagal effects of spinal anesthesia assessed by heart rate variability analysis. *Anesth Analg* 80:315, 1995.
20. Gratadour P, Viale JP, Parlow J, et al. Sympathovagal effects of spinal anesthesia assessed by the spontaneous cardiac baroreflex. *Anesthesiology* 87:1359, 1997.
21. Kimura T, Komatsu T, Hirabayashi A, et al. Autonomic imbalance of the heart during total spinal anesthesia evaluated by spectral analysis of heart rate variability. *Anesthesiology* 80:694, 1994.
22. Pollard JB. Cardiac arrest during spinal anesthesia: Common mechanisms and strategies for prevention. *Anesth Analg* 92:252, 2001.
23. Oberg B, Thoren P. Studies on left ventricular receptors, signalling in non-medullated vagal afferents. *Acta Physiol Scand* 85:145, 1972.
24. Oberg B, Thoren P. Increased activity in left ventricular receptors during hemorrhage or occlusion of caval veins in the cat. A possible cause of the vaso-vagal reaction. *Acta Physiol Scand* 85:164, 1972.
25. Baron JF, Decaux-Jacolot A, Edouard A, et al. Influence of venous return on baroreflex control of heart rate during lumbar epidural anesthesia in humans. *Anesthesiology* 64:188, 1986.
26. Jacobsen J, Sofelt S, Brocks V, et al. Reduced left ventricular diameters at onset of bradycardia during epidural anaesthesia. *Acta Anaesthesiol Scand* 36:831, 1992.
27. Caplan RA, Ward RJ, Posner K, et al. Unexpected cardiac arrest during spinal anesthesia: A closed claims analysis of predisposing factors. *Anesthesiology* 68:5, 1988.
28. Sivarajan M, Amory DW, Lindbloom LE, et al. Systemic and regional blood-flow changes during spinal anesthesia in the rhesus monkey. *Anesthesiology* 43:78, 1975.
29. Blomberg S, Emanuelsson H, Kvist H, et al. Effects of thoracic epidural anesthesia on coronary arteries and arterioles in patients with coronary artery disease. *Anesthesiology* 73:840, 1990.
30. Blomberg S, Emanuelsson H, Ricksten SE. Thoracic epidural anesthesia and central hemodynamics in patients with unstable angina pectoris. *Anesth Analg* 69:558, 1989.
31. Stanley GD, Pierce ET, Moore WJ, et al. Spinal anesthesia reduces oxygen consumption in diabetic patients prior to peripheral vascular surgery. *Reg Anesth* 22:53, 1997.
32. Butterworth J. Physiology of spinal anesthesia: what are the implications for management? *Reg Anesth Pain Med* 23:370, 1998.
33. Ng K, Parsons J, Cyna AM, et al. Spinal versus epidural anaesthesia for caesarean section. *Cochrane Database Syst Rev* 2:CD003765, 2004.
34. Bonica JJ, Berges PU, Morikawa K. Circulatory effects of peridural block. I. Effects of level of analgesia and dose of lidocaine. *Anesthesiology* 33:619, 1970.
35. Jorfeldt L, Lofstrom B, Pernow B, et al. The effect of local anaesthetics on the central circulation and respiration in man and dog. *Acta Anaesthesiol Scand* 12:153, 1968.
36. Bonica JJ, Kennedy WF Jr, Ward RJ, et al. A comparison of the effects of high subarachnoid and epidural anesthesia. *Acta Anaesthesiol Scand Suppl* 23:429, 1966.
37. Bonica JJ, Akamatsu TJ, Berges PU, et al. Circulatory effects of peridural block. II. Effects of epinephrine. *Anesthesiology* 34:514, 1971.
38. Sundberg A, Wattwil M, Arvill A. Respiratory effects of high thoracic epidural anaesthesia. *Acta Anaesthesiol Scand* 30:215, 1986.
39. Conn DA, Moffat AC, McCallum GD, et al. Changes in pulmonary function tests during spinal anaesthesia for caesarean section. *Int J Obstet Anesth* 2:12, 1993.
40. Yun E, Topulos GP, Body SC, et al. Pulmonary function changes during epidural anesthesia for cesarean delivery. *Anesth Analg* 82:750, 1996.
41. Reber A, Bein T, Hogman M, et al. Lung aeration and pulmonary gas exchange during lumbar epidural anaesthesia and in the lithotomy position in elderly patients. *Anaesthesia* 53:854, 1998.

42. Sakura S, Saito Y, Kosaka Y. The effects of epidural anesthesia on ventilatory response to hypercapnia and hypoxia in elderly patients. *Anesth Analg* 82:306, 1996.

43. Groeben H, Schwalen A, Irsfeld S, et al. Pulmonary sympathetic denervation does not increase airway resistance in patients with chronic obstructive pulmonary disease (COPD). *Acta Anaesthesiol Scand* 39:523, 1995.

44. Ballantyne JC, Carr DB, deFerranti S, et al. The comparative effects of postoperative analgesic therapies on pulmonary outcome: Cumulative meta-analyses of randomized, controlled trials. *Anesth Analg* 86:598, 1998.

45. Eappen S, Kissin I. Effect of subarachnoid bupivacaine block on anesthetic requirements for thiopental in rats. *Anesthesiology* 88:1036, 1998.

46. Hodgson PS, Liu SS, Gras TW. Does epidural anesthesia have general anesthetic effects? A prospective, randomized, double-blind, placebo-controlled trial. *Anesthesiology* 91:1687, 1999.

47. Tverskoy M, Fleyshman G, Bachrak L, et al. Effect of bupivacaine-induced spinal block on the hypnotic requirement of propofol. *Anaesthesia* 51:652, 1996.

48. Gentili M, Huu PC, Enel D, et al. Sedation depends on the level of sensory block induced by spinal anaesthesia. *Br J Anaesth* 81:970, 1998.

49. Hahnenkamp K, Herroeder S, Hollmann MW. Regional anaesthesia, local anaesthetics and the surgical stress response. *Best Pract Res Clin Anaesthesiol* 18:509, 2004.

50. Rutberg H, Hakanson E, Anderberg B, et al. Effects of the extradural administration of morphine, or bupivacaine, on the endocrine response to upper abdominal surgery. *Br J Anaesth* 56:233, 1984.

51. Lattermann R, Carli F, Wykes L, et al. Perioperative glucose infusion and the catabolic response to surgery: The effect of epidural block. *Anesth Analg* 96:555, 2003.

52. Lee TW, Grocott HP, Schwinn D, et al. High spinal anesthesia for cardiac surgery: Effects on beta-adrenergic receptor function, stress response, and hemodynamics. *Anesthesiology* 98:499, 2003.

53. Kouraklis G, Glinavou A, Raftopoulos L, et al. Epidural analgesia attenuates the systemic stress response to upper abdominal surgery: A randomized trial. *Int Surg* 85:353, 2000.

54. Treschan TA, Taguchi A, Ali SZ, et al. The effects of epidural and general anesthesia on tissue oxygenation. *Anesth Analg* 96:1553, 2003.

55. Kabon B, Fleischmann E, Treschan T, et al. Thoracic epidural anesthesia increases tissue oxygenation during major abdominal surgery. *Anesth Analg* 97:1812, 2003.

56. Pflug AE, Halter JB. Effect of spinal anesthesia on adrenergic tone and the neuroendocrine responses to surgical stress in humans. *Anesthesiology* 55:120, 1981.

57. Halter JB, Pflug AE. Effect of sympathetic blockade by spinal anesthesia on pancreatic islet function in man. *Am J Physiol* 239:E150, 1980.

58. Liu SS, McDonald SB. Current issues in spinal anesthesia. *Anesthesiology* 94:888, 2001.

59. Frank SM, Beattie C, Christopherson R, et al. Epidural versus general anesthesia, ambient operating room temperature, and patient age as predictors of inadvertent hypothermia. *Anesthesiology* 77:252, 1992.

60. Frank SM, Shir Y, Raja SN, et al. Core hypothermia and skin-surface temperature gradients. Epidural versus general anesthesia and the effects of age. *Anesthesiology* 80:502, 1994.

61. Frank SM, Nguyen JM, Garcia CM, et al. Temperature monitoring practices during regional anesthesia. *Anesth Analg* 88:373, 1999.

62. Cattaneo CG, Frank SM, Hesel TW, et al. The accuracy and precision of body temperature monitoring methods during regional and general anesthesia. *Anesth Analg* 90:938, 2000.

63. Sessler DI. Perioperative heat balance. *Anesthesiology* 92:578, 2000.

64. Matsukawa T, Sessler DI, Christensen R, et al. Heat flow and distribution during epidural anesthesia. *Anesthesiology* 83:961, 1995.

65. Kurz A, Sessler DI, Schroeder M, et al. Thermoregulatory response thresholds during spinal anesthesia. *Anesth Analg* 77:721, 1993.

66. Ozaki M, Kurz A, Sessler DI, et al. Thermoregulatory thresholds during epidural and spinal anesthesia. *Anesthesiology* 81:282, 1994.

67. Kim JS, Ikeda T, Sessler DI, et al. Epidural anesthesia reduces the gain and maximum intensity of shivering. *Anesthesiology* 88:851, 1998.

68. Saito T, Sessler DI, Fujita K, et al. Thermoregulatory effects of spinal and epidural anesthesia during cesarean delivery. *Reg Anesth Pain Med* 23:418, 1998.

69. Frank SM, El-Rahmany HK, Cattaneo CG, et al. Predictors of hypothermia during spinal anesthesia. *Anesthesiology* 92:1330, 2000.

70. Leslie K, Sessler DI. Reduction in the shivering threshold is proportional to spinal block height. *Anesthesiology* 84:1327, 1996.

71. Szmuk P, Ezri T, Sessler DI, et al. Spinal anesthesia speeds active postoperative rewarming. *Anesthesiology* 87:1050, 1997.

72. Rodgers A, Walker N, Schug S, et al. Reduction of postoperative mortality and morbidity with epidural or spinal anaesthesia: results from overview of randomised trials. *BMJ* 321:1493, 2000.

73. Tuman KJ, McCarthy RJ, March RJ, et al. Effects of epidural anesthesia and analgesia on coagulation and outcome after major vascular surgery. *Anesth Analg* 73:696, 1991.

74. Bredbacka S, Blomback M, Hagnevik K, et al. Per- and postoperative changes in coagulation and fibrinolytic variables during abdominal hysterectomy under epidural or general anaesthesia. *Acta Anaesthesiol Scand* 30:204, 1986.

75. Donadoni R, Baele G, Devulder J, et al. Coagulation and fibrinolytic parameters in patients undergoing total hip replacement: Influence of the anaesthesia technique. *Acta Anaesthesiol Scand* 33:588, 1989.

76. Henny CP, Odoom JA, ten Cate H, et al. Effects of extradural bupivacaine on the haemostatic system. *Br J Anaesth* 58:301, 1986.

77. Modig J, Karlstrom G. Intra- and post-operative blood loss and haemodynamics in total hip replacement when performed under lumbar epidural versus general anaesthesia. *Eur J Anaesthesiol* 4:345, 1987.

78. Kehlet H. Modification of responses to surgery by neural blockade. In: Cousins MJ, Bridenbaugh PO, eds, *Neural Blockade in Clinical Anesthesia and Management of Pain*, 3rd ed. Philadelphia, PA: Lippincott-Raven, 1998, p 129.

79. Sharrock NE, Beksac B, Flynn E, et al. Hypotensive epidural anaesthesia in patients with preoperative renal dysfunction undergoing total hip replacement. *Br J Anaesth* 96:207, 2006.

80. Mulroy MF. Hernia surgery, anesthetic technique, and urinary retention-apples, oranges, and kumquats? *Reg Anesth Pain Med* 27:587, 2002.

81. Kuipers PW, Kamphuis ET, van Venrooij GE, et al. Intrathecal opioids and lower urinary tract function: A urodynamic evaluation. *Anesthesiology* 100:1497, 2004.

82. Steinbrook RA. Epidural anesthesia and gastrointestinal motility. *Anesth Analg* 86:837, 1998.

83. Gould TH, Grace K, Thorne G, et al. Effect of thoracic epidural anaesthesia on colonic blood flow. *Br J Anaesth* 89:446, 2002.

84. Johansson K, Ahn H, Lindhagen J, et al. Effect of epidural anaesthesia on intestinal blood flow. *Br J Surg* 75:73, 1988.

85. Mallinder PA, Hall JE, Bergin FG, et al. A comparison of opiate- and epidural-induced alterations in splanchnic blood flow using intra-operative gastric tonometry. *Anaesthesia* 55:659, 2000.

86. Sielenkamper AW, Eicker K, Van Aken H. Thoracic epidural anesthesia increases mucosal perfusion in ileum of rats. *Anesthesiology* 93:844, 2000.

87. Adolphs J, Schmidt DK, Mousa SA, et al. Thoracic epidural anesthesia attenuates hemorrhage-induced impairment of intestinal perfusion in rats. *Anesthesiology* 99:685, 2003.

88. Michelet P, D'Journo XB, Roch A, et al. Perioperative risk factors for anastomotic leakage after esophagectomy: influence of thoracic epidural analgesia. *Chest* 128:3461, 2005.

89. Holte K, Kehlet H. Epidural analgesia and risk of anastomotic leakage. *Reg Anesth Pain Med* 26:111, 2001.

90. Fotiadis RJ, Badvie S, Weston MD, et al. Epidural analgesia in gastrointestinal surgery. *Br J Surg* 91:828, 2004.

91. Whelan E, Wood AJ, Shay S, et al. Lack of effect of spinal anesthesia on drug metabolism. *Anesth Analg* 69:307, 1989.

92. Ray DC, Robbins AG, Howie AF, et al. Effect of spinal anaesthesia on plasma concentrations of glutathione S-transferase. *Br J Anaesth* 88:285, 2002.

Contraindications To Neuraxial Anesthesia

Nollag O'Rourke
Khadija Khan
David L. Hepner

CHAPTER

5

INTRODUCTION

Neuraxial anesthesia and analgesia are widely used due to multiple benefits, including venous thromboembolism prevention, early discharge, improved comfort, and postoperative pain management. In addition, many patients desire to remain awake for their surgical procedures, and long-term analgesia with tunneled epidural catheters is becoming more common for chronic pain patients and for palliative care in the cancer patient.[1] Although serious complications after regional anesthesia are rare (less than 0.1%), epidural abscess and hematoma, radiculopathy, cauda equina syndrome, and even paraplegia have been attributed to neuraxial techniques (see Chap. 6).[2,3] Therefore, it is essential for the practitioner of regional anesthesia not only to understand the implications of neuraxial techniques on certain physiologic and pathologic conditions, but also to understand the implications of these processes on neuraxial techniques.

This chapter will review conditions that may pose relative contraindications to neuraxial techniques. Even though there are very few, if any, absolute contraindications to neuraxial techniques, there are many pathologic states for which the initiation of neuraxial anesthesia/analgesia is considered controversial. It is the goal of this chapter to review evidence-based medicine surrounding these controversies. A thorough understanding of the risks of neuraxial anesthesia in the presence of pathologic states is essential to the risk/benefit analysis for individual patients.

ABSOLUTE CONTRAINDICATIONS

▶ Coagulopathy

Disseminated intravascular coagulation (DIC) is characterized by widespread activation of coagulation as a result of a disease process, leading to intravascular (IV) deposition of fibrin, depletion of platelets and coagulation factors, and suppression of anticoagulants (i.e., antithrombin III, protein C and S, and tissue factor-pathway inhibitor).[4] In addition, fibrinolysis is impaired with the end result being severe bleeding, and thrombosis of small and midsize vessels.[4] Conditions associated with DIC are listed in Box 5-1.

Laboratory findings include a platelet count below $100 \times 10^3/mm^3$, prolonged prothrombin time (PT) and activated plasma thromboplastin time (aPTT), the presence of fibrin degradation products or D-dimers in plasma, and low levels of fibrinogen and antithrombin III.[4] Treatment includes the

---

Box 5-1

Conditions Associated with DIC

▶ Sepsis

▶ Trauma

▶ Organ destruction

　▶ Pancreatitis

▶ Malignancy

▶ Obstetric conditions

　▶ Placental abruption

　▶ Amniotic fluid embolism

　▶ HELLP syndrome

▶ Vascular abnormalities

　▶ Hemangioma

　▶ Aneurysm

▶ Liver failure

▶ Transfusion related

　▶ Massive transfusion

　▶ Transfusion reaction

correction of the underlying cause, and the use of blood products to replace coagulation components. Although neuraxial techniques are contraindicated in the setting of frank DIC, DIC may develop after an epidural catheter has been placed. Different views have been advocated as to when to remove these catheters. Some recommend the catheter be removed provided there is no evidence of bleeding around the epidural catheter insertion site,[5] while others have recommended that the epidural catheter remain in situ until the coagulopathy has resolved.[3] Of note, epidural hematomas have been reported to occur at the time of epidural catheter withdrawal in patients with altered coagulation.[6] No matter what approach is chosen, it is important to aggressively correct the coagulopathy by treating the underlying cause and administering blood products, perform thorough neurologic checks to detect early spinal cord compression from a spinal-epidural hematoma, and avoid injecting neuraxial local anesthetics as this may blunt early signs of cord compression.

▶ Septic Shock

Sepsis represents a generalized systemic inflammatory response to infection and results in failure of organ perfusion and widespread tissue injury. It is usually subdivided into *early hyperdynamic* and *late hypovolemic* phases.[7] The early hyperdynamic phase is characterized by hypotension, hypoperfusion, low systemic vascular resistance (SVR), and increased cardiac output.[7] The late phase is characterized by decreased cardiac output, increased peripheral vascular resistance, oliguria, and myocardial depression. A coagulopathy often develops with the presence of fibrin degradation products. An additional concern is the dissemination of IV pathologic organisms to the cerebrospinal fluid (CSF) or epidural space.

The decision to perform neuraxial anesthesia in a patient with frank sepsis must include a very thorough risk-benefit analysis. Neuraxial techniques are usually avoided unless there is a compelling reason to perform them. For example, the use of spinal anesthesia following failed intubation in a parturient with frank sepsis has been reported.[8] The authors concluded that if systemic infection is viewed as an absolute contraindication to neuraxial anesthesia, some patients may be inadvertently exposed to potentially greater risks associated with failed tracheal intubation.[8]

Should a regional technique be planned in the presence of systemic infection, prior treatment with an antibiotic is indicated, as this is likely to prevent seeding into the CSF. A slow-onset neuraxial technique is preferred, as worsening hypotension may occur due to relative dehydration and decreased SVR. Aggressive and early treatment with intravenous fluids and direct-acting vasopressors, such as neosynephrine and epinephrine, are essential to the management of patients with this life-threatening condition.

RELATIVE CONTRAINDICATIONS

▶ Septicemia

The Febrile Patient

Infection and fever are common clinical problems in fields such as obstetric anesthesia, where common bacterial and viral infections are often present at the time of a planned neuraxial technique. Controversy exists regarding the use of neuraxial anesthesia in bacteremic patients because of the possibility of "seeding" the epidural or subarachnoid space, with resultant meningitis or a spinal-epidural abscess (see Chap. 6). A single study in rats has explored the link among *Escherichia coli* bacteremia, spinal anesthesia, and meningitis.[9] Meningitis developed in bacteremic rats following dural puncture, but not in bacteremic rats that did not receive a dural puncture or healthy rats that received a dural puncture.[9] Of note, antibiotic treatment prior to the dural puncture prevented CSF infection in all bacteremic rats following dural puncture. However, the application of these results to the human clinical situation is unclear for a number of reasons. The dural tear was made with a 26-gauge needle that is relatively much larger in rats than humans, and the rats showed signs of overt septic shock. Septic shock is clinically not comparable to the low-grade fever due to bacteremia or viremia that commonly occurs during infections. In addition, *E. coli* is not usually the causative organism in documented infections associated with neuraxial anesthesia. Finally, local anesthetics have bacteriostatic properties, which may be clinically significant.

Human studies are even more conflicting. Although there are many reports of meningitis or epidural abscess after the administration of spinal, epidural, or combined spinal-epidural techniques,[10–12] there is no evidence for a cause and effect relationship. In some cases, identification of the causative bacteria suggests that lapses in sterile technique, rather than bloodborne pathogens, were probably responsible for the infection. Unfortunately, any serious neurologic complication is likely to be attributed to the neuraxial technique.

It is safe to conclude that there is no substantial evidence of a definite link between neuraxial techniques performed in the setting of bacteremia and the subsequent development of meningitis or epidural abscess. Indeed, a large retrospective study of over 10,000 patients who received spinal anesthesia found no single case of meningitis.[13] This finding is reassuring, given that many of these cases were in the obstetric setting where there is a high incidence of transient bacteremia coupled with a relatively high rate of maternal infection.[14] Data from the obstetric anesthesia literature support the safety of neuraxial techniques in the presence of an intra-amniotic infection.[15] Although most of the patients in this report did not receive antibiotics prior to the neuraxial technique, common practice supports the use of antibiotics prior to needle insertion.[16]

In summary, while there are no definite guidelines to aid the decision as to whether to perform neuraxial anesthesia in the febrile patient, most authorities would agree that it is safe to administer neuraxial anesthesia in the setting of mild bacteremia or maternal systemic infection following the initiation of antibiotic therapy. However, it seems wise to avoid neuraxial techniques in patients with clinical signs of frank sepsis.

Viral Infections

Herpes Simplex Virus. Herpes simplex virus 2 (HSV-2) is the most common sexually transmitted viral disease. An estimated 45 million people in the United States are affected.[17] Five to ten percent of women experience symptomatic recurrent genital herpes during pregnancy, and 25% of these will have an HSV-2 outbreak during the last month of pregnancy.[17]

There has been much concern and controversy surrounding the use of neuraxial anesthesia in patients with HSV-2 infection during pregnancy due to the theoretical risk of inoculation of virus into the central nervous system (CNS), resulting in meningitis or encephalitis. Since primary infection causes viremia, and may present with constitutional symptoms and genital lesions, neuraxial anesthesia during a primary infection could potentially transmit viral particles from the mother's blood into the CNS. Of note, cauda equina syndrome is an uncommon complication of primary HSV-2 infection. Secondary HSV-2 infection manifests as recurrent genital lesions in the absence of constitutional symptoms, and there are no viral antigens in the blood due to the presence of maternal antibodies. There are no reports of septic or neurologic complications related to neuraxial anesthesia in the presence of secondary infection.[18] Although it appears prudent to avoid neuraxial anesthesia in the setting of primary HSV-2, most patients have a silent primary infection followed years later by genital lesions. Occasionally, it may be difficult to differentiate between primary and secondary infections (Table 5-1). Most anesthesiologists feel comfortable initiating neuraxial anesthesia in patients with genital lesions without constitutional symptoms.

Varicella Zoster Virus. The primary infection commonly known as *chicken pox* or *varicella* is characterized by fever, malaise, and a maculopapular rash that becomes vesicular. In children the infection is usually benign and self-limited. Although only 2% of all cases occur in adulthood, severe complications of primary varicella zoster virus (VZV) infection, such as encephalitis and pneumonitis, are more common in adults.[19] With reactivation, VZV produces a vesicular erythematous rash localized to one or more dermatomes that is known as herpes zoster. Postherpetic neuralgia, characterized by chronic pain, develops in many patients following reactivation of VZV and is not related to neuraxial techniques (see Chap. 17).

Table 5-1

Comparison of Primary and Recurrent HSV-2 Infections

	Primary Infection	Recurrent Infection
Immunology	No prior antibodies	Antibodies present from prior genital outbreaks
Symptoms	Malaise, myalgia, and fevers more likely to be present	Less common and severe
Genital lesions	Appear 2–14 days following constitutional symptoms or may not appear at all	Always present
Viral shedding	Present even in the absence of symptoms	Less likely
Neonatal risk	Very high	Low
Treatment	Acyclovir markedly reduces viral shedding	Acyclovir may be beneficial
Neuraxial techniques	Potential for inoculation into the CNS	No contraindication Avoid the lesion

The presence of active lesions at the site of insertion is considered a relative contraindication to neuraxial techniques. Controversy exists, however, if no active lesions occur at the entry site. Because VZV infection is uncommon in adulthood, no evidence-based anesthesia guidelines exist, although several recommendations can be found in the literature. Patients presenting with acute cutaneous VZV may be viremic for up to 2 weeks after the onset of the syndrome, and although caution should be exercised, neuraxial compared to general anesthesia is likely to reduce the risk of varicella pneumonia should anesthesia be needed.[20] The CNS is the most common site of involvement besides the skin, and acute cerebellar ataxia, encephalitis, aseptic meningitis, and Guillain-Barré syndrome have been reported.[20] Therefore, should neuraxial anesthesia be used in the presence of VZV, meticulous neurologic examination should be performed and early antiviral therapy should be considered.[20] The use of a small bore pencil-point needle may be advantageous because of the potential advantage of introducing fewer virus particles into the CNS.

Human Immunodeficiency Virus. The human immunodeficiency virus (HIV) pandemic has spread to every country in the world and has infected 56 million people worldwide, including 20 million people who have already died. An estimated 1.1 million people in the United States have been infected with HIV, with women being the fastest growing group of new cases. Women of childbearing age constitute a large percentage of these new cases.[21] It was initially thought that performance of a neuraxial technique would risk the spread of the disease to the CNS. HIV, however, is a neurotrophic virus with low infectivity and early spread to the CNS, and several studies have shown that neuraxial anesthetic techniques do not accelerate the progression to the CNS.[22] It is now well accepted that HIV infection does not contraindicate the use of neuraxial anesthesia provided that a thorough neurologic and hematologic evaluation has been performed (Box 5-2). Hematologic pathology is common in patients with HIV. The estimated incidence of anemia is 75%. Thrombocytopenia, defined as platelet count less than $100 \times 10^3/mm^3$, is also common with a reported incidence of 5–15% (see "Thrombocytopenia," below).[23] Careful physical examination, documentation of preexisting neurologic deficits, and careful monitoring for the resolution of blockade should be undertaken. Patients should also be evaluated for the presence of other opportunistic or sexually transmitted infections. Current or prior use of HIV-related therapies may have implications for the performance of neuraxial techniques (Box 5-3).

Strict attention to aseptic technique is of utmost importance because of the state of immunosuppression. To date, no studies have documented immunosuppressive changes or infectious sequelae as a result of neuraxial anesthesia.

Box 5-2

Neuraxial Anesthetic Implications of HIV

- Blood/body fluid exposure
  - Potential for acquiring disease
  - Concurrent sexually transmitted disease
- Peripheral neuropathy
  - Thorough neurologic examination
- Substance abuse
  - Medication adjustment
- AIDS-related dementia
  - Informed consent may be difficult
  - Mental status changes with opioids
- Cardiomyopathy
  - Potential for cardiovascular collapse
- Nephropathy
  - Potential for renal failure and fluid overload
- Hematologic disease
  - Thrombocytopenia and bleeding diathesis
- Antiviral medications
  - Drug interactions

Box 5-3

Neuraxial Anesthetic Implications of Antiretroviral Drug Therapy

- Potential for drug interactions
- Thrombocytopenia
  - Potential contraindication for regional anesthesia
- Neutropenia
  - Potential for opportunistic infections during the performance of neuraxial techniques
- Electrolyte abnormalities
  - Electrocardiogram abnormalities
- Hepatic failure
  - Drug-dose adjustment
- Peripheral neuropathy
  - Thorough neurologic check prior to neuraxial techniques
- Cardiac arrhythmias
  - May be worsened with profound sympathectomy

However, localized and deep track infections have been reported in HIV-infected patients with chronic indwelling epidural catheters used for pain management.[24] Complications that occur as a result of neuraxial techniques may also present a challenge for the practitioner of neuraxial anesthesia. For example, should headache occur after a neuraxial technique, diseases commonly present in immunosuppressed HIV patients should be considered. If a postdural puncture headache is high in the differential diagnosis, initial therapies should be conservative, including bed rest, analgesics, oral hydration, and caffeinated products. Should this management fail, an epidural blood patch can be considered. CNS HIV infection occurs early in the disease, and, therefore, an epidural blood patch is unlikely to alter the course of CNS infection. The absence of adverse events following an epidural blood patch in HIV-positive patients has been reported.[25,26] Therefore, alternatives such as the use of extradural saline or heterologous HIV-negative blood do not seem indicated.[25]

▶ Preexisting Central Nervous System Disease

Multiple Sclerosis

Multiple sclerosis (MS) is the most common autoimmune inflammatory demyelinating disease of the CNS, and primarily affects women of Northern European decent who are of childbearing age. Two general patterns of MS have been identified: an exacerbating remitting form in which attacks appear abruptly and resolve over several months, and a chronic progressive pattern.[27] Common symptoms of MS include sensory disturbance in the limbs, visual loss, motor weakness, diplopia, gait disturbance, and bladder and bowel dysfunction. There is currently no curative treatment for MS. Immunosuppressive therapies, such as corticosteroids, may hasten recovery from a relapse but do not alter the overall course of the disease. Human interferon (IFN) beta is the first therapeutic agent to convincingly reduce the MS relapse rate and retard disability.[28]

Historically, central conduction blockade, especially spinal anesthesia, has been implicated in the exacerbation of MS. It has been speculated that local anesthetic neurotoxicity may be more likely in demyelinated nerves. However, these studies are very small, and a cause and effect relationship is not proven.[29] Theoretically, epidural anesthesia may be less of a risk, as concentrations of local anesthetic in the white matter of the spinal cord are lower than with spinal anesthesia.[30]

Many studies have supported the safe use of epidural analgesia in patients with MS. Neither breast-feeding nor epidural analgesia appear to have an adverse effect on the rate of relapse or on the progression of disability in MS.[31]

Relapse rates were similar in pregnant women who received epidural analgesia for vaginal delivery compared to those who received local infiltration.[30] Interestingly, all the women who had postpartum relapses received epidural bupivacaine concentrations greater than 2.5 g/mL. The authors suggested that higher concentrations, or prolonged administration of epidural analgesia, where local anesthetic concentration in the CSF increases, may lead to an increase in relapse rate.[30]

Although there are few reports on the use of spinal anesthesia in patients with MS, its use can be considered with low doses of local anesthetic given the relatively short duration of surgery in patients receiving spinal anesthesia, the avoidance of repeated doses of local anesthetic, and the low CSF concentration. In addition, the use of spinal anesthesia has been noted to improve bladder spasticity present in some patients with MS.[32] Several issues are important to remember when considering the use of neuraxial techniques in patients with MS, including a preanesthetic evaluation of the existing neurologic symptoms and the sparing of local anesthetic dose with the addition of opioids (Box 5-4). In addition, patients should be counseled that the effect of neuraxial analgesia and anesthesia on the course of MS has not been rigorously studied and is, therefore, largely unknown.

Neural Tube Defects: Spina Bifida

The incidence of neural tube defects (NTD) is highly variable and depends on ethnic and geographic factors, with the highest rates found in Ireland, Great Britain, Pakistan, India, and Egypt. The overall incidence of NTD in the United States is 1 per 1000 births, second only to cardiac malformations as the

---

Box 5-4

Neuraxial Anesthetic Considerations in MS

▶ Document preexisting neurologic disease
▶ Informed consent
   ▶ Increased relapse rate postpartum
   ▶ Unknown effect of anesthetic
▶ No contraindication to neuraxial techniques
   ▶ Opioid use in neuraxial techniques
   Minimize local anesthetic use
   Minimal motor blockade
▶ Spinal anesthesia can be used
   Low doses of local anesthetic
   Avoid repeated doses of local anesthetics
   Decrease muscle spasticity

most prevalent congenital anomaly, and results from failure of the neural arch to close normally between 25 and 28 days after conception.[33] Spina bifida is a condition which results when the bony vertebrae fail to enclose the neural elements in the bony canal, and there are varying degrees of failed closure.

Spina bifida cystica consists of myelomeningocele and meningocele. *Myelomeningocele,* the most severe form of spina bifida, results from herniation of the meninges, and consists of the neural elements going through the defect in the bony vertebrae. The protruding membranous sac contains meninges, CSF, nerve roots, and dysplastic spinal cord. In some cases there may be no membrane, but only a fully exposed section of the spinal cord. Disturbances during earlier stages of neural tube formation, canalization, and retrogressive differentiation may result in lesions that may be covered by skin. Patients with myelomeningocele always exhibit some degree of paralysis and loss of sensation below the damaged vertebrae. The amount of disability depends largely on vertebral level and the degree of nerve damage. The majority of patients with myelomeningocele also have hydrocephalus and Chiari II malformations.[34]

The rarest type of spina bifida, *meningocele,* involves only the meninges, which protrude through the vertebral defect. The meninges form a fluid-filled sac that is usually covered with skin, the spinal cord is normal, and affected people are usually asymptomatic. Spina bifida occulta is defined as failure of closure of the neural arch without herniation of the meninges or neural tissues. Usually spina bifida occulta is a minor defect involving one vertebra, typically L5-S1. It occurs so commonly in the general population (5–36%) that it is considered a normal variant.[35] In a small number of people, spina bifida occulta is more extensive with either a bigger vertebral split, or the involvement of two or more vertebrae. There may be visible signs on the skin, such as a mole or nevus (i.e., birthmark), a dimple or sinus, or a patch of hair. This type of spina bifida occulta is significant, as there may be associated scoliosis or other neurologic abnormalities that should be evaluated.

Congenital tethering or stretching of the spinal cord occurs when the cord is attached to an abnormal structure in the lumbar spine. Abnormal fixation of the spinal cord results in traction on the neural tissue, which, in turn, leads to ischemia and progressive neurologic deterioration. There is a thick filum terminale or low-lying conus medullaris. The conus medullaris terminates at a level below the L1-L2 intervertebral space. A widened or more caudal termination of the subarachnoid space can be associated with this abnormality. Spinal cord tethering occurs in almost all cases of spina bifida cystica and in some cases of spina bifida occulta.[36]

Management of Patients with Spina Bifida Oculta.
Neuraxial anesthesia for patients with spina bifida occulta does not usually pose any problems as in most cases the underlying anomaly is limited to a single vertebrae with normal underlying neural structures. Also, the most common site for spina bifida occulta lesions is the L5-S1 vertebral level, which is below the insertion site for most epidural or spinal procedures. If a neuraxial block is performed at the level of an occulta lesion, there is an increased risk of dural puncture due to the absence of lamina and variable formation of the ligamentum flavum at the site.[37] For the same reasons, an epidural injection at the level of an occulta lesion may result in a patchy or higher than normal blockade. Radiologic investigation can be performed for patients with spina bifida occulta and overlying superficial lesions, in order to determine if an underlying cord abnormality is present. If plain film abnormalities are present, magnetic resonance imaging (MRI) is the single most effective imaging modality for both initial diagnosis and preoperative evaluation.

Management of Patients with Spinal Bifida Cystica.
Patients with severe spina bifida cystica may have neuropathic bladder or more severe urologic problems, abnormal pelvic growth, and differential spinal growth causing scoliosis and resulting in restrictive lung disease. They may also have sensory and motor impairment below the level of the lesion. Therefore, evaluation of these patients prior to attempting a neuraxial technique should include the determination of the level of the lesion, whether scoliosis and kyphosis are present, residual function below the level of the lesion, and whether corrective surgery has been performed, including shunt placement. In addition, respiratory function, especially if severe lumbar or thoracic vertebral deviations are present, and renal function should be evaluated and imaging studies obtained (Box 5-5). A thorough discussion with the patient is recommended, providing informed consent to any neuraxial technique and a realistic expectation of achievable analgesia. A deficiency of the dorsal interspinous layer of ligaments may complicate localization of the epidural space when the loss-of-resistance technique is used.[38] Similar to patients with spina bifida occulta with underlying cord abnormalities, patients with spina bifida cystica have an increased risk of dural puncture, especially when anesthesia is initiated at the level of the defect. Therefore, it is best to use an intervertebral space below the level of the lesion or corrective surgery, as this will decrease the risk of injury because of a tethered spinal cord with a low-lying conus medullaris. There is also an increased risk of abnormal spread of local anesthetic due to alteration in structure of the epidural space, resulting in either excessive cranial or inadequate caudal spread. Neuraxial anesthesia behaves unpredictably even after successful neonatal lumbosacral meningocele repair; the onset may be faster, and a lower dose of analgesic drug may be necessary.[39] Additional methods of pain relief, such as systemic opioids or pudendal block, have also been recommended for inadequate caudal blockade.[39]

Neuraxial Anesthetic Considerations in Patients with Spina Bifida Cystica

▸ Evaluate the level of the lesion
  ▸ Motor and sensory deficits
  ▸ Residual function below the affected level
▸ Evaluate for evidence of scoliosis or kyphosis
  ▸ Examination of the back
  ▸ Imaging studies
  ▸ Prior corrective surgery
▸ Evaluate pulmonary function
  ▸ Restrictive lung disease
▸ Evaluate renal function
▸ Provide adequate informed consent
  ▸ More difficult to achieve analgesia
  ▸ Increased incidence of complications

Intracranial Neoplasm

Brain tumors encompass neoplasms that originate in the brain itself (primary brain tumors) or metastasize to the brain (secondary brain tumors). Gliomas account for over 80% of primary CNS malignancies. Brain metastases are the most common form of intracranial tumor, accounting for more than one-half of brain tumors in the adult.[40] The presence of an intracranial neoplasm has serious implications for the anesthetic management of labor and delivery. In patients with an intracranial mass lesion and raised intracranial pressure (ICP), CSF pressure may rise with painful contractions and increase the risk of brain herniation. The provision of adequate pain relief during labor reduces the risk to the mother by providing a pain-free second stage, and allowing for an instrumental vaginal delivery in order to avoid pushing. Alternatively, cesarean delivery may be appropiate.[41] The choice of anesthesia, however, is controversial (Table 5-2). Lumbar puncture is usually contraindicated in patients with increased ICP or space-occupying lesions because lumbar CSF drainage can increase the pressure gradient between the supratentorial and infratentorial compartments and thus result in rapid herniation.[42] Epidural anesthesia may also be dangerous in patients with space-occupying lesions, not only because of the risks associated with accidental dural puncture, but also because epidural drug and fluid injection can increase ICP.[43] Despite these risks, there are reports of successful use of epidural anesthesia in parturients with intracranial neoplasms.[44] Spinal anesthesia has also been described for emergency cesarean delivery in a patient with symptoms of raised ICP due to a glioblastoma.[45] The rationale is that small bore, pencil-point needles cause minimal to no CSF leakage, even when used in association with mildly increased ICP. Although some anesthesiologists may advocate general anesthesia because of the risk of brain herniation, general anesthesia is also not without risks. Increased ICP may occur with induction and intubation, and emergence. Therefore, a very careful risk-benefit analysis should be conducted prior to deciding on a particular anesthetic technique.

Hydrocephalus with Shunt

Hydrocephalus may be congenital and present at birth, or it may be acquired and arise later in life. Congenital hydrocephalus can be due to blockage at the aqueduct (aqueductal stenosis), congenital anomalies such as a Chiari malformation or Dandy Walker malformation, or secondary to an inflammatory process when premature birth causes bleeding within the brain. The treatment for this condition is placement of a lumboperitoneal, ventriculoperitoneal, or ventriculoatrial shunt.

Table 5-2

Anesthetic Considerations of Patients with Increased ICP

Neuraxial Anesthesia	General Anesthesia
May attenuate the increased ICP that results from painful uterine contractions	Induction, airway manipulation, and emergence may increase ICP
Dural breach may increase the supratentorial-infratentorial pressure gradient and result in brain herniation	Some drugs such as succinylcholine may increase ICP
Epidural drug injection may increase ICP	

Neuraxial anesthesia has been safely used for the management of patients with a shunt without complications.[46,47] Although some have argued that radiologic studies should be performed in order to ascertain the exact location of the shunt prior to initiating a neuraxial technique,[48] others have performed neuraxial techniques safely without the aid of imaging studies.[46] There are no reported cases of trauma to the spinal portion of a lumboperitoneal shunt. Shunts are typically located at a low intervertebral space (L3-L4 or L4-L5) and the tubing runs laterally to the peritoneum.[46] Common sense dictates the insertion of the needle at an intervertebral space below or above the scar, depending on the location of the shunt. There is also concern that drugs in the CSF may leak into the atrium or peritoneum, depending on the shunt type.[47] Therefore, theoretically, a single-shot spinal is not the preferred neuraxial technique. Because of the risk of shunt infection, it has been recommended that prophylactic antibiotics be administered prior to initiating neuraxial techniques.[47]

Symptoms of shunt failure, such as headache and increased ICP, may be confused with postdural puncture headache.[49] Safe and successful performance of an epidural blood patch has been reported in a patient with a lumboperitoneal shunt.[47] Although there are no reported cases of patients with third ventriculostomy receiving neuraxial techniques, neuraxial anesthesia is not contraindicated and the decision as to the type of anesthesia should be based on surgical considerations and the neurologic status of the patient.[50]

▶ Neuraxial Anesthesia and Anticoagulation

Anticoagulation increases the risk of spinal-epidural hematoma after neuraxial anesthesia (see Chap. 6). Neuraxial anesthesia in the presence of anticoagulation has been addressed by a consensus conference of the American Society of Regional Anesthesia and Pain Medicine (ASRA) and this information is summarized later.[51] As always, the decision to perform neuraxial anesthesia in the presence of anticoagulation should use a risk-benefit analysis. If the risk level warrants it, frequent lower extremity neurologic assessment should be performed during neuraxial anesthesia/analgesia and for a period of time after catheter removal. Consideration should be given to using low concentration local anesthetic techniques, when possible, to facilitate neurologic assessment.

Antiplatelet Drugs

Platelets are instrumental in primary hemostasis, leading to a platelet plug, and providing the membrane surface on which activation of the clotting cascade occurs. Therefore, any platelet abnormality secondary to disease or medication has the potential to lead to significant bleeding complications, including a spinal-epidural hematoma. There are multiple antiplatelet agents including aspirin (ASA), nonsteroidal anti-inflammatory drugs (NSAIDs), thienopyridines (ticlopidine and clopidogrel), and GP IIb-IIIa receptor antagonists (abciximab, eptifibatide, and tirofiban).

ASA and NSAIDs impair platelet aggregation by inhibiting cyclooxygenase (COX) and preventing the formation of thromboxane, which is a potent platelet aggregator (Table 5-3). While the action of ASA on platelet COX is permanent, lasting the life span of the platelet (7–10 days), the effect of other NSAIDs is shorter (3 days). COX consists of two different enzymes: COX-1 is a constitutive enzyme and COX-2 is an inducible isoform.[52] COX-1 is present in platelets, whereas COX-2 is not. The anti-inflammatory and analgesic properties of the COX-2 inhibitors, celecoxib, and valdecoxib, are attributed to the decreased synthesis of prostaglandin H_2 by selectively inhibiting COX-2.[52]

The thienopyridines exert their antiplatelet effect by irreversible inhibition of adenosine diphosphate (ADP). These drugs inhibit platelet fibrinogen binding and subsequent platelet-platelet interaction.[51,53] Ticlopidine has a longer effect on platelet function and should be stopped 10–14 days prior to surgery, whereas clopidogrel should be discontinued 7 days prior to surgery.[51]

Platelet GP IIb-IIIa receptor antagonists inhibit platelet aggregation by interfering with the binding of fibrinogen and von Willebrand factor (vWF) to GP IIb-IIIa receptor sites on activated platelets.[54] The platelet function returns to normal about 8 h after discontinuation of eptifibatide and tirofiban, and 24–48 h after abciximab.[51]

Neuraxial analgesia performed in the presence of ASA and NSAIDs alone is considered safe, as the risk of spinal-epidural hematoma in these patients is low.[51] A retrospective analysis of 61 case reports of epidural hematoma and neuraxial techniques found that most cases (68%) occurred in patients with impaired coagulation.[3] Three cases followed neuraxial techniques performed in the presence of a single antiplatelet agent, such as ASA, ticlopidine, or indomethacin. However, no specific details were given about each individual case.[3] The concurrent use of antiplatelet therapy and other medications that affect clotting may increase the risk of bleeding and, therefore, caution should be exercised.

Thienopyridines and neuraxial anesthesia should be approached with more caution. These agents, unlike ASA and NSAIDs, also affect primary platelet aggregation to the subendothelium, thus preventing hemostatic plug formation and the effects on platelet function are irreversible.[51] Therefore, the use of neuraxial techniques should be avoided until there is platelet recovery. Platelet GP IIb-IIIa receptor antagonists block the final common pathway to

Table 5-3

Neuraxial Techniques and Antiplatelet Agents

Antiplatelet Drug	Mechanism of Action	Anesthetic Management
ASA	Irreversible inhibition of platelet COX	No contraindications Avoid combination of antiplatelet agents
NSAIDs	Inhibit platelet COX Prevents thromboxane A2 synthesis	No contraindications Avoid combination of antiplatelet agents
COX-2 inhibitors	Selective inhibition of COX-2	No contraindications
Thienopyridines Clopidogrel Ticlopidine	Inhibit ADP-mediated platelet aggregation	Avoid for 7 days Avoid for 14 days
Glycoprotein IIb-IIIa receptor antagonists Abciximab Eptifibatide Tirofiban	Inhibit binding of vWF and fibrinogen to receptor sites	Avoid for 8 h Avoid for 8 h Avoid for 2 days

platelet aggregation for a short period of time (hours) and neuraxial techniques are contraindicated during this period.

Heparin

Heparin is a negatively charged, water-soluble acid. Its anticoagulant effect is due to a unique pentasaccharide sequence. The pentasaccharide binds to antithrombin III and accelerates the inactivation of factors II, IX, X, XI, and XII (Fig. 5-1). While long saccharide chains are needed to inhibit factor II, those with less than 18 saccharide units inhibit factor X.[55] The biological half-life of heparin is dose and molecular size dependent and ranges from 1 to 2 h for intravenous unfractionated heparin, and from 3 to 6 h for low molecular weight heparins (LMWH).[55] Unfractionated heparin's anticoagulant effect is monitored with the aPTT. Patients on heparin for more than 4 days should also have a platelet count measured due to the possibility of heparin-induced thrombocytopenia.[56] Subcutaneous (SQ) prophylactic unfractionated heparin (5000 U twice a day for deep venous thrombosis prophylaxis) is unlikely to cause an increase in the aPTT, and is not a contraindication to neuraxial techniques (Table 5-4).[51] Epidural catheter placement or removal should be delayed for at least 2–4 h following the discontinuation of therapeutic doses of unfractionated heparin. Confirmation of a return to normal hemostatic function with an aPTT is indicated. When intravenous unfractionated heparin is used intraoperatively, administration should be delayed for at least 1 h after a neuraxial technique. The same guidelines should be used for epidural catheter removal, as it has been suggested that catheter removal is as traumatic as catheter placement.[3]

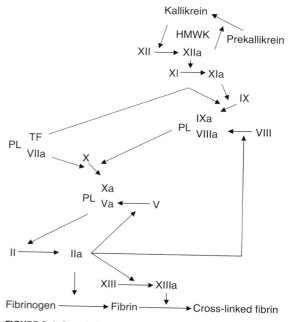

FIGURE 5-1. Coagulation cascade. PL, phospholipid; HMWK, high molecular weight kininogen; and TF, tissue factor.

Table 5-4

Neuraxial Anesthetic Considerations with Unfractionated Heparin

Heparin Dose/Type Therapy	Anesthetic Considerations
5000 units SQ twice a day (prophylactic dose)	No contraindication to neuraxial technique Better to perform neuraxial procedure before heparin dose Avoid other medications that impair coagulation
High SQ doses (>5000 U SQ twice a day)	Anticoagulation response unpredictable Check aPTT prior to performing neuraxial technique
Therapeutic heparin (aPTT 60–80 s)	Neuraxial anesthesia contraindicated Stop heparin for 2–4 h and recheck aPTT before initiating neuraxial anesthesia
Intraoperative heparinization (5000–10,000 U IV bolus)	Wait at least 1 h after neuraxial technique
Heparin therapy > 4 days	Check platelet count

LMWH differs from unfractioned heparin biochemically and pharmacologically (Table 5-5).[57] It has a greater inhibitory effect against factor Xa than against thrombin because of its shorter chain length. It has greater bioavailability and a longer half-life than unfractionated heparin.[57] After a SQ dose of LMWH, the peak anti-Xa activity occurs at 3–4 h and decreases to 50% of peak activity by 12 h. LMWH is excreted by the kidney and the half-life is increased in patients with obesity or renal failure.[57] The aPTT is not a sensitive laboratory measurement of LMWH activity. The anti-Xa level measures its anticoagulant effect, but is not predictive of bleeding complications.[51]

There have been 60 reported cases of epidural hematoma associated with neuraxial techniques and LMWH since its introduction in 1993.[58] Plausible explanations include high doses of LMWH, twice a day dosing, and the performance of neuraxial techniques during the time of peak LMWH activity. These cases were the driving force behind the ASRA consensus conference on neuraxial anesthesia and anticoagulation, first convened in 1998, and updated in 2002.[51] Key points of these guidelines include the delay of neuraxial techniques for at least 10–12 h following the administration of a prophylactic dose of LMWH, and 24 h after a therapeutic dose (Box 5-6). Spinal anesthesia is preferred as it is less traumatic than epidural anesthesia. Anti-Xa activity measurement is not recommended because it has not been standardized. It is the authors' belief that neuraxial techniques should be avoided in the presence of increased anti-Xa activity, but that normal activity in the setting of recent LMWH administration does not mean that neuraxial techniques can be safely performed.

Fondaparinux, a new anticoagulant, is a synthetic pentasaccharide that selectively binds to antithrombin, thus inducing a conformational change that significantly increases the antifactor Xa activity without inhibition of factor IIa.[59] It is not associated with thrombocytopenia because it does not cross-react with antibodies against heparin-platelet factor 4 complexes. Unlike other factor Xa antagonists, it has a very long half-life (18 h) and it may take up to 96–120 h to completely eliminate this agent from the circulation.[59] Until further data are available, neuraxial anesthesia should be avoided in patients receiving this medication for at least 4 days after the last dose. There are reported cases of fondaparinux administered 2 h after an atraumatic single spinal needle pass or epidural catheter removal without adverse outcomes.[51]

Table 5-5

Comparison of Unfractionated Heparin and LMWH

	Unfractionated Heparin	LMWH
Antifactor Xa-II ratio	1:1	>2:1
Bioavailability	Around 30%	Close to 100%
Half-life	1–2 h	3–6 h
Measurement of activity	aPTT	Anti-Xa activity
Clearance	Saturable cellular mechanism	Renal

Box 5-6

Anesthetic Considerations with LMWH

- Peak onset is at 3–6 h after dosing
  - Worst time to perform neuraxial techniques
- 50% anti-Xa level at 12 h
  - Best to avoid neuraxial techniques
  - Single-shot spinal technique is preferred
  - Careful neurologic follow-up
- Plasma half-life increases with obesity and renal failure
- Prophylactic doses
  - Enoxaparin 30 mg twice a day
  - Enoxaparin 40 mg once a day
  - Wait at least 10–12 h
- Therapeutic doses
  - Enoxaparin 1 mg/kg twice a day
  - Enoxaparin 1.5 mg/kg once a day
  - Wait at least 24 h
- No need to check anti-Xa level
- Dose LMWH 2 h after epidural catheter removal

Table 5-6

Vitamin-K-Dependent Factor Half-lives

Factors	Half-life (h)
VII	6
IX	24
X	24–36
II	60–72

factors to bind calcium, thereby leading to decreased formation of thrombin. The PT is primarily related to factor VII and X levels. The initial increase in PT (standardized as the international normalized ratio [INR]) following the initiation of warfarin therapy reflects the inhibition of factor VII activity, the vitamin-K-dependent factor with the shortest half-life. The full anticoagulant effect of warfarin takes several days and depends on the respective half-lives of factors II, IX, and X (Table 5-6).[51,60] The opposite happens on discontinuation of warfarin therapy, when the normalization of the INR reflects return of factor VII activity before full recovery of the other vitamin-K-dependent factors. For any given elevated INR, coagulation is more likely to be impaired when recovering from the effects of anticoagulation than when initiating anticoagulation.

In anticipation of surgery, warfarin should be discontinued 4–5 days prior to procedures and the INR measured on the day of surgery (Table 5-7).[61] Normalization of the INR is recommended prior to the performance of neuraxial techniques. It is considered appropriate to perform neuraxial techniques at the beginning of warfarin anticoagulation provided that a

Warfarin

Warfarin blocks the vitamin-K-dependent gamma-carboxylation of factors II, VII, IX, X, and anticoagulant proteins C and S. This leads to the inability of the clotting

Table 5-7

Neuraxial Anesthetic Considerations with Warfarin

Warfarin Dose/Type Therapy	Anesthetic Considerations
Single low dose (≤ 5 mg) less than 24 h from neuraxial technique Minimal increase in INR	Permissible to perform neuraxial techniques Avoid other medications that affect coagulation
Therapeutic doses INR > 1.4	Discontinue 4–5 days prior to neuraxial technique Recheck PT, confirm return to normal hemostasis
Anticoagulation with abnormal INR	Coagulation more likely to be impaired with decreasing INR Careful neurologic evaluation in the presence of epidural catheters Hold warfarin if INR > 3 INR ≤ 1.4 prior to catheter removal

single low dose has been administered less than 24 h prior to the block.[51] Patients on low-dose warfarin (5 mg or less) with an indwelling epidural catheter should have daily measurements of INR until catheter removal. Warfarin should be reduced or withheld if the INR is greater than 3.[51] The catheter is removed once the INR value is less than 1.5. This number is based on data from trials that correlated hemostasis with factor activity levels greater than 40%.[51,60]

Fibrinolytic Drugs

The fibrinolytic system keeps clot formation in check by degrading cross-linked fibrin into fibrin split products.[62] An endogenous tissue-type plasminogen activator catalyses the formation of plasmin from plasminogen, which in turn degrades fibrin and procoagulant factors V and VIII. In addition, the degradation products of fibrinogen and fibrin also possess significant anticoagulation properties.[51] Exogenous plasminogen activators accelerate the formation of plasmin, and hence fibrin breakdown.[62] Unfortunately, these exogenous medications do not differentiate the fibrin of a thrombus from that of a hemostatic plug and have the potential to lead to an epidural hematoma if neuraxial anesthesia is initiated in the presence of these drugs. In addition, patients who receive fibrinolytic drugs are also likely to have impaired primary and secondary hemostasis due to the concomitant use of intravenous heparin and antiplatelet agents.

Current recommendations involve the avoidance of exogenous plasminogen activators for 10 days following neuraxial techniques.[51] However, a risk-benefit analysis in a patient with an acute myocardial infarct may determine the benefit of these medications even in the presence of recent trauma to noncompressible vessels. Regular neurologic examinations (at least every 2 h) are mandatory. There are currently no recommendations as to a safe medication administration-neuraxial anesthesia interval, nor are there recommendations regarding when an epidural catheter can be safely removed following unanticipated use of these medications. The 2003 ASRA consensus conference suggests that measurement of fibrinogen level may guide decision making, as it is one of the last clotting factors to recover.[51] It is important to understand that even though the half-life of fibrinolytic drugs is short (as short as 10–20 min for urokinase), the thrombolytic and anticoagulant effect of these medications may last for days.

▶ Thrombocytopenia and Thrombasthenia

Thrombocytopenia is caused by a variety of physiologic and pathologic conditions and is a relative contraindication to neuraxial anesthesia. Common causes of thrombocytopenia are outlined in Box 5-7. There are little data to support the

---

Box 5-7

Common Causes of Thrombocytopenia

- Gestational thrombocytopenia
- ITP
- Other immune disorders
  - Systemic lupus erythematous
  - Antiphospholipid syndrome
- Preeclampsia
- TTP
- HUS
- DIC
- Drug induced
  - HIT
- Type IIb vWD

---

notion that neuraxial techniques be avoided at any one absolute platelet count. Beilin et al. reviewed the medical records of 30 parturients with platelet counts between 69 and $98 \times 10^3/mm^3$ who received epidural analgesia without any complications.[63] Twenty women had gestational thrombocytopenia, six preeclampsia, three immune thrombocytopenia purpura, and one an infection. Most anesthesiologists feel comfortable initiating neuraxial anesthesia in these patients as long as the platelet count is greater than $70,000 \times 10^3/mm^3$, and there is no evidence of bleeding.[64] The etiology of the thrombocytopenia, the trend in the platelet number, and the history and physical examination are more important than the absolute platelet count per se. Having said this, most anesthesiologists are reluctant to perform a neuraxial technique if the platelet count is under $70 \times 10^3/mm^3$ unless there is a compelling indication to do so based on a risk-benefit analysis. A spinal technique is less traumatic than an epidural technique, and is preferred once the platelet count is under $70 \times 10^3/mm^3$. Soft, flexible catheters are preferred for an epidural technique as they have a lower incidence of venous cannulation.

Thrombocytopenia in Pregnancy

Thrombocytopenia, defined as a platelet count below $100 \times 10^3/mm^3$, is found in 10% of pregnant females. Thrombocytopenia is usually mild with platelet counts ranging from 70 to $150 \times 10^3/mm^3$, past medical history is not significant for bleeding, and there is not an increased risk of maternal or fetal bleeding complications. Neuraxial techniques are not contraindicated in these otherwise healthy patients without any signs or symptoms of platelet dysfunction.[64]

Immune thrombocytopenic purpura (ITP) is the most common cause of thrombocytopenia in the general population, and is especially common in woman of childbearing age. The pathogenesis is immunologically mediated via IgG antiplatelet antibodies that recognize platelet membrane glycoproteins. This leads to increased platelet destruction by the reticuloendothelial system, particularly the spleen, with older platelets being more likely to be destroyed.[65] Platelet function is usually normal despite a lower platelet count. Symptoms range from none, to a history of easy bruising, petechiae, epistaxis, and gingival bleeding. The decision to perform neuraxial anesthesia is based on the platelet count and the history and physical examination. Some authors consider a platelet count of $50 \times 10^3/mm^3$ adequate for the initiation of neuraxial techniques provided that there is no clinical evidence of bleeding complications.[64] A single-shot spinal technique is preferred due to its less traumatic nature when compared to an epidural technique. If an epidural technique is chosen, a flexible and soft catheter is preferred to decrease the risk of venous cannulation.

Preeclampsia affects 6% of all pregnancies and accounts for 21% of cases of maternal thrombocytopenia.[66] Thrombocytopenia may be the earliest clinical feature in some patients, even before hypertension or proteinuria develops. It is usually moderate and is present in 15% of preeclamptic patients.[67] Platelet counts that are trending downward may be an indication of worsening disease and the need for delivery. The platelet count may decrease to a nadir 24–48 h postpartum, but clinical manifestations usually resolve after delivery. There is no absolute platelet count number that precludes the placement of an epidural catheter. The decision to perform a neuraxial technique is based on bleeding history, the platelet count trend, the airway examination, and the likelihood of cesarean delivery.

HELLP syndrome is characterized by **h**emolysis, **e**levated **l**iver enzymes, and a **l**ow **p**latelet count. It occurs in up to 10% of pregnancies complicated by severe preeclampsia, usually presents in the second or third trimester or the postpartum period, and may be life threatening.[67] Of note, it may occur in parturients with no other signs of preeclampsia, and one or all of the components of the HELLP syndrome may be present. The HELLP syndrome per se is not a contraindication to neuraxial anesthesia; however, thrombocytopenia or the presence of a coagulopathy may influence the decision of whether to perform a neuraxial technique. A coagulopathy is not usually present unless the platelet count is less than $100 \times 10^3/mm^3$. Other coagulation factors may be affected following microangiopathic platelet destruction and therefore, PT, aPTT, and fibrinogen levels should be monitored once the platelet count is under $100 \times 10^3/mm^3$.

Thrombocytopenia Purpura

Microangiopathic hemolytic anemia, thrombocytopenia, and multiorgan failure are common features of thrombotic thrombocytopenia purpura (TTP) and hemolytic uremic syndrome (HUS).[68] Other clinical manifestations include neurologic abnormalities, which are more common and severe in TTP, fever, and renal dysfunction. Renal dysfunction is more severe in HUS compared to TTP. The thrombocytopenia is caused by intravascular platelet aggregation, and it may be difficult to differentiate TTP and HUS from other causes of thrombocytopenia unless accompanying signs and symptoms are present.[68] Neuraxial anesthesia should be approached with caution in these patients. Platelet count less than $100 \times 10^3/mm^3$, functional platelet defects, prolonged PT, and decreased coagulation factor activity may be present. DIC is rarely associated with TTP and HUS.

Drug-Induced Thrombocytopenia

There are multiple drugs that can trigger an immune-mediated thrombocytopenia. Drug-dependent antibodies against platelets are formed after the binding of the drug to a platelet-membrane molecule by complement activation.[69] Thrombocytopenia occurs suddenly and in isolation, and recovers 5–7 days after the discontinuation of the offending drug. Drugs most commonly associated with thrombocytopenia include quinidine, quinine, rifampin, and trimethoprim-sulfamethoxazole.[69] The most likely drug during the perioperative period is heparin. Heparin-induced thrombocytopenia (HIT) is mediated via IgG and IgM antibodies, and occurs in up to 5% of patients receiving heparin for longer than 5 days.[56] HIT may also be triggered by heparin-coated IV catheters or heparin flush solutions. Although more common with unfractionated heparin, there is also cross-reactivity with LMWH. The clinical manifestations vary, and HIT may present with bleeding or thrombosis due to intravascular platelet aggregation. Immediate removal of heparin is likely to reverse the thrombocytopenia in less than 1 week. Avoidance of drugs known to cause thrombocytopenia in individual patients, and normalization of the platelet count are necessary prior to the performance of neuraxial techniques.

Thrombasthenia

Glanzmann's thrombasthenia (GT) is an autosomal recessive disease characterized by a qualitative or quantitative defect in platelet membrane glycoprotein IIb-IIIa.[70] This glycoprotein binds to fibrinogen and vWF and mediates platelet aggregation with activators such as collagen, ADP, epinephrine, arachidonic acid, and thrombin.[69] There are two types of GT: type I and type II. While both types are characterized by a deficiency of glycoprotein IIb-IIIa, type I is more severe and is accompanied by low levels of fibrinogen. Mucocutaneous bleeding is more severe with type I, and the disorder is confirmed by platelets that do not aggregate in the presence of activators such as epinephrine. Acquired GT is rare and is characterized by normally expressed glycoprotein IIb-IIIa that is nonfunctional due to autoantibodies.[71]

Bernard-Soulier syndrome is another disease characterized by abnormal platelet aggregation as a result of abnormal adhesion. It is an autosomal recessive disorder with quantitative or qualitative abnormality in glycoprotein Ib-V-IX, an active receptor for vWF.[72] Similar to GT, the syndrome presents with mucocutaneous bleeding. The ristocetin-induced platelet aggregation (RIPA) test, which measures the ability of vWF to support aggregation, is abnormal. Platelet aggregation to agonists that require fibrinogen for binding is abnormal in patients with GT, but unchanged in those with Bernard-Soulier syndrome.[72]

There are no reports in the anesthesia literature of patients with GT or Bernard-Soulier syndrome receiving neuraxial techniques. In part, this may be due to the rarity of these disorders. In addition, most of these patients have a history of mucocutaneous bleeding consistent with a platelet abnormality, and most anesthesiologists avoid neuraxial techniques in these patients. The treatment of choice is platelet transfusion, but repeated transfusions predispose to the development of antiplatelet antibodies making it difficult to predict which patients will respond.

Measurement of Platelet Function

Although the bleeding time is likely to be increased in patients with abnormal platelet function, bleeding time determination has many limitations. It is operator dependent and difficult to standardize and reproduce. The thromboelastogram (TEG) provides a global assessment of coagulation, including clotting factor and platelet function, and their interaction.[73] TEG can determine the clot strength, the rate of clot formation and strengthening, and fibrinolysis. TEG values include R time (time to first clot formation), K time and α angle (rate of clot strengthening), MA (maximum strength of developed clot), and LY30 (percent lysis at 30 min after MA is reached) (Fig. 5-2).[73] K time, α angle, and MA are more specific for fibrinogen activity and platelet function and are used to assess the baseline clot strength as well as the change in response to platelet transfusions. In addition, there is a strong correlation between the MA and the platelet count. Platelet counts above $75 \times 10^3/mm^3$ are associated with a normal MA.[73]

The platelet function analyzer (PFA-100) is a relatively new technique for differentiating normal from abnormal platelet function and evaluating primary hemostasis.[74] It measures the time required for whole blood to occlude an aperture of a bioactive membrane coated with the platelet

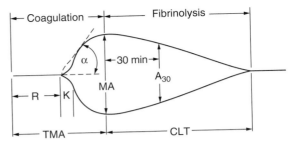

FIGURE 5-2. Thromboelastograph tracing. R time = time to first clot formation, K time = time to 20 mm, α angle = rate of clot strengthening, A = amplitude, maximum amplitude (MA) = maximum strength of developed clot, A_{30} = amplitude of tracing 30 min after MA is reached, TMA = time to maximum amplitude, and CLT = clot lysis time (time from MA until A = 2 mm). LY30 (percent lysis at 30 min after MA is reached) is calculated as A_{30}/MA.

agonists epinephrine and ADP (closure time).[74] Although an increased aperture time correlates with decreased platelet function, it is difficult to differentiate a quantitative from a qualitative defect. The PFA, however, can be used to follow the response to platelet transfusion in patients with thrombasthenia. Similar to TEG, the closure time of the PFA-100 correlates with the platelet count. A platelet count greater than $70 \times 10^3/mm^3$ is associated with a normal closure time.[74] Results from TEG and PFA-100 further support the notion that a platelet count greater than $75 \times 10^3/mm^3$, in the absence of significant findings on history and physical examination, is likely to be associated with normal platelet function and, therefore, normal primary hemostasis. Thus, it would seem reasonable to proceed with neuraxial anesthesia if the TEG or PFA results are normal.

▶ Inherited Hemorrhagic Disorders

von Willebrand's Disease

von Willebrand's disease (vWD) is the most common inherited hemorrhagic disorder to affect both sexes. The exact prevalence of the disease is not known because of variable expressivity and reduced penetrance, but it has been estimated to be present in 2–3% of the general population.[75] It is characterized by quantitatively decreased (type 1 and type 3) or qualitatively abnormal vWF (type 2; Table 5-8). There is a defect in platelet interaction with the subendothelium (adhesion) and with other platelets (aggregation). In addition, vWF carries factor VIII in the circulation, and protects it from inactivation and clearance.[75] Therefore, patients with vWD also have a defect in fibrin formation. Patients with vWD present with signs of platelet impairment manifested as mucocutaneous bleeding, including epistaxis, gingival bleeding, easy bruising, and menorrhagia.

Table 5-8

Classification of vWD

Type	vWF	Factor VIII	Quantitative vs. Qualitative	Prevalence in Patients with vWD
1	Decreased	Decreased	Quantity	60–80%
2A	Decreased	Decreased	Quality	15–30% of all type 2
2B	Low to low normal	Low to low normal	Quality	15–30% of all type 2
2M	Low to low normal	Low to low normal	Quality	15–30% of all type 2
2N	Low to low normal	Decreased	Quality	15–30% of all type 2
3	Markedly decreased or absent	Markedly decreased	Quantity	5–10%

Type 1 vWD is the most common type and has an autosomal dominant inheritance. It is the milder form of the disease, and accounts for 70% of all cases. There is a decrease in plasma levels of vWF and factor VIII.[75] It is usually responsive to desmopressin (DDAVP), which increases the release of vWF from platelets and endothelial cells. Symptoms usually improve during pregnancy due to the physiologic increase in plasma factor VIII and vWF.[76]

Type 2 vWD also has an autosomal dominant mode of inheritance, but with a qualitative abnormality of vWF. It accounts for up to 20–30% of all cases of vWD, and is characterized by various subtypes. Type 2A vWD has an absence of large and intermediate size multimers and RIPA. Type 2B vWD has an absence of large size multimers, and the interaction between platelets and vWF is increased. Thrombocytopenia is a unique feature of this type of vWD, but does not predict clinical severity. Type 2M vWD has normal size multimers but with decreased platelet-dependent vWF function. Type 2N vWD has a defect in the binding of factor VIII to vWF.[75]

Type 3 vWD has an autosomal recessive mode of inheritance and is rarely seen. It is the more severe form of vWD and is characterized by a minimal amount of vWF and low plasma levels of factor VIII.[75] It usually presents with severe bleeding, is not responsive to DDAVP, and does not improve with pregnancy.

All patients with a history resembling vWD should have coagulation screening tests, including platelet count, PT, and aPTT to rule out other causes of bleeding. Specialized testing for vWD is important to confirm the diagnosis, and to establish a proper subclassification and treatment options. The ristocetin cofactor activity assay (vWF:RCo) measures vWF binding to platelet GpIb or vWF activity. Plasma vWF antigen (vWF:Ag) quantifies the deficiency of vWD, and factor VIII activity is measured in a functional assay. The RIPA test assesses the ability of the platelet-associated vWF to support aggregation. Gel electrophoresis aids in delineation of the vWF multimer structure.[75]

DDAVP is a synthetic analog of antidiuretic hormone and transiently increases the levels of factor VIII and vWF by causing their release from the endothelial cells (Table 5-9).[77] It is most effective for type 1 vWD with a response rate of approximately 80%. The response with type 2 vWD is unpredictable. DDAVP is contraindicated in cases of type 2B disease as it can precipitate or worsen thrombocytopenia. There is no response in patients with type 3 disease as there is minimal if any vWF. DDAVP is administered intravenously at a dose of 0.2–0.4 μg/kg body weight over 30 min. The plasma factor VIII and vWF plasma levels increase three to five times, and remain elevated for 8–10 h after DDAVP administration.[77] Repeat doses are recommended every 12–24 h. Antihemophilic factor/ vWF complex (Humate P) is a heat inactivated concentrate that contains more vWF activity than factor VIII (2.5:1 IU) and is indicated for type 3 and some cases of type 2 vWD.[77] Factor VIII plasma levels should be monitored during therapy, as this is the main predictor of surgical hemostasis. Peak plasma levels of factor VIII are achieved after 6–8 h of treatment.

The management of a patient with vWD is best performed with a multidisciplinary approach that includes the surgeon/obstetrician, hematologist, and anesthesiologist. There is a direct correlation among vWF:Ag, vWF:RCo, and factor VIII levels and normal hemostasis, and it is often difficult to decide whether to perform neuraxial techniques for these patients. Neuraxial techniques are contraindicated if the coagulation screen is abnormal, as in cases with more severe types of vWD where the vWF is markedly reduced or abnormal. There are several reports of neuraxial anesthesia administered to patients with mild forms of type 1 vWD without any complications following normalization of factor VIII and vWF plasma levels during pregnancy or after DDAVP treatment.[76,78] Of note, it is important to understand

Table 5-9

Treatment of vWD

Type	Bleeding	Pregnancy	DDAVP Response	Treatment
1	Mild	Improve	Good	DDAVP
2A	Variable	Minimal change	Variable	DDAVP or factor VIII concentrate*
2B	Thrombocytopenia likely to worsen bleeding	Worsen	Likely to worsen thrombocytopenia	Factor VIII concentrate
2M	Variable	Minimal change	Variable	DDAVP or factor VIII concentrate*
2N	Variable	Minimal change	Variable	DDAVP or factor VIII concentrate*
3	Severe	No change	No response	Factor VIII concentrate

*DDAVP trial is recommended after initial diagnosis, as the response is variable.

that while type 1 vWD may be corrected temporarily during pregnancy or with DDAVP, the level of vWD decreases after the delivery of the placenta or 8–10 h following DDAVP therapy. This has some implications in the delivery of neuraxial techniques, as the removal of an epidural catheter may occur at the time when vWF and factor VIII levels are decreasing.

Factor Deficiencies

Common factor deficiencies include factors VIII, IX, and XI. Hemophilia A and B are X-linked diseases associated with deficiencies of factors VIII and IX, respectively. The diseases are present almost exclusively in males (1/10,000), and carrier females are usually free of any bleeding complications. Unlike platelet disorders, bleeding is usually deep, causing hemarthrosis.[79] Factor XI deficiency has an autosomal recessive mode of inheritance and is common in Ashkenazi Jews. Bleeding complications are more common in females, including menorrhagia and postpartum hemorrhage.[76] All of these factor deficiencies are associated with an elevated aPTT that is highly suggestive of an abnormality in the intrinsic pathway, as these factors are essential to the activation of factor Xa, which in turn converts prothrombin to thrombin (Fig. 5-1).

Neuraxial techniques can be used in carriers of hemophilia that have normal factor levels and are free of bleeding complications. Although neuraxial techniques are best avoided in homozygous patients with known factor deficiencies, there are reported cases of neuraxial techniques in patients with normal aPTT and factor levels after replacement therapy.[80] In addition, there is a report of two pregnant patients with mild to moderate factor XI deficiency and a normal aPTT who received neuraxial techniques without any complications.[79] Of note, factor XI is one of the few factors that decreases as pregnancy progresses. It is important to understand that isolated case reports of neuraxial techniques in these patients should not be equated with safety, as epidural hematoma has a low prevalence in the general population (1:150,000–1:220,000).[3] Factor XII deficiency leads to an elevated aPTT without any known bleeding complications. Patients with this factor deficiency should have a complete hematologic workup to rule out other causes of elevated aPTT, and neuraxial techniques are permissible in the absence of bleeding tendencies.

Antiphospholipid Antibodies

Lupus anticoagulants (LAC) and anticardiolipin antibodies (ACA) are autoantibodies against phospholipid-protein complexes and may result in abnormal platelet aggregation and thrombocytopenia. In addition, circulating LACs interfere with phospholipid-dependent coagulation tests resulting in prolongation of the aPTT.[81] LAC elevates aPTT in vitro, but increases clotting in vivo and, therefore, patients with LAC are more likely to experience a thrombotic event than abnormal bleeding.[82] Interaction of these antibodies with phospholipids of the platelet membranes may contribute to venous, arterial, and placental thrombosis.

The challenge arises when these patients are treated with heparin to prevent these complications, as the aPTT is likely to remain elevated even after heparin has been discontinued. If the decision is made to perform a neuraxial technique, blood heparin assays, activated clotting test, or thrombin time have been used to monitor the heparin levels. The determination of baseline aPTT levels is recommended prior to initiating heparin anticoagulation.[81] Another option is to check anti-Xa levels, but controversy exists regarding the use of anti-Xa monitoring to predict heparin response. The abnormal phospholipid that contributes to this artificially elevated aPTT can be confirmed by measuring ACA with an enzyme-linked immunosorbent assay (ELISA).[82] A careful history and physical examination, as well as the determination of the platelet count and PT are important to rule out any other coagulopathy.

Neuraxial Anesthesia or Catheter Insertion Under General Anesthesia

There is a great deal of controversy over the insertion of subarachnoid or epidural catheters, or the initiation of neuraxial anesthesia while patients are undergoing general anesthesia. While most series have demonstrated an absence of neurologic injury when patients received intrathecal opioid injection,[83] spinal drainage,[84] or lumbar epidural catheters under general anesthesia,[85] the incidence of neurologic complications related to neuraxial techniques is too small to allow determination of actual risk of this practice.[85] Neuraxial anesthesia for children may only be possible under heavy sedation or general anesthesia; however, in adults it is usually possible to perform these techniques with minimal to no sedation.[86] Serious complications during neuraxial anesthesia are more likely to occur after a paresthesia during needle puncture, or with pain during the injection of local anesthetics.[2] Closed claims analysis demonstrated that 39% of lumbosacral nerve root injuries were associated with paresthesia during needle insertion, and another 13% were associated with pain during drug injection.[87] Cases of permanent loss of cervical spinal cord function due to direct spinal cord injection of local anesthetics when interscalene blocks were performed under general anesthesia have been reported.[88] Therefore, close communication with the patient is essential in order to recognize a paresthesia during needle insertion or pain during injection of a drug. Rosenquist and Birnbach have argued that the risk-benefit ratio does not support the use of neuraxial techniques under general anesthesia, even when performed at the lumbar level.[86] There is a wide vertebral level range at which the spinal cord terminates, and anesthesiologists often inaccurately identify specific lumbar interspaces (see Chap. 1).[89] Current data support the practice of inserting needles and catheters into the epidural or subarachnoid space of adults with minimal to no sedation in order to recognize pain or paresthesias during needle or catheter placement, or drug injection.

Neuraxial Techniques Following Dural Puncture or Epidural Blood Patch

It has been postulated that a previous epidural blood patch for a postdural puncture headache may lead to obliteration of the epidural space. Reorganization of the blood clot has been hypothesized to cause fibrous tissue formation around the dura, leading to obstruction to spread of local anesthetics in the epidural space.[90] Some authors have reported that previous dural puncture was associated with a higher incidence of subsequent inadequate epidural anesthesia, requiring larger doses of local anesthetics.[91,92] Possible explanations for this observation include the presence of a preexisting abnormality in the epidural space causing difficulty with the initial epidural technique (resulting in breach of the dura), or that dural puncture may result in rearrangement of dural architecture, resulting in changes in the epidural space.

In contrast to the above reports, other authors have reported successful epidural analgesia following a previous dural tap or epidural blood patch.[93,94] These studies found no association between a history of prior epidural blood patch and subsequent unsuccessful neuraxial anesthesia. The history of a prior dural puncture, however, was reported to increase the likelihood of a subsequent puncture.[93]

Because the data are conflicting as to the subsequent effects of prior dural puncture and epidural blood patch, it may be prudent to disclose to patients that a prior dural puncture may be associated with more difficult initiation of epidural anesthesia, with an increased likelihood of inadvertent dural puncture and inadequate or failed anesthesia.

Gross Anatomic Abnormalities

Previous Spinal Surgery

Harrington originally described the use of distraction and compression rods for the treatment of scoliosis in 1962.[95] Current surgical techniques employ Harrington, Luque, and Cotrell-Doubousset metal rods. Common to these rods is the removal of spinous processes and interspinous ligaments, the decortication of vertebrae, and the placement of bone graft material over the vertebrae.[96]

Although neuraxial anesthesia is not contraindicated in patients with prior spinal instrumentation, technical difficulty due to fused areas from scar tissue or bone grafting are often encountered.[96] Other problems that may contribute to a greater degree of difficulty performing neuraxial techniques include further degenerative spine changes below the area of fusion, the involvement of the L4 and L5 vertebral levels in up to 20% of patients, and the possibility of an injury to the ligamentum flavum during the surgical procedure, resulting in adhesions in the epidural space.[96] Potential problems include the inability to locate the epidural space (see Chap. 2), limited spread of local anesthetic above the level of the spinal fusion, and an increased incidence of dural puncture. In a small series of nine patients with Harrington rods receiving epidural analgesia for labor, successful analgesia was achieved in seven patients despite close to 50% (4/9) having some of the complications mentioned earlier.[96] Although these patients suffer from postdural puncture headache following an unintentional dural breech, an epidural blood patch will be as difficult as the original technique and there is the possibility that the epidural space has been obliterated.

Conventional radiographs and a copy of the surgical report are helpful prior to initiating neuraxial anesthesia in patients with any type of rods.[97] Anteroposterior and lateral radiographs demonstrate the position of the spinal elements, the instrumentation itself, the presence of graft material, and evidence of gross anatomic abnormalities. A spinal technique may be preferred over an epidural, as it is less likely to be affected by distortions of the epidural space, has a more specific endpoint, and is more reliable. Should an extended period of analgesia or anesthesia be required, the use of a continuous spinal catheter following intentional or unintentional dural breech has been described.[97,98] Ultrasonography has been suggested as an aid to identify landmarks and locate the midline.[97] The rod and the vertebra to which it is anchored are usually positioned in the midline; however, this may not be true in the middle part of the rod, as the vertebral column may be significantly displaced laterally.[97] Interestingly, the rods may be the only visible image on the ultrasound to aid midline location.

In conclusion, neuraxial techniques can be offered to patients with prior spinal instrumentation. These patients may be reluctant to accept neuraxial techniques due to anxiety, back pain, or simply because they have been told to avoid any instrumentation of their back. Reassurance that these techniques are safe and generally effective is very important, while at the same time disclosing the increased incidence of complications.

► Lower Back Disease

Neuraxial anesthesia is often performed in patients with known back disease, ranging from commonly occurring low back pain without any anatomic etiology, to lumbar spinal stenosis. Other common causes of low back pain include spondylolisthesis and herniated disc. A thorough history and physical examination is important in order to identify any preexisting muscular or neurologic disease prior to an attempted neuraxial technique. Although permanent neurologic injury as a result of a neuraxial technique is very low, ranging from 0.01 to 0.03% (see Chap. 6),[99] any undocumented pathology prior to a needle insertion may be attributed to the neuraxial technique.

There has been significant controversy in the obstetric literature regarding epidural techniques and postpartum backache. Even though retrospective reviews have demonstrated an association,[100] prospective studies have demonstrated that the majority of parturients had similar back pain during pregnancy and prior to the epidural technique.[101] Furthermore, the incidence of postpartum back pain was similar regardless of the performance or avoidance of neuraxial techniques.[101]

A paresthesia is often present following a spinal needle insertion into the subarachnoid space or during epidural catheter advancement. Although a paresthesia is more common in patients with known spine pathology or complaints, it is not associated with any long-term neurologic condition.[102] However, extreme caution should be exercised in the presence of a paresthesia during needle or catheter insertion. A persistent, recurrent, or reproducible paresthesia, or pain during injection is more likely to be associated with a lasting radiculopathy in the same distribution.[2] Variable distribution of medication in the epidural space,[103] and delayed onset of anesthesia have been demonstrated in patients with sciatica.[104] Delayed onset of anesthesia occurs when comparing patients with known spinal pathology to healthy patients, as well as between affected and unaffected nerves and nerve roots in patients with known pathology.

Regional techniques are not contraindicated in the presence of back pain and are not likely to exacerbate it. A careful history and physical examination will most likely demonstrate that the cause of back pain is not of neurologic origin. Sciatica may occur in the presence of lumbar disc herniation with radicular symptoms, and patients should be informed that neuraxial techniques might reproduce these symptoms. An imaging study such as a MRI is helpful in the presence of radicular symptoms and will help identify the location of the injury. The L4-L5 and L5-S1 interspaces are implicated in over 95% of cases of lumbar spine pathology,[105] and it is best to perform a neuraxial technique at a different interspace. Finally, it is important to discuss with patients that any significant pathology in the lumbar spine may result in a technically more difficult neuraxial procedure, with the possibility of reproducing pathologic symptoms, and inadequate anesthesia due to uneven distribution of medication in the epidural space.

► Localized Infection

The administration of neuraxial techniques in patients with a localized infection, particularly near the site of skin puncture, has been viewed with some skepticism. There is a concern that spinal-epidural abscess or spinal meningitis may result.[9,106,107] While hematogenous spread of the localized infection to the CSF has been implicated as a possible cause of meningitis and spinal-epidural abscess,[106,107] direct inoculation of bacteria at the time of block initiation may also account for neuraxial infection.[106] Epidural anesthesia has been used in the presence of distant abscesses or infected wounds without any complications.[108] Of note, deep or superficial epidural infections are more likely in patients on intensive care units, with long duration of epidural catheterization, receiving immunosuppression or low-dose anticoagulation, or with diabetes or cancer.[106,109] Other identifiable risk factors include chronic renal failure, steroid administration, herpes zoster, and rheumatoid arthritis.[110] Therefore, these factors should be taken into consideration when deciding whether to use neuraxial techniques in patients who are febrile or with a localized infection. Specifically, any sign of infection in close proximity to the insertion site should be viewed as a relative contraindications to neuraxial techniques.[108,111]

There are a number of steps that are recommended in order to avoid contamination during epidural catheter insertion (see Chap. 2). Adequate time must be allowed for drying of skin preparation fluid, the number of attempts should be minimized, and the catheter site should be covered with a clear occlusive dressing at the time of insertion.[110] It is important to examine catheters daily, remove them if there is any sign of infection at the puncture site, and maintain a high index of suspicion for an epidural abscess when caring for patients whose epidural catheters were placed at the time of a localized infection or a febrile episode. In addition, there should be a low threshold for suspicion of an epidural abscess in the presence of neurologic signs. A MRI scan should be obtained and antibiotics that cover the most common organism, *Staphylococcus aureus,* should be initiated (see Chap. 6).[106] This will enable prompt diagnosis and treatment with reduced likelihood of permanent neurologic sequelae.

A risk-benefit analysis should be conducted in patients with a localized infection before initiating neuraxial anesthesia and this should be discussed with the patient. The risk factors that increase the risk of an epidural abscess in predisposed patients should be taken into consideration. The use of antibiotics prior to a neuraxial technique is currently recommended in patients with evidence of a localized infection. Although there is no evidence for a cause and effect relationship between neuraxial techniques and meningitis or epidural abscesses in these patients, any serious neurologic complication may be attributed to the neuraxial technique. The initiation of neuraxial analgesia for the treatment of acute pain from herpes zoster infection is discussed in Chap. 17.

▶ Preload-Dependent Conditions

Central neuraxial techniques lead to decreased preload and afterload secondary to sympathetic blockade and its associated venous and arterial dilation (see Chap. 4).[112] Therefore, patients with conditions such as aortic stenosis (AS) and hypertrophic cardiomyopathy (idiopathic hypertrophic subaortic stenosis [IHSS]), which are associated with a fixed or dynamic left ventricular outflow tract obstruction, are likely to deteriorate under these conditions.

Box 5-8

Changes Associated with AS and Anesthetic Considerations

▶ Fixed stroke volume
  ▶ Avoid decreases in preload
  ▶ Avoid tachycardia
▶ Compensatory left ventricular concentric hypertrophy
  ▶ Avoid decreases in afterload
  ▶ A slowly titrated regional anesthetic is permissible
  ▶ Direct-acting vasopressor to restore SVR
    ▶ Phenylephrine
  ▶ Avoid aggressive fluid resuscitation
▶ Dependent on atrial contraction to maintain preload
  ▶ Maintain normal sinus rhythm

Aortic Stenosis

Patients with AS have compensatory left ventricular concentric hypertrophy and a fixed stroke volume (Box 5-8). Decreased afterload exacerbates the left ventricular outflow tract gradient and decreases diastolic pressure (upstream coronary artery perfusion pressure).[113] Decreased preload leads to decreased stroke volume. Tachycardia decreases left ventricular filling time and also results in decreased stroke volume. Patients with AS have a noncompliant left ventricle and are more dependent on atrial contraction to maintain preload. Patients are at increased risk for myocardial ischemia because perfusion of the endocardium is decreased in the hypertrophied heart. Therefore, decreases in afterload and preload, and tachycardia (or a heart rhythm other than sinus) lead to a decreased cardiac output and coronary artery perfusion pressure, which lead to myocardial ischemia, worsening ventricular function, further decreases in coronary artery perfusion pressure, worsening ischemia, and so on.

The acute sympathectomy induced by the rapid induction of neuraxial anesthesia may cause acute decompensation in the patient with AS by acutely decreasing preload and afterload. Therefore, a single-shot spinal anesthetic is contraindicated. A carefully titrated neuraxial anesthetic is necessary in patients with AS to avoid the sudden decrease in preload and SVR. A slowly titrated neuraxial technique with continuous monitoring and maintenance of arterial and right atrial pressure or central volume status is permissible.

It is preferable to administer a direct-acting vasopressor to restore the SVR, rather than an intravenous fluid bolus, as this may precipitate left ventricular failure.[114] Phenylephrine is the vasoconstrictor of choice should hypotension develop, as it does not increase heart rate or contractility. A slowly titrated epidural technique may be used safely, especially in patients with mild to moderate disease for whom low thoracic blockade is adequate.[115] Other options include a combined spinal-epidural or continuous spinal technique with a gradual onset of a sympathectomy, allowing for careful titration of vasopressors, and minimal fluid resuscitation based on left atrial pressures measured via a central venous or pulmonary artery catheter.[116,117] The safe use of continuous spinal anesthesia has been described in patients with severe AS scheduled for hip surgery. Blood and pulmonary artery pressure and cardiac output measurements, calculated SVR, and sensory level were used to guide the infusion of subarachnoid local anesthetics.[117]

Obstructive Hypertrophic Cardiomyopathy

Obstructive hypertrophic cardiomyopathy, sometimes referred to as IHSS, is characterized by left ventricular and interventricular septum hypertrophy leading to obstruction of the left ventricular outflow tract during systole.[112,118] Similar to the management of AS, it is essential to maintain preload and afterload and avoid tachycardia. Reduction in preload and afterload increases the left ventricular outflow tract gradient and decreases left ventricular filling, conditions that may lead to hypotension and ischemia.[118] Tachycardia and enhanced contractility also worsen dynamic left ventricular outflow obstruction. Neuraxial anesthesia is relatively contraindicated in these patients because the rapid onset of sympathetic blockade decreases both preload and afterload, especially after a single-shot spinal technique. Epidural and combined spinal-epidural techniques, however, have been used safely in these patients.[118,119] The goals are to maintain euvolemia, vascular resistance, and sinus rhythm, conditions that are accomplished with a slowly titrated neuraxial technique. Neuraxial labor analgesia may be initiated with intrathecal opioid only (no local anesthetic), followed by an infusion of epidural local anesthetic. Invasive blood pressure and central pressure monitoring via a central or pulmonary artery catheter are recommended in more severe cases. Hypotension may be best treated with incremental intravenous doses of phenylephrine.

▶ Lack of Consent

The concept of informed consent is a hallmark of modern medical ethics and is firmly grounded in the principle of respect for autonomy.[120] The two key elements for informed consent are patient understanding of the risks and benefits of a particular procedure, and physician recommendation regarding the best available options.[120] However, patients may not be able to provide consent due to an altered mental status, even when a neuraxial technique may be in the best interests of the patient. Therefore, implied consent is used in cases where there is a medical emergency, in patients with an altered mental status, and where the health-care proxy is unavailable. The anesthesiologist is choosing the best available option based on scientific information and what is in the patient's best interests.

Some have argued that patients in severe pain may be unable to provide informed consent.[120] However, others have demonstrated that even patients with significant labor pain were satisfied with the level of informed consent provided by the anesthesiologist.[121] Interestingly, patients felt that all neuraxial technique-related complications should be disclosed, regardless of severity or risk.[121] It has also been argued that beneficence provides a moral requirement to relieve pain and, therefore, relieving the pain is more important than the informed consent per se unless there is explicit patient refusal.[122] Although the use of sedatives or analgesics for premedication does not appear to interfere with the informed consent process as long as the patient is not too sedated to conduct an intelligible conversation,[120] common sense dictates that the consent be obtained prior to the administration of these medications, if possible. Parents should be able to provide consent for minors, and emancipated minors should be able to provide consent themselves.[120] Health-care proxy consent is allowable in cases where there has been a proven lack of patient competency. However, the issue of competency should not be dealt with at the time of the informed consent process. Should the health-care proxy be unavailable, the best interests of the patient should be taken into account, balancing the risks and benefits of neuraxial techniques.[120]

Informed consent is more than signing a piece of paper for medicolegal protection. The patient should understand the risks and benefits of neuraxial techniques compared to other options, and be directed toward the best and safest technique.

SUMMARY

Neuraxial anesthesia techniques have numerous benefits and are well accepted, especially for certain surgical procedures or patient populations. In addition, neuraxial anesthesia is now safer than ever before. Major complications are very unusual. Certain patient characteristics, however, may increase the risks associated with neuraxial anesthesia, and may even pose major risks to the patient. An example is the introduction of LMWH in the early 1990s that led to multiple cases of epidural hematoma. Therefore, it is essential to recognize and understand the multiple circumstances where a neuraxial anesthesia technique needs to be tailored to certain physiologic or pathologic states, or when it should be avoided altogether. As is true for almost all medical decision-making, a thorough knowledge of the risks and benefits of the procedure and disease state is necessary to make the best possible decision.

REFERENCES

1. Kopacz D, Neal JM. Regional anesthesia and pain medicine: Residency training—the year 2000. *Reg Anesth Pain Med* 27:9, 2002.
2. Auroy Y, Narchi P, Messiah A, et al. Serious complications related to regional anesthesia: Results of a prospective survey in France. *Anesthesiology* 87:479, 1997.
3. Vandermeulen EP, Van Anken H, Vermylen J. Anticoagulants and spinal-epidural anesthesia. *Anesth Analg* 79:1165, 1994.
4. Levi M, Ten Cate H. Current concepts: Disseminated intravascular coagulation. *N Engl J Med* 341:586, 1999.
5. Sprung J, Cheng EY, Patel S. When to remove an epidural catheter in a parturient with disseminated intravascular coagulation. *Reg Anesth* 17:351, 1992.
6. Okuda Y, Kitajima T. Epidural hematoma in a parturient who developed disseminated intravascular coagulation after epidural anesthesia. *Reg Anesth Pain Med* 26:383, 2001.
7. Kuczkowski KM, Reisner LS. Anesthetic management of the parturient with fever and infection. *Can J Anaesth* 15:409, 2003.
8. Hinchliffe D, Norris A. Management of failed intubation in a septic parturient. *Br J Anaesth* 89:328, 2002.
9. Carp H, Bailey S. The association between meningitis and dural puncture in bacteremic rats. *Anesthesiology* 76:739, 1992.
10. Lee JJ, Parry H. Bacterial meningitis following spinal anaesthesia for caesarean section. *Br J Anaesth* 66:383, 1991.
11. Kee WD, Jones MR, Thomas P, et al. Extradural abscess complicating extradural anaesthesia for caesarean section. *Br J Anaesth* 69:647, 1992.
12. Bouhemad B, Dounas M, Mercier FJ, et al. Bacterial meningitis following combined spinal-epidural analgesia for labour. *Anaesthesia* 53:292, 1998.
13. Vandam LD, Dripps RD. Long-term follow-up of patients who received 10,098 spinal anesthetics. IV. *JAMA* 172:1483, 1960.
14. Blanco JD, Gibbs RS, Castaneda YS. Bacteremia in obstetrics: Clinical course. *Obstet Gynecol* 58:621, 1981.
15. Bader AM, Gilbertson L, Kirz L, et al. Regional anesthesia in women with chorioamnionitis. *Reg Anesth* 17:84, 1992.
16. Beilin Y, Bodian CA, Haddad EM, et al. Practice patterns of anesthesiologists regarding situations in obstetric anesthesia where clinical management is controversial. *Anesth Analg* 83:735, 1996.
17. Corey L, Handsfield HH. Genital herpes and public health: Addressing a global problem. *JAMA* 283:791, 2000.
18. Bader AM, Camann WR, Datta S. Anesthesia for cesarean delivery in patients with herpes simplex virus type-2 infections. *Reg Anesth* 15:261, 1990.
19. Enders G, Miller E, Cradock-Watson J, et al. Consequences of varicella and herpes zoster in pregnancy: Prospective study of 1739 cases. *Lancet* 343:1548, 1994.
20. Brown NW, Parsons AP, Kam PC. Anaesthetic considerations in a parturient with varicella presenting for Caesarean section. *Anaesthesia* 58:1092, 2003.
21. Adler MW. ABC of AIDS. Development of the epidemic. *BMJ* 294:1083, 1987.
22. Greene ER Jr. Spinal and epidural anesthesia in patients with the acquired immunodeficiency syndrome. *Anesth Analg* 65:1090, 1986.
23. Kain ZN, Mayes LC, Pakes J, et al. Thrombocytopenia in pregnant women who use cocaine. *Am J Obstet Gynecol* 173:885, 1995.
24. Du Pen SL, Peterson DG, Williams A, et al. Infection during chronic epidural catheterization: Diagnosis and treatment. *Anesthesiology* 73:905, 1990.
25. Gibbons JJ. Post-dural puncture headache in the HIV-positive patient. *Anesthesiology* 74:953, 1991.
26. Tom DJ, Gulevich SJ, Shapiro HM, et al. Epidural blood patch in the HIV-positive patient. Review of clinical experience. San Diego HIV Neurobehavioral Research Center. *Anesthesiology* 76:943, 1992.
27. Rutschmann OT, McCrory DC, Matchar DB, et al. Immunization and MS: A summary of published evidence and recommendations. *Neurology* 59:1837, 2002.
28. Johnson KP. The historical development of interferons as multiple sclerosis therapies. *J Mol Med* 75:89, 1997.
29. Bamford C, Sibley W, Laguna J. Anesthesia in multiple sclerosis. *Can J Neurol Sci* 5:41, 1978.
30. Bader AM, Hunt CO, Datta S, et al. Anesthesia for the obstetric patient with multiple sclerosis. *J Clin Anesth* 1:21, 1988.
31. Confavreux C, Hutchinson M, Hours MM, et al. Rate of pregnancy-related relapse in multiple sclerosis. Pregnancy in Multiple Sclerosis Group. *N Engl J Med* 339:285, 1998.
32. Dalmas AF, Texier C, Ducloy-Bouthors AS, et al. Obstetrical analgesia and anaesthesia in multiple sclerosis. *Ann Fr Anesth Reanim* 22:861, 2003.
33. Harmon JP, Hiett AK, Palmer CG, et al. Prenatal ultrasound detection of isolated neural tube defects: Is cytogenetic evaluation warranted? *Obstet Gynecol* 86:595, 1995.
34. Fishman MA. Recent clinical advances in the treatment of dysraphic states. *Pediatr Clin North Am* 23:517, 1976.
35. Avrahami E, Frishman E, Fridman Z, et al. Spina bifida occulta of S1 is not an innocent finding. *Spine* 19:12, 1994.
36. Rekate HL. Neurosurgical management of a child with spina bifida. In: Rekate HL, ed, *Comprehensive Management of Spina Bifida*. Boca Raton, FL: CRC Press, 1991, p. 93.
37. McGrady EM, Davis AG. Spina bifida occulta and epidural anaesthesia. *Anaesthesia* 43:867, 1988.
38. Tidmarsh MD, May AE. Epidural anaesthesia and neural tube defects. *Int J Obstet Anesth* 7:111, 1998.
39. Vaagenes P, Fjaerestad I. Epidural block during labour in a patient with spina bifida cystica. *Anaesthesia* 36:299, 1981.
40. Surawicz TS, McCarthy BJ, Kupelian V, et al. Descriptive epidemiology of primary brain and CNS tumors: Results from the Central Brain Tumor Registry of the United States, 1990–1994. *Neuro-oncol* 1:14, 1999.
41. Finfer SR. Management of labour and delivery in patients with intracranial neoplasms. *Br J Anaesth* 67:784, 1991.
42. Su TM, Lan CM, Yang LC, et al. Brain tumor presenting with fatal herniation following delivery under epidural anesthesia. *Anesthesiology* 96:508, 2002.
43. Grocott HP, Mutch WA. Epidural anesthesia and acutely increased intracranial pressure. Lumbar epidural space hydrodynamics in a porcine model. *Anesthesiology* 85:1086, 1996.
44. Goroszeniuk T, Howard RS, Wright JT. The management of labour using continuous lumbar epidural analgesia in a patient with a malignant cerebral tumour. *Anaesthesia* 41:1128, 1986.

45. Atanassoff PG, Alon E, Weiss BM, et al. Spinal anaesthesia for cae-sarean section in a patient with brain neoplasma. *Can J Anaesth* 41:163, 1994.

46. Bedard JM, Richardson MG, Wissler RN. Epidural anesthesia in a parturient with a lumboperitoneal shunt. *Anesthesiology* 90:621, 1999.

47. Kaul B, Vallejo MC, Ramanathan S, et al. Accidental spinal anal-gesia in the presence of a lumboperitoneal shunt in an obese par-turient receiving enoxaparin therapy. *Anesth Analg* 95:441, 2002.

48. Abouleish E, Ali V, Tang RA. Benign intracranial hypertension and anesthesia for cesarean section. *Anesthesiology* 63:705, 1985.

49. Wisoff JH, Kratzert KJ, Handwerker SM, et al. Pregnancy in patients with cerebrospinal fluid shunts: Report of a series and review of the literature. *Neurosurgery* 29:827, 1991.

50. Littleford JA, Brockhurst NJ, Bernstein EP, et al. Obstetrical anesthesia for a parturient with a ventriculoperitoneal shunt and third ventriculostomy. *Can J Anaesth* 46:1057, 1999.

51. Horlocker TT, Wedel DJ, Benzon H, et al. Regional anesthesia in the anticoagulated patient: Defining the risks (the second ASRA Consensus Conference on Neuraxial Anesthesia and Anticoagulation). *Reg Anesth Pain Med* 28:172, 2003.

52. Catella-Lawson F, Reilly MP, Kapoor SC, et al. Cyclooxygenase inhibitors and the antiplatelet effects of aspirin. *N Engl J Med* 345:1809, 2001.

53. Taniuchi M, Kurz HI, Lasala JM. Randomized comparison of ticlopidine and clopidogrel after intracoronary stent implanta-tion in a broad patient population. *Circulation* 104:539, 2001.

54. Mondoro TH, White MM, Jennings LK. Active GPIIb-IIIa con-formations that link ligand interaction with cytoskeletal reor-ganization. *Blood* 96:2487, 2000.

55. Hirsh J, Bates SM. The emerging role of low-molecular-weight heparin in cardiovascular medicine. *Prog Cardiovasc Dis* 42:235, 2000.

56. McCrae KR, Bussel JB, Mannucci PM, et al. Platelets: An update on diagnosis and management of thrombocytopenic disorders. *Hematology* 282, 2001.

57. Aguilar D, Goldhaber SZ. Clinical uses of low-molecular-weight heparins. *Chest* 115:1418, 1999.

58. Wedel DJ. Anticoagulation and regional anesthesia. *Anesth Analg* 96:114S, 2003.

59. Buller HR, Davidson BL, Decousus H, et al. Subcutaneous fonda-parinux versus intravenous unfractionated heparin in the initial treatment of pulmonary embolism. *N Engl J Med* 349:1695, 2003.

60. Xi M, Beguin S, Hemker HC. The relative importance of the fac-tors II, VII, IX and X for the prothrombinase activity in plasma of orally anticoagulated patients. *Thromb Haemost* 62:788, 1989.

61. Kearon C, Hirsh J. Management of anticoagulation before and after elective surgery. *N Engl J Med* 336:1506, 1997.

62. Levine GN, Ali MN, Schafer AI. Antithrombotic therapy in patients with acute coronary syndromes. *Arch Intern Med* 161:937, 2001.

63. Beilin Y, Zahn J, Comerford M. Safe epidural analgesia in thirty parturients with platelet counts between 69,000 and 98,000 mm-3. *Anesth Analg* 85:385, 1997.

64. Douglas MJ. Platelets, the parturient and regional anesthesia. *Int J Obstet Anesth* 10:113, 2001.

65. Johnson JR, Samuels P. Review of autoimmune thrombocytope-nia: Pathogenesis, diagnosis, and management in pregnancy. *Clin Obstet Gynecol* 42:317, 1999.

66. Kam PCA, Thompson SA, Liew ACS. Thrombocytopenia in the parturient. *Anaesthesia* 59:255, 2004.

67. Anonymous. Report of the National High Blood Pressure Education Program Working Group on High Blood Pressure in Pregnancy. *Am J Obstet Gynecol* 183:S1, 2000.

68. Esplin MS, Branch DW. Diagnosis and management of throm-botic microangiopathies during pregnancy. *Clin Obstet Gynecol* 42:360, 1999.

69. George JN. Platelets. *Lancet* 355:1531, 2000.

70. Uzunlar HI, Eroglu A, Senel AC, et al. A patient with Glanzmann's thrombasthenia for emergent abdominal surgery. *Anesth Analg* 99:1258, 2004.

71. Tholouli E, Hay CRM, O'Gorman P, et al. Acquired Glanzmann's thrombasthenia without thrombocytopenia: A severe acquired autoimmune bleeding disorder. *Br J Haematol* 127:209, 2004.

72. Fausett B, Silver RM. Congenital disorders of platelet function. *Clin Obstet Gynecol* 42:390, 1999.

73. Sharma SK, Philip J, Whitten CW, et al. Assessment of changes in coagulation in parturients with preeclampsia using throm-boelastography. *Anesthesiology* 90:385, 1999.

74. Vincelot A, Nathan N, Collet D, et al. Platelet function during pregnancy: An evaluation using the PFA-100 analyser. *Br J Anaesth* 87:890, 2001.

75. Nichols WC, Ginsburg D. von Willebrand disease. *Medicine* 76:1, 1997.

76. Kadir RA, Lee CA, Sabin CA, et al. Pregnancy in women with von Willebrand's disease or factor XI deficiency. *Br J Obstet Gynaecol* 105:314, 1998.

77. Mannucci PM. Treatment of von Willebrand's disease. *N Engl J Med* 351:683, 2004.

78. Cohen S, Daitch JS, Amar D, et al. Epidural analgesia for labor and delivery in a patient with von Willebrand's disease. *Reg Anesth* 14:95, 1989.

79. Kadir RA, Aledort LM. Obstetrical and gynaecological bleeding: A common presenting symptom. *Clin Lab Haematol* 22:12, 2000.

80. Hack G, Hofmann P, Brackmann HH, et al. Regional anaesthe-sia in haemophiliacs. *Anaesth Intensive Care* 15:45, 1980.

81. Fahy BG, Malinow AM. Anesthesia with antiphospholipid anti-bodies: Anesthetic management of a parturient with lupus anti-coagulant and anticardiolipin antibody. *J Clin Anesth* 8:49, 1996.

82. Levy RA, de Meis E, Pierangeli S. An adapted ELISA method for differentiating pathogenic from nonpathogenic aPL by a beta 2 glycoprotein I dependency anticardiolipin assay. *Thromb Res* 114:573, 2004.

83. Gwirtz KH, Young JV, Byers RS, et al. The safety and efficacy of intrathecal opioid analgesia for acute postoperative pain: Seven years' experience with 5969 surgical patients at Indiana University Hospital. *Anesth Analg* 88:599, 1999.

84. Grady RE, Horlocker T, Brown RD, et al. Neurologic complications after placement of cerebrospinal fluid drainage catheters and nee-dles in anesthetized patients: Implications for regional anesthesia. Mayo Perioperative Outcomes Group. *Anesth Analg* 88:388, 1999.

85. Horlocker TT, Abel MD, Messick JM, et al. Small risk of serious neurologic complications related to lumbar epidural catheter placement in anesthetized patients. *Anesth Analg* 96:1547, 2003.

86. Rosenquist RW, Birnbach DJ. Epidural insertion in anesthetized adults: Will your patients thank you? *Anesth Analg* 96:1545, 2003.

87. Cheney FW, Domino KB, Caplan RA, et al. Nerve injury associ-ated with anesthesia: A closed claims analysis. *Anesthesiology* 90:1062, 1999.

88. Benumof JL. Permanent loss of cervical spinal cord function associated with interscalene block performed under general anesthesia. *Anesthesiology* 93:1541, 2000.

89. Broadbent CR, Maxwell WB, Ferrie R, et al. Ability of anaesthetists to identify a marked lumbar interspace. *Anaesthesia* 55:1122, 2000.

90. Rainbird A, Pfitzner J. Restricted spread of analgesia following epidural blood patch. Case report with a review of possible complications. *Anaesthesia* 38:48, 1983.

91. Ong BY, Graham CR, Ringaert KRA, et al. Impaired epidural analgesia after dural puncture with and without subsequent blood patch. *Anesth Analg* 70:76, 1990.

92. Duffy PJ, Crosby ET. The epidural blood patch. Resolving the controversies. *Can J Anaesth* 46:878, 1999.

93. Blanche R, Eisenach JC, Tuttle R, et al. Previous wet tap does not reduce success rate of labor epidural analgesia. *Anesth Analg* 79:291, 1994.

94. Hebl JR, Horlocker TT, Chantigian RC, et al. Epidural anesthesia and analgesia are not impaired after dural puncture with or without epidural blood patch. *Anesth Analg* 89:390, 1999.

95. Harrington PR. Treatment of scoliosis. Correction and internal fixation by spine instrumentation. *J Bone Joint Surg* 44A:591, 1962.

96. Crosby ET, Halpern SH. Obstetric epidural anaesthesia in patients with Harrington instrumentation. *Can J Anaesth* 36:693, 1989.

97. Yeo ST, French R. Combined spinal-epidural in the obstetric patient with Harrington rods assisted by ultrasonography. *Br J Anaesth* 83:670, 1999.

98. Moran DH, Johnson MD. Continuous spinal anesthesia with combined hyperbaric and isobaric bupivacaine in a patient with scoliosis. *Anesth Analg* 70:445, 1990.

99. Tsen LC. Neurologic complications of labor analgesia and anesthesia. *Int Anesthesiol Clin* 40:67, 2002.

100. MacArthur C, Lewis M, Knox EG, et al. Epidural anaesthesia and long term backache after childbirth. *BMJ* 301:9, 1990.

101. Russell R, Dundas R, Reynolds F. Long term backache after childbirth: Prospective search for causative factors. *BMJ* 312:1384, 1996.

102. Tetzlaff JE, Dilger JA, Wu C, et al. Influence of lumbar spine pathology on the incidence of paresthesia during spinal anesthesia. *Reg Anesth Pain Med* 23:560, 1998.

103. Miller DC. Epiduralgrams: Characteristics of contrast flow within the epidural space. *Pain Med* 2:247, 2001.

104. Benzon HT, Braunschweig R, Molloy RE. Delayed onset of epidural anesthesia in patients with back pain. *Anesth Analg* 60:874, 1981.

105. Jonsson B, Stromqvist B. Symptoms and signs in degeneration of the lumbar spine. A prospective, consecutive study of 300 operated patients. *J Bone Joint Surg Br* 75:381, 1993.

106. Brookman CA, Rutledge ML. Epidural abscess: Case report and literature review. *Reg Anesth Pain Med* 25:428, 2000.

107. Roberts SP, Petts HV. Meningitis after obstetric spinal anaesthesia. *Anaesthesia* 45:376, 1990.

108. Jakobsen KB, Christensen MK, Carlsson PS. Extradural anaesthesia for repeated surgical treatment in the presence of infection. *Br J Anaesth* 75:536, 1995.

109. Wang LP, Hauerberg J, Schmidt JF. Incidence of spinal epidural abscess after epidural analgesia: A national 1-year survey. *Anesthesiology* 91:1928, 1999.

110. Philips JMG, Stedeford JC, Hartsilver E, et al. Epidural abscess complicating insertion of epidural catheters. *Br J Anaesth* 89:778, 2002.

111. Carson D, Wildsmith JA. The risk of extradural abscess. *Br J Anaesth* 75:520, 1995.

112. Kuczkowski KM. Labor analgesia for the parturient with cardiac disease: What does an obstetrician need to know? *Acta Obstet Gynecol Scand* 83:223, 2004.

113. Pittard A, Vucevic M. Regional anaesthesia with a subarachnoid microcatheter for caeserean section in a parturient with aortic stenosis. *Anaesthesia* 53:169, 1998.

114. Brighouse D. Anaesthesia for caesarian section in patients with aortic stenosis: The case for regional anesthesia. *Anaesthesia* 53:107, 1998.

115. Brian JE, Seifen AB, Clark RB, et al. Aortic stenosis, cesarean delivery, and epidural anesthesia. *J Clin Anesth* 7:264, 1995.

116. VanHelder T, Smedstad KG. Combined spinal epidural anaesthesia in a primigravida with valvular heart disease. *Can J Anaesth* 45:488, 1998.

117. Collard CD, Eappen S, Lynch EP, et al. Continuous spinal anesthesia with invasive hemodynamic monitoring for surgical repair of the hip in two patients with severe aortic stenosis. *Anesth Analg* 81:195, 1995.

118. Autore C, Brauneis S, Apponi F, et al. Epidural anesthesia for cesarean section in patients with hypertrophic cardiomyopathy: A report of three cases. *Anesthesiology* 92:286, 1999.

119. Ho KM, Kee WD, Poon MC. Combined spinal and epidural anesthesia in a parturient with idiopathic hypertrophic subaortic stenosis. *Anesthesiology* 87:168, 1997.

120. Hoehner PJ. Ethical aspects of informed consent in obstetric anesthesia: New challenges and solutions. *J Clin Anesth* 15:587, 2003.

121. Pattee C, Ballantyne M, Milne B. Epidural analgesia for labour and delivery. Informed consent issues. *Can J Anaesth* 44:918, 1997.

122. Post LF, Blustein J, Gordon E, et al. Pain, ethics, culture, and informed consent to relief. *J Law Med Ethics* 24:348, 1996.

Complications and Side Effects of Central Neuraxial Techniques

Eric Cappiello
Lawrence C. Tsen

CHAPTER

6

INTRODUCTION

In 1899, just 14 years after the first recorded intrathecal administration of a local anesthetic (LA), the German surgeon August Bier reported a series of six patients who experienced pain, vomiting, and postoperative headaches following intrathecal cocaine.[1] The high incidence of such complications following spinal anesthesia, attributed primarily to the use of wide bore needles and the LA cocaine, threatened to derail the interest of the medical community and public in central neuraxial techniques. With advances in equipment, techniques, medications, and experience, the risk-benefit ratio for central neuraxial techniques has improved considerably; these techniques now comprise a large percentage of the diagnostic, therapeutic, analgesic, and anesthetic methods used by anesthesiologists. Neuraxial techniques are associated with side effects and complications, as are all medical procedures, and these should be considered when consulting with patients and surgeons, planning an anesthetic, and considering preventative and treatment strategies. Awareness, prevention, diagnosis, and treatment are the foundations for the safe provision of neuraxial techniques.

The incidence of specific side effects and complications, preventative strategies, differential diagnosis, and treatment will be discussed. For the purposes of this chapter, complications of neuraxial anesthesia have been arbitrarily divided into minor and major based on the likelihood of death or permanent disability. This is not to suggest that seemingly minor complications cannot result in significant morbidity or mortality.

INCIDENCE OF COMPLICATIONS AFTER NEURAXIAL ANESTHESIA

Permanent neurologic injury associated with central neuraxial blockade is fortunately extremely rare and for this reason the true incidence is difficult to determine. In prospective and retrospective surveys evaluating approximately 90,000 patients collectively, the incidence of persistent neurologic sequelae varies between 0.01 and 0.03%.[2–4] Auroy et al.[5] performed a multicenter prospective survey over a 5-month period in France; 40,640 spinal and 30,413 epidural anesthetics were performed and neurologists examined all deficits lasting more than 2 days. The incidence of cardiac arrest and neurologic complications, although very low, was significantly higher after spinal than epidural anesthesia (Fig. 6-1) Nineteen of 34 patients who developed a radiculopathy, cauda equina syndrome (CES), or paraplegia recovered completely within 3 months. Common findings among patients diagnosed with radiculopathy were the presence of pain on injection ($n = 2$), paresthesia during dural puncture ($n = 19$), or the use of hyperbaric 5% lidocaine ($n = 9$). A subsequent multicenter prospective survey conducted by Auroy et al.[6] over a 10-month period used a 24-h telephone hotline for the reporting of complications occurring after regional anesthetics. A total of 41,079 spinal and 35,293 epidural anesthetics were performed, which resulted in 31 and 7 serious events following spinal and epidural techniques, respectively. The incidence of cardiac arrest ($n = 10$) and neurologic complications ($n = 14$) was again very low; however, more common following spinal anesthesia (Fig. 6-1).

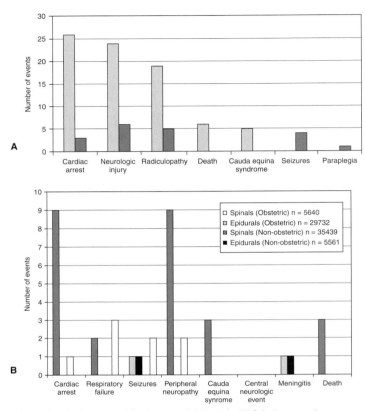

FIGURE 6-1. Serious event following neuraxial blockade. (A) Spinal compared to epidural anesthesia. (B) Nonobstetric spinal compared to epidural anesthesia and obstetric spinal compared to epidural anesthesia. *Adapted from Auroy Y, Narchi P, Messiah A, et al. Serious complications related to regional anesthesia: Results of a prospective survey in France. Anesthesiology 87:479, 1997; Auroy Y, Benhamou D, Bargues L, et al. Major complications of regional anesthesia in France: The SOS Regional Anesthesia Hotline Service. Anesthesiology 97:1274, 2002.*

The American Society of Anesthesiologist's (ASA) closed claims project has reported the analysis of regional anesthesia claims on several occasions.[7,8] Cheney et al.[7] reported on the 4183 claims in the ASA's closed claims database in 1999. Six hundred and seventy claims for anesthesia-related nerve injury were evaluated (16% of total claims), of which 189 claims involved damage to the lumbosacral roots or spinal cord (Fig. 6-2). Lumbosacral root injuries were predominantly related to the use of regional anesthetic techniques and frequently associated with paresthesias during needle or catheter placement or pain on injection. In 2004, Lee et al.[8] observed that the incidence of claims for neurologic deficits following neuraxial techniques was proportionally higher in the obstetric population (Box 6-1).

Lee et al., however, reported that claims filed for permanent and severe deficits following obstetric neuraxial techniques were less common, a finding that has been corroborated in

Box 6-1

Closed Claims Related to Regional Anesthesia from 1980 to 1999

Total regional anesthesia claims	1005
Number of obstetric neuraxial block claims	368
Percentage of obstetric claims related to neuraxial block	51%
Number of nonobstetric neuraxial block claims	453
Percentage of nonobstetric claims related to neuraxial block	41%

Source: Data from Ref. 8.

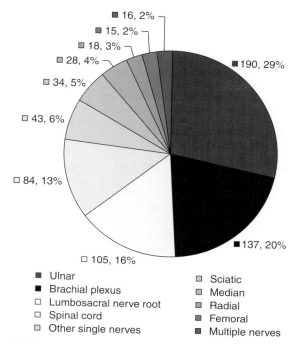

FIGURE 6-2. Anesthesia-related nerve injury: number of claims in ASA's closed claims database (1999). There were 4183 total claims and 670 nerve injury claims. Numbers indicate number of claims and percentages indicate percentage of total nerve injury claims. *Adapted from Cheney FW, Domino KB, Caplan RA, et al. Nerve injury associated with anesthesia: A closed claims analysis. Anesthesiology 90:1062, 1999.*

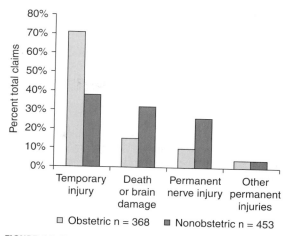

FIGURE 6-3. Neuraxial anesthesia-related claims in the ASA's closed claims database: obstetric compared to nonobstetric claims. *Adapted from Lee LA, Posner KL, Domino KB, et al. Injuries associated with regional anesthesia in the 1980s and 1990s: A closed claims analysis. Anesthesiology 101:143, 2004.*

other studies (Fig. 6-3). A retrospective review of 505,000 obstetric epidural procedures identified three serious complications involving more than a single peripheral nerve[9]: one patient had permanent paraplegia (possibly caused by arachnoiditis), and the neurologic deficits in two further patients, resulting from an epidural hematoma and abscess, resolved after surgical decompression.[10] In a prospective study, Wong et al.[11] interviewed all the women who delivered at a single institution over a 1-year period on postpartum day 1 (N = 6048). Women who reported symptoms of lumbosacral spine or lower extremity nerve injuries were examined by a physiatrist; 56 women (0.92%) were diagnosed with a nerve injury, of which only one injury could be attributed to neuraxial anesthesia. The authors concluded that the use of intrapartum neuraxial blockade was not associated with risk of nerve injury. Similarly, Sartore et al.[12] observed 70 matched pairs of primiparous women who labored with or without epidural analgesia and found that epidural analgesia was not associated with symptoms related to perineal trauma and pelvic floor muscle weakness.

Despite the perception that neurologic dysfunction following central neuraxial techniques is causally related to complications with the technique, the true etiology is often multifactorial and difficult to identify for several reasons. First, central and peripheral neurologic dysfunction occur de novo; spinal-epidural abscesses, hematomas, and vascular accidents occur spontaneously. Second, repetitive subclinical trauma due to activities of daily life or other events, such as labor and delivery, may cause strain to the ligaments, discs, and bony structures of the back and ultimately manifest as deficits.[13] Third, disease states, such as diabetes or previously undiagnosed or latent progressive neurologic diseases such as multiple sclerosis or amyotrophic lateral sclerosis, may coincidentally be associated with the perioperative development of new neurologic signs or symptoms. Alternatively, surgical stress may influence the progression of these diseases in the postoperative period. Fourth, surgical misadventures due to nerve traction, stretching, or transection, intra- or postoperative positioning and padding, and ischemia related to pneumatic tourniquet use can result in neurologic dysfunction. For example, recent cadaveric dissections have demonstrated that the location of the ilioinguinal and iliohypogastric nerves places them at greater risk for direct instrumental injury during abdominal and pelvic surgery than previously believed.[14] Finally, inappropriate casts, splints, or dressings, and the casual positioning of partially insensate extremities of sedated patients in the postoperative period may lead to nerve compression injuries. These considerations are made particularly relevant given the types of patients and applications for which neuraxial techniques are indicated; blocks for acute and chronic pain, thoracic surgery, orthopedic surgery, and obstetric labor and delivery.

EVALUATION OF NEUROLOGIC DYSFUNCTION AFTER NEURAXIAL ANESTHESIA

The mechanisms of neurologic injury are often unclear or multifactorial; therefore, the etiologic investigation into neurologic complications following neuraxial techniques should be directed toward timely diagnosis and therapy, rather than finding fault. The importance of this should be underscored, as the reversibility of some neurologic injury is directly related to timely diagnosis and treatment, and the window of opportunity may be small. When neurologic complaints are detected after neuraxial anesthesia the anesthesiologist is usually notified first. He or she should evaluate the patient in a timely manner, consider the differential diagnosis, and decide whether further consultation or imaging studies are necessary. Peripheral neurologic injury is not uncommon following surgery and anesthesia and needs to be differentiated from central neuraxial injury. Knowledge of the normal motor, muscle stretch reflex, and sensory innervation of the lower trunk and extremities significantly aids in determining the location and severity of a lesion.

▶ Evaluating Neurologic Complaints

A good neurologic examination can be brief yet comprehensive; the goal is to determine the location, the extent, and the reversibility of the dysfunction within the nervous system. Deficits can involve anything from the brain to muscle. A brief historic review and examination of the patient's overall medical and mental status including medications, consciousness, orientation, attention, motivational tone, and affect/mood can rule out certain global pathologies. Cerebral involvement can be signaled by cranial nerves deficits, whereas cerebellar, pyramidal, and extrapyramidal involvement can be evaluated by heel-to-shin, heel-to-toe walking, and balance maneuvers. Spinal cord and peripheral nerve pathology should be evaluated by testing motor, reflex, and sensory functions, starting proximally and working distally; recording such findings can assist in determining the etiology of the deficit, communicating deficits to consultants, and documenting appropriate evaluation and follow-up.

Motor Function

Evaluation of motor function is important to delineating the location and cause of injury. Observation of muscle bulk and tone may help distinguish acute pathology versus chronic pathology. Most polyneuropathies selectively involve longer nerve fibers, preferentially affecting the distal muscles of the legs; in the mildest cases, only the intrinsic foot muscles may be affected. Power in the basic muscle groups should be assessed and recorded on a functional 5-unit scale: 5/5 = full power, 4/5 = movement against some resistance, 3/5 = movement against gravity, 2/5 = movement with gravity eliminated, 1/5 = trace movement, 0/5 = no visible movement. Having the patient stand on one foot or tiptoe walk may elicit subtle weakness in the powerful leg muscles, such as the hip abductors and ankle plantar flexors. Table 6-1 lists the innervation of the major motor muscle groups of the lower extremity.

Muscle Stretch Reflex Function

The absence of muscle stretch reflexes suggests pathology of either the sensory afferents or motor efferents subserving the reflex arc. Reflexes are examined for response, reproducibility, and symmetry, and recorded on a scale of 4 units: 4/4 = hyperreflexia with clonus, 3/4 = hyperreflexia, 2/4 = normal, 1/4 = diminished (normal when symmetric), 0/4 = absent. The root origins of common lower extremity reflexes are noted in Table 6-1.

Sensory Function

Although a thorough neurologic examination includes vibration and joint position testing, the response to light touch, deep pressure, pinprick, and temperature at strategic sites on the lower extremities can be easily accomplished with readily available tools and may help determine the possible locations of the deficit (Table 6-2).

▶ Diagnostic Tests

After documenting the presence and extent of a neurologic deficit, additional diagnostic modalities may be used if a progressive or concerning lesion is suspected. Consultation with neurologists, neurosurgeons, or physiatrists may be indicated. Magnetic resonance imaging (MRI) is becoming the neurodiagnostic modality of choice and has advantages over computed tomography (CT scan) in evaluating disorders where bony artifacts (brainstem and spinal cord) can occur. Unfortunately, MRI is often negative in inflammatory, ischemic, traction-induced, and even some metastatic lesions. Gadolinium, a paramagnetic contrast material, can enhance MRI information and is especially useful when meningeal inflammation is suspected.

An electroencephalogram (EEG) measures cerebral cortex (principally gray matter or neuronal) electrical activity and may help differentiate cortical from subcortical pathology, especially in the absence of MRI or CT scan evidence (e.g., early stroke, seizure, and metabolic disorders). Electromyography (EMG) measures the physiologic function

Table 6-1

Lumbosacral Nerve Root Innervation

Root	Muscle	Reflex Affected	Motor Weakness	Paresthesia
L1, L2	Iliopsoas		Hip flexion	Groin, anterior thigh
L3	Adductors longus, brevis, magnus, and minimus	± Knee jerk	Hip adduction	Anterior knee and anterior lower leg
L3, L4	Quadriceps femoris	± Knee jerk	Knee extension	
L4	Tibialis anterior	Knee jerk	Knee extension	Medial lower leg and ankle
L5	Extensor hallucis longus, brevis Extensor digitorum longus, brevis	Hamstring jerk	Toe extension (dorsiflexion)	Anterolateral lower leg and dorsum of foot
L5	Gluteus medius		Hip abduction	
L5, S1	Semitendinosus Semimembranosus Biceps femoris	Knee flexion		
S1	Gastrocnemius Soleus	Ankle jerk	Ankle flexion (plantar flexion) Foot eversion	Sole and lateral border of foot and ankle
S1	Flexor digiti brevis		Toe flexion (plantar flexion)	

of the motor unit (anterior horn cell, axon, neuromuscular junction, and muscle fibers), and can help distinguish nerve, neuromuscular junction, or muscle pathology, and may help locate the lesion within the motor unit and be useful in predicting prognosis.[15]

Table 6-2

Testing Locations for Determining Innervation Level

Dermatomal Level	Testing Location
L1	Inguinal crease
L2	Anterior thigh
L3	Medial knee
L4	Medial malleolus
L5	Dorsum web between great and second toe
S1	Lateral heel
S2	Medial popliteal fossa

A discussion of specific neurologic deficits is outside the scope of this chapter; however, more detailed resources exist.[16] Expert consultation may be warranted for all but the simplest diagnoses. Although acute compressive or stretch injuries generally recover over time, patients may require splinting and/or physical therapy during the recovery period in order to prevent secondary injury.

MINOR COMPLICATIONS

▶ Backache

Backache is among the most common symptoms experienced in adults; approximately 70% complain of backache sometime in their lifetime. Symptoms are common in particular patient populations; for example, during pregnancy and after delivery when exaggerated lumbar lordosis, ligamentous laxity, and poor body mechanics contribute to musculoskeletal pain. Because of the temporal association to neuraxial anesthesia, anesthesiologists are often called on to evaluate postpartum and postoperative back pain; a complete differential diagnosis of back pain should be considered (Table 6-3).

Table 6-3

Causes of Back Pain

General Classification	Specific Disorder
Mechanical disorders	Degenerative disc disease
	Herniated discs
	Muscular or ligamentous strain (pregnancy)
	Facet arthropathy
	Spinal stenosis
	Myelopathy
	Spondylolysis/spondylolisthesis
	Failed back syndrome
Developmental disorders	Sacral agenesis
	Scheuermann's kyphosis
	Scoliosis
Inflammatory and infectious disorders	Ankylosing spondylitis
	Discitis
	Osteoporosis
	Sacroiliitis
	Arachnoiditis
Tumors	Osteoid osteomas
	Osteoblastomas
	Aneurysmal bone cysts
	Granulomas
	Enchondromas
	Hemangiomas
	Osteosarcomas
	Myelomas
	Chordomas
Trauma	Dislocations and fractures
	Skin/subcutaneous tissue injuries
	Ligamentous injuries
	Musculoskeletal injuries
	Spinal cord, root, or nerve injury
	Blood supply injuries (ischemic or compressive)
Neuraxial blockade	Local tenderness due to tissue trauma
	Chemical inflammation (LA, cleaning solution, contaminants)
	Skin site infection
	Neuroma formation
	Direct spinal cord, root, or nerve injury
	Epidural abscess
	Epidural hematoma

Central neuraxial techniques have been associated with localized tenderness from soft tissue trauma irrespective of whether a paramedian or midline approach is used. A lower incidence has been observed after spinal compared to epidural techniques, perhaps owing to the smaller needle size, the single bolus administration of medications, and the infrequent use of catheters with spinal anesthesia. A persistent discrete tender spot at the insertion site may be caused by the formation of a peripheral neuroma.

Burning or deep aching back pain has been described after epidural 2-chloroprocaine. The preservative ethylene-diaminetetraacetic acid (EDTA) was believed to be the responsible agent.[17] It has been hypothesized that EDTA leaks into the paraspinous tissue, binds calcium, and results in paraspinous muscle spasm lasting up to 36 h. Stevens et al. observed that patients experienced less back pain with smaller volumes of 2-chloroprocaine (less than 20 mL), the removal of EDTA, the pH adjustment to a higher value, or the use of a LA other than 2-chloroprocaine.[17] Transient neurologic syndrome (TNS) is another cause of neuraxial-related backache and is discussed in further detail later in this chapter.

The use of epidural techniques for labor and delivery may be the best vindication for neuraxial techniques not directly being associated with musculoskeletal back pain. Several studies have indicated almost identical rates of new backache up to 6 months postpartum in those who did and did not receive epidural analgesia for labor.[18,19] Loughnan et al. performed a randomized controlled comparison of backache after epidural and meperidine labor analgesia.[20] Using an intent-to-treat analysis, similar prevalence rates of postpartum backache were observed in the epidural (48%, $n = 301$) and meperidine (50%, $n = 310$) groups; a further analysis which excluded patients with back pain prior to delivery noted that the incidence of new postpartum back pain was 29 and 28% in the epidural and meperidine groups, respectively. As musculoskeletal pain often represents muscular strain, conservative treatment with over-the-counter analgesics, heat, and rest is recommended. Should symptoms become more severe and signs more progressive, other etiologies such as epidural abscess, hematoma, or other incidental pathology (e.g., spinal tumor, sacroiliitis, osteomyelitis, and thrombophlebitis) should be considered.

Bradycardia

Bradycardia associated with central neuraxial blockade is discussed in detail in Chap. 4. Bradycardia following central neuraxial blockade is often accompanied by hypotension and may result from normal compensatory mechanisms of arterial and venous baroreceptors. In addition, blockade of the preganglionic cardiac accelerator

---

Box 6-2

Risk Factors for Bradycardia Following Spinal and Epidural Techniques

Moderate Bradycardia (40–50 bpm)

▶ Baseline HR < 60 bpm
▶ Male gender
▶ Age < 37 years
▶ Nonemergency surgical status
▶ Beta-blockade use
▶ Case duration

Severe Bradycardia (<40 bpm)

▶ Baseline HR < 60 bpm
▶ Male gender

Source: Data from Ref. 21.

---

fibers (T1 to T5) and reduction in venous return, resulting in decreased right atrial stretch receptor afferent activity, may contribute to bradycardia. Risk factors for bradycardia are listed in Box 6-2.

Lesser et al.[21] evaluated the incidence of bradycardia in 6663 nonobstetric patients, older than the age of 12 years, undergoing either spinal or epidural anesthesia. *Moderate bradycardia*, defined as a heart rate (HR) between 40 and 50 beats per minute (bpm), occurred in 9.5% of the cases, and was associated with baseline HR of less than 60 bpm, age younger than 37 years, male gender, nonemergency surgical status, presence of β-adrenergic blocker use, and case duration. *Severe bradycardia*, defined as HR less than 40 bpm, occurred in 0.7% of the cases, and was associated with baseline HR of less than 60 bpm and the male gender.

Severe bradycardia following spinal anesthesia may be accompanied by cardiac arrest (see "Cardiac Arrest," later). However, when detected early, bradycardia usually responds to intravenous (IV) atropine 0.4 mg; when accompanied by hypotension, the use of ephedrine 10 mg IV may be beneficial, as a rapidly beating, but empty, heart will not result in increased cardiac output. On rare occasion, epinephrine, dopamine, and isoproterenol may be required and titrated to effect.

Hearing Loss

An association between central neuraxial techniques, especially spinal anesthesia, and audiometrically documented hearing loss has been demonstrated. Usually in the low-frequency range (125–500 Hz), which accounts for the typical subclinical presentation, speech frequency (500–2000 Hz) loss has been described as well.[22] Overall, an incidence between 0.4 and 40% of transient hearing loss (*hypoacusis*) following spinal techniques has been observed, but less than 25% are clinically noticeable, and the duration of hearing loss is usually less than 1 week.[22] Young people are more often affected than the elderly.[23]

The postulated theory for hearing loss with spinal anesthesia involves the loss of cerebrospinal fluid (CSF). Alterations in CSF pressure are transmitted to the perilymph (the fluid in the outer scala) by direct communication via the cochlear aqueduct. Endolymph (fluid in scala media), which has an indirect communication via the endolymphatic duct embedded in the dura mater, responds to changes in CSF pressure much more slowly. This imbalance in pressures causes distortion of the basilar membrane, subsequent disruption of hair cell function, and ultimately hearing deficits.

Consistent with this mechanism, the size and design of the needle appears to play a role in the incidence of hearing loss. In a study comparing 22- and 26-gauge needles, 13/14 patients versus 4/14 patients, respectively, had hearing loss across the audible and low-frequency ranges.[24] Because larger needles have been associated with a greater incidence of hearing impairment, hearing loss would be expected to occur with a dural puncture with an epidural needle, although to date this has not been reported. Uncomplicated epidural anesthesia has not been associated with hearing impairment.

Spinal anesthesia-associated hypoacusis improves after an epidural blood patch (EBP). In one prospective study of 15 patients, 12 patients had significant hearing improvement as documented by audiometric testing performed 1 h prior to and following an EBP.[25] Improvement in both groups was also observed in changing from a sitting to a supine position. The literature to date appears to indicate that, without treatment, hearing impairment improves over time. However, as with other neurologic impairments caused by dural puncture and CSF loss, should the impairment be disabling or not improving, an EBP should be strongly considered.

▶ Horner Syndrome

Horner syndrome, which includes the symptoms of ptosis, miosis, enophthalmos, and anhidrosis, is caused by blockade of preganglionic sympathetic fibers from the first three to five thoracic spinal segments and accompanies 1–4% of epidural blocks.[26] Due to the sensitivity of the smaller diameter and more easily blocked sympathetic fibers, even dilute solutions of LAs, injected distant from the upper thoracic spine, have been observed to cause the syndrome. However, symptoms can also be associated with unintentional high or total spinal (see "Total Spinal Anesthesia," later) or subdural blockade. Although sometimes annoying, symptoms abate without sequelae over time.

▶ Hypotension

Hypotension following central neuraxial blockade is among the most commonly observed complications. The mechanisms of hypotension associated with central neuraxial blockade are discussed in detail in Chap. 4. Defined by a reduction in systolic, diastolic, or mean blood pressures by 20–30%, hypotension following neuraxial blockade has been observed to occur in 30–90% of cases. Hypotension may be exacerbated by bradycardia (see "Bradycardia," earlier). It is associated with high thoracic levels of spinal blockade, age greater than 40 years, obesity, concurrent general and neuraxial anesthesia, coexisting β-adrenergic blockade, hypovolemia, and the addition of phenylephrine to the LA (Table 6-4).[27,28]

Nausea, vomiting, light-headedness, and complaints of difficulty breathing are common presenting symptoms of hypotension. Severe hypotension may result in arrhythmias, heart block, ischemia, and cardiac collapse. Symptomatic hypotension is usually readily amenable to treatment; however, in certain patients hypotension is the harbinger of rapid and profound decompensation (e.g., aortic stenosis). In parturients, severe or sustained maternal hypotension can lead to impaired uterine and intervillous blood flow, resulting in fetal hypoxia, acidosis, and neonatal depression.

Table 6-4

Variables Associated with Increased Odds for Developing Hypotension Following Neuraxial Blockade

Variable	Odds Ratio
Peak block height ≥ T5	3.8
Chronic alcohol consumption	3.1
Emergency surgery	2.84
Age ≥ 40 years	2.5
Baseline SBP < 120 mmHg	2.4
History of hypertension	2.2
Combination of spinal and general*	1.9
Spinal puncture at or above L2-L3 interspace	1.8
Addition of phenylephrine to the LA solution	1.6
Body mass index	1.08±

Abbreviation: SBP = systolic blood pressure.
*Compared to spinal anesthesia alone ± per 1 kg/m² increases in BMI.
Source: Data from Refs. 27, 28.

Box 6-3

Prevention and Treatment of Neuraxial Blockade-induced Hypotension

Prophylaxis	Treatment
Intravascular volume expansion (colloid > crystalloid)	Intravascular volume expansion (colloid > crystalloid)
Vasopressor IV dose (ephedrine 5–10 mg, phenylephrine 40–80 µg)	Vasopressor IV dose (ephedrine 5–10 mg, phenylephrine 40–80 µg, epinephrine 0.1 µg/kg)
Smaller dose of intrathecal/epidural LA	
Substitution of opioid for LA	
Slow titration of epidural LA	
Wrapping the legs (thromboembolic stockings, inflatable splints or boots) or elevating the legs	
Beach chair position	Trendelenburg or "leg up" position to improve blood flow to heart/brain

---

Diverse methods have been used with variable success in an attempt to reduce the incidence and severity of hypotension following neuraxial blockade. These include prophylactic intravascular volume expansion and vasopressor use, limiting blockade to one side and limiting unnecessarily high blockade, and also includes nonpharmacologic methods such as abdominal or medical anti-shock trousers (MAST) trousers, or manipulating bed and body positions (Box 6-3).

The beach chair position, for example, may limit venous pooling and high sympathetic blockade, and uterine displacement in parturients significantly reduces hypotension, particularly after the 20th gestational week. Limiting the subarachnoid or epidural dose may result in less hypotension. For example, combined spinal-epidural anesthesia can be initiated with a low spinal dose and augmented with epidural doses, if necessary, after blood pressure equilibration.[29] The substitution of opioids for LAs in the intrathecal space may reduce the incidence and degree of hypotension, but does not entirely eliminate it.[30]

Volume expansion with crystalloid solutions before the initiation of neuraxial blockade may reduce the incidence and severity of hypotension; however, the effect is often minimal, despite volumes as large as 20 mL/kg over 20 min.[31,32] This poor response is likely secondary to the pharmacokinetics of IV crystalloid solution, as solutions rapidly redistribute to the extracellular compartment.[33] Crystalloid infusion administered at the time of initiation of blockade resulted in higher cardiac output and less nausea and vomiting when compared to an infusion 20 min before block initiation.[32,34] Again, this may be explained by the difference in crystalloid pharmacokinetics when administered before and after neuraxial blockade: crystalloid is more likely to remain in the intravascular compartment if administered in the face of hypovolemia (induced by the block), rather than during normovolemia (before the block).

In contrast to crystalloid solutions, colloid solutions administered before initiating neuraxial anesthesia are more effective in preventing hypotension. This is likely secondary to their longer intravascular half-life.[33] Variations among colloids, including molecular size and weight, colloid oncotic pressure, and side effects may influence their selection and ultimate effect on hypotension.

Vasopressors are commonly used to prevent and treat hypotension. Ephedrine and phenylephrine are among the most commonly used agents. Although both agents have been used prophylactically prior to central neuraxial techniques, their effectiveness is variable. This is most likely based on differences in the timing, method, and dose of administration; for example, single bolus dose or continuous infusion before or after initiation of the blockade, and the patient's baseline cardiovascular and volume status. Reflex tachycardia or bradycardia may occur. Although a combination of agents may have superior action over ephedrine or phenylephrine alone, this has yet to be demonstrated consistently. Overall, the most practical course of action may be to chose an agent or combination of agents depending on patient variables (e.g., blood pressure, HR, estimated volume status, and chronic medications), that will treat the hypotension with the least amount of undesirable side effects. A reasonable vasopressor algorithm incorporates a single prophylactic dose of ephedrine or phenylephrine timed to correspond to the expected onset of the sympathectomy, with subsequent treatment based on HR, blood pressure, and symptoms (Table 6-5); if a single agent does not work, larger doses may be used; however, alternative drugs should be readily available, as a combination of agents may work better given their different alpha- and beta-receptor stimulation characteristics (Table 6-6).

▶ Nausea and Vomiting

Perioperative nausea and vomiting (PONV) is a common complication of both neuraxial and general anesthesia. A number of different risk factors and mechanisms have been

Table 6-5

Hypotension Treatment Algorithm

HR (bpm)	MAP	Symptom	Treatment
<45	Within 20% of baseline	Asymptomatic	Atropine 0.4 mg IV or ephedrine 5–10 mg
<100	Within 20% of baseline	Symptomatic	Ephedrine 5–10 mg IV
<100	Below 20% of baseline	Asymptomatic	Ephedrine 5–10 mg IV
>100	Below 20% of baseline	Symptomatic	Phenylephrine 40–80 μg IV

Abbreviation: MAP = mean arterial pressure.

Box 6-4

Risk Factors for PONV

Patient Factor

- Female gender
- History of PONV
- History of motion sickness
- Pain
- Anxiety
- Nonsmoking status
- Gastric distention
- Increased intracranial pressure
- Hypoglycemia

Surgical Factor

- Long surgical duration
- Specific surgeries (intra-abdominal, major gynecologic, laparoscopic, breast, ENT, strabismus)

Anesthetic Factor

- Volatile anesthetics
- Nitrous oxide
- Opioids
- Neostigmine
- Hypotension (especially following neuraxial techniques)
- Hypoxemia

Abbreviation: ENT = ear, nose, throat.

associated with PONV (Box 6-4) and the incidence varies widely among different patient populations. Stimulation of the chemoreceptor trigger zone (CTZ) receptor(s) appears to be a common, although not exclusive, pathway for the production of PONV. Four major receptor systems of the CTZ may be involved: dopaminergic (D2), cholinergic (muscarinic), histaminergic (H1), and the serotonergic (5-HT$_3$) receptors. PONV following neuraxial techniques has been associated with the onset of hypotension and the use of neuraxial opioids.

Hypotension, a common complication of epidural and spinal anesthesia, may present as nausea. Believed related to hypoxemia or hypoperfusion of the CTZ, the administration of oxygen has been noted to decrease the incidence of emesis despite the presence of hypotension.[35] Correction of hypotension, however, remains the recommended and most effective therapy. Although small doses of fentanyl have been observed to improve analgesia and result in less nausea when compared to IV ondansetron during cesarean delivery,[36] certain opioids, particularly morphine, have been associated with both early and late PONV, perhaps related to systemic and CSF diffusion of opioids, respectively. Intrathecal morphine-associated PONV does not appear to be dose related.[37]

Table 6-6

Relative α- and β-Adrenergic Activity of Vasopressors

Drug	Alpha (vasoconstriction)	Beta (cardiac inotropic and chronotropic)
Ephedrine (5–10 mg bolus)	+	+
Phenylephrine (40–80 μg bolus)	++	−
Methoxamine (0.2–0.5 mg bolus)	++	−
Dopamine (low dose ~ 2–10 μg/kg/min)	−	+
Dopamine (~5–20 μg/kg/min)	++	+++
Dobutamine (2–3 μg/kg/min)	+	+++
Norepinephrine (0.05–0.15 μg/kg/min)	+++	+
Epinephrine (0.1 μg/kg bolus; 0.05–0.5 μg/kg/min)	+++	+++

Table 6-7

Antiemetics for Treatment of PONV*

Agent	Early Nausea	Late Nausea	Early Vomiting	Late Vomiting
Droperidol 0.5–0.75 mg	4.8 (3.0–12)	11 (6.9–25)	10 (4.6–51)	3.4 (2.4–5.7)
Droperidol 1–1.25 mg	6.1 (4.5–9.4)	6.8 (5.2–9.7)	7.6 (5.8–11)	8.2 (5.6–15)
Droperidol 1.5–2.5 mg	5.9 (3.8–13)	5.8 (3.8–12)	6.9 (4.7–13)	7.1 (4.2–23)
Dexamethasone 8 mg	5 (2.2–21)	4.3 (2.3–26)	3.6 (2.3–8)	4.3 (2.6–12)
Ondansetron 1 mg	21 (9–infinity)		9 (5.3–30)	15 (8–210)
Ondansetron 4 mg	5.6 (4–9)	4.6 (4–5.5)	5.5 (4.4–7.5)	6.4 (5.3–7.9)
Ondansetron 8 mg	11 (4.2–infinity)	6.4 (4.6–10)	6.4 (4.7–10)	5.0 (4–6.7)
Metoclopramide 10 mg	16 (7.5–210)	12 (6–1587)	9.1 (5.5–27)	10 (6–41)
Scopolamine 0.2 mg transdermal	6.3 (3.7–25)	4.3 (2.9–8.3)	12.5 (6.7–infinity)	5.6 (4–9.1)

*Table presented as number needed to treat (NNT) and 95% confidence interval (CI). Early = 0–6 h, late = 0–24 h.
Source: Data from Refs. 39 to 43.

Regardless of etiology, a multimodal approach to therapy is recommended due to the multifactorial nature of PONV.[38] Included in this approach is the use of antiemetics (Table 6-7),[39–43] hydration, effective analgesia, anxiolytics, intraoperative supplemental oxygen, and nonpharmacologic techniques (e.g., acupuncture, acupressure, and hypnosis). The combination of antiemetic agents has greater efficacy with similar side effect profiles than monotherapy in preventing both early and late PONV.[38] The combination of a 5-HT$_3$-receptor antagonist with droperidol or dexamethasone has been noted to be particularly efficacious. Unfortunately, droperidol has recently been removed from many hospital formularies due to a Food and Drug Administration (FDA) "black box" warning noting an association between droperidol and cardiac arrhythmias. Although this association is still being questioned, current access to droperidol has been severely limited.

Pneumocephalus

Pneumocephalus, or intracranial air, may result when air is inadvertently injected intrathecally during attempted identification of the epidural space using the loss-of-resistance to air technique, or when air is not cleared from the syringe prior to intrathecal injection. Although the incidence is unknown, a number of cases have been reported in the literature.[44] The most frequent symptom of pneumocephalus is a severe, generalized headache immediately following a dural puncture or when changing to an upright position. Pneumocephalus can also be associated with nausea, vomiting, and alterations in consciousness and mental status.[44]

CT scan or a plain film of the head will often reveal the presence of the air in the ventricles. The symptoms usually resolve over a period of hours as the air is absorbed; however, therapy with 100% oxygen or a hyperbaric chamber has been used to decrease the duration of symptoms when large amounts of air or significant symptoms are present.

Postdural Puncture Headache

Postdural puncture headache (PDPH) is a common complication of neuraxial techniques. It may follow a deliberate or accidental breach of the dura mater, recognized or unrecognized, and occurs with an estimated incidence of less than 3%. The postulated mechanism by which symptoms occur is loss of CSF through the dural rent, resulting in traction on intracranial structures and referred pain via the trigeminal (frontal region) and the glossopharyngeal, vagus, and cervical nerves (occiput region).[45] A second mechanism may be related to reflex cerebral vasodilation and increased cerebral blood flow to compensate for the increased volume loss of CSF, resulting in a vascular-type headache.

PDPH most commonly presents within 15–48 h of the dural puncture. The majority of patients complain of a fronto-occipital headache that worsens on standing and improves on lying supine. Tinnitus, low-frequency hearing loss, diplopia, photophobia, nausea, and vomiting may accompany PDPH. The onset of cranial nerve involvement, including double vision and hearing changes, should prompt expeditious evaluation and treatment. The incidence of PDPH is directly related to needle size and type (see Chap. 2). Smaller-gauge, pencil-point needles result in a lower incidence of PDPH compared to larger-gauge, cutting needles. Several other factors have been associated with an increased incidence of PDPH, including younger age, female gender, using a loss-of-resistance to air (vs. saline) technique to identify the epidural space, cephalad or caudad orientation of the needle bevel, a midline (vs. paramedian) approach to the dural sac, and less operator experience with neuraxial techniques (Table 6-8).

PDPH typically resolves spontaneously: approximately 72% resolve within 7 days. However, the headache can persist for months and even years.[45] Symptomatic improvement can be obtained through the use of conservative measures, including assuming a recumbent position, hydration, oral analgesics, and caffeine (Table 6-9). Fioricet and Fiorinal are oral products that contain caffeine. Additional treatment modalities have been described, including abdominal binders, drugs that cause vasoconstriction (e.g., aminophylline and sumatriptan), and agents placed in the epidural space (e.g., albumin, dextran, fibrin glue, and Gelfoam); however, many of these techniques have not been robustly evaluated and some appear to offer only limited success. If symptoms interfere with the activities of daily living, an EBP should be considered.

An EBP is the current gold standard therapy for PDPH. The efficacy of the first blood patch is 70–98%.[46] Autologous blood is injected into the epidural space. The mechanisms by which an EBP relieves a PDPH are believed to be dural compression with translocation of CSF to the intracranial compartment and the formation of a clot that diminishes the CSF egress. Subarachnoid and epidural

pressures are transiently elevated for approximately 20 min after an EBP and the mass effect of the blood resolves over several hours.

An EBP is performed under strict aseptic conditions and ideally with two practitioners (Table 6-10). Other causes of headache should be ruled out before initiating an EBP. Following a discussion of therapeutic options, and the risks and benefits of an EBP, informed written consent should be obtained. Standard monitors (e.g., blood pressure monitor and pulse oximetry) are placed and an IV line is started; the IV is used to administer fluids, small doses of anxiolytics or analgesics, and any other medications should hypotension, bradycardia, or other complications occur. The patient should be placed in the lateral recumbent position to minimize positional headache and limit patient movement, especially if anxiolytics or analgesics are given. The arm with the IV is ideally placed in the nondependent position, as it is easier to perform venipuncture and obtain autologous blood from the dependent arm. A venipuncture site should be identified, prepared with disinfectant, and draped in a sterile fashion. As blood injected into the lumbar epidural space preferentially spreads in the cephalad direction, the interspace where the presumed dural puncture occurred or one interspace caudal to this space, should be identified and prepared in a sterile fashion. The identification is optimally performed with a loss-of-resistance to sterile saline, as a pneumocephalus through the dural rent may occur if air is used. Once the epidural space is located, the blood sample (10–20 mL) is obtained and injected slowly through the epidural needle, stopping if the patient reports moderate, persistent back pain or radicular pain. The blood sample should not be obtained until the epidural space is identified, as difficulties in locating the epidural space may occur, and the blood may clot. Moreover, if dural puncture occurs, the practitioner may wish to delay the EBP for 24 h. Proceeding immediately with the EBP may be less effective and may result in arachnoiditis from a moderate amount of blood passing into the intrathecal sac. Following the EBP, the patient should be placed in the recumbent, supine position with a pillow under the knees. The amount of time the patient should remain in this position is controversial, but usually varies between 30 and 120 min.

The ideal blood patch volume and timing after dural puncture are under investigation, but appear to be 15–20 mL and greater than 24 h, respectively. The use of saline or blood in a prophylactic manner has met with only limited success.[47] Follow-up visits and phone calls should be made until resolution of symptoms, and the patient should be instructed to avoid straining or lifting heavy objects for the next several days, to increase fluid intake (caffeinated beverages, avoidance of alcohol), and to call the anesthesiologist

Table 6-8

Risk Factors for PDPH

Category	Risk Factor
Practitioner	Limited neuraxial technique experience
	Fatigue (higher incidence on night shifts)
Technique	Larger-gauge needle
	Cutting needle (vs. pencil-point needle)
	Loss-of-resistance to air (vs. saline)
	Cephalad or caudal (vs. lateral) orientation of needle
	Midline approach (vs. paramedian) approach (controversial)
Patient	Younger age
	Female gender

Table 6-9

Treatment Options for PDPH

Therapy	Agent/Dose	Comment
Psychologic support		Validation of symptoms and involvement in resolution important
Bedrest		Symptomatic relief, not preventative or therapeutic
Abdominal binder		Impractical and limited benefit
Hydration	Oral or IV fluids	Avoid alcohol, limited benefit
Caffeine	1. Caffeine sodium benzoate IV 500 mg in lactated Ringers 1 L over 4 h 2. Caffeinated beverages 3. Fioricet and Fiorinal	Promotes constriction of dilated cerebral vessels
Analgesics	1. Fioricet 1–2 tabs q 4 h, not to exceed 6 tabs q 24 h* 2. Fiorinal 1–2 tabs q 4 h, not to exceed 6 tabs q 24 h* 3. Percocet 4. NSAIDs	
Alternative medications	1. Aminophylline 100 mg PO bid (extended release) or 225 mg q 8 h × 3–5 d 2. Sumatriptan 10 mg PO tid for up to 96 h 3. Adrenocorticotropic hormone	Works by vasoconstriction Works by vasoconstriction Experience limited, may not be uniformly effective
EBP	Autologous blood, 10–20 mL, drawn aseptically	Prophylactic use controversial Performed with loss-of-resistance to saline (to avoid pneumocephalus). Decubitus position for 1–2 h following EBP may be of benefit
Epidural saline injection	Preservative-free saline, 30–40 mL; some follow with infusion of 40 mL/h over 12–24 h	May offer transient relief
Epidural albumin, dextran, fibrin glue, or gelatin powder (Gelfoam)		Experience limited, may require placement under direct observation

*Fioricet (butalbital 50 mg, acetaminophen 325 mg, and caffeine 40 mg). Fiorinal (butalbital 50 mg, aspirin 325 mg, and caffeine 40 mg).

if fever, erythema, and/or persistent drainage from the epidural skin puncture site develops. Furthermore, the patient should be instructed to immediately return to the hospital or an emergency department if she develops weakness, paralysis, or bladder or bowel dysfunction. An EBP may be repeated after 24–48 h if the cure is incomplete or the headache recurs. However, failure of the second patch should prompt a more concerted review of other possible headache etiologies, including cerebral venous thrombosis, pituitary apoplexy, intracranial tumors, migraine and other nonspecific headaches, and chemical or infective meningitis.

▶ Pruritus

Neuraxial opioids cause pruritus. The incidence is as high as 30–100% and is more commonly observed when opioids are administered in the intrathecal space versus epidural space.

Table 6-10

Technique for EBP

Timetable	Procedure	Comment
Preparation	1. Confirmation of PDPH 2. Informed consent	Consider migraine, tension, or caffeine-withdrawal headache, hypertensive disorders, infectious diseases, dural venous sinus thrombosis, intracranial pathology, pneumocephalus
Procedure	1. IV line placement 2. Monitors placed 3. Consider anxiolytic or analgesics (midazolam 1–2 mg, fentanyl 25–100 µg, IV) 4. Patient positioned in lateral recumbent position with IV arm in nondependent position 5. Venipuncture site identified, prepared aseptically, and draped 6. Vertebral interspace where dural rent occurred is identified, aseptically prepared, and draped 7. Epidural space identified with loss-of-resistance to saline technique 8. Venipuncture performed and autologous blood obtained (10–20 mL) 9. Administration of blood, stopping if moderate back discomfort or radicular pain occurs	All procedures should be performed under strict aseptic conditions
Postprocedure	1. Written instructions for contact and care given 2. Follow-up visits or phone calls until resolution	Patients must be instructed to return to the hospital if worsening back pain, sensory or motor weakness, or bladder/bowel dysfunction develops

Pruritus is typically self-limited and may be generalized or localized to regions of the nose, face, and chest. Opioid-induced pruritus appears to be influenced by the particular combination of LAs and opioids; of interest, the addition of epinephrine to an opioid-LA combination appears to augment the degree of pruritus.[48] Concomitant injection of LAs decreases the incidence and severity. Pruritus does not represent an allergic reaction; therefore, if flushing, urticaria, rhinitis, bronchoconstriction, or cardiac symptoms also occur, a LA or other drug-induced allergic reaction should be considered (see "Allergy to Local Anesthetics," later).

The cause of neuraxial opioid-induced pruritus is not known, although multiple theories have been proposed. These include mu receptor stimulation at the medullary dorsal horn, antagonism of inhibitory transmitters, and activation of an "itch center" in the central nervous system (CNS).[49] Pharmacologic treatment for pruritus includes opioid antagonists, agonist-antagonists, antihistamines, nonsteroidal anti-inflammatory drugs (NSAIDs), propofol, droperidol, and a scopolamine patch (Table 6-11).[49] Serotonin antagonists, for example, ondansetron, have been observed to significantly reduce the incidence of intrathecal morphine-induced pruritus.[50] While opioid antagonists, such as naltrexone or naloxone, or partial agonist-antagonists, such as nalbuphine, represent the most effective treatment of pruritus, the use of these agents, either as a single bolus or continuous infusion, may result in analgesia reversal as well. Antihistamines are often prescribed, but are largely ineffective because the mechanism of pruritus is not histamine related.

▶ Shivering

Shivering may be associated with neuraxial anesthesia with an incidence as high as 20–61%.[51] The onset of shivering may occur within minutes of initiation of neuraxial blockade. It is uncomfortable for patients and may interfere with the use of automated blood pressure cuffs, pulse oximetry, and electrocardiography. The etiology is unclear, but may involve a differential inhibition of spinal cord afferent thermoreceptors and redistribution of body heat (see Chap. 4).[52]

Table 6-11

Pharmacologic Treatments for Pruritus

Agent	Mechanism	Postulated Site of Action	Dose	Efficacy	Note
Ondansetron	Antagonize 5-HT$_3$ receptor	Medullary dorsal horn, nucleus trigeminus	0.1 mg/kg or 8 mg IV	Multiple studies show efficacy	Additional antiemetic effect
Propofol	Depress posterior horn transmission	Medullary dorsal horn	10 mg IV × 2 30 mg IV over 24 h	Studies conflicting	Sedation minimal at low doses, monitoring advised if infusion used
NSAIDs: Diclofenac and tenoxicam	Inhibit cyclo-oxygenase and reduce PGE$_1$ and PGE$_2$; may modulate the perception of pruritus	Endoplasmic reticulum of macrophages	Diclofenac 100 mg PR, tenoxicam 20 mg IV	Studies show some efficacy	
Nalbuphine	Antagonize mu receptor	Medullary dorsal horn, nucleus trigeminus	3–10 mg IV	Studies show efficacy	Drowsiness at higher doses; greater efficacy than propofol, naloxone, or diphenhydramine
Naltrexone	Antagonize mu receptor	Medullary dorsal horn, nucleus trigeminus	6–9 mg PO	Studies show efficacy	Higher doses may create need for rescue analgesia
Naloxone	Antagonize mu receptor	Medullary dorsal horn, nucleus trigeminus	Up to 2 µg/kg/h	Studies show efficacy	At higher doses may create need for rescue analgesia
Diphenhydramine	Antagonize histamine-1	CNS and periphery	25–50 mg IV/IM/PO	Studies note limited efficacy for neuraxial opioid-induced pruritus	Neuraxial opioid pruritus not histamine related; pruritus relieved by sedation
Droperidol	Neuroleptic agent, weakly antagonizes 5-HT$_3$ receptor	Medullary dorsal horn, nucleus trigeminus	1.25–5 mg IV	Studies conflicting	Higher doses associated with sedation, FDA black box warning due to ECG changes

Abbreviations: PGE$_1$ = prostaglandin E$_1$, PGE$_2$ = prostaglandin E$_2$

Shivering has been treated with IV meperidine, clonidine, doxapram, ketanserin, and alfentanil with similar efficacy (Table 6-12).[53] Recently, Kasai et al. have described the novel use of amino acid infusions to alter the thermoregulatory response to spinal anesthesia.[54] In addition, the use of neuraxial epinephrine or opioids, or warming the LA solution to body temperature, may reduce the incidence of shivering.[51]

▶ Urinary Retention

The ability to void is controlled by a complex relationship among neurotransmitters, neural circuits, and smooth and striated muscles[55] and these may be altered by neuraxial anesthesia (see Chap. 10). Although the inability to void is commonly associated with neuraxial LAs or opioids, the incidence following general anesthesia may be greater. In a meta-analysis

Table 6-12

Treatment Options for Shivering

Medication	Dosage	Relative Benefit	NNT
Nefopam	7–11 mg (0.1–0.15 mg/kg)	2.62	3
Tramadol	0.5 mg/kg	1.77	3
Tramadol	3 mg/kg	2.50	1.7
Meperidine	12.5–35 mg	1.67	3
Clonidine	65–220 µg	1.32	3.7*
Clonidine	140–150 µg	1.83	3.7*
Clonidine	220–300 µg	1.61	3.7*

Abbreviations: NNT = numbers needed to treat.
*Data from all clonidine trials combined.
Source: Data from Ref. 53.

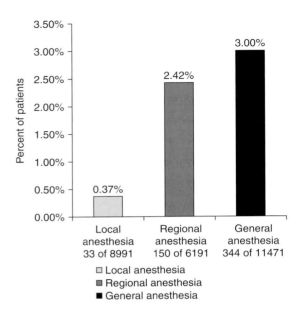

FIGURE 6-4. Incidence of urinary retention in an observational study (*N* = 26,653) comparing local anesthesia, regional anesthesia, and general anesthesia. *Adapted from Jensen P, Mikkelsen T, Kehlet H. Postherniorrhaphy urinary retention effect of local, regional, and general anesthesia: A review. Reg Anesth Pain Med 27:612, 2002.*

comparing local, regional, and general anesthesia, Jensen et al.[56] found that urinary retention occurred at a higher rate after general anesthesia compared to local and regional anesthesia in patients undergoing herniorrhaphy (Fig. 6-4). Not surprisingly, urinary retention has been observed more frequently following gynecologic and urologic surgery, or a difficult vaginal instrumental delivery with or without neuraxial analgesia, where the sacral nerves necessary for urinary function may be affected. In addition, advanced patient age, male gender (controversial), increased duration of surgery, overdistention of the bladder, increased sympathetic stimulation via pain and anxiety, and previous voiding problems can all contribute to increased postoperative urinary retention.[57]

The mechanism by which LAs affect urinary retention is blockade of the sacral nerve roots, of which S2 is of particular importance. Efferent and afferent pathways pass through the S2, S3, and S4 spinal nerve roots to control the detrusor muscle (responsible for urine storage and micturition), internal urethral sphincter, and the external urethral sphincter function. In contrast to LAs, opioids may affect bladder function at both central and peripheral sites. Opioids cause the detrusor muscle and the urethral sphincter to become nonsynchronized, resulting in urinary retention. This effect appears mediated by mu or delta opioid receptors and is reversible with naloxone.[58]

Urinary retention usually resolves with time, often following almost complete sensory and motor blockade recovery.[59] Overdistention of the bladder, however, can permanently injure the detrusor muscle. Therefore, care should be taken to minimize fluid administration, or an indwelling bladder catheter should be used if large amounts of fluid are administered or blockade is prolonged. In patients without a catheter, regular assessment of bladder volume should be made, with catheterization, if necessary. If the ability to void does not return in a timely fashion, a consultation with a urologist should be considered. Similarly, if urinary incontinence occurs, the preanesthetic baseline bladder function, the possibility of overflow incontinence, and more serious entities such as a hematoma or CES should be considered.

MAJOR COMPLICATIONS

Major complications from neuraxial techniques encompass a spectrum of entities. Fortunately, most major complications are rare, but may result in permanent adverse sequelae. Often, the impact of the complication depends on a timely assessment and response. Major complications include neurologic dysfunction, allergy to LAs, anterior spinal artery syndrome (ASAS), direct trauma, drug toxicity, infection, hematoma, and total spinal anesthesia (Table 6-13).

► Allergy to Local Anesthetics

The vast majority of "allergies" to LAs are the result of vasovagal reactions, systemic epinephrine responses, anxiety

Table 6-13

Major Complications of Neuraxial Anesthesia

	TNS	CES	TM	ASAS	Arachnoiditis	Epidural Hematoma	Epidural Abscess
Signs and symptoms	Pain in the lower back and/or buttocks with or without radiation to one or both legs	Pain in the low back	Pain with motor weakness and sensory alterations	Painless loss of motor and sensory function	Pain in the back that increases with activity	Pain or pressure in the back with progressive motor or sensory blockade	Pain in the back that is tender on palpitation accompanied by sensory or motor deficits, and fever
	Describe pain as burning, cramping, or aching	Unilateral or bilateral sciatica, variable lower extremity motor and sensory loss (particularly in the saddle region)	Allodynia (a heightened sensitivity to touch)	Preservation of vibration and joint position appreciation	Variable leg pain, and other sensory and motor abnormalities	Radicular pain, or increasing blockade	Radicular pain
		Bladder and bowel dysfunction	Bladder and bowel dysfunction			Bladder and bowel dysfunction	Bladder and bowel dysfunction
Cause	All contemporary LAs	Ischemic compression by a hematoma or abscess, or direct neurotoxicity, possibly due to prolonged neuro tissue exposure to high doses or concentrations of LAs solutions	Exact cause is unknown, however, viral, infectious, abnormal immune reactions (e.g., lupus), ischemia, and multifocal neurologic diseases (e.g., multiple sclerosis), neuraxial techniques have also been implicated [0]	Hypotension, disruption of blood supply, vasoconstrictors or vasospasm	Disinfectants, LAs, contrast media, blood, infectious sources, vasoconstrictors, hemorrhage, multiple spinal surgeries	May occur spontaneously, after trauma or after instrumentation; higher risk if the patient is anticoagulated with abnormal coagulation status at the time of instrumentation or catheter removal	Bacterial, immunocompromised patients are at higher risk, nonsterile techniques involving the epidural or intrathecal space

(Continued)

Table 6-13

Major Complications of Neuraxial Anesthesia (Continued)

	TNS	CES	TM	ASAS	Arachnoiditis	Epidural Hematoma	Epidural Abscess
Testing	None	MRI studies	MRI or a myelogram				
	MRI or a myelogram	MRI and angiogram					
	MRI	MRI					
	Consults Anesthesiologist	Neurologist and/or neuro-surgeon	Neurologist	Neurologist	Neurologist	Neurologist and/or neurosurgeon	Neurologist and/or neurosurgeon
Onset	12–24 h after surgery	Symptoms have been known to develop acutely (hours to days) or subacutely (1–2 weeks)	Following insult whether surgical or traumatic	May occur years following the precipitating cause	May occur spontaneously, 0–2 days after insult	2–7 days after instrumentation	
Treatment	NSAIDs	Opioids	Heat	Muscle relaxants			
Leg elevation	Little clinical data exist on recovery or therapy although high-dose corticosteroids have been used	Corticosteroids (although no clinical data exist)					

Pain management, physiotherapy, exercise, and psychotherapy is often recommended	Correction of any existing hypotension, correction of vasospasm, physiotherapy, exercise	Pain management, physiotherapy, exercise, and psychotherapy is often recommended, steroid injections and electrical stimulation may be helpful, surgical intervention usually not helpful	Surgical decompression is usually indicated and neurologic outcome is better if decompression occurs within 6–12 h of onset of symptoms	IV antibiotics, percutaneous drainage, laminotomy with washout of the epidural space, and laminectomy		
Recovery Full	Little clinical data exist on recovery	Begins within 2–12 weeks of the onset of symptoms and may continue for up to 2 years; no improvement within the first 3–6 months, significant recovery is unlikely	Variable, may have full recovery, partial, or none	Does not improve significantly with treatment, chronic pain disorder that is not progressive	Variable and dependent on extent of neurologic involvement and treatment	Variable, dependent on extent of neurologic involvement and treatment
Duration Symptoms last for 6 h to 7 days	Variable	Variable	Variable	Incurable	Variable	Variable

attacks, and systemic toxic reactions to LAs, often reported after dental or minor office procedures (Table 6-14).

True allergic reactions to LAs do occur, but often consist of hypersensitivity reactions limited to redness or edema of the skin or mucous membranes. Occasionally, more serious symptoms, such as anaphylaxis or anaphylactoid reactions, may occur. The incidence of serious anaphylactic or anaphylactoid reactions to LAs is estimated to range from 1 in 3500 to 13,000 cases.[60] Less than 3% of cases of intraoperative anaphylaxis are believed to be caused by LAs.[60] Significantly higher rates are estimated for muscle relaxants (69%), latex (12%), and antibiotics (8%).[60]

Most type I (IgE)-mediated allergic reactions occur with ester linkage-type LAs (e.g., procaine, chloroprocaine, tetracaine, and benzocaine) due to previous exposures to para-aminobenzoic acid (PABA)-containing products in the environment, including lotions, sunscreens, cosmetics, foodstuffs, sulfonamide agents, and methylparaben (a preservative).[61] Allergies to amide LAs are extremely rare, but have been reported. The most common immune-mediated LA reaction is a delayed, type IV hypersensitivity reaction or contact dermatitis. There is no cross-reactivity between amide and ester LAs, except in cases where the allergen is a preservative. Cross-reactivity can occur between ester LAs, but this is uncommon among amide LAs. Management strategies for patients with a history of LA allergies are listed in Table 6-15 and should be based on the patient's particular allergy history.

Management of allergic reactions to LAs mimics the management of any anaphylactic reaction, and includes removing (if possible) the presumptive agent, early administration of epinephrine (5–10 µg and 100–500 µg IV boluses for hypotension and cardiovascular collapse, respectively), and airway support with 100% oxygen and intubation, if necessary. IV administration of histamine-1 and -2 blockers (diphenhydramine 0.5–1 mg/kg and ranitidine 150 mg, respectively), bronchodilators (albuterol and ipratropium bromide), and corticosteroids (hydrocortisone 1–5 mg/kg) should be considered. The presence of serum tryptase, a mast cell protease, can confirm an anaphylactic reaction, and the offending drug can be identified by skin prick testing, intradermal testing, or serologic testing.[60]

Table 6-14

Differentiating Alleged Allergies to LAs

	Allergy	Epinephrine Absorption	Vasovagal Reaction	LA Toxicity
Dermatologic	Hives Pruritus Angioedema	Diaphoresis	Diaphoresis Paler	Numbness of lips and tongue
Neurologic		Headache Tremors Anxiety Weakness Cerebral hemorrhage	Tremors Anxiety Weakness Tunnel vision Dizziness Loss of consciousness	Fine tremors of face and hands Excitation Double vision Grand mal seizures Coma
Cardiac	Hypotension Shock	Hypertension Tachycardia Palpitations Cardiac arrhythmias Cardiac arrest	Hypotension Bradycardia	Hypotension Cardiac arrhythmias Cardiac arrest
Respiratory	Bronchospasm Rhinorrhea	Tachypnea	Tachypnea	Apnea
General			Nausea Emesis	Nausea Emesis

Table 6-15

LA Selection Algorithms Based on Allergy History

Reaction	Avoid	Use
Allergy to ester LA	Avoid ester LA	Amide LA without paraben or sulfite antioxidants
Allergy to methyl- and propylparaben: (PABA) products	Avoid ester LA	Amide LA without paraben or sulfite antioxidants
Allergy to sulfonamides and sulfite antioxidants	Avoid ester LA	Amide LA without paraben or sulfite antioxidants
Allergy to amide LA	Avoid amide LA	Ester LA

▶ Cardiac Arrest

Cardiac arrest following central neuraxial blockade is not an infrequent event. It is often preceded by bradycardia and hypotension (Fig. 6-5) and is associated with a blockade of the preganglionic cardiac accelerator fibers (T1 to T5) and a reduction in venous return. In a prospective study by Auroy et al.[5] of 103,730 regional anesthetics, 26 spinal and 3 epidural anesthesia cases resulted in cardiac arrest (Fig. 6-1A). The incidence of cardiac arrest during spinal anesthesia (6.4 per 10,000) was statistically higher when compared to all other regional techniques (1 per 10,000), as was the number that resulted in fatalities. In a more recent prospective study involving 158,083 regional anesthesia cases, Auroy et al. reported 10 spinal anesthesia cases and no epidural anesthesia cases associated with cardiac arrest (Fig. 6-1B).[6] The incidence of cardiac arrest during spinal anesthesia was 2.5 per 10,000.[6] Caplan et al.[62] reviewed 14 closed insurance claim cases of sudden cardiac arrest following spinal anesthesia in which only one of eight survivors was able to conduct independent daily living activities, and identified two associated patterns. First, the use of sufficient sedation to produce a sleep-like state may have masked the degree of respiratory insufficiency and cyanosis; this may have contributed to the cardiac arrest. Second, inadequate central venous filling, despite the administration of α-adrenergic agonists and intravascular volume, and position changes, may have contributed to reduced organ perfusion, increased arrest duration, and increased neurologic damage.

Pollard, in evaluating the circulatory alterations associated with spinal and epidural anesthesia, suggests that vigilance, volume administration prior to neuraxial blockade and as a replacement for surgical fluid loss, and early treatment of bradycardia are important elements in avoiding cardiac arrest.[63,64] Treatment of neuraxial anesthesia-associated bradycardia (see "Bradycardia," earlier) should begin with an aggressive stepwise escalation of therapy with atropine (0.4–0.6 mg), ephedrine (25–50 mg), and the early administration of epinephrine (0.2–0.3 mg). The use of epinephrine in the setting of profound bradycardia or cardiac arrest may be critical for maintaining the necessary coronary perfusion pressure gradient of 15–20 mmHg.[65] In response to recent animal evidence that suggests vasopressin may be superior to epinephrine, especially in the setting of cardiopulmonary resuscitation (CPR) during epidural anesthesia,[66] the most current advanced cardiovascular life support (ACLS) protocol for cardiac arrest supports the use of epinephrine 1 mg IV, every 3–5 min or vasopressin 40 units IV as a single, one-time dose. Regardless of the perceived causes of the cardiac arrest, an expedited examination of the patient and an event analysis preceding the arrest, should be conducted to evaluate

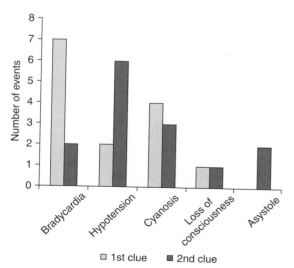

FIGURE 6-5. Early (first and second) clinical signs associated with 14 cardiac arrests during spinal anesthesia. *Adapted from Caplan RA, Ward RJ, Posner K, et al. Unexpected cardiac arrest during spinal anesthesia: A closed claims analysis of predisposing factors. Anesthesiology 68:5, 1988.*

Box 6-5

Potentially Reversible Causes of Cardiac Arrest

Hypovolemia	Tablets (drug overdose, accidents)
Hypoxia	Tamponade, cardiac
Hydrogen ion—acidosis	Tension pneumothorax
Hyper-/hypokalemia, other metabolic disorders	Thrombosis, coronary (acute)
Hypothermia	Thrombosis, pulmonary (embolism)
Hypo-/hyperglycemia	Trauma

Source: Data from Ref. 87.

---

other potentially reversible causes (Box 6-5); and all appropriate ACLS measures should be instituted.

Direct Trauma

Incorrect appreciation of the angle of needle insertion or the vertebral level of spinal or epidural needle placement, or intentional cervical, thoracic, or high lumbar epidural needle and catheter placement may result in direct trauma to the spinal cord and nerve roots. As an indirect measure of trauma, a paresthesia on needle or catheter placement appears to be a frequent occurrence, but an infrequent cause of permanent or disabling neurologic injury. The incidence of transient paresthesias on placement of epidural catheters vary from 5 to 25%.[67] In a retrospective study of 4767 spinal anesthetics, 298 (6.3%) patients reported paresthesias on placement, but only 6 patients had persistent paresthesias postoperatively.[68]

The presence of paresthesias and severe lancinating pain in the dermatomes adjacent to, or below, the site of puncture during needle placement should not, however, be dismissed lightly. Permanent injury with deficits having the same distribution as the elicited paresthesia have been observed.[5,7,69] Reynolds reported a series of seven patients who experienced pain on insertion of the spinal needle at the L2-L3 interspace.[70] CSF was free flowing in all cases, and in all but one patient, adequate surgical anesthesia ensued. Unilateral sensory loss persisted in all patients, accompanied by foot drop and urinary symptoms in six and three patients, respectively. MRI demonstrated small unilateral fluid collections, consistent with a hemorrhage or an infarct, in the conus of the spinal cord. These findings suggest that spinal cord damage may occur with needle placement.

Should a paresthesia persist on needle entry or catheter placement, the drug should not be injected and consideration should be given to reinsertion in another interspace or abandonment of the technique. Of interest, the mere presence of a catheter in the spinal or epidural space may present a source of trauma;[68] whether this trauma is related to inflammation or demyelination, as observed in animal models,[71] or the pooling of concentrated solutions of LAs, is unclear.

Taken together, these findings suggest that initiation of central neuraxial anesthesia in adult patients who are heavily sedated or undergoing a general anesthetic should be performed with extreme care. Often the best guide to an improperly placed needle is a conscious and communicating patient.

Drug Toxicity

Toxicity is defined as the capacity to cause injury. Although drug toxicity can be produced through the incorrect use of agents or methods of delivery, even the correct use of agents in the proper doses and correct delivery methods may result in injury. Laboratory and clinical evidence confirm that LAs, even at established clinical doses, are potentially toxic to the nerve itself;[72,73] systemic toxicity with LAs occurs as well.

Direct Histopathologic Nerve Injury

Symptoms ranging from prolonged blockade to permanent neurologic sequelae have been associated with spinal and epidural LA use. Whether this represents a progression of the same pathogenic process is unclear and controversial. Direct evidence does exist; however, LAs can cause direct nervous tissue changes. Lambert et al.,[74] in isolated desheathed amphibian nerve studies, demonstrated irreversible conduction blockade following exposure to 0.5% tetracaine and 5% lidocaine with and without dextrose. Kirihara et al.[75] found that epidural lidocaine was associated with less severe histopathologic changes than spinal lidocaine in a nonpregnant rat model. Finally, using a nonpregnant rabbit model, Yamashita et al.[76] found that histopathologic changes to the spinal cord occurred in the following order: 10% lidocaine = 2% tetracaine > 2% bupivacaine > 2% ropivacaine.

Transient Neurologic Syndrome. TNS, historically referred to as transient radicular irritation (TRI) or postspinal pain syndrome (PSPS), is usually defined as pain in the lower back and/or buttocks, with or without radiation to one or both legs after uneventful resolution of spinal anesthesia (see Chap. 11).[77] Typically, the symptoms last for approximately 1 week. In a meta-analysis of randomized controlled studies evaluating TNS, Eberhart et al.[78] reviewed

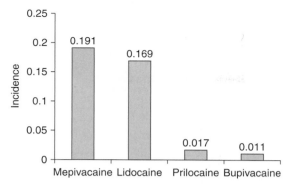

FIGURE 6-6. Incidence of transient neurologic symptoms after intrathecal LAs. *Adapted from Eberhart LH, Morin AM, Kranke P, et al. Transient neurologic symptoms after spinal anesthesia. A quantitative systematic overview (meta-analysis) of randomized controlled studies. Anaesthesist 51:539, 2002.*

2813 patients from 29 studies. The incidence of TNS was found to be highest after mepivacaine and lidocaine, and lowest after bupivacaine (Fig. 6-6). LA baricity and concentration, and the addition of vasoconstrictors and glucose, had no apparent influence on the incidence of TNS. All contemporary LAs, including ropivacaine and levobupivacaine, have been associated with TNS.

Cauda Equina Syndrome. The cauda equina is comprised of nerve roots caudal to the termination of the spinal cord and is particularly susceptible to trauma due to a poorly developed epineurium and relative hypovascularity. CES is an uncommon entity caused by trauma, lumbar disc disease, tumors, ankylosing spondylitis, and abscesses. The syndrome produces complaints of low back pain, unilateral or bilateral sciatica, bladder and bowel dysfunction, and variable lower extremity motor and sensory loss (particularly in the saddle region). Ischemic compression by a hematoma or abscess, or direct neurotoxicity may cause CES following central neuraxial techniques. Prolonged exposure of nerve tissue to high doses or concentrations of LA solutions have been associated with direct neurotoxicity and CES as described earlier. The clinical scenario of high dose or concentration exposure may follow both single dose and continuous spinal anesthesia, intended epidural anesthesia with inadvertent intrathecal injection, and repeated intrathecal injection after a failed spinal block.[79,80] Symptoms consistent with CES should prompt early consultation by neurologists and/or neurosurgeons, with possible MRI studies. Little clinical data exist on recovery or therapy, although high-dose corticosteroids have been used.

Transverse Myelitis. Transverse myelitis (TM) is a neurologic disorder caused by inflammation (myelitis) across the width (transverse) of the spinal cord that occurs in individuals of both genders and all ages.[81] The incidence is unknown; however, an estimated 1400 new cases are diagnosed each year in the United States. Similar to CES, the exact cause of TM is unknown. Viral, bacterial, abnormal immune reactions (e.g., lupus), ischemia, and multifocal neurologic diseases (e.g., multiple sclerosis) have been associated with the development of TM. Neuraxial techniques have also been implicated.[81] TM may occur at all spinal cord levels and symptoms depend on the exact segment involved. In most cases, however, four classic features are involved, including pain, motor weakness, sensory alterations, and bowel and bladder dysfunction. Pain is the presenting symptom in approximately 30–50% of all patients with TM and allodynia; a heightened sensitivity to touch may also be present. Symptoms have been known to develop acutely (hours to days) or subacutely (1–2 weeks).

The diagnosis of TM is made by eliminating other potential causes, including herniated discs, tumors, stenosis, or abscesses, and other autoimmune disorders. A MRI or myelogram (injecting dye into the intrathecal sac) is often performed. Although no clinical data exist on the value of corticosteroids on the course of TM, these drugs are often prescribed in the belief that autoimmune mechanisms are responsible. Partial or complete spontaneous recovery has been reported, although ventilation dependency, spasticity, and permanent disability may occur. Recovery begins within 2–12 weeks of onset and continues for up to 2 years. If no improvement is witnessed within the first 3–6 months, significant recovery is unlikely. Single, recurrent and relapsing cases of TM have been reported.

Arachnoiditis. Disinfectants, LAs, contrast media, blood, infectious sources, vasoconstrictors, and hemorrhage may cause arachnoiditis, a very rare, inflammatory disorder of the arachnoid membranes which surround and protect the spinal cord and cauda equina.[82] The thickened, fibrotic, and constrictive membranes which result can sometimes be identified by myelography or MRI.[83] Although it has been hypothesized that arachnoiditis can be caused by the inadvertent intrathecal injection of large doses of chloroprocaine formulated with the preservative sodium metabisulfite, this theory has been recently questioned.[84]

Patients with arachnoiditis typically report back pain that increases with activity, variable leg pain, and other sensory and motor abnormalities that typically do not progress. IV corticosteroids, nonsteroidal anti-inflammatory agents, and antibiotics may reduce the inflammatory response associated with arachnoiditis; however, significant improvement is unlikely.[82] The overall outcome is usually poor, and management is limited to chronic pain management and physiotherapy.

Systemic Toxicity/Inadvertent Intravascular Injection

The intravascular injection or absorption of LAs can result in systemic toxicity. Rapid intravascular absorption may follow trauma to the epidural vessels; this trauma is a common occurrence during initiation of the epidural and spinal anesthesia and may be influenced by pregnancy, patient positioning, and technique. Intravascular injection may also occur after the inadvertent placement of an epidural catheter or needle into a blood vessel, or the migration of a catheter into a vessel. Pregnancy and the seated position (vs. a lateral or lateral head-down position), results in engorgement of the epidural venous plexus, making it significantly more vulnerable to needle trauma (Fig. 6-7). [85,86] Techniques associated with less vessel trauma include the injection of 3–10 mL of normal saline through the epidural needle prior to the catheter passage, use of soft-tip flexible catheters, and limiting catheter insertion into the epidural space to no more than 5 cm. LA absorption and toxicity can be further reduced by the avoidance of direct administration of LA through the epidural needle, the use of appropriate concentrations of LA, aspiration and injection in 3–5 mL increments, the

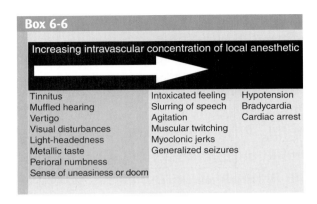

administration of an epidural test dose (see Chap. 2), and maintenance of a high index of suspicion.

The clinical signs and symptoms of LA toxicity are related to the specific agent administered, the rate of administration, and the resulting plasma concentration (see Chap. 3; Box 6-6). Lower plasma concentrations of LAs affect the CNS while higher concentrations are toxic to the cardiovascular system. Tinnitus, muffled hearing, vertigo, visual disturbances, light-headedness, a metallic taste sensation, perioral numbness, and a sense of uneasiness or doom are early signs associated with subtoxic plasma concentrations of all LAs.[87] This can progress to an intoxicated feeling, slurring of speech, agitation, muscular twitching, myoclonic jerks, and generalized seizures as plasma concentrations increase. Even higher plasma concentrations lead to cardiovascular manifestations, including hypotension, bradycardia, and ultimately cardiac arrest. While symptoms and signs of toxicity typically follow this progression, severe toxicity can also present as sudden onset of convulsions or cardiac arrest. This is particularly true following the inadvertent intravascular injection of a large LA bolus, especially those with a narrow therapeutic index, for example, bupivacaine.

The initial symptoms of LA toxicity are caused by blockade of inhibitory neurons within the cortical structures of the brain. Coma occurs as plasma concentrations increase and excitatory neurons are blocked.[88] Respiratory acidosis appears to decrease the dose of LAs required to induce seizures by several mechanisms. These include increased cerebral blood flow and thus LA delivery to the brain, increased concentration of ionized drug in the brain, and by a direct excitatory effect on subcortical structures.[89] With increasing plasma concentrations, CNS changes are followed by, and may even produce, cardiac arrhythmias.[90] Cardiac collapse may follow from direct inhibition of the sodium, potassium, and calcium channels in the myocardium.[91] More potent LAs are generally associated

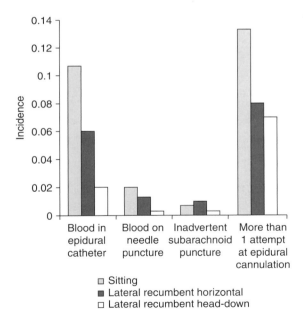

FIGURE 6-7. Incidence of epidural blood vessel trauma and inadvertent dural puncture: patients in sitting compared to lateral recumbent horizontal, and lateral recumbent, head-down positions. *Adapted from Bahar M, Chanimov M, Cohen ML, et al. Lateral recumbent head-down posture for epidural catheter insertion reduces intravascular injection. Can J Anaesth 48:48, 2001.*

with greater cardiotoxicity due to enhanced binding and slower dissociation from these channels. The new amide LAs ropivacaine and levobupivacaine (both formulated as S-enantiomers) appear to have less cardiotoxicity compared to racemic bupivacaine, despite questions regarding potency.[92] Whether these differences are enough to justify their routine use is based on the way they are used (single large boluses for peripheral blocks vs. smaller central neuraxial block doses), drug concentration, and acquisition costs.

Treatment of LA toxicity should include calling for assistance, providing oxygen and assisting ventilation (possibly intubating to protect the airway), terminating convulsions (although most are self-limiting), and supporting the circulation (Box 6-7). Cardiovascular support may require the use of α-adrenergic agonists, inotropic agents, phosphodiesterase III inhibitors such as amrinone and milrinone, and ultimately, cardiopulmonary bypass.[93] Various arrhythmic agents once believed to be helpful in the setting of LA toxicity, such as amiodarone and nicardipine, which can decrease cardiac contractility, and even lidocaine, which can worsen a cardiac block, are undergoing reevaluation. A novel, investigational treatment for LA-induced cardiovascular toxicity is the use of a lipid emulsion to bind free LA agents. Weinberg et al.[94] demonstrated the value of this modality in promoting recovery and survival from bupivacaine-induced cardiac arrest in a dog model.

▶ Infection

Bacterial infection following neuraxial techniques may present as a localized skin infection, an abscess, meningitis, or arachnoiditis. Infection can be introduced by the equipment or solutions from the skin or through a hematogenous route. The most common source of bacterial infection at both skin and deep sites is the patient's own skin flora, comprised predominantly of staphylococcal species, especially *Staphylococcus aureus* and *Staphylococcus epidermidis*. Spread from oropharyngeal droplets of health-care providers may also occur. Four cases of *Streptococcus viridans* meningitis following spinal anesthesia in patients cared for by an anesthesiologist with recurrent pharyngitis' who did not wear a mask during the procedures' have been reported. This suggests that face masks should be part of an aseptic insertion protocol (see Chap. 2). Attention to the selection and proper use of skin disinfection solutions has been advocated, including the avoidance of multiuse bottles of disinfection solutions,[95] and the use of alcohol-based solutions, which appear to have more effective bactericidal activity than povidone iodine.[96,97] Finally, the use of a "no touch technique,"

Box 6-7

Treatment of Acute Systemic LA Toxicity

1. Halt further LA administration
2. Place patient in the supine position (left lateral tilt if pregnant)
3. Call for assistance and additional equipment, including airway and code carts
4. Apply standard monitoring
5. Review and support the ABCs
   a. Airway:
      i. Establish a clear airway using a jaw thrust or chin lift if necessary
      ii. Establish suctioning capability if possible
   b. Breathing
      i. Apply oxygen with a face mask
      ii. Provide artificial ventilation if necessary with mask ventilation. Intubation should be considered if mask ventilation is inadequate, if patient is at risk of gastric content aspiration, or for better ventilatory control
      iii. Consider a muscle relaxant such as succinylcholine 50 mg IV. Muscle relaxants may eliminate the outward signs of a seizure; however, cerebral hypermetabolism may still occur, thus anticonvulsants should be considered
   c. Circulation
      i. Increase IV fluids if hypotension is present
      ii. Establish electrocardiographic monitoring. Prolonged PR, QRS, and QT intervals, reentrant tachycardias with aberrant conduction and atrioventricular dissociation may herald pending cardiovascular collapse. Avoid class 1B antidysrhythmic agents (phenytoin, mexiletine, tocainide) as they may worsen toxicity. Consider amrinone (2 mg/kg) or milrinone (0.2 mg/kg) IV
      iii. Consider vasopressor and inotropic support. Atropine 0.4 mg IV for bradycardia, ephedrine 10–20 mg for hypotension, epinephrine (titrated) for profound cardiovascular collapse
      iv. Institute CPR and consider cardiopulmonary bypass if complete cardiovascular collapse. Expect a prolonged course of resuscitation
6. Consider seizure control with midazolam 1–5 mg IV, diazepam 5–10 mg, thiopental 50–100 mg IV, or propofol (20–50 mg). Avoid phenytoin, as it may potentiate LA toxicity

where only the introducer and not the shaft of the spinal needle is touched, has been suggested. Should an infection occur, bacteriophage typing of skin swabs and the catheter tip may be useful to determine the potential source of infection.

Approximately 2–5% of skin sites become inflamed when an epidural catheter remains in place longer than 24 h. While this inflammation may not represent an infection, the colonization rate of catheter tips has been noted to increase dramatically with the presence of inflammation in an intensive care unit setting.[98] Higher catheter tip colonization rates have been associated with more than one skin puncture within an interspace, catheterization beyond 48 h, and morbid obesity. Culture positive tips, however, may represent contamination of the catheter on removal and have been found to have no association with type of surgery, type of antibiotics used, patient gender or age, duration of catheter placement, or maximum body temperature.[99] In contrast, cellulitis or purulent discharge from the neuraxial puncture site should prompt the removal of the catheter and culturing the catheter tip and skin swabs. Until a definitive microbiologic diagnosis is made, empiric antibiotic therapy should be started with an agent with known coverage for *S. aureus*.

Spinal-Epidural Abscess

An epidural abscess is a rare complication, even in patients who are immunocompromised, bacteremic, or in intensive care unit settings. In a prospective study conducted in Denmark, all nine epidural abscesses found following the placement of 17,372 epidural catheters were in elderly patients of whom eight were immunocompromised. Bader, et al.[100] examined the use of regional anesthesia in 293 women with chorioamnionitis. Forty-three patients had received antibiotics prior to needle or catheter placement. No patients in the study, including those with documented bacteremia, had infectious neuraxial complications. Finally, Du Pen et al.[101] followed 350 cancer patients with chronic, tunneled epidural catheters and found epidural and deep track catheter-related infections on an average of 1 in every 1702 days in the 19 patients who developed infections. The infections resolved with catheter removal and antibiotics in all patients, and 15 patients had catheters replaced with no recurrent infections.

An abscess often presents with backache that is tender on palpitation and accompanied by radicular pain, sensory or motor deficits, and fever. The limited ability to expand within the epidural space may result in segmental compromise to the spinal cord or its vascular supply. Initial evaluation is best with a MRI with contrast. Therapeutic options range from IV antibiotics, percutaneous drainage, laminotomy with washout of the epidural space, and laminectomy.

The presence of neurologic deficits should encourage a more aggressive surgical response.[102]

Meningitis

Meningitis may be caused by bacterial, viral, or chemical entities. Most cases are bacterial and nosocomial in origin, associated with organisms found in the nasal, oropharyngeal, and vaginal passages, not on the skin. Common pathogens include *Neisseria meningitides*, *Streptococcus pneumoniae*, and *Haemophilus influenzae*. Although all central neuraxial techniques have been associated with meningitis, the occurrence is rare. A dural puncture has been hypothesized to allow passage of blood borne pathogens across the blood-brain barrier; however, even in settings where bacteremia is common (e.g., chorioamnionitis), lumbar puncture and epidural anesthesia are rarely associated with meningitis.

Carp and Bailey,[103] in a rat model, found that only when dural punctures were performed in the presence of a moderate level of bacteremia did meningitis result. The creation of a dural puncture without the presence of bacteremia, and vice versa, did not result in meningitis. In addition, even in the presence of bacteremia, if antibiotics (for which the bacterial colonies had a known sensitivity) were given immediately prior to the dural puncture, the risk of meningitis appeared to be eliminated. Although some methodological issues prevent an exact clinical correlation, these results suggest that appropriate antibiotic coverage in the setting of an infection can allow for the safe use of neuraxial techniques even in patients at risk for bacteremia.

Signs and symptoms of meningitis include headache, nausea, vomiting, photophobia, Kernig's sign, nuchal rigidity, and fever (Table 6-16).[43,104] Nuchal rigidity and the elicited signs of Kernig and Brudzinski have all been noted to be poor diagnostic signs of meningitis.[104]

The diagnosis is confirmed via a dural puncture for CSF examination and culture. Treatment with antibiotic therapy usually results in full recovery. Chemical, or aseptic, meningitis has symptoms similar to infectious meningitis, has been observed with all central neuraxial techniques, and is often attributed to inflammation created by skin preparation disinfectants contaminating the CSF.

▶ Subdural Anesthesia

The subdural injection of LAs can sometimes be distinguished from spinal and epidural injection by the resulting patchy block with higher than expected cephalad spread. In addition, mild to moderate hypotension is often observed, as the LA blocks sympathetic outflow to the heart and vessels (Table 6-17).

Table 6-16

Signs and Symptoms of Meningitis

Description	Sign or Symptom*
Classic triad (percentage presenting with symptom)	Nuchal rigidity (94%); sensitivity = 30%, LR = 0.94
	High temperature (81–85%)
	Altered mentation (83%)
Neurologic	Headache, photophobia, seizures, focal neurologic deficits, papilledema, hearing loss (late finding)
Nonneurologic	Nausea, emesis, rash, joint pain
Elicited signs	Kernig's sign; sensitivity = 5%, LR = 0.97
	Brudzinski's sign; sensitivity = 5%, LR = 0.97

*LR is likelihood ratio for a positive test result. Kernig's sign (inability to straighten the lower leg when the hip is flexed 90 degrees). Brudzinski's sign (neck flexion results in hip and knee flexion).
Source: Data from Refs. 43, 104.

The resulting block is often associated with an inadequate degree of analgesia or anesthesia in the lower extremities, and with variable sensory and motor changes in the upper extremities. The cephalad spread may create a sensation of dyspnea, facial and corneal anesthesia, and Horner syndrome (anhydrosis, enophthalmos, ptosis, and miosis). The estimated incidence of subdural blockade is 1 in 2000 attempted epidural blocks. Several predisposing factors have been suggested, including prior dural puncture and the rotation of an epidural needle during identification of the epidural space and placement of the epidural catheter.[105]

Treatment is similar to total spinal blockade (see "Total Spinal Anesthesia," below), with attention to basic resuscitation, consideration of oxygenation and possibly airway protection, and vasopressor and fluid support.

▶ Total Spinal Anesthesia

Total spinal anesthesia in current practice is an unplanned event which occurs in approximately 1 in 1400 attempted epidural blocks, but may complicate both spinal and epidural anesthesia.[106] Although onset of total spinal anesthesia usually

---

Table 6-17

Signs and Symptoms of a Subdural Blockade

Nerve	Sign or Symptom
Sympathetic	Minimal to moderate degree of hypotension
Sensory	Higher than expected level of sensory blockade
	Blockade often bilateral, but can be asymmetric
	Sensory changes occur over 10–20 min
	Patchy, variable quality of blockade
	Poor caudal spread with sacral sparing
	Horner syndrome, facial and corneal anesthesia
	Sense of dyspnea
Motor	Higher than expected level of motor blockade, including upper extremities
	Motor blockade of variable density

Signs and Symptoms of Total Spinal Blockade*

▸ Rapid sympathetic, sensory, and motor blockade

▸ Bradycardia and hypotension

▸ Dyspnea with difficulty swallowing

▸ Limited ability to phonate

▸ Unconsciousness

▸ Respiratory depression with respiratory muscle and diaphragm paralysis

▸ Brainstem and cerebral hypoperfusion

*Symptoms and signs may occur simultaneously, rather than sequentially; unconsciousness and respiratory depression may be the initial signs.

occurs within a few minutes of LA administration, total spinal anesthesia may also occur 30–40 min later with changes in patient position, particularly with longer-acting agents. Total spinal blockade manifests with rapidly ascending sensory and motor changes, bradycardia and hypotension, dyspnea with difficulty swallowing, and limited ability to phonate (Box 6-8). Unconsciousness and respiratory depression may soon follow; respiratory muscle paralysis, direct brainstem depression, or severe cerebral hypoperfusion leading to ischemia of the brainstem respiratory centers may all contribute to respiratory depression. On occasion, following a large dose of LA in the intrathecal space, unconsciousness and respiratory depression are the first indications of a total spinal blockade.

Total spinal blockade may result from the inadvertent intrathecal or subdural administration of an epidural dose of LA secondary to misplacement or migration of an epidural needle or catheter, translocation of epidural medications through an intentional or unintentional dural hole, or the use of very large doses of LA injected into the epidural space. Total spinal anesthesia has also been observed with multicompartment epidural catheters (the orifices are in multiple compartments), or with the bolus administration of LAs or saline through an epidural catheter following an intrathecal injection as part of a combined spinal-epidural technique. Presumably, injecting fluid into the epidural space compresses the dural sac and encourages the cephalad spread of spinal anesthetics.[107] Finally, total spinal anesthesia is more likely to occur when spinal anesthesia is attempted after failed epidural blockade.[108]

Total spinal anesthesia can usually be avoided with close attention to the initial LA injection and all subsequent injections. With single-dose spinal techniques using hyperbaric solutions, maintenance of the thoracic curvature in a slightly higher position may limit excessive cephalad spread. Aspiration, use of epidural test doses, and incremental injection regimens are safe practices with catheter-based techniques. Unusual patient complaints or response to LA injection should prompt consideration of catheter removal and replacement. Management of total spinal anesthesia consists of basic resuscitation support (airway, breathing, and circulation), early provision of oxygen with a low threshold for airway protection via intubation, and vasopressor and fluid support. If the patient is stable, sedation may be added until the block regresses.

▸ Vascular Trauma

Anterior Spinal Artery Syndrome

Despite multiple feeder and radicular arteries, the blood supply to the spinal cord is tenuous in certain regions. A single midline spinal artery is responsible for supplying the majority of the anterior spinal cord; by contrast, a pair of arteries supply the posterior aspects (see Chap. 1). These three longitudinal arteries receive their principal blood supply from six to seven feeder arteries, with the largest being the radicularis magna (artery of Adamkiewicz) to the anterior spinal artery. This artery shares the responsibility for the blood flow to the spinal conus with two branches of the internal iliac arteries, the iliolumbar and the lateral sacral arteries. In an estimated 85% of the population, the artery of Adamkiewicz arises from the aorta between T9 and L2 and supplies the majority of the conus; when the takeoff is higher, the contribution of the iliac arteries is greater. The spinal conus is at risk for ischemia when iliac artery blood flow is reduced or ceases during certain operations, such as an aortobifemoral bypass surgery, a gravid hysterectomy, or operative procedures associated with massive blood loss. The development of ASAS probably requires concomitant vascular disease and a reduction in spinal blood flow through obstruction, compression, or arterial hypotension.[109] Increases in CSF or spinal venous pressure by spinal stenosis, intraspinal tumors, or intraspinal collagen deposits have also been implicated.

Thrombosis or spasm of the anterior spinal artery classically affects the motor, pain, and temperature sensation fibers found in the anterior two-thirds of the spinal cord. The resulting syndrome presents as painless loss of motor and sensory function with the preservation of vibration and joint position appreciation, which are carried by posterior column fibers.

Persistent hypotension induced by neuraxial anesthesia has been implicated as a contributing factor in some cases of ASAS. Theoretically, neuraxial vasopressors could also affect spinal cord blood flow, but this has not been validated. Should signs and symptoms consistent with ASAS occur, correction of any existing hypotension and a consultation with a neurologist are indicated. MRI and angiogram analysis may reveal spinal cord infarction.[109]

Spinal/Subdural/Epidural Hematoma

Although the bony vertebrae serve to protect the spinal cord from trauma, on rare occasions, entrapment of space-occupying lesions (e.g., abscesses and hematomas) within the vertebral canal may lead to direct spinal cord or cauda equina compression and/or ischemia. Epidural hematomas occur spontaneously in normal or hematologically altered patients (as a result of coagulopathy or anticoagulant therapy), even without instrumentation. As such, existing or induced hemostatic abnormalities must be carefully considered in terms of significance, severity, reversibility, and perceived risks and benefits prior to the use of various anesthetic options (see Chap. 5).

Although the exact incidence of hematomas associated with neuraxial blockade is unknown, it has been estimated to be less than 1 in 150,000 and less than 1 in 220,000 epidural and spinal anesthetics, respectively.[110] Review of case reports also suggests that the risk of hematoma is higher with epidural techniques.[111] Fifteen of 61 reported cases of spinal hematoma from 1906 to 1994 were associated with spinal anesthesia, while the remaining 46 cases involved epidural anesthesia. Moreover, in 15 of the 32 patients with an indwelling epidural catheter, the spinal hematoma occurred immediately after the removal of the epidural catheter. Although patient, technique selection, and reporting bias may have influenced this summary report, it is likely that the larger needle and frequent use of a catheter associated with the epidural technique results in increased trauma to blood vessels.

In the case report review by Vandermeulen et al. cited earlier, hemostatic abnormalities were present in 68% of the cases, and 25% of the patients had needle or catheter insertions that were difficult or bloody.[111] Although there are no data to support mandatory cancellation of an operative procedure following traumatic initiation of neuraxial blockade, direct communication with the surgeon, an assessment of risks and benefits, as well as frequent neurologic checks of the lower extremities may be warranted. The report of the second ASRA Consensus Conference on Neuraxial Anesthesia and Anticoagulation[112] evaluated the available evidence and provided recommendations on the use of various types of medications that can affect coagulation, tests, and outcomes (Tables 5-3, 5-4, and 5-7).

Of additional concern is the restoration of adequate hemostasis following cessation of anticoagulation. Because clotting factors are differentially affected following the onset versus the recovery from anticoagulation, equivalent coagulation testing results may not represent equivalent coagulation function (see Chap. 5).[112] Moreover, the concurrent use of more than one anticoagulant agent, compared to single agent therapy, makes the integrity of the coagulation system less predictable. Therefore, coagulation status should be optimized at the time of initiation of the neuraxial technique and catheter removal in anticoagulated patients, and sensory and motor function neurologic testing should be frequently and routinely performed during catheter maintenance and immediately after catheter removal.

Early signs of spinal cord compression include progressive motor or sensory blockade and complaints of back pain or pressure (Table 6-13). The onset of bowel or bladder incontinence or urinary retention, radicular pain, or increasing blockade or neurologic deficits warrants a consultation with a neurologist and/or neurosurgeon. Space-occupying lesions are best confirmed by urgent MRI scanning as they are initially undetectable on plain radiographs and CT scans do not reliably distinguish hematoma from adjacent bone. Surgical decompression is usually indicated and neurologic outcome is better if decompression occurs within 6–12 h of onset of symptoms.[111]

SUMMARY

Complications following spinal, epidural, and combined spinal-epidural techniques are diverse and include major or minor, acute or progressive, and remittent or persistent injuries. Often the sequelae and overall outcome is dependent on the clinician's response. Knowledge of potential complications and defined algorithms for response are essential to optimal management and mitigation of adverse outcomes. Ross[113] noted in reviewing obstetric anesthesia closed claims, that most of the claims were for "minor" injuries and the establishment of good rapport, involvement in (patient) education, and provision of realistic risks, benefits, and expectations may lead to the best overall outcomes. Awareness, prevention, diagnosis, and treatment of complications are the foundations for the safe provision of neuraxial techniques.

REFERENCES

1. Van Zundert A, Goerig M. August Bier 1861-1949. A tribute to a great surgeon who contributed much to the development of modern anesthesia on the 50th anniversary of his death. *Reg Anesth Pain Med* 25:26, 2000.
2. Usubiaga JE. Neurological complications following epidural anesthesia. *Int Anesthesiol Clin* 13:1, 1975.
3. Kane RE. Neurologic deficits following epidural or spinal anesthesia. *Anesth Analg* 60:150, 1981.

4. Phillips OC, Ebner H, Nelson AT, et al. Neurologic complications following spinal anesthesia with lidocaine: A prospective review of 10,440 cases. *Anesthesiology* 30:284, 1969.

5. Auroy Y, Narchi P, Messiah A, et al. Serious complications related to regional anesthesia: Results of a prospective survey in France. *Anesthesiology* 87:479, 1997.

6. Auroy Y, Benhamou D, Bargues L, et al. Major complications of regional anesthesia in France: The SOS Regional Anesthesia Hotline Service. *Anesthesiology* 97:1274, 2002.

7. Cheney FW, Domino KB, Caplan RA, et al. Nerve injury associated with anesthesia: A closed claims analysis. *Anesthesiology* 90:1062, 1999.

8. Lee LA, Posner KL, Domino KB, et al. Injuries associated with regional anesthesia in the 1980s and 1990s: A closed claims analysis. *Anesthesiology* 101:143, 2004.

9. Scott DB, Hibbard BM. Serious non-fatal complications associated with extradural block in obstetric practice. *Br J Anaesth* 64:537, 1990.

10. Scott DB. Epidural blockade. In: Rogers MC, Tinker JH, Covino BG, et al., eds, *Principles and Practice of Anesthesiology*. St. Louis, MO: Mosby-Year Book, 1993, p. 1307.

11. Wong CA, Scavone BM, Dugan S, et al. Incidence of postpartum lumbosacral spine and lower extremity nerve injuries. *Obstet Gynecol* 101:279, 2003.

12. Sartore A, Pregazzi R, Bortoli P, et al. Effects of epidural analgesia during labor on pelvic floor function after vaginal delivery. *Acta Obstet Gynecol Scand* 82:143, 2003.

13. Snooks SJ, Swash M, Mathers SE, et al. Effect of vaginal delivery on the pelvic floor. *Br J Surg* 77:1358, 1990.

14. Whiteside JL, Barber MD, Walters MD, et al. Anatomy of ilioinguinal and iliohypogastric nerves in relation to trocar placement and low transverse incisions. *Am J Obstet Gynecol* 189:1574, 2003.

15. Aminoff MJ. Electrophysiologic testing for the diagnosis of peripheral nerve injuries. *Anesthesiology* 100:1298, 2004.

16. Tsen LC. Neurologic complications of labor analgesia and anesthesia. *Int Anesthesiol Clin* 40:67, 2002.

17. Stevens RA, Urmey WF, Urquhart BL, et al. Back pain after epidural anesthesia with chloroprocaine. *Anesthesiology* 78:492, 1993.

18. Dickinson JE, Paech MJ, McDonald SJ, et al. The impact of intrapartum analgesia on labour and delivery outcomes in nulliparous women. *Aust N Z J Obstet Gynaecol* 42:59, 2002.

19. Breen TW, Ransil BJ, Groves PA, et al. Factors associated with back pain after childbirth. *Anesthesiology* 81:29, 1994.

20. Loughnan BA, Carli F, Romney M, et al. Epidural analgesia and backache: A randomized controlled comparison with intramuscular meperidine for analgesia during labour. *Br J Anaesth* 89:466, 2002.

21. Lesser JB, Sanborn KV, Valskys R, et al. Severe bradycardia during spinal and epidural anesthesia recorded by an anesthesia information management system. *Anesthesiology* 99:859, 2003.

22. Sprung J, Bourke DL, Contreras MG, et al. Perioperative hearing impairment. *Anesthesiology* 98:241, 2003.

23. Gultekin S, Ozcan S. Does hearing loss after spinal anesthesia differ between young and elderly patients? *Anesth Analg* 94:1318, 2002.

24. Fog J, Wang LP, Sundberg A, et al. Hearing loss after spinal anesthesia is related to needle size. *Anesth Analg* 70:517, 1990.

25. Lybecker H, Andersen T, Helbo-Hansen HS. The effect of epidural blood patch on hearing loss in patients with severe postdural puncture headache. *J Clin Anesth* 7:457, 1995.

26. Day CJ, Shutt LE. Auditory, ocular, and facial complications of central neural block. A review of possible mechanisms. *Reg Anesth* 21:197, 1996.

27. Carpenter RL, Caplan RA, Brown DL, et al. Incidence and risk factors for side effects of spinal anesthesia. *Anesthesiology* 76:906, 1992.

28. Hartmann B, Junger A, Klasen J, et al. The incidence and risk factors for hypotension after spinal anesthesia induction: An analysis with automated data collection. *Anesth Analg* 94:1521, 2002.

29. Vercauteren MP, Coppejans HC, Hoffmann VH, et al. Prevention of hypotension by a single 5-mg dose of ephedrine during small-dose spinal anesthesia in prehydrated cesarean delivery patients. *Anesth Analg* 90:324, 2000.

30. Sia AT, Chong JL, Tay DH, et al. Intrathecal sufentanil as the sole agent in combined spinal-epidural analgesia for the ambulatory parturient. *Can J Anaesth* 45:620, 1998.

31. Park GE, Hauch MA, Curlin F, et al. The effects of varying volumes of crystalloid administration before cesarean delivery on maternal hemodynamics and colloid osmotic pressure. *Anesth Analg* 83:299, 1996.

32. Morgan PJ, Halpern SH, Tarshis J. The effects of an increase of central blood volume before spinal anesthesia for cesarean delivery: A qualitative systematic review. *Anesth Analg* 92:997, 2001.

33. Ueyama H, He YL, Tanigami H, et al. Effects of crystalloid and colloid preload on blood volume in the parturient undergoing spinal anesthesia for elective Cesarean section. *Anesthesiology* 91:1571, 1999.

34. Mojica JL, Melendez HJ, Bautista LE. The timing of intravenous crystalloid administration and incidence of cardiovascular side effects during spinal anesthesia: The results from a randomized controlled trial. *Anesth Analg* 94:432, 2002.

35. Ratra CK, Badola RP, Bhargava KP. A study of factors concerned in emesis during spinal anaesthesia. *Br J Anaesth* 44:1208, 1972.

36. Manullang TR, Viscomi CM, Pace NL. Intrathecal fentanyl is superior to intravenous ondansetron for the prevention of perioperative nausea during cesarean delivery with spinal anesthesia. *Anesth Analg* 90:1162, 2000.

37. Palmer CM, Emerson S, Volgoropolous D, et al. Dose-response relationship of intrathecal morphine for postcesarean analgesia. *Anesthesiology* 90:437, 1999.

38. Habib AS, Gan TJ. Evidence-based management of postoperative nausea and vomiting: A review. *Can J Anaesth* 51:326, 2004.

39. Henzi I, Sonderegger J, Tramer MR. Efficacy, dose-response, and adverse effects of droperidol for prevention of postoperative nausea and vomiting. *Can J Anaesth* 47:537, 2000.

40. Tramer MR, Moore RA, Reynolds DJ, et al. A quantitative systematic review of ondansetron in treatment of established postoperative nausea and vomiting. *BMJ* 314:1088, 1997.

41. Henzi I, Walder B, Tramer MR. Dexamethasone for the prevention of postoperative nausea and vomiting: A quantitative systematic review. *Anesth Analg* 90:186, 2000.

42. Kranke P, Morin AM, Roewer N, et al. The efficacy and safety of transdermal scopolamine for the prevention of postoperative nausea and vomiting: A quantitative systematic review. *Anesth Analg* 95:133, 2002.

43. Attia J, Hatala R, Cook DJ, et al. The rational clinical examination. Does this adult patient have acute meningitis? *JAMA* 282:175, 1999.

44. Shenouda PE, Cunningham BJ. Assessing the superiority of saline versus air for use in the epidural loss-of-resistance technique: A literature review. *Reg Anesth Pain Med* 28:48, 2003.

45. Turnbull DK, Shepherd DB. Post-dural puncture headache: Pathogenesis, prevention and treatment. *Br J Anaesth* 91:718, 2003.

46. Duffy PJ, Crosby ET. The epidural blood patch. Resolving the controversies. *Can J Anaesth* 46:878, 1999.

47. Scavone BM, Wong CA, Sullivan JT, et al. Efficacy of a prophylactic epidural blood patch in preventing post dural puncture headache in parturients after inadvertent dural puncture. *Anesthesiology* 101:1422, 2004.

48. Douglas MJ, Kim JH, Ross PL, et al. The effect of epinephrine in local anaesthetic on epidural morphine-induced pruritus. *Can Anaesth Soc J* 33:737, 1986.

49. Szarvas S, Harmon D, Murphy D. Neuraxial opioid-induced pruritus: A review. *J Clin Anesth* 15:234, 2003.

50. Yeh HM, Chen LK, Lin CJ, et al. Prophylactic intravenous ondansetron reduces the incidence of intrathecal morphine-induced pruritus in patients undergoing cesarean delivery. *Anesth Analg* 91:172, 2000.

51. Shehabi Y, Gatt S, Buckman T, et al. Effect of adrenaline, fentanyl and warming of injectate on shivering following extradural analgesia in labour. *Anaesth Intensive Care* 18:31, 1990.

52. Sessler DI. Perioperative heat balance. *Anesthesiology* 92:578, 2000.

53. Kranke P, Eberhart LH, Roewer N, et al. Pharmacological treatment of postoperative shivering: A quantitative systematic review of randomized controlled trials. *Anesth Analg* 94:453, 2002.

54. Kasai T, Nakajima Y, Matsukawa T, et al. Effect of preoperative amino acid infusion on thermoregulatory response during spinal anaesthesia. *Br J Anaesth* 90:58, 2003.

55. de Groat WC, Yoshimura N. Pharmacology of the lower urinary tract. *Annu Rev Pharmacol Toxicol* 41:691, 2001.

56. Jensen P, Mikkelsen T, Kehlet H. Postherniorrhaphy urinary retention effect of local, regional, and general anesthesia: A review. *Reg Anesth Pain Med* 27:612, 2002.

57. Tammela T. Postoperative urinary retention: Why the patient cannot void. *Scand J Urol Nephrol Suppl* 175:75, 1995.

58. Kuipers PW, Kamphuis ET, van Venrooij GE, et al. Intrathecal opioids and lower urinary tract function: A urodynamic evaluation. *Anesthesiology* 100:1497, 1995.

59. Tsen LC, Schultz R, Martin R, et al. Intrathecal low-dose bupivacaine versus lidocaine for in vitro fertilization procedures. *Reg Anesth Pain Med* 26:52, 2001.

60. Hepner DL, Castells MC. Anaphylaxis during the perioperative period. *Anesth Analg* 97:1381, 2003.

61. Finucane BT. Allergies to local anesthetics: The real truth. *Can J Anaesth* 50:869, 2003.

62. Caplan RA, Ward RJ, Posner K, et al. Unexpected cardiac arrest during spinal anesthesia: A closed claims analysis of predisposing factors. *Anesthesiology* 68:5, 1988.

63. Pollard JB. Cardiac arrest during spinal anesthesia: Common mechanisms and strategies for prevention. *Anesth Analg* 92:252, 2001.

64. Pollard JB. Common mechanisms and strategies for prevention and treatment of cardiac arrest during epidural anesthesia. *J Clin Anesth* 14:52, 2002.

65. Rosenberg JM, Wahr JA, Sung CH, et al. Coronary perfusion pressure during cardiopulmonary resuscitation after spinal anesthesia in dogs. *Anesth Analg* 82:84, 1996.

66. Krismer AC, Hogan QH, Wenzel V, et al. The efficacy of epinephrine or vasopressin for resuscitation during epidural anesthesia. *Anesth Analg* 93:734, 2001.

67. Ong BY, Cohen MM, Esmail A, et al. Paresthesias and motor dysfunction after labor and delivery. *Anesth Analg* 66:18, 1987.

68. Horlocker TT, McGregor DG, Matsushige DK, et al. A retrospective review of 4767 consecutive spinal anesthetics: Central nervous system complications. Perioperative Outcomes Group. *Anesth Analg* 84:578, 1997.

69. Oswalt K. Medical/legal issues in regional anesthesia. *Am Soc Reg Anesth News* 4, 1989.

70. Reynolds F. Damage to the conus medullaris following spinal anaesthesia. *Anaesthesia* 56:238, 2001.

71. Myers RR, Sommer C. Methodology for spinal neurotoxicity studies. *Reg Anesth* 18:439, 1993.

72. Ready LB, Plumer MH, Haschke RH, et al. Neurotoxicity of intrathecal local anesthetics in rabbits. *Anesthesiology* 63:364, 1985.

73. Rigler ML, Drasner K, Krejcie TC, et al. Cauda equina syndrome after continuous spinal anesthesia. *Anesth Analg* 72:275, 1991.

74. Lambert LA, Lambert DH, Strichartz GR. Irreversible conduction block in isolated nerve by high concentrations of local anesthetics. *Anesthesiology* 80:1082, 1994.

75. Kirihara Y, Saito Y, Hashimotoa K, et al. Comparative neurotoxicity of intrathecal and epidural lidocaine. *Anesthesiology* 99:961, 2003.

76. Yamashita A, Matsumoto M, Matsumoto S, et al. A comparison of the neurotoxic effects on the spinal cord of tetracaine, lidocaine, bupivacaine, and ropivacaine administered intrathecally in rabbits. *Anesth Analg* 97:512, 2003.

77. Pinczower GR, Chadwick HS, Woodland R, et al. Bilateral leg pain following lidocaine spinal anaesthesia. *Can J Anaesth* 42:217, 1995.

78. Eberhart LH, Morin AM, Kranke P, et al. Transient neurologic symptoms after spinal anesthesia. A quantitative systematic overview (meta-analysis) of randomized controlled studies [German]. *Anaesthesist* 51:539, 2002.

79. Lambert DH, Hurley RJ. Cauda equina syndrome and continuous spinal anesthesia. *Anesth Analg* 72:817, 1991.

80. Drasner K, Rigler ML, Sessler DI, et al. Cauda equina syndrome following intended epidural anesthesia. *Anesthesiology* 77:582, 1992.

81. Krishnan C, Kaplin AI, Deshpande DM, et al. Transverse myelitis: Pathogenesis, diagnosis and treatment. *Front Biosci* 9:1483, 2004.

82. Aldrete JA. Neurologic deficits and arachnoiditis following neuroaxial anesthesia. *Acta Anaesthesiol Scand* 47:3, 2003.

83. Chiapparini L, Sghirlanzoni A, Pareyson D, et al. Imaging and outcome in severe complications of lumbar epidural anaesthesia: Report of 16 cases. *Neuroradiology* 42:564, 2000.

84. Taniguchi M, Bollen AW, Drasner K. Sodium bisulfite: Scapegoat for chloroprocaine neurotoxicity? *Anesthesiology* 100:85, 2004.

85. Igarashi T, Hirabayashi Y, Shimizu R, et al. The fiberscopic findings of the epidural space in pregnant women. *Anesthesiology* 92:1631, 2000.

86. Bahar M, Chanimov M, Cohen ML, et al. Lateral recumbent head-down posture for epidural catheter insertion reduces intravascular injection. *Can J Anaesth* 48:48, 2001.

87. Hazinski MF, Cummins RO, Field JM. *Handbook of Emergency Cardiovascular Care for Healthcare Providers.* Dallas, TX: American Heart Association, 2004.

88. Zink W, Graf BM. Toxicology of local anesthetics. Clinical, therapeutic and pathological mechanisms [German]. *Anaesthesist* 52:1102, 2003.

89. Englesson S, Matousek M. Central nervous system effects of local anaesthetic agents. *Br J Anaesth* 47(Suppl):241, 1975.

90. de La Coussaye JE, Aya AG, Eledjam JJ. Neurally-mediated cardiotoxicity of local anesthetics: Direct effect of seizures or of local anesthetics? *Anesthesiology* 98:1295, 2003.

91. McCaslin PP, Butterworth J. Bupivacaine suppresses [Ca(2+)](i) oscillations in neonatal rat cardiomyocytes with increased extracellular K+ and is reversed with increased extracellular Mg(2+). *Anesth Analg* 91:82, 2000.

92. Ohmura S, Kawada M, Ohta T, et al. Systemic toxicity and resuscitation in bupivacaine-, levobupivacaine-, or ropivacaine-infused rats. *Anesth Analg* 93:743, 2001.

93. Hirabayashi Y, Igarashi T, Saitoh K, et al. Comparison of the effects of amrinone, milrinone and olprinone in reversing bupivacaine-induced cardiovascular depression. *Acta Anaesthesiol Scand* 44:1128, 2000.

94. Weinberg G, Ripper R, Feinstein DL, et al. Lipid emulsion infusion rescues dogs from bupivacaine-induced cardiac toxicity. *Reg Anesth Pain Med* 28:198, 2003.

95. Birnbach DJ, Stein DJ, Murray O, et al. Povidone iodine and skin disinfection before initiation of epidural anesthesia. *Anesthesiology* 88:668, 1998.

96. Birnbach DJ, Meadows W, Stein DJ, et al. Comparison of povidone iodine and DuraPrep, an iodophor-in-isopropyl alcohol solution, for skin disinfection prior to epidural catheter insertion in parturients. *Anesthesiology* 98:164, 2003.

97. Yentur EA, Luleci N, Topcu I, et al. Is skin disinfection with 10% povidone iodine sufficient to prevent epidural needle and catheter contamination? *Reg Anesth Pain Med* 28:389, 2003.

98. Darchy B, Forceville X, Bavoux E, et al. Clinical and bacteriologic survey of epidural analgesia in patients in the intensive care unit. *Anesthesiology* 85:988, 1996.

99. Kostopanagiotou G, Kyroudi S, Panidis D, et al. Epidural catheter colonization is not associated with infection. *Surg Infect* (Larchmt) 3:359, 2002.

100. Bader AM, Gilbertson L, Kirz L, et al. Regional anesthesia in women with chorioamnionitis. *Reg Anesth* 17:84, 1992.

101. Du Pen SL, Peterson DG, Williams A, et al. Infection during chronic epidural catheterization: Diagnosis and treatment. *Anesthesiology* 73:905, 1990.

102. Parkinson JF, Sekhon LH. Surgical management of spinal epidural abscess: Selection of approach based on MRI appearance. *J Clin Neurosci* 11:130, 2004.

103. Carp H, Bailey S. The association between meningitis and dural puncture in bacteremic rats. *Anesthesiology* 76:739, 1992.

104. Thomas KE, Hasbun R, Jekel J, et al. The diagnostic accuracy of Kernig's sign, Brudzinski's sign, and nuchal rigidity in adults with suspected meningitis. *Clin Infect Dis* 35:46, 2002.

105. Collier CB. Accidental subdural block: Four more cases and a radiographic review. *Anaesth Intensive Care* 20:215, 1992.

106. Paech MJ, Godkin R, Webster S. Complications of obstetric epidural analgesia and anaesthesia: A prospective analysis of 10,995 cases. *Int J Obstet Anesth* 7:5, 1998.

107. Park PC, Berry PD, Larson MD. Total spinal anesthesia following epidural saline injection after prolonged epidural anesthesia. *Anesthesiology* 89:1267, 1998.

108. Furst SR, Reisner LS. Risk of high spinal anesthesia following failed epidural block for cesarean delivery. *J Clin Anesth* 7:71, 1995.

109. Hong DK, Lawrence HM. Anterior spinal artery syndrome following total hip arthroplasty under epidural anaesthesia. *Anaesth Intensive Care* 29:62, 2001.

110. Tryba M. Epidural regional anesthesia and low molecular weight heparin: Pro (German). *Anasth Intensivmed Notfallmed Schemerzther* 28:179, 1993.

111. Vandermeulen EP, Van Aken H, Vermylen J. Anticoagulants and spinal-epidural anesthesia. *Anesth Analg* 79:1165, 1994.

112. Horlocker TT, Wedel DJ, Benzon H, et al. Regional anesthesia in the anticoagulated patient: Defining the risks (the Second ASRA Consensus Conference on Neuraxial Anesthesia and Anticoagulation). *Reg Anesth Pain Med* 28:172, 2003.

113. Ross BK. ASA closed claims in obstetrics: Lessons learned. *Anesthesiol Clin North America* 21:183, 2003.

Central Neuraxial Blockade for Lower Extremity Major Orthopedic Surgery

Robert Doty, Jr.
Radha Sukhani

INTRODUCTION

Neuraxial block techniques are widely used for lower extremity major orthopedic surgery and offer several benefits compared to general anesthesia (GA). One of the most important is the ability to provide extended postoperative pain control that is superior to that provided by systemic opioids alone. The majority of patients undergoing major orthopedic procedures are elderly and they often have coexisting medical conditions. The choice of the appropriate neuraxial blockade technique for these patients is often determined by their physical status and the complexity of the planned surgical procedure. Optimal perioperative management requires consideration of several factors, including medical risks, susceptibility to venous thromboembolism (VTE), blood loss and potential fluid shifts, effective postoperative pain control allowing early initiation of physical therapy and rehabilitation, and the rare, but possible, risk of perioperative neurologic injury. This chapter focuses on these clinical issues, which are important to the perioperative management of patients undergoing lower extremity major orthopedic surgery.

ANESTHETIC CHOICES AND OUTCOME: NEURAXIAL VERSUS GENERAL ANESTHESIA

The patient population presenting for lower extremity major orthopedic procedures is changing as older and sicker patients with serious coexisting medical problems undergo elective and urgent/emergency surgery in increasing numbers. Two important considerations for the anesthesiologist providing perioperative care to this patient population are (1) the prevalence of coexisting medical morbidities, specifically cardiac, pulmonary, cerebral, and neuropsychiatric disease, diabetes, and renal dysfunction; and (2) the risk of postoperative cardiac morbidity and mortality, and deep venous thrombosis (DVT) with risk for fatal pulmonary embolism (PE).

There has been a considerable debate as to whether or not the type of anesthesia (regional vs. general) influences postoperative outcomes in patients undergoing major surgery, including risk for myocardial ischemia/infarction, VTE/PE, and postoperative cognitive dysfunction (POCD). The reduced incidence of DVT with epidural anesthesia and analgesia is well documented in patients undergoing hip and knee replacement surgery.[1,2] Perioperative epidural analgesia extended for more than 24 h after surgery results in a significant reduction in myocardial ischemia in patients following major general and hip surgery.[3] The incidence of early cognitive dysfunction during the first 7 postoperative days has also been shown to be significantly lower in patients receiving regional compared to GA.[4]

Together, these clinical studies support beneficial effects of regional anesthesia on specific organ systems. Whether these beneficial effects translate to improved overall short- and long-term outcomes is controversial. A recent meta-analysis of a large number of clinical trials, and review of a large body of literature, suggests that neuraxial anesthesia (NA) and postoperative epidural analgesia provide superior pain control, and reduce mortality and other serious complications in patients undergoing major general and orthopedic surgery compared to GA.[5–9] The evidence from the published studies that favors the use of regional anesthesia with respect to postoperative outcomes in patients undergoing various major surgeries is summarized in the following paragraphs.

Overall Morbidity and Mortality

Comorbidities, including cardiac disease, hypertension, and diabetes mellitus, have a major impact on postoperative mortality. In a recent case-controlled study of risk factors for perioperative complications after uncemented total knee arthroplasty, identified risk factors included concomitant cardiac and neuropsychiatric disease, advanced age (greater than 70 years), American Society of Anesthesiologists physical status (ASA PS) greater than or equal to 3, and general (vs. regional) anesthesia.[10] Elderly patients undergoing hip fracture surgery are at especially high risk for perioperative myocardial ischemia with a reported incidence in the range of 35–42%.[11–13]

Two major causes of morbidity and mortality following major total joint arthroplasty are myocardial ischemia/infarction and VTE, including risk for fatal PE.[11,14,15] In a prospective review over a 10-year period of 10,244 patients who underwent primary total hip or knee arthroplasty, the overall incidence of serious complications within 30 postoperative days was 2.2%.[14] These included myocardial infarction 0.4%, PE 0.7%, DVT 1.5%, and death 0.5%. Most adverse events increased in frequency with older age (greater than 70 years). Myocardial infarction was more common in male patients. Overall frequency of adverse events was not different between patient populations undergoing total hip arthroplasty (THA) and total knee arthroplasty (TKA). However, the incidence of PE was higher in patients undergoing TKA.[14]

A meta-analysis of 141 trials (9559 patients) in all types of surgery in which patients were allocated to any anesthetic that included neuraxial blockade compared to GA concluded that overall mortality was reduced by about a third (neuraxial blockade 103 deaths/4871 patients vs. GA 144 deaths/4688 patients).[7]

Myocardial Ischemia and Infarction

Epidural anesthesia continued postoperatively for more than 24 h significantly reduced the incidence of postoperative myocardial infarction in a systematic review of 17 randomized-controlled trials which included 1173 patients.[3] The overall postoperative myocardial infarction rate was 6.3%, with a lower rate in the epidural group, and a rate difference of −3.8% (95% confidence interval −7.4 to −0.2%). Compared to conventional intramuscular opioids, continuous epidural analgesia (CEA) initiated at the time of hospital admission was associated with a lower incidence of perioperative adverse cardiac events in elderly hip fracture patients at high risk for coronary artery disease (conventional analgesia 7 of 34 vs. epidural analgesia 0 of 34 adverse cardiac events).[9]

Table 7-1

Prevalence of VTE after Orthopedic Surgery in Patients Without Thromboembolic Prophylaxis*

Surgical Procedure	VTE		PE	
	Total (%)	Proximal (%)	Total (%)	Fatal (%)
THA	45–57	23–36	0.7–30	0.1–0.4
TKA	40–84	9–20	1.8–7	0.2–0.7
Hip fracture surgery	30–60	17–36	4.3–24	3.6–12.9

*Data from clinical trials in which mandatory postoperative venography was performed.
Data from Ref. 6.

Venous Thromboembolism

Asymptomatic VTE is common following major lower extremity orthopedic surgery or trauma. Perioperative thromboprophylaxis using anticoagulants influences anesthetic choices, as well as the management of neuraxial catheters for postoperative analgesia. Safe application of central neuraxial blocks requires that anesthesiologists be familiar with the prevalence and risk factors for VTE in different surgical populations, and the recommended thromboprophylactic regimens so that the risks and benefits of different anesthetic techniques can be weighed and the appropriate anesthetic choices and perioperative care plan can be implemented.

The prevalence of DVT at 7–14 days after THA, TKA, and hip fracture surgery is 50–60% (Table 7-1).[15] The risk of DVT is increased in the presence of coexisting medical conditions (Box 7-1).[15,16] In a case-controlled study of patients undergoing THA or TKA, obesity (body mass index [BMI] greater than 30 kg/m²), ASA PS greater than or equal to 3, and lack of thromboprophylaxis were found to be the risk factors for clinically relevant VTE events.[16]

In comparison to GA and postoperative systemic opioid analgesia, NA and extended epidural analgesia reduces the incidence of DVT and PE (Table 7-2).[1,2,7,17]

Recommended Pharmacologic Thromboprophylaxis

Because of a high risk for postoperative VTE, primary prophylaxis with anticoagulants is recommended and is cost-effective in patients undergoing THA, TKA, and surgery for hip fracture.[15,18] Several anticoagulant-based prophylaxis

Box 7-1

Risk factors for VTE

Primary hypercoagulable states

▸ Protein C and S deficiency

▸ Antithrombin 3 deficiency

Secondary hypercoagulable states

▸ Bed rest or immobility > 5 days

▸ Obesity

▸ Fracture of the pelvis, hip, or leg

▸ History of myocardial infarction

▸ History of congestive heart failure

▸ Malignancy

▸ Hormone replacement therapy

▸ Prior history of thromboembolism

▸ Varicose veins

▸ History of smoking

▸ Major surgery

Box 7-2

Recommendations for Thromboprophylaxis for Major Orthopedic Surgery

Elective hip or knee replacement

▸ LMWH—12–24 h after surgery or 4–6 h after surgery at half the high-risk dose, or adjusted dose warfarin (INR range 2.0–3.0) starting preoperatively or immediately after surgery

▸ Anticoagulant thromboprophylaxis is recommended for 7–10 days

▸ Adjunct prophylaxis with elastic stockings and intermittent pneumatic compression

Hip fracture surgery

▸ LMWH or adjusted dose warfarin (as above) postoperatively. Initiate this preoperatively if surgery is delayed > 24 h

▸ Low-dose unfractionated heparin (5000 U SQ every 12 h) is an alternate option but efficacy data are limited

▸ Consider prophylactic inferior vena cava filter in patients who are at high risk for postoperative bleeding from anticoagulant-based thromboprophylaxis

Abbreviation: INR = international normalized ratio.
Data from Ref. 1.

regimens have been studied. The prophylaxis regimens recommended by the 2001 American College of Chest Physicians Consensus Committee are used most commonly.[15,19] These recommendations are outlined in Box 7-2.

Neuraxial blockade and anticoagulant thromboprophylaxis can be used concomitantly. However, safe application of NA and analgesia in the anticoagulated patient requires appropriate timing of the neuraxial procedure and neuraxial catheter removal relative to the timing of anticoagulant drug administration. The American Society of Regional Anesthesia "Consensus Statements on Neuraxial Anesthesia and Anticoagulation" addresses this issue[20] (see Chap. 5).

▸ **Intraoperative Blood Loss**

Epidural anesthesia, when compared to GA, is associated with a decrease in intraoperative blood loss during orthopedic, as well as other surgical procedures. The presumed

Table 7-2

Incidence of DVT and PE: GA vs. NA

Author (Reference Number)	Number of Patients	DVT Incidence (%)		PE Incidence (%)	
		GA	NA	GA	NA
Modig [1]	60	77	40	33	10
Jorgensen [2]	48	59	18	4	0
Rodgers [7]	9559	4.5	3	1.4	0.6
Sorenson [17]	246	45	17	–	–

Data from Refs. 1, 2, 7, and 17.

mechanisms of blood loss reduction with neuraxial blockade are: decrease in mean arterial blood pressure, redistribution of blood away from the nondependent surgical site, and decrease in venous pressure due to elimination of positive pressure ventilation. In a meta-analysis of 141 trials (9559 patients undergoing various major surgeries), use of neuraxial blockade was associated with 50% reduction in transfusion requirements.[7]

Postoperative Delirium and Cognitive Dysfunction

Postoperative cognitive dysfunction is common in the elderly and comprises a wide variety of disorders including impairment of cognitive function, dementia, and delirium. POCD, especially delirium, is associated with an increased mortality and prolonged hospital stay.[21] In hip fracture patients, the incidence of perioperative delirium ranges from 28 to 41%. Delirium at admission (before surgery) is associated with poor physical and functional outcomes postoperatively, and is an important predictor of postoperative mortality.[21,22] Postoperative delirium, lasting greater than 6 weeks, predicts poor long-term functional outcome after hip fracture surgery because it significantly impacts the ability to live independently.[22] Several preoperative, intraoperative, and postoperative factors have been incriminated in the etiology of POCD, including advanced age (age greater than 70 years), preexisting cognitive impairment, alcohol abuse, electrolyte imbalance, prolonged surgery, psychoactive medications, postoperative sepsis, and pulmonary complications.[23] In a multicenter international study of early and long-term POCD in elderly patients after major abdominal and orthopedic surgery, perioperative hypotension and hypoxemia were not found to be significant risk factors.[24] Compared to GA, regional anesthesia does not reduce the incidence of delayed (3 months) POCD. It does, however, reduce the incidence of early POCD and delirium that contributes to increased early morbidity and prolonged hospital stay.[22,24]

Stress Response to Surgery

Reductions in postoperative cardiac-, pulmonary-, and coagulation-related morbidity in patients treated with epidural anesthesia and postoperative analgesia have been attributed to the blunting of the surgical stress response.[25] Release of neuroendocrine hormones associated with the surgical stress response may alter myocardial oxygen supply/demand dynamics, enhance development of a hypercoagulable state, inhibit fibrinolysis, and contribute to postoperative immunosuppression and infection.[26] Intraoperative use of epidural anesthesia and postoperative analgesia with local

anesthetics for surgical procedures below the umbilicus achieves complete somatic and sympathetic block, thus, completely suppressing the stress response.[21,25,26] Epidural opioids administered alone attenuate the stress response but are not as effective as epidural local anesthetics.[26]

Functional Recovery and Rehabilitation

Optimal pain control using regional anesthesia techniques (continuous epidural anesthesia and analgesia or continuous femoral nerve block) accelerates functional recuperation and shortens hospital stay following major knee surgery by allowing early intense rehabilitation using continuous passive motion and physical therapy.[27]

Quality of Postoperative Analgesia

Epidural analgesia, regardless of the analgesic agent (local anesthetic or local anesthetic plus opioid or opioid alone) or location of the epidural catheter provides superior postoperative analgesia when compared to systemic opioids.[19]

In summary, the impact of NA/analgesia techniques on postoperative outcomes with respect to mortality and life-threatening events need to be defined further. However, recent evidence supports improved outcomes with respect to overall morbidity.[19–22] Furthermore, pain control is more effective with the use of epidural analgesia.[19] Recent emphasis on adequate pain control with the introduction of Joint Commission on Accreditation of Healthcare Organizations (JCAHO) guidelines for the assessment of pain as the "fifth vital sign" supports the use of neuraxial and other regional anesthesia modalities for the treatment of pain associated with orthopedic surgery.[28] A recent survey of 464 orthopedic surgeons (the hip and knee surgery database) who performed 9327 total hip and 13,846 total knee arthroplasties found the use of spinal or epidural anesthesia increased from 34 to 46% for total hip, and 43 to 54% for total knee arthroplasties between 1996 and 2001.[9] Ninety-nine percent of patients who received NA also received some type of anticoagulant thromboprophylaxis.

NEURAXIAL ANESTHETIC TECHNIQUES

Neuraxial blockade can be used as a sole anesthetic, as a supplement to GA (integrated epidural-general anesthesia [EGA]) or for providing prolonged postoperative analgesia. Until recently, spinal and epidural blocks have been the standard neuraxial techniques for lower extremity orthopedic surgery. Over the last decade, however, combined spinal-epidural anesthesia (CSE) has evolved as an optimal NA technique for orthopedic surgery. In a prospective study that compared CSE with spinal or epidural blockade for major orthopedic surgery of the lower extremity, latency to surgical anesthesia and intraoperative surgical conditions provided by spinal and CSE anesthesia were comparable, and both were superior to that provided by epidural blockade.[29] CSE combines the advantages of spinal and epidural anesthesia and mitigates the disadvantages. Limitations of CSE can largely be overcome with increased experience with the technique. The advantages of CSE are summarized in Box 2-8.

Although CSE is gaining popularity as an ideal NA technique for major orthopedic surgery, there are clinical situations for which spinal or epidural anesthesia may be more appropriate. Important determinants of the choice of a particular neuraxial technique include the complexity and duration of surgery, potential for significant blood loss and large fluid shifts, patient preference, need for prolonged postoperative analgesia, and the type and timing of the administration of anticoagulant thromboprophylaxis.

At the authors' institution, spinal or CSE anesthesia are the preferred neuraxial techniques when the surgery is to be performed under neuraxial blockade without supplemental GA. Epidural anesthesia, on the other hand, is used as a component of integrated EGA.

Integrated Epidural-General Anesthesia

Longer and more complicated procedures such as revision arthroplasty, acetabular bone grafting and reconstructive surgery with risk of injury to pelvic structures, and insertion of long stem femoral prosthesis that are associated with major blood loss and fluid shifts, are suitable procedures for integrated EGA. The integrated approach allows for a reduction in the requirements of general anesthetics and opioids and ensures optimal postoperative epidural analgesia with improved recovery and rehabilitation.

An epidural technique is an appropriate choice when using an integrated approach because the cephalad level of block can be controlled more predictably compared to a CSE technique. One of the major concerns for the anesthesiologist when using an integrated approach is hypotension associated with induction of GA, as well as during the periods of major intraoperative blood loss. The induction of GA in patients undergoing THA with an epidural block up to the T10 level increases the odds of developing clinically relevant hypotension (EGA 41% vs. epidural anesthesia 23%). The cumulative frequency of hypotension throughout the surgical procedure is also higher with EGA.[30] The extent of sympathetic denervation with neuraxial blocks (epidural or spinal) is related to the cephalad level of sensory blockade. Restricting the cephalad level of blockade to the lower thoracic dermatomes may avoid major cardiovascular depression by preserving compensatory mechanisms: (1) reflex increase

---

Box 7-3

Factors Contributing to Hemodynamic Depression During Integrated EGA

Depression of baroreceptor activity

▷ Cardiac sympathectomy—block of cardioaccelerator fibers

▷ Depression of central vasomotor efferent activity

▷ Direct myocardial depression

▷ Reduction in venous return associated with mechanical ventilation

---

in efferent sympathetic activity with reflex vasoconstriction above the level of block and (2) compensatory increase in the activity of the unblocked splanchnic nerves (T6 to L1) with increase in catecholamine release from the adrenal medulla.[31]

Several factors contribute to an increased risk of hemodynamic depression in patients receiving EGA (Box 7-3).[31–33] Cardiovascular depression, associated with intraoperative blood loss and major fluid shifts, is more profound with EGA. Patients with a history of chronic hypertension, especially those being treated with angiotensin-converting enzyme (ACE) inhibitors and diuretics, are particularly susceptible to hypotension at induction of anesthesia. The renin-angiotensin system (RAS) contribution to blood pressure control becomes important when the sympathetic nervous system is blocked by epidural anesthesia and GA. Angiotensin II, in addition to direct vasoconstrictor action, enhances peripheral effects of norepinephrine.[34,35]

Optimizing Integrated Epidural-General Anesthesia

Optimal management of EGA requires ensuring: (1) adequate, but not an excessive, level of epidural blockade for surgery, (2) use of appropriate doses of inhalation and intravenous anesthetics/opioids to ensure amnesia during surgery, and (3) maintenance of optimal intravascular volume.

Level of Epidural Block: Hemodynamic depression associated with epidural anesthesia can be minimized by the following:

▶ Avoid the bolus administration of large doses of short- and intermediate-acting local anesthetics that may produce profound sympathetic blockade at induction.

▶ Establish the desired level of epidural anesthesia by slow incremental doses of a long-acting local anesthetic. The epidural distribution of local anesthetic and resultant sympathetic block is enhanced in the elderly because the intervertebral foramina are narrow and local anesthetic loss from the epidural to paravertebral space is decreased. Typically, 10–12 mL of 0.5% bupivacaine (50–70 mg) will achieve a low thoracic level (T8 to T10) of epidural anesthesia after lumbar epidural injection.

▶ Maintain the desired level of epidural block by the administration of a continuous infusion of a long-acting agent such as bupivacaine, levobupivacaine, or ropivacaine. An infusion of 0.5% bupivacaine 5–6 mL/h (25–30 mg/h) is optimal to provide an adequate level of anesthesia and muscle relaxation without resulting in an unacceptably high level of blockade during surgery.

▶ If muscle relaxants are used during EGA, the epidural concentration can be reduced to an analgesic concentration, for example, 0.25% bupivacaine. This will reduce requirements for the GA component and maintain an adequate level of analgesia at emergence.

▶ Ensure adequate intravascular volume and preload prior to induction of GA by adequate hydration and maintenance of appropriate patient position to maximize venous return.

Use of Appropriate Dose of Inhalation and Intravenous Anesthetics. Appropriate conduct of EGA ensures rapid recovery and excellent postoperative analgesia with minimal respiratory depression. With the integrated technique, the general anesthetic component is added to provide amnesia, patient comfort or immobility, and when necessary, mechanical ventilation of the lungs. Patients require low end-tidal concentrations of volatile agents during EGA.[33] NA also markedly potentiates the effects of sedatives. Doses of midazolam and thiopental required to induce sedation or hypnosis are approximately 50% lower during NA.[36,37] Lidocaine epidural anesthesia has been shown to reduce the minimal alveolar concentration (MAC) of sevoflurane from 1.18 to 0.52%.[33] The observed decrease in MAC seen with epidural anesthesia has been attributed to "deafferentation" via the inhibition of tonic afferent spinal nerve signaling to the brain and the spinal cord. Since volatile anesthetic agents produce dose-dependent cardiovascular depression, the use of lower doses improves hemodynamic stability during EGA.

Optimizing Intravascular volume (Preload). Reflex tachycardia in response to decreased preload may be absent even when the level of epidural blockade is too low to involve cardiac accelerator fibers.[32] Lumbar epidural anesthesia enhances vagal tone mainly through a decrease in venous return, and changes in venous return may modify the heart rate. The heart rate decreases as venous return decreases; and absolute bradycardia indicates a marked reduction (greater than or equal to 25%) in venous return, such as that following acute blood loss or the head-up position.[31] Cardiovascular instability, in association with uncorrected

hypovolemia, is more profound in the presence of neuraxial block, and bradycardia is a danger signal as it represents a critical reduction of venous return and cardiac filling.[38]

Most patients receiving EGA will have clinically significant hypotension at induction of GA. The appropriate interventions include intravenous fluids, elevation of the legs, or slight head-down tilt to promote venous return, and incremental doses of an appropriate inotropic drug (Box 7-4). Phenylephrine in small bolus doses (50–100 µg) can be helpful if ephedrine alone does not produce the desired result. A pure alpha agonist (vasoconstrictor) such as phenylephrine may not be suitable primary intervention because it increases the mean arterial pressure at the expense of cardiac output.[39]

Epinephrine Test Dose and Integrated Epidural-General Anesthesia

The traditional epidural test dose may be less reliable in the anesthetized patient as the patient cannot report subjective symptoms of local anesthetic toxicity, and the hemodynamic responses to systemic epinephrine may be attenuated. At one MAC, halothane and isoflurane attenuate intrinsic hemodynamic variability and interfere with the expected heart rate response, as well as the blood pressure response to epinephrine (Box 7-5).[40,41] In addition, there is a progressive decline with age in the chronotropic response to epinephrine and a false negative epinephrine test dose may occur in the elderly (greater than 60 years of age).[42]

Box 7-4

Interventions for Hypotension Associated with Integrated EGA

▷ Intravenous crystalloids/colloids administration

▷ Promote venous return

  ▷ Leg elevation

  ▷ Slight head-down tilt

▷ Intravenous ephedrine 10–20 mg

▷ Intravenous phenylephrine if heart rate > 90 bpm

Severe hypotension with bradycardia
(Indicates critical reduction in venous return)

▷ Rapid restoration of intravascular volume with crystalloids/colloids/blood

▷ IV ephedrine, if unresponsive prompt administration IV epinephrine 50–100 µg increments

Note: Monitor central venous pressure when major fluid shifts are expected.

Acute and chronic use of β-adrenergic blockers also reduces the heart rate changes observed after intravenous epinephrine injection.[43,44] Recommendations for the safe administration of continuous epidural local anesthetics for epidural anesthesia are listed in Box 7-6.

Choice of Local Anesthetics for Continuous Epidural Anesthesia and Analgesia

Longer-acting local anesthetics such as bupivacaine, levobupivacaine, and ropivacaine provide the flexibility of potent analgesia with minimal postoperative motor block and low risk of tachyphylaxis (a potential problem with intermediate duration local anesthetics, such as lidocaine). Epidural levobupivacaine and bupivacaine are nearly equipotent in the labor analgesia pain model, and ropivacaine is 40–60% less potent.[45,46] In patients undergoing THA, the clinical profile of epidural anesthesia produced by 0.5% levobupivacaine has been shown to be similar to that produced by the same concentration of ropivacaine and

bupivacaine, with no difference in the total volume of local anesthetic solution required to complete the surgery.[47] Ropivacaine, however, produces a less intense motor block than either bupivacaine or levobupivacaine. Patient-controlled epidural analgesia (PCEA) infusions of 0.125% levobupivacaine or bupivacaine, or 0.2% ropivacaine provided comparable pain relief with similar motor recovery profiles for analgesia for the first 12 h following surgery.[47] Dose-dependent improvement in the quality of postoperative analgesia was reported when three concentrations of epidural levobupivacaine (0.0625, 0.125, and 0.25%) were compared following major orthopedic surgery. However, motor block was also directly related to concentration.[48] To provide optimal postoperative epidural analgesia with minimal motor block, it is preferable to use dilute solutions of local anesthetic such as 0.0625% bupivacaine or levobupivacaine, or 0.2% ropivacaine in conjunction with opioids.

▶ ### Spinal Anesthesia

Spinal anesthesia is a suitable neuraxial technique for surgical procedures outlined in Box 7-7. A major advantage of spinal anesthesia is profound sensory and motor block with a small amount of local anesthetic drug. Of concern is the risk of hypotension due to a limited reserve for hemodynamic compensation and a tendency to more extensive anesthetic spread in the elderly resulting in a higher level of blockade. Cardiac arrest and death have also been reported in elderly patients during spinal anesthesia for hip arthroplasty.[49–51] In a large survey of complications of regional anesthesia, the incidence of cardiac arrest associated with spinal anesthesia was 2.5/10,000 (9/35,439) cases.[50] In comparison there were no cases of cardiac arrest among the 5561 cases of epidural anesthesia. There were three fatalities among the nine patients who suffered cardiac arrest, all three occurring in elderly patients (greater than 80 years) who were undergoing hip surgery.[50] The identifiable risk factors for catastrophic hemodynamic events in patients undergoing surgery under spinal anesthesia are old age, use of a large dose of local anesthetic, high block level, preoperative fasting and hypovolemia, preoperative antihypertensive therapy, intraoperative bleeding, position change, and application of bone cement. Steps that can be undertaken to increase the safety margin of spinal anesthesia in elderly orthopedic patients are listed in Box 7-8.

Choice of Local Anesthetic Drug, Dose, and Baricity

The major determinants of the spread of local anesthetic in cerebrospinal fluid (CSF) and the extent of blockade are total dose of the local anesthetic drug, conformation of the spinal canal (presence of kyphosis, lordosis), baricity, position of the patient immediately after injection of hyperbaric and hypobaric solutions, and CSF volume in the lumbosacral dural sac.[52,53] Local anesthetic dose, baricity, and patient position can be manipulated to achieve the desired cephalad level of blockade. The determinants of the duration of the block are the choice of drug, dose, and the addition of adjuvants (vasoconstrictors, opioids, and alpha-2 agonists).

Isobaric Local Anesthetics. Isobaric solutions of local anesthetics in moderate doses are ideal for providing low thoracic (T8 to T10) spinal blockade appropriate for lower extremity orthopedic surgery. A major advantage of isobaric solutions is that a change in the position of the patient (common practice during orthopedic surgery) has minimal effect on the distribution of the local anesthetic and, therefore, the cephalad spread of spinal anesthesia.

Factors that influence the cephalad level of anesthesia with isobaric solutions include the vertebral level of the spinal injection, total dose of local anesthetic, as well as body habitus. In a prospective study that compared three doses of 0.5% plain bupivacaine (15, 20, and 25 mg) in ASA PS 1 orthopedic patients between 20 and 60 years of age, interindividual variability of the cephalad extent of anesthesia was greater in the 20 and 25 mg dose groups compared to the 15 mg group (Fig. 7-1).[54]

Obesity enhances the spread of isobaric spinal local anesthetics. More extensive cephalad spread of sensory block was found to occur in patients with increased BMI compared to patients with normal BMI after injection of 15 mg of 0.5% plain (in saline) bupivacaine at the L3-L4 and L4-L5 interspace.[55] The mean sensory levels for patients with

---

Box 7-8

Increasing the Safety Margin of Spinal Anesthesia in Elderly Orthopedic Patients

▷ Aim for a cephalad level of block lower than a midthoracic level:

  ▷ Select appropriate local anesthetic dose (e.g., 10–15 mg of bupivacaine)

  ▷ Use isobaric rather than hyperbaric solutions

  ▷ Use lower doses in patients with high BMI

  ▷ Use a lower lumbar interspace for local anesthetic injection

▷ Ensure euvolemic state

▷ Avoid sudden position change; specifically avoid the head-up position

▷ Minimize or avoid the use of local anesthetic adjuncts, such as epinephrine and clonidine

▷ Consider the use of CSA to facilitate administration of incremental doses of local anesthetics in high-risk elderly

---

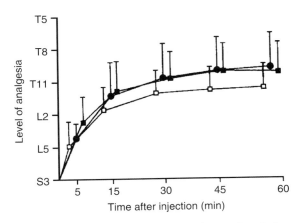

FIGURE 7-1. Cephalad level pinprick analgesia (mean and standard deviation) as a function of time following the intrathecal injection of plain 0.5% bupivacaine 3 mL (☐), 4 mL (●), and 5 mL (■) at L4-L5 vertebral interspace. The maximum cephalad level of analgesia in the 3 mL (15 mg) group was T12 ± 2 dermatomal levels and that in the 4 mL (20 mg) and 5 mL (25 mg) groups was T10 ± 3 dermatomal levels. *Used with permission from Taivainen T, Tuominen M, Rosenberg PH. Spread of spinal anesthesia using various doses of plain 0.5% bupivacaine injected at the L IV-V interspace. Acta Anesthesiol Scand 33:652, 1989.*

normal BMI for the L3-L4 and L4-L5 injection levels were T9 and T11, and for patients with high BMI the sensory levels were T4 and T8, respectively.

Hypobaric Local Anesthetics. Hypobaric local anesthetics are selectively distributed to the nondependent side after subarachnoid injection and are, therefore, suitable for hip surgery in the lateral decubitus position. Two advantages of hypobaric spinal anesthesia are: (1) spinal anesthesia is induced in the operative (lateral decubitus) position, thus requiring no further movement of the anesthetized patient, and (2) a slight head-down position keeps the level of blockade from rising and, at the same time, improves venous return and hemodynamic stability. The position of the patient during, and 20–30 min after injection influences the distribution of hypobaric local anesthetic. The head-up position during this time interval may produce an undesirably high level of sensory and sympathetic block. The local anesthetic dose and patient's position, therefore, should be carefully adjusted to prevent excessive cephalad spread.

Preparation of a hypobaric solution requires that the local anesthetic solution be diluted to a concentration below 0.33%. Therefore, only local anesthetics of high potency, such as bupivacaine and tetracaine, which can reliably produce sensory and motor block at these lower concentrations, are appropriate for hypobaric spinal anesthesia. Clinical studies using hypobaric solutions are limited. In one study a slow injection (25 s) compared to a fast injection (10 s) of hypobaric tetracaine 10 mg resulted in a differential block between dependent and nondependent sides with lower level of spinal anesthesia that was of longer duration.[56] Conversely, in another study, no difference in sensory levels between the two sides occurred when hypobaric bupivacaine 15 mg (0.33% solution) was injected either by slow or fast injection in patients undergoing THA.[57]

Comparison of Hypobaric Versus Isobaric Solutions. The defining limit between hypobaric and isobaric local anesthetic solutions has been considered a baricity of 0.9990. A 0.5% solution of commercially available plain bupivacaine for epidural anesthesia has a baricity of 0.999343 ± 0.000004 g/mL at 37°C. When mixed with CSF, the resultant baricity of 0.5% bupivacaine is 0.998876 making it slightly hypobaric at body temperature.[58] Intrathecal injection of plain 0.5% bupivacaine solution in the sitting position results in sensory levels which are one to two segments higher than the sensory levels resulting from the injection of the same dose with patient in the lateral decubitus position.[59] In a recent study, the anesthetic and hemodynamic effects of isobaric and hypobaric bupivacaine 0.5% were compared in patients undergoing THA in the lateral position. The isobaric solution contained 0.5% bupivacaine 3.5 mL (17.5 mg) mixed with normal saline to a final concentration of 0.3%,

and the hypobaric solution contained 0.5% bupivacaine 3.5 mL (17.5 mg) mixed with sterile water to a final concentration of 0.3%. No difference in the quality of motor block was noted and the hemodynamic changes were similar. The use of a hypobaric solution, however, prolonged sensory regression to the L2 dermatome and significantly delayed the time to use of first analgesic. The authors concluded that a longer duration of analgesia of 45 min, noted with the hypobaric solution, was clinically relevant.[58] The baricities of the two solutions, however, were almost identical: 0.9967 (hypobaric) versus 0.9988 (isobaric).

Local Anesthetic Dose. Hyperbaric solutions of local anesthetics gravitate to the thoracic spine concavity. Consequently, increasing the dose may not increase the level of blockade higher than T4. The level of anesthesia with hyperbaric and hypobaric solutions is primarily dependent on patient position. In general, blockade level is directly related to dose when isobaric solutions of local anesthetics are used for spinal anesthesia.

Duration of Spinal Anesthesia

Primary determinants of duration of spinal anesthesia are the local anesthetic drug, the dose, and the supplemental adjuvants used. Since the duration of surgery for most major lower extremity orthopedic surgeries is greater than 2 h, appropriate local anesthetics choices are bupivacaine, ropivacaine, levobupivacaine, and tetracaine. Equal doses of hyperbaric preparations of tetracaine and bupivacaine produce comparable levels of anesthesia. Tetracaine, however, results in prolonged motor block compared to bupivacaine even though the time to four-segment sensory block regression has been shown to be similar with the two drugs.[60] Because of the delay in recovery of lower lumbar and sacral anesthesia, tetracaine is a suitable spinal local anesthetic for surgeries of longer duration at or below the knee.

Anesthetic Adjuvants

Intrathecal analgesic adjuvants serve to decrease the dose of local anesthetics, prolong duration of anesthesia, and provide prolonged postoperative analgesia.

Vasoconstrictors. Both epinephrine (0.1–0.5 mg) and phenylephrine (0.5–5 mg) have been used to prolong the duration of spinal anesthesia in a dose-dependent manner.[61] Vasoconstrictors have the dual effect of decreasing the vascular uptake of local anesthetics, and having direct analgesic effect via α-adrenergic stimulation. The most commonly used vasoconstrictor is epinephrine 0.1–0.2 mg. When added to lidocaine or bupivacaine, epinephrine prolongs anesthesia in the lumbosacral segments, although the time to two-segment regression is not altered.[61–63] Adding epinephrine to tetracaine prolongs the duration of anesthesia by 25–53%.[61]

Opioids. Intrathecal lipophilic opioids such as fentanyl and sufentanil produce selective spinal analgesia (see Chap. 12). Sufentanil is highly lipid soluble, has a large volume of distribution, and therefore, has a low spinal selectivity making it less suitable as an anesthetic adjuvant for spinal anesthesia. Fentanyl is less lipid soluble, has a relatively higher spinal selectivity, and provides dose-dependent analgesia when injected intrathecally.

Fentanyl has been combined with subtherapeutic doses of local anesthetics to provide surgical anesthesia. A "minidose" of plain bupivacaine 4 mg in combination with fentanyl 20 μg provided satisfactory spinal anesthesia for surgical repair of hip fracture in the elderly.[64] The combination caused dramatically less hypotension than plain bupivacaine 10 mg, and nearly eliminated the need for vasopressor support of blood pressure. The number of study subjects, however, was too small to evaluate the failure rate of the minidose technique. In our experience, a bupivacaine dose less than 8 mg does not consistently produce a reliable level of neuraxial blockade or duration of spinal anesthesia for surgical repair of traumatic hip fracture.

Adrenergic Agonists. When used in conjunction with intrathecal local anesthetics, clonidine prolongs the duration of anesthesia and postoperative analgesia. The effect is attributed to altered disposition of local anesthetic, or from direct α_2-adrenergic stimulation in the substantia gelatinosa of the spinal cord.[65] Duration of spinal anesthesia has been shown to increase more than twofold when clonidine 150 μg is administered in conjunction with intrathecal bupivacaine 5 mg, or with epidural bupivacaine 50 mg in patients undergoing lower extremity orthopedic surgery. Intrathecal clonidine, but not epidural clonidine, decreases the mean arterial blood pressure.[65] Hypotension and bradycardia, the major side effects of intrathecal clonidine, make it an unsuitable adjuvant for neuraxial blocks in high-risk elderly patients.

▶ Continuous Spinal Anesthesia

Continuous spinal anesthesia (CSA) uses an indwelling subarachnoid catheter and permits fractionation of the local anesthetic dose to achieve the desired level of surgical anesthesia. In comparison to single-dose spinal anesthesia, CSA offers several advantages: titration of the block level and duration of the spinal anesthesia, hemodynamic stability, and the ability to provide postoperative analgesia. CSA is specifically beneficial in elderly or debilitated orthopedic patients who will not

tolerate the hemodynamic instability inherent to single-dose spinal anesthesia.[66,67] The use of CSA, however, introduces increased risk and technical difficulties in placing an intrathecal catheter, and potential neurologic sequelae.[68,69] In a retrospective comparative analysis of 603 CSA compared to 4767 single-dose spinal anesthetics, Horlocker et al. reported an increased frequency of traumatic (bloody) taps, paresthesias, postdural puncture headache, and finally, a higher frequency of temporary or permanent neurologic deficits in patients who received a continuous spinal catheter (Table 7-3).[69,70] The authors proposed that CSA should be reserved for high-risk patients who would benefit from fractionation of the local anesthetic dose and the hemodynamic stability associated with the technique. The total local anesthetic dose and concentration administered during CSA should be carefully monitored to limit the potentially neurotoxic effects of large doses of local anesthetics administered intrathecally.

Maldistribution of a large dose of concentrated local anesthetics is the widely accepted mechanism of neurologic sequelae following CSA.[71,72] The recommendations that have been proposed to minimize the neurologic sequelae following CSA are outlined in Box 7-9.

CSA Equipment, Technique, and Local Anesthetic Dose Guidelines

Microcatheters for CSA are not available in the United States. These catheters were withdrawn from the market following reports of cauda equina syndrome associated with their use, which was attributed to local anesthetic neurotoxicity from sacral maldistribution of the drug (see Chap. 6). Macrocatheters (19- to 20-gauge), primarily multiport epidural

Table 7-3		
Neurologic Complications: Single Dose vs. CSA		
Complication	% Patients	
	Single Dose (n = 4767)	CSA (n = 603)
Traumatic (bloody) taps	3.3	8.3
Paresthesia during procedure	6.3	17.2
Postdural puncture headache	1.3	9.6
Neurologic sequelae (persistent paresthesia)	0.12	0.5
Cauda equina syndrome	0	0.16 (1 patient)
Data from Refs. 69, 70.		

> **Box 7-9**
>
> ### Recommendations for Minimizing Neurologic Sequelae following CSA
>
> ▸ Limit catheter insertion to 2 cm into the intrathecal space to avoid caudad catheter misdirection and sacral pooling
>
> ▸ In case of inadequate block level, change the baricity of the local anesthetic, or patient position instead of adding more local anesthetic of the same baricity
>
> ▸ Place the patient in 5- to 10-degree Trendelenburg position to minimize sacral pooling of the local anesthetic
>
> ▸ If bupivacaine or tetracaine 20–25 mg fails to produce the desired level of block, abandon the technique

catheters placed via an 18-gauge Tuohy needle using a standard epidural kit, are more commonly used for CSA.

The use of a subarachnoid catheter, and the ability to repeatedly administer local anesthetic, eliminates the need to use intrathecal epinephrine. Spinal anesthesia can be initiated with isobaric bupivacaine or tetracaine in concentrations of 0.25–0.5%. The administration of local anesthetic drug is done by titration, for example, 5 mg is administered initially and the level of sensory block is checked at 10 min. This is followed by 2.5 mg increments of drug every 5 min until the appropriate sensory level of surgical anesthesia, and adequate motor block, are achieved. If this does not occur after a maximum dose of 15 mg has been administered, the following steps should be undertaken[82]:

1. Place the patient in a slight Trendelenburg position.

2. Change the baricity of the injected local anesthetic to a hyperbaric solution.

3. Administer the additional hyperbaric local anesthetic in 2.5 mg increments every 5 min to a maximum dose of 25 mg.

4. Consider CSA to be a failure, and abandon it when bupivacaine or tetracaine 25 mg have failed to achieve the appropriate sensory and motor block for surgery.

▸ Combined Spinal-Epidural Anesthesia

Combined spinal-epidural anesthesia is an ideal neuraxial block technique for orthopedic surgery of the lower extremities because it provides a rapid onset of profound motor and sensory block, avoids high sensory block (provided local anesthetic dose and baricity are appropriately selected), and allows for prolonged surgical anesthesia and postoperative analgesia.

Potential Pitfalls of Combined Spinal-Epidural Anesthesia

Although several techniques have been described, a single insertion needle-through-needle technique is most commonly used for CSE anesthesia. The epidural space is identified, a small-gauge (24- to 27-gauge) pencil-point spinal needle is passed beyond the tip of epidural needle tip into the subarachnoid space, the spinal needle is withdrawn after subarachnoid local anesthetic injection, and the epidural catheter is then inserted (see Chap. 2). Potential problems with the needle-through-needle CSE technique are discussed in the following paragraphs.

Failure to Locate the Subarachnoid Space. Earlier publications reported a high rate of failed spinal anesthesia during CSE anesthesia. More recent reports, however, suggest a failure rate of 1–5%.[73–75] Two important causes of failure to locate the subarachnoid space are: (1) the spinal needle is too short or (2) deviation of the spinal needle from the midline. Clinical studies using a needle-through-needle technique indicate that the epidural space depth in the midline ranges between 3 and 17 mm, with a distance greater than 10 mm in 15% of patients, and greater than 13 mm in 3% of patients. A spinal needle of appropriate length, which extends 15 mm beyond the tip of epidural needle, should reduce the risk of failed dural puncture. Spinal needle deviation from the midline lengthens the epidural needle tip to dural distance. The dural sac in the lumbar region is triangular in shape with a narrow apex pointing posteriorly. Therefore, a small degree of lateral needle deflection can miss the dural sac.

Inadequate Spinal Anesthesia Component. Partial loss of local anesthetic intended for the subarachnoid space may result in an inadequate spinal anesthesia component. Contributing factors include poor spinal needle stabilization because the spinal needle is anchored only by dura mater and is subject to movement and displacement, high internal resistance of long, small-gauge spinal needles leading to leakage of local anesthetic at the needle hub during rapid injection, and injection into the anterior epidural space (the pencil-point spinal needle may indent the dura mater causing apposition of the posterior and anterior dura mater with needle tip passing beyond the dural sac into the anterior epidural space). Tips for preventing failure of the spinal component are discussed in Chap. 2.

Failed or Incomplete Epidural Component. In a large prospective survey of 25,000 cases, 11% of the epidural catheters were clearly not in the epidural space based on testing with a local anesthetic bolus.[75] The incidence of a failed epidural catheter with a CSE technique has been reported to be lower than that following an epidural technique used alone.[76,77] The possibility of having a misplaced epidural catheter secondary to a false loss-of-resistance is uncommon during CSE because a successful subarachnoid puncture confirms correct needle placement in the epidural space.

Interpretation of the Epidural Test Dose. Establishing a subarachnoid block prior to epidural catheter placement introduces difficulty with the interpretation of the traditional epidural test dose (epinephrine-containing local anesthetic) to rule out inadvertent intravascular or subarachnoid placement of the epidural catheter tip. A T5 or higher sensory block level results in attenuation of both the heart rate and blood pressure responses to the intravascular injection of epinephrine. Lidocaine 45 mg is unreliable and unsafe for use as an intrathecal test dose in the presence of preexisting subarachnoid block from the spinal local anesthetic component of CSE anesthesia. Problems with the test dose during the CSE technique has led to a greater reliance on the negative aspiration test and local anesthetic dose fractionation. A continuous infusion of local anesthetic is another safe approach to prevent sudden high level of block in the event the epidural catheter has migrated into the subarachnoid space, or to prevent a high blood level of local anesthetic in the event the epidural catheter has migrated into the intravascular space.

Risk of Subarachnoid Catheter Migration. Theoretically, the epidural catheter may enter the subarachnoid space through the dural puncture made by the spinal needle or through an unrecognized dural tear made by the tip of the epidural needle. Epiduroscopy studies done on cadavers suggest that the likelihood of subarachnoid catheter migration is minimal through the dural punctures made by 25- or 26-gauge spinal needle.[78] This risk, however, was found to be high (45%) when the dural puncture was made with a 17- to 18-gauge epidural needles. Subarachnoid catheter placement during CSE is more likely to occur during the procedure and subsequent catheter migration is rare. Rawal et al. reported more than 26,000 cases of CSE without any recognized intrathecal catheter migration.[79]

Drug Flux Across the Dura Mater During Combined Spinal-Epidural Anesthesia. There is a potential risk of drug flux from the epidural to subarachnoid space via the dural puncture made by the spinal needle. In vitro studies on meningeal tissue from monkeys have demonstrated that the magnitude of flux through the needle puncture is directly related to the spinal needle diameter.[80] The in vitro model examining drug flux has limitations in that the dynamics of the epidural-dural gradient cannot be reproduced. The subarachnoid–epidural pressure gradient of 5–15 cm of water in the clinical setting prevents drug flux into the subarachnoid space. During the initial phase of a large bolus of epidural drug administration, however, the epidural pressure may exceed subarachnoid pressure, allowing drug flux to occur into the subarachnoid space. The most marked clinical effect is likely to occur when there is a dural puncture with a large needle, for example, a 17-gauge Tuohy needle, followed by the administration of a high concentration of local anesthetic drug or hydrophilic opioid. To minimize high CSF levels of local anesthetics and opioids during CSE anesthesia, epidural drugs should be administered via a continuous infusion rather than as high concentration boluses.

Subarachnoid Component of Combined Spinal-Epidural Anesthesia

The outcome of subarachnoid block during CSE anesthesia may be altered by patient position, local anesthetic dose, and baricity. The authors prefer performing the CSE technique in the sitting position because identification of the midline is easier, CSF pressure is higher, and CSF flow is faster. This may reduce the risk of failure of the spinal component. The baricity of the subarachnoid local anesthetic becomes important when the sitting position is used. A delay in assuming the supine position after hyperbaric local anesthetic injection may lead to an inadequate level of sensory block. Isobaric solutions of local anesthetics prevent this scenario because the spread of local anesthetic is less posture dependent. It must be noted, however, that isobaric solutions of bupivacaine (0.5 or 0.75% plain solutions) are slightly hypobaric at body temperature and if the patient sits too long (e.g., difficult epidural catheter placement), a higher than expected level of subarachnoid block may occur.

Subarachnoid Local Anesthetic Dose. CSE anesthesia can be performed with a low dose, or a full dose, of subarachnoid local anesthetic. A low dose (sequential CSE anesthesia) allows neuraxial blockade to be restricted to the lowest dermatome level needed, thereby minimizing the extent of sympathetic block. For sequential CSE anesthesia, an intentionally low dose of subarachnoid local anesthetic is injected, and the block is subsequently (15–20 min later) extended with incremental doses of epidural local anesthetic until a desired level of block is obtained. This adds to the safety of the neuraxial technique in patients at high risk for hypotension, for example, patients with underlying cardiac disease; obese, fragile, elderly, diabetic (autonomic neuropathy) patients; and patients with a history of hypertension on multiple antihypertensive medications, specifically ACE inhibitors. The disadvantage of sequential CSE is that it may

Summary of CSE Technique

Sequential CSE

▶ Subarachnoid component—low dose of desired local anesthetic (e.g., bupivacaine or tetracaine 5 mg)

▶ Epidural component—test dose: check maximum level of sensory block (after 15–20 min). Administer 3 mL increments of desired long-acting local anesthetic until satisfactory level of block occurs

▶ Start a continuous infusion (e.g., 20–30 mg/h [4–6 mL] of 0.5% bupivacaine)

Full-dose CSE

▶ Subarachnoid component—full subarachnoid dose of desired local anesthetic (e.g., bupivacaine or tetracaine 8–12.5 mg)

▶ Epidural component—test dose: check maximum level of sensory block (after 15–20 min). Adequate block level—initiate continuous infusion of long-acting local anesthetic. Inadequate block level—administer 3 mL increments of desired local anesthetic until satisfactory level, followed by a continuous infusion as above. Delay the continuous infusion if patient is hemodynamically unstable

Inadvertent dural puncture by epidural needle

▶ Place the epidural catheter one to two intervertebral spaces higher

▶ Administer local anesthetics and opioids via infusion to minimize drug flux across dural puncture

take as long to attain the desired level of surgical anesthesia as conventional epidural anesthesia.

A full dose of local anesthetic for the subarachnoid component of CSE anesthesia is the more common practice as it allows rapid onset of the desired level of surgical anesthesia. When selecting the local anesthetic dose for the subarachnoid component of CSE anesthesia, one must be aware that the subarachnoid block induced during the CSE procedure produces greater sensorimotor anesthesia and prolonged recovery compared with "single-shot" spinal anesthesia. There is also a higher incidence of hypotension and vasopressor use despite using identical doses and baricity of local anesthetics.[81,82] Several possible reasons exist for this observation. The volume of the lumbar intrathecal compartment depends on the balance between the CSF and subatmospheric epidural pressure.

Insertion of the epidural needle disrupts this relationship as epidural pressure becomes equal to atmospheric pressure. Additionally, air or saline introduced into the epidural space using the loss-of-resistance technique may result in dural compression and reduction of the lumbosacral CSF volume.[81] At the authors' institution, full-dose CSE anesthesia is performed with plain 0.5% (isobaric) bupivacaine 8–12.5 mg (the lower dose for elderly and obese patients). Typically, this dose produces a T7 to T10 level of sensory block that is appropriate for lower extremity orthopedic surgery (Box 7-10).

Epidural Component of Combined Spinal-Epidural Anesthesia

Early in the development of CSE anesthesia it was recognized that the maximum level of sensory block was rapidly extended by epidural injection of a relatively small dose of local anesthetic.[83] Several studies examined the impact of saline versus local anesthetic injection on block extension following CSE anesthesia.[83–86] The results were conflicting, probably because the timing of the epidural "top-up" with respect to subarachnoid local anesthetic administration was variable among the different studies. The block extension produced by an early (within 15–20 min of subarachnoid dose) top-up with saline, during the period the subarachnoid block is evolving, occurs from the volume effect of dural compression (Fig. 7-2). Evaluation of the volume

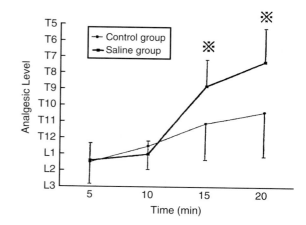

FIGURE 7-2. Changes in the analgesic levels during CSE anesthesia after epidural injection of saline or nothing (control). The control group received no further epidural saline injection. The saline group received saline 10 mL through an epidural catheter at the L2-L3 or L3-L4 interspaces 10 min after spinal anesthesia. *Significantly different vs. control group ($P < 0.05$). *Used with permission from Takiguchi T, Okano T, Egawa H. The effect of epidural saline injection on analgesic level during combined spinal-epidural anesthesia assessed clinically and myelographically. Anesth Analg 85:1097, 1997.*

effect produced by the epidural injection of 10 mL of saline using myelography has demonstrated a 25% reduction in the diameter of the lumbar subarachnoid compartment with a concurrent rise in the level of the contrast medium by two vertebral levels.[86] This volume effect does not play a significant role in the extension of sensory block during CSE anesthesia once the maximum sensory level from the spinal component of the block is established.[86,87]

INTRAOPERATIVE CONCERNS AND NEURAXIAL ANESTHESIA

▶ Tourniquet Pain and Neuraxial Blockade

Pneumatic tourniquets are commonly used during extremity surgery to provide a bloodless surgical field and minimize blood loss. Tourniquet pain may occur during spinal and epidural anesthesia despite an adequate level of sensory block, with a higher frequency during epidural anesthesia.[88–90] Tourniquet pain/discomfort usually appears 45–60 min after tourniquet inflation, increases in intensity over time, and may be associated with an increase in heart rate and blood pressure. Tourniquet pain associated with spinal anesthesia has been related to the dose, type, and baricity of the local anesthetic, and to the level of the sensory block.[89–92]

The mechanism of tourniquet pain is poorly understood. It is speculated that during spinal anesthesia, both A-delta fibers (mediating fast pain) and C fibers (mediating slow pain) are inhibited. As the concentration of local anesthetic in the CSF declines over time, C fibers may become unblocked earlier than A-delta fibers resulting in tourniquet pain despite an otherwise satisfactory level of sensory blockade.[89] In vitro studies suggest that C fibers are more resistant to local anesthetic-induced conduction blockade than the larger A-delta fibers, and the differential blockade is more marked with tetracaine than with bupivacaine.[93] In patients undergoing lower extremity orthopedic surgery, the incidence of tourniquet pain was higher with 15 mg of plain intrathecal tetracaine (60%) compared to an equivalent dose of plain bupivacaine (25%).[89] Epidural and intrathecal morphine delayed the onset and decreased the incidence of tourniquet pain, but not its severity.[94,95] Clinical strategies to minimize tourniquet pain are listed in Box 7-11.

▶ Blood Conservation

Blood loss associated with total hip and knee arthroplasty can be substantial. Large variations in perioperative blood transfusion have been observed following total hip and knee arthroplasties among different institutions.[96] A survey of 330 orthopedic surgeons in the United States about the

---

Box 7-11

Clinical Strategies to Minimize Tourniquet Pain

▶ Use bupivacaine vs. tetracaine for neuraxial blocks

▶ Use isobaric vs. hyperbaric solution for subarachnoid block

▶ Use intrathecal or epidural opioids

▶ Definitive treatment: release the tourniquet for 5 min allowing limb reperfusion between 1 and 2 h of tourniquet inflation

---

transfusion requirements following lower extremity total joint arthroplasty in 9482 patients (hip replacement 3920 and knee replacement 5562), revealed several important findings[96]:

▶ Blood transfusion was required in 46% of patients (57% in THA and 39% in TKA).

▶ Amongst those transfused 66% received autologous blood and 34% received allogeneic blood.

▶ The most important predictors of allogeneic blood transfusion were low baseline (preoperative) hemoglobin and lack of predonated autologous blood units.

▶ There was significant waste of predonated autologous blood and 45% of the 9920 predonated units were not used.

▶ Of the patients who received predonated autologous blood, 9% required additional transfusion with allogeneic blood.

▶ The highest prevalence of transfusions was in patients who underwent revision hip arthroplasty (autologous blood 32% and allogeneic blood 37%) and those who underwent bilateral TKA (autologous blood 44% and allogeneic blood 28%).

The risks of allogeneic blood product transfusion include infection, immunosuppression, transfusion reactions, and transfusion-related lung injury. Therefore, both preoperative and intraoperative strategies have been used to minimize allogeneic blood transfusions[97] (Box 7-12).

Preoperative Strategies

Preoperative autologous blood donation (PABD) and erythropoietin are effective preoperative strategies to minimize allogeneic blood transfusions. Routine PABD prior to major orthopedic surgery leads to increased costs, over collection, preoperative anemia, and wastage of autologous units.[98,99] Additionally, patients participating in PABD programs may be over transfused because of the use of more liberal criteria

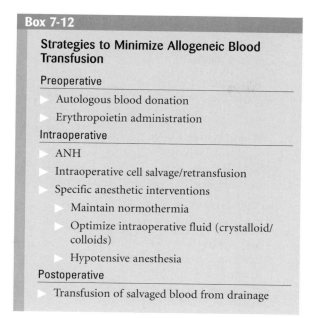

Box 7-12

Strategies to Minimize Allogeneic Blood Transfusion

Preoperative

▷ Autologous blood donation

▷ Erythropoietin administration

Intraoperative

▷ ANH

▷ Intraoperative cell salvage/retransfusion

▷ Specific anesthetic interventions

  ▷ Maintain normothermia

  ▷ Optimize intraoperative fluid (crystalloid/colloids)

  ▷ Hypotensive anesthesia

Postoperative

▷ Transfusion of salvaged blood from drainage

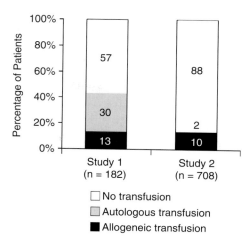

FIGURE 7-3. Observational study of perioperative management of autologous and allogenic blood transfusion. Preoperative interventions in study group 1 included 2 units of autologous blood donation (PABD) and oral iron therapy for baseline Hct > 33%. Interventions in study group 2 were as follows: erythropoietin was administered to anemic patients (baseline Hct ≤ 37%). PABD was used only for patient with baseline Hct between 37 and 39%. Patients with baseline Hct > 39% received neither PABD nor erythropoietin. Change in policy from the study 1 to 2 resulted in a reduction of overall transfusions from 43 to 12%. There was a 15-fold reduction in autologous transfusion rate and no significant change in the rate of allogeneic transfusion. *Used with permission from Couvert C, Laffon M, Baud A, et al. A restrictive use of both autologous donation and recombinant human erythropoietin is an efficient policy for primary total hip or knee arthroplasty. Anesth Analg 99:262, 2004.*

for transfusion. The difference in transfusion practices accounts for marked variation (53–81%) in perioperative blood transfusions during hip and knee arthroplasties amongst different institutions.[96] An appropriate selection of patients who will benefit from PABD and/or erythropoietin can minimize the transfusion rates for both allogeneic and autologous blood and minimize overall costs. In a prospective observational study of 708 patients undergoing primary total hip and knee arthroplasties, a marked decrease in transfusion rates occurred using the following predefined criteria for PABD and erythropoietin administration[100] (Fig. 7-3). Erythropoietin was administered to anemic patients (baseline hematocrit [Hct] less than or equal to 37%). PABD was used only for patients with baseline Hct between 37 and 39%. Patients with baseline Hct greater than 39% received neither PABD nor erythropoietin. The cost of preoperative erythropoietin (three doses) is comparable to PABD, and side effects such as hypertension and thrombotic events are uncommon with limited doses.

Intraoperative Strategies

Several intraoperative strategies are used to lower the incidence of allogeneic transfusion (Box 7-12). Acute normovolemic hemodilution (ANH) is considered a low cost and patient friendly alternative to PABD. Potential risks of ANH are related to a decrease in hemoglobin concentration and the use of specific replacement fluids to maintain normovolemia. Judicious fluid therapy using appropriate volumes of colloids and crystalloids minimizes the risk of coagulopathy

during ANH. Elderly patients and patients with coronary artery disease have been shown to tolerate moderate degrees of ANH.[97]

Intraoperative cell salvage and retransfusion of washed red cells is widely used for orthopedic procedures expected to have large blood loss (greater than or equal to 1000 mL). Safe application of this modality requires periodic monitoring of acid-base and electrolyte status, specifically when multiple units of salvaged red cells are being transfused. Transfusion of saline-washed red cells produces hyperchloremic metabolic acidosis and a decrease in calcium and magnesium concentrations.[101] To prevent the risk of air embolism the bags containing the processed red blood cell suspension should be deaired and transfused without pressurization.

Experience with the use of antifibrinolytic agents, such as aprotinin and tranexamic acid, to minimize blood loss and thereby allogeneic blood transfusion for major orthopedic surgery is very limited. Although aprotinin decreased blood loss and transfusion requirements in patients undergoing complicated hip surgery, it is unclear whether the small reduction in blood loss justifies the high cost and risks associated with its use.[102]

Hypothermia compromises blood coagulation and platelet function and maintenance of normothermia in patients undergoing total hip replacement has been shown to reduce blood loss and allogeneic blood transfusion.[103]

Moderate degrees of hypotension (mean arterial pressure 60–70 mmHg) are commonly used to minimize intraoperative blood loss. However, safety and efficacy of hypotensive anesthesia with mean arterial pressure lower than this range has not been well studied in elderly patients with coexisting cardiovascular disease. Furthermore, decreasing mean arterial pressures from 60–70 mmHg, to approximately 50 mmHg, appears to be of limited benefit with respect to surgical blood loss and allogeneic transfusion requirements.[97]

▶ Treatment of Neuraxial Blockade-Induced Hypotension

Hypotension is the most common physiologic effect of central neuraxial blockade, and is primarily the result of sympathetic blockade causing arterial and venous dilation with functional hypovolemia (see Chap. 4). Depending on the criteria used to define hypotension, the reported incidence of hypotension following spinal anesthesia ranges from 5 to 33%.[104–106] The incidence is higher if hypotension is defined as systolic blood pressure less than 90 mmHg, and relatively lower if defined as a mean arterial pressure decrease greater than 30% from baseline. The incidence of hypotension following spinal anesthesia is higher in the elderly, especially those undergoing surgery for fractured femur.[107,108] Risk factors for hypotension are outlined in Box 7-13 and are discussed in detail in Chap. 6.

The strategies which have been used for prevention and/or treatment of hypotension induced by neuraxial blocks include: (1) prehydration with crystalloids or colloids to increase the circulating blood volume and cardiac output, and (2) pharmacologic reversal of the reduction in systemic vascular resistance by the use of a vasopressor agent. In a prospective randomized trial of patients greater than 60 years of age undergoing elective THA, no prehydration versus prehydration with 500 mL of crystalloid or colloid solution (administered over 10 min immediately before initiation of spinal anesthesia) was not associated with a greater degree of hypotension or a need for vasopressor therapy.[109] Administration of 8 mL/kg of colloid following induction of spinal anesthesia in patients with fracture of the femoral neck resulted in a decrease in systemic vascular resistance, and no change in cardiac output despite an increase in central venous pressure (CVP).[110] These observations suggest that volume expansion alone is not consistently effective in attenuating spinal anesthesia-induced hypotension in the elderly. Additionally, volume loading in elderly patients

---

Box 7-13

Risk Factors for Hypotension following Neuraxial Blocks

Patient factors

▷ Baseline systolic blood pressure < 120 mmHg

▷ ASA PS ≥ 3

▷ History of hypertension

▷ Antihypertensive medications, especially ACE inhibitors

▷ Chronic alcohol consumption

Anesthetic factors

▷ Spinal anesthesia at or above L2-L3 interspace

▷ Peak block height higher than T5

▷ Addition of vasoconstrictors and alpha-2 agonists to spinal local anesthetics

▷ Combination of spinal anesthesia and GA

Data from Refs. 34, 104, and 106.

---

with limited cardiac reserve increases the risk of fluid overload, hemodilution, and cardiovascular complications.

The alternative strategy for prevention and treatment of neuraxial block-induced hypotension is administration of vasopressor agents. In contrast to intravascular volume loading, which does not reverse decreases in systemic vascular resistance, α-adrenergic agonists, such as metaraminol and phenylephrine, reliably prevent or reverse decreases in blood pressure by increasing systemic vascular resistance. In elderly patients undergoing emergency hip fracture surgery, intramuscular methoxamine (10 mg) administered prior to spinal anesthesia resulted in greater hemodynamic stability compared to intravenous administration of 500 mL 6% hetastarch or crystalloid solution.[108,110] Metaraminol use was associated with an increase in systemic vascular resistance index, whereas colloid infusion increased CVP without significantly increasing the cardiac index. Ephedrine, a mixed α- and β-adrenergic agent, is the most frequently used vasopressor for treating neuraxial block-induced hypotension. The hemodynamic effects, of ephedrine, however, are dependent on the maintenance of intravascular volume with intravenous fluids. In comparison, metaraminol is less dependent on the intravenous volume loading for its action.[110]

Prophylactic administration of alpha agonists for prevention of spinal anesthesia-induced hypotension carries the risk of drug-induced hypertension in patients with preexisting hypertension. Administration of intramuscular phenylephrine 3 mg before tetracaine spinal anesthesia to T7 level in patients greater than 65 years of age for hip fracture surgery resulted in hypertension in 7% of normotensive and 13% of hypertensive patients.[111] Prophylactic α-adrenergic agonists should, therefore, be used with caution in elderly patients with a history of hypertension. α-Adrenergic agonists are also inappropriate for treating hypotension associated with bradycardia during spinal anesthesia.

To summarize, crystalloid and colloid preloading for prevention of neuraxial blockade-induced hypotension is of questionable benefit. Prophylactic administration of α-adrenergic agonists carries the risk of hypertension in patients with a preexisting history of hypertension. Optimal therapy for hypotension consists of alpha agonists for hypotension without bradycardia, mixed alpha and beta agonists, such as ephedrine, plus intravenous fluids for hypotension with moderate bradycardia, and epinephrine plus intravenous fluids for hypotension with severe bradycardia.

▶ Bone Cement and Intraoperative Embolism

Increased intramedullary pressure, induced by mechanical compression of the femoral canal by femoral stem insertion during THA, is considered the underlying mechanism for intraoperative embolization.[112,113] Disruption of the thin walled blood vessels in the medullary canal by compressive loads allows the intravasation of marrow, fat, and bone debris, which embolizes throughout the venous system. Migration of the bone marrow elements in the draining veins activates the coagulation cascade and, in combination with venous stasis, leads to the manifestation of bone cement implantation syndrome. The clinical manifestations vary, and include acute hypotension, hypoxemia, cardiac arrest, sudden death, postoperative neurologic sequelae, and DVT.[112–115]

The high incidence of VTE during THA can be attributed to the combination of occlusion of the femoral vein, endothelial lesions, and embolization of tissue thromboplastin with bone marrow debris. Prophylaxis against fat and marrow embolism using a bone marrow vacuum cementing technique has been shown to reduce the incidence of DVT following THA.[116]

The role of changes in intermedullary pressure in the genesis of intraoperative embolism has been well studied. The operative techniques known to reduce the risk of embolization include insertion of the femoral stem without cement, pulsatile lavage prior to application of cement, distal venting of the femur prior to cement application, and bone marrow vacuum cementing technique.[114,117,118] The modified surgical techniques using noncemented prostheses or bone marrow vacuum cementing have been shown to have the greatest efficacy in reducing the incidence of embolic phenomena.[117,118]

The hemodynamic and pulmonary changes associated with embolization may be subclinical in patients with good cardiopulmonary reserve. However, life-threatening cardiopulmonary sequelae may occur in patients whose hemodynamic compensatory mechanisms are compromised because of preexisting cardiopulmonary disease or extensive sympathetic blockade secondary to high neuraxial blockade. In these high-risk patients, consideration should be given to using surgical techniques that minimize embolization as well as neuraxial techniques that minimize sympathectomy.

POSTOPERATIVE NEURAXIAL ANALGESIA

Effective management of postoperative pain allows expeditious implementation of physical therapy and rehabilitation following major lower extremity orthopedic surgery. Clinical evidence supports a correlation between the quality of postoperative analgesia and immediate and long-term functional outcome following major orthopedic surgery.[27,119] Patients undergoing TKA with continuous epidural anesthesia/analgesia experience a more complete and faster rehabilitation compared to those given intravenous patient-controlled analgesia (PCA).[119] The incidence of side effects with CEA, however, is higher compared to those associated with continuous femoral nerve blockade. Patients undergoing hip surgery (THA or hip fracture surgery) experience severe pain during the first 24 h postoperatively, and have been shown to have adequate pain relief following a single dose of intrathecal morphine.[120,121] Concern over the risk of epidural hematoma from the indwelling epidural catheter with concomitant use of anticoagulation for thromboprophylaxis has limited the application of CEA for extended (greater than 24 h) postoperative analgesia in patients undergoing lower extremity major joint surgery.

Extended postoperative neuraxial analgesia is also a concern in patients at risk for compartment syndrome. Pain and aggravation of pain by passive muscle stretching is the most sensitive, and often the only, clinical finding before the onset of ischemic dysfunction in muscles and nerves in the presence of compartment syndrome.[122] Following surgical treatment of tibial plateau or shaft fractures (a surgical condition at high risk for compartment syndrome), patients who received postoperative epidural analgesia were found to have a four-time higher risk of neurologic complications compared to those receiving systemic opioids.[123] Therefore, if compartment syndrome is a significant risk, extended CEA for postoperative pain should be avoided.

▶ Continuous Epidural Analgesia

Postoperative CEA can be provided with dilute solutions of long-acting local anesthetics or opioids, or more commonly, a combination of the two. Dilute solutions (0.05–0.2%) of local anesthetics such as bupivacaine or ropivacaine administered as a continuous infusion, with the option of PCEA, are ideal. Low concentrations of long-acting local anesthetics combined with low concentrations of epidural morphine or other opioids minimize hemodynamic depression and motor blockade, and facilitate ambulation. Ropivacaine has the advantage of reduced motor blockade, greater selectivity for blocking A-delta and C fibers, and decreased cardiotoxicity.[124,125] Higher blood levels of local anesthetics should be expected in elderly and frail patients; therefore, the dose should be reduced accordingly. Details on the selection and dose of local anesthetics and adjuvants for postoperative analgesia are discussed in Chap. 16.

▶ Subarachnoid Opioid Analgesia

Pain after THA and femoral neck fracture surgery can be effectively controlled by adding a small dose (e.g., 0.2 mg) of intrathecal preservative-free morphine sulfate (ITMS) to the spinal anesthetic drug, followed by postoperative intravenous patient-controlled analgesia (PCA).[126] ITMS has an opioid sparing effect (reduction in the 24-h PCA morphine requirement) in patients undergoing hip surgery. In patients undergoing TKA, ITMS improves pain scores but fails to reduce the opioid consumption, suggesting that ITMS may not be a suitable postoperative analgesic intervention for knee arthroplasty. ITMS is an effective alternative to extended CEA in the following clinical situations (Box 7-14):

1. Primary THA, especially those using small incisions and muscle sparing techniques.

2. Patients scheduled for early ambulation and rehabilitation (*Fast Track* hip arthroplasty). Residual motor weakness associated with epidural local anesthetics may interfere with early rehabilitative efforts.

3. Patients at high risk for deep vein thrombosis who have been placed on low molecular weight heparin (LMWH),

or other forms of anticoagulation that contraindicates the use of an indwelling epidural catheter.

ITMS has a dose-dependent analgesic and side effect profile. The side effects (nausea, vomiting, pruritus, and respiratory depression) decrease with lower doses (less than or equal to 0.1 mg), but the quality and duration of analgesia deteriorates accordingly.[121] The optimal dose of ITMS for pain control after THA has been studied extensively.[121,126–128] ITMS 0.1–0.2 mg provides the best balance between analgesic efficacy and side effect profile. ITMS 0.2 mg usually provides adequate pain relief for approximately 8 h following hip arthroplasty. Since elderly patients (greater than 80 years) were not included in most of the studies that examined ITMS dose response, caution should be exercised when extrapolating the findings of these studies to elderly patients or sick patients (ASA PS greater than 3).

▶ Extended Release Morphine Epidural Analgesia

The ideal analgesic regimen for management of postoperative lower extremity major orthopedic procedure pain should provide uninterrupted pain relief (no analgesic gaps) and be compatible with adjunct therapies, for example, anticoagulant thromboprophylaxis. Conventional CEA uses a mixture of local anesthetic and opioid and has several limitations[75] outlined in Box 7-15. Most of the limitations of CEA are related to the presence of the indwelling epidural catheter. The advent of aggressive perioperative anticoagulant thromboprophylaxis in patients undergoing lower extremity major orthopedic surgery, particularly total hip or knee arthroplasties, has resulted in a decrease in the use of CEA.

Box 7-14

Intrathecal Morphine Sulfate Analgesia

Candidates

▶ THA

▶ "Fast track" arthroplasty (early ambulation)

▶ High risk of thromboembolism (early anticoagulation)

Technique

▶ ITMS combined with local anesthetic spinal anesthesia

▶ 0.1–0.2 mg

Box 7-15

Limitations of CEA (Mixture of Local Anesthetic and Opioid)

▶ High incidence (up to 80%) of analgesic gaps

▶ Epidural catheter failure/malfunction rate = 20–25%

▶ High resource utilization (labor intensive)

▶ Motor weakness of lower extremities (lumbar > thoracic epidural analgesia)

▶ Risk of epidural hematoma with concomitant anticoagulant thromboprophylaxis

▶ Patient activity impaired by epidural catheter connected to an infusion device

Data from Ref. 75.

Box 7-16

Epidural Sustained Release Morphine: Dosing Guidelines and Clinical Management

▶ Site of administrations: DepoDur is recommended for lumbar epidural administration only*

▶ Dose:

  ▶ Lower extremity major orthopedic surgery—15 mg

  ▶ Elderly patients (age ≥ 65)—10 mg

▶ Confirm epidural catheter placement before sustained release morphine administration†

▶ Timing: administer sustained release morphine > 15 min after local anesthetic epidural test dose

▶ After morphine administration, do not inject any other epidural drugs and remove the epidural catheter

▶ Monitoring: guidelines for sustained release morphine should mimic those for epidural morphine, but should be continued for 48 h‡

*Currently there is no clinical experience with DepoDur injected at more cephalad epidural levels.
†Subarachnoid administration of the drug may result in prolonged/profound respiratory depression.
‡The adverse event profile for DepoDur is the same as conventional epidural morphine, but of longer duration after a single dose.

Sustained release liposome encapsulated morphine (DepoDur, Endopharmaceuticals, Inc.), recently made available in the United States, provides 48 h of postoperative analgesia with a single epidural dose for patients undergoing total hip or knee arthroplasty. This extended delivery of epidural morphine eliminates the need for an indwelling epidural catheter and infusion device. A recent study compared single doses of sustained release morphine (15, 20, or 25 mg) to placebo (preservative-free saline), administered before the induction of general or NA for THA. The placebo group required much higher amounts of intravenous fentanyl during the first 48 h postoperatively compared to the sustained release morphine groups, with 25% of the morphine patients requiring no supplemental intravenous fentanyl.[129]

The experience with sustained release lysosomal morphine is currently limited, but the concept appears promising in simplifying and improving the postoperative analgesia regimens for lower extremity major orthopedic surgery. The adverse event profile of sustained release morphine is similar to that of conventional epidural morphine, necessitating monitoring the patient for potential respiratory depression

for the period of the drug's duration, that is, 48 h. Also, as with conventional epidural morphine, the concurrent use of other central nervous system depressants (e.g., sedatives, hypnotics, and tranquilizers) increases the risk of respiratory depression, hypotension, and profound sedation.

The safety and efficacy of sustained release morphine when used in conjunction with epidural local anesthetics has not yet been studied. Administration of sustained release morphine within 3 min of an epidural test dose (lidocaine 3 mL with epinephrine 1:200,000) increases the bioavailability of the morphine. The current recommendation, therefore, is to administer the sustained release morphine at least 15 min after the epidural local anesthetic test dose. Based on the limited published data, guidelines have been compiled for DepoDur administration at the authors' institution (Box 7-16).

POSTOPERATIVE CONCERNS AND NEURAXIAL ANESTHESIA

▶ Neurologic Deficit Following Major Orthopedic Surgery

Although rare, NA techniques carry a potential risk of nerve injuries such as segmental neuropathy, cauda equina syndrome, and conus medullaris syndrome.[49,50,129,130] Nerve injuries in patients undergoing lower extremity orthopedic surgery can also occur from surgical- and patient-related factors (Box 7-17). The overall incidence of nerve injury following total hip or knee arthroplasty varies widely based on the underlying surgical pathology. A meta-analysis of 34,335 total hip arthroplasties (primary and revision) identified 359 (1%) nerve palsies.[131] The prevalence of nerve palsy in primary total hip arthroplasties was 0.9%. Surgical risk factors for postoperative nerve injury are listed in Table 7-4.

The vast majority of nerve injuries following THA involve the sciatic nerve (80%), followed in frequency by injury to the femoral (0.1–0.4%), and obturator or gluteal nerve (0.01%).[131] In most reports of sciatic nerve injury,

Table 7-4

Surgical Risk Factors: Postoperative Nerve Injury Following THA

Surgical Risk Factor	Prevalence Ratio
Primary vs. revision arthroplasty	1:3
Male vs. female	1:2
Osteoarthritis vs. congenital dysplasia	1:2

Data from Ref. 132.

Box 7-17

Anesthetic-, Surgical-, and Patient-related Causes of Postoperative Neurologic Deficits

Anesthesia related

- Epidural space-occupying lesion—hematoma, abscess
- Local anesthetic neurotoxicity (e.g., cauda equina syndrome)
- Needle trauma—segmental neuropathy, conus medullaris syndrome

Surgery related

- Retractor-induced stretch, compression, or ischemia
- Compression by subgluteal hematoma
- Positional injury—compression and stretching (e.g., abduction splint-related peroneal nerve injury)

Patient related

- Preexisting lesion—tumor, vascular anomaly, or congenital cyst
- Preexisting subclinical neuropathy
  - Alcoholic neuropathy
  - Diabetic neuropathy
  - Proximal compressive neuropathy—spinal stenosis

regardless of the cause, the common peroneal component is involved more frequently and sustains greater damage than the tibial component. The susceptibility of the common peroneal division to injury has been attributed to several of its anatomic features:

1. The common peroneal division is composed of fewer and larger fasciculi with less connective tissue compared to the tibial division. Nerves with large and tightly packed fasciculi are more vulnerable to mechanical injury than those in which the fasciculi are smaller and more loosely dispersed in a larger amount of connective tissue.

2. Compared to the tibial component, the peroneal component of the sciatic nerve is relatively fixed at two points—at the level of the sciatic notch and at the neck of the fibula. Therefore, it is more vulnerable to stretch injury.

3. The peroneal component lies lateral to the to the tibial component, and is therefore more vulnerable to surgical

injury such as traction, pressure injury from retractors, or heat injury from extruded bone cement.[131,132]

Anesthesia-Related Neurologic Deficits

Local Anesthetic Neurotoxicity. The nerve roots of the cauda equina in the subarachnoid space are poorly myelinated and particularly vulnerable to chemical damage by local anesthetics. Local anesthetic toxicity is dose related (volume X concentration). Local anesthetic neurotoxicity presenting as cauda equine syndrome has been reported following subarachnoid injection of high doses of lidocaine, tetracaine, and chloroprocaine (for example, the inadvertent subarachnoid injection of a large volume of local anesthetic solution intended for the epidural space)[133,134] (see Chap. 6). To reduce the incidence of neurotoxicity, the recommended concentration and dose of subarachnoid local anesthetics should not be exceeded.

Mechanical Trauma to Nerve Tissue. Needle contact with neural elements elicits a paresthesia. It has been speculated that the frequency of procedural paresthesia is higher following the use of atraumatic, pencil-point spinal needles for single-shot spinal or CSE anesthesia.[135] An atraumatic needle is expected to indent the dura mater before its tip enters the subarachnoid space. The chances of needle-nerve contact and, therefore, paresthesia increases because the needle tip penetrates further into the subarachnoid space. There is a correlation between painful procedural paresthesias and subsequent neurologic sequelae.[49,50,70,136]

Needle trauma localized to a nerve root of the cauda equina may produce limited segmental symptoms (radiculopathy). This is the most common cause of postoperative neurologic sequelae presenting with symptoms of paresthesia, dysesthesia, and rarely, motor deficit. In contrast, injury to the conus medullaris produces extensive damage with devastating clinical symptoms. Reynolds reported seven cases of conus medullaris injury following a single-shot spinal or CSE anesthesia using an atraumatic spinal needle.[130] All patients were women and each reported procedural paresthesia. Foot drop occurred in six patients, urinary retention in three patients, and all had persistent unilateral sensory loss along the distribution of L4 to S1 dermatomes. Magnetic resonance imaging (MRI) demonstrated syrinx formation at the level of the conus medullaris in six patients.

The incidence of radiculopathy following spinal anesthesia ranges from 0.2 to 1/1000.[49,50,70,135] Injury to the conus medullaris is rare, with one study citing the incidence as 2/41,950 cases.[136] Since the clinical outcome of conus medullaris injury is devastating, every precaution should be undertaken to prevent this injury. The site of lumbar puncture for spinal anesthesia should be distal to the conus medullaris. Therefore, the anesthesiologist should be cognizant of two anatomic pitfalls (see Chap. 1):

1. The level of the termination of the spinal cord—MRI studies suggest that the spinal cord ends distal to the L1 vertebra in 2% of cases.[135,137]

2. Intercristal line (Tuffier's line)—The line joining the highest point of the iliac crests is commonly used to identify the appropriate vertebral interspace (L3-L4 or L4-L5) for lumbar puncture. Inaccuracies in identifying the appropriate lumbar interspace have been demonstrated to occur in the hands of experienced anesthesiologists.[138] In 67% of cases, the marked space was one to three interspaces higher than the intended interspace. This inaccuracy was more likely in elderly female women with osteoporosis and in obese patients.

Pitfalls in identifying the correct interspace and variations in the anatomy with respect to the site of termination of the spinal cord introduce a finite risk of serious mechanical injury to the conus medullaris or the cauda equina in the vicinity of the conus medullaris. Recommendations for prevention of neurologic injuries in association with spinal anesthesia are outlined in Box 7-18.

Management of Postoperative Neuropathies

All patients undergoing major lower extremity procedures should be routinely evaluated postoperatively for peripheral nerve function. Judicious selection of local anesthetic drug

---

Box 7-18

Recommendation for Prevention of Neurologic Injuries Associated with Spinal Anesthesia

▶ Use the recommended dose/concentration of local anesthetics

▶ Minimize local anesthetic dose/concentration in patients with subclinical neuropathy. Avoid epinephrine in these patients

▶ Select a lower interspace for lumbar puncture in elderly females and obese patients

▶ Pay attention to procedural paresthesias

　▶ Lancinating paresthesia: move to lower interspace

　▶ Persistent paresthesia: abandon subarachnoid block

　▶ Mild to moderate paresthesia: readjust the needle proceed with caution seeking patient input. *Do not inject if paresthesia persists*

---

and dose used for neuraxial analgesia will prevent undue delays in the initial postoperative evaluation. At the authors' institution, a maintenance infusion of epidural local anesthetic (long-acting agent, e.g., bupivacaine) is discontinued 30 min prior to the end of surgery. This allows return of motor function of the lower extremities within an hour after the end of the procedure.

The peroneal and tibial components of the sciatic nerve should be examined separately. Motor function is evaluated by checking active plantar flexion (tibial nerve) and active dorsiflexion (peroneal nerve). If a central neuraxial space-occupying lesion is suspected, an immediate MRI and neurosurgical consult are indicated. If a peripheral neuropathy is discovered, a neurology consult should be obtained to confirm the distribution of motor and sensory deficits and assist in localizing the nerve injury with electrodiagnostic studies. The short head of the biceps femoris is the only muscle in the thigh that is innervated by the peroneal nerve. Electromyographic findings suggestive of denervation of this muscle indicate that injury to the sciatic nerve has occurred at the level of the proximal thigh.

SUMMARY

Recent evidence suggests that neuraxial anesthesia (NA) and analgesia for lower extremity major orthopedic surgery improve perioperative outcomes with respect to morbidity and optimal pain control. The outcomes with respect to mortality and life-threatening events need to be defined further.

Spinal and epidural NA have been the standard neuraxial techniques for major lower extremity orthopedic surgery. Over the last decade, CSE anesthesia has evolved as an ideal neuraxial technique for these procedures. The majority of patients presenting for major lower extremity orthopedic surgery are the elderly and many have multiple coexisting medical conditions. Ensuring hemodynamic stability in these high-risk patients requires selection of the appropriate neuraxial technique with a focus on maintaining a safe and desirable level of blockade, and limiting extensive sympathectomy.

To provide safe perioperative care the anesthesiologist should be attentive to several clinical issues, including the selection of an appropriate local anesthetic drug, dose, and baricity, treatment of hypotension, optimal management fluid therapy (including allogeneic blood products), and provision for appropriate postoperative analgesia. Finally, safe application of neuraxial blockade requires awareness of perioperative risks associated with the use of anticoagulant-based thromboprophylaxis, and potential neurologic injuries associated with neuraxial block techniques and surgical procedures.

REFERENCES

1. Modig J, Borg T, Karlstrom G, et al. Thromboembolism after total hip replacement: Role of epidural and general anesthesia. *Anesth Analg* 62:174, 1983.

2. Jorgensen L, Rasmussen L, Nielsen P, et al. Antithrombotic efficacy of continuous extradural analgesia after knee replacement. *Br J Anaesth* 66:8, 1991.

3. Beattie WS, Badner NH, Choi P, et al. Epidural analgesia reduces postoperative myocardial infarction: A meta analysis. *Anesth Analg* 93:853, 2001.

4. Rasmussen LS, Johnson T, Kuipers HM, et al. Does anesthesia cause postoperative cognitive dysfunction? A randomized study of regional versus general anesthesia in 438 elderly patients. *Acta Anesthesiol Scand* 47:260, 2003.

5. Block BM, Liu SS, Rowlingson AJ, et al. Efficacy of postoperative epidural analgesia: A meta-analysis. *JAMA* 290:2455, 2003.

6. Liu S, Carpenter RL, Neal JM. Epidural anesthesia and analgesia: Their role in postoperative outcome. *Anesthesiology* 82:1474, 1995.

7. Rodgers A, Walker N, Schug S, et al. Reduction of postoperative mortality and morbidity with epidural or spinal anesthesia: Results from overview of randomized trials. *BMJ* 321:1, 2000.

8. Moraca RJ, Sheldon DG, Thirlby RC. The role of epidural anesthesia and analgesia in surgical practice. *Ann Surg* 238:663, 2003.

9. Matot I, Oppenheim-Eden A, Ratrot R, et al. Preoperative cardiac events in elderly patients with hip fracture randomized to epidural or conventional analgesia. *Anesthesiology* 98:156, 2003.

10. Perka C, Arnold U, Buttgereit F. Influencing factors on perioperative morbidity in knee arthroplasty. *Clin Orthop* 378:183, 2000.

11. Marsch SCU, Schaefer HG, Skarvan K, et al. Perioperative myocardial ischemia in patients undergoing elective hip arthroplasty during lumbar regional anesthesia. *Anesthesiology* 76:518, 1992.

12. Scheinin H, Virtanen T, Kentala E, et al. Epidural infusion of bupivacaine and fentanyl reduces perioperative myocardial ischemia in elderly patients with hip fracture: A randomized controlled trial. *Acta Anesthesiol Scand* 44:1061, 2000.

13. Juelsgaard P, Sand NPR, Felsby S, et al. Perioperative myocardial ischemia in patients undergoing surgery for fractured hip randomized to incremental spinal, single dose or general anesthesia. *Eur J Anaesthesiol* 15:656, 1998.

14. Mantilla CB, Horlocker TT, Schroeder DR, et al. Frequency of myocardial infarction, pulmonary embolism, deep venous thrombosis, and death following primary hip or knee arthroplasty. *Anesthesiology* 96:1140, 2002.

15. Geerts WH, Heit JA, Clagett GP, et al. Prevention of venous thromboembolism. *Chest* 119:132S, 2001.

16. Mantilla CB, Horlocker TT, Schroeder DR, et al. Risk factors for clinically relevant pulmonary embolism and deep venous thrombosis in patients undergoing primary hip or knee arthroplasty. *Anesthesiology* 99:552, 2003.

17. Sorenson R, Pace N, Anesthetic techniques during surgical repair of femoral neck fractures. *Anesthesiology* 77:1095, 1992.

18. Mohr DN, Silverstein MD, Ilstrup DM, et al. Venous thromboembolism associated with hip and knee arthroplasty: Current prophylactic practices and outcomes. *Mayo Clin Proc* 67:861, 1992.

19. Anderson FA, Hirsh J, White K, et al. Temporal trends in prevention of venous thromboembolism following primary total hip or knee arthroplasty 1996–2001. *Chest* 124:349S, 2003.

20. Horlocker TT, Wedel DJ, Benzon H, et al. Regional anesthesia in the anticoagulated patient: Defining the risks. *Reg Anesth Pain Med* 29(Suppl 1):1, 2004.

21. Marcantonio ER, Goldman L, Mangione CM, et al. A clinical prediction rule for delirium after non-cardiac surgery. *JAMA* 27:134, 1994.

22. Zakriya K, Sieber FE, Christmas C, et al. Brief postoperative delirium in hip fracture patients affects functional outcome at three months. *Anesth Analg* 98:1798, 2004.

23. Wu CL, Hsu W, Richman JM, et al. Postoperative cognitive function as an outcome of regional anesthesia and analgesia. *Reg Anesth Pain Med* 29:257, 2004.

24. Moller JT, Cluitmans P, Rasmussen LS, et al. Long-term postoperative cognitive dysfunction in the elderly. ISPOCD1 study. *Lancet* 351:857, 1998.

25. Kehlet H, Holte K. Effect of postoperative analgesia on surgical outcome. *Br J Anaesth* 87:67, 2001.

26. Kehlet H. Modification of response to surgery by neural blockade: Clinical implications. In: Cousins MJ, Bridenbough PO, eds, *Neural Blockade in Clinical Anesthesia and Management of Pain*, 3rd ed. Philadelphia, PA: JB Lippincott, 1998, p. 129.

27. Capdevila X, Barthelet Y, Biboulet P, et al. Effects of perioperative analgesic technique on the surgical outcome and duration of rehabilitation after major knee surgery. *Anesthesiology* 91:8, 1999.

28. Philips DM. JCAHO pain management standards are unveiled. *JAMA* 284:428, 2000.

29. Holmstrom B, Laugaland K, Rawal N, et al. Combined spinal epidural block versus spinal and epidural block for orthopedic surgery. *Can J Anaesth* 40:601, 1993.

30. Borghi B, Casati A, Iuorio S, et al. Frequency of hypotension and bradycardia during general anesthesia, epidural anesthesia, or integrated epidural–general anesthesia for total hip replacement. *J Clin Anesth* 14:102, 2002.

31. Cousins MJ, Veering BT. Epidural neural blockade. In: Cousins MJ, Bridenbaugh PO, eds, *Neural Blockade in Clinical Anesthesia and Management of Pain*, 3rd ed. Philadelphia, PA: Lippincott-Raven, 1998, p. 243.

32. Baron JF, Decaux-Jacolot A, Edouard A, et al. Influence of venous return on baroreflex control of HR during lumbar epidural anesthesia in humans. *Anesthesiology* 64:188, 1986.

33. Hodgson PS, Liu SS, Gras TW. Does epidural anesthesia have general anesthetic effects? A prospective randomized, double-blind placebo-controlled trial. *Anesthesiology* 91:1687, 1999.

34. Colson P, Ryckwaert F, Coriat P. Renin angiotensin system antagonists and anesthesia. *Anesth Analg* 89:1143, 1999.

35. Eyraud D, Mouren S, Teugels K, et al. Treating anesthesia-induced hypotension by angiotensin II in patients chronically treated with angiotensin-converting enzyme inhibitors. *Anesth Analg* 86:259, 1998.

36. Tverskoy M, Shagal M, Finger J, et al. Subarachnoid bupivacaine blockade decreases midazolam and thiopental hypnotic requirements. *J Clin Anesth* 6:487, 1994.

37. Tverskoy M, Shifrin V, Finger J, et al. Effect of epidural bupivacaine block on midazolam hypnotic requirements. *Reg Anesth* 21:209, 1996.

38. Sander-Jensen K, Marving J, Secher M, et al. Does the decrease in heart rate prevent a detrimental decrease in end systolic volume during central hypovolemia in men? *J Vasc Dis* 687, 1990.

39. Goertz AW, Seeling W, Heinrich H., et al. Effect of phenylephrine bolus administration on left ventricular function during

thoracic and lumbar epidural anesthesia combined with general anesthesia. *Anesth Analg* 76(3):541, 1993.

40. Liu SS, Carpenter RL. Hemodynamic responses to intravascular injection of epinephrine-containing epidural test doses in adults during general anesthesia. *Anesthesiology* 84:81, 1996.

41. Tanaka M, Takahashi S, Kondo T, et al. Efficacy of simulated epidural test doses in adult patients anesthetized with isoflurane: A dose-response study. *Anesth Analg* 81:987, 1995.

42. Guinard JP, Mulroy MF, Carpenter RL. Aging reduces the reliability of epidural epinephrine test doses. *Reg Anesth* 20:193, 1995.

43. Guinard JP, Mulroy MF, Carpenter RL, et al. Test doses: Optimal epinephrine content with and without acute beta-adrenergic blockade. *Anesthesiology* 73:386, 1990.

44. Mulroy MF, Norris MC, Liu SS. Safety steps for epidural injection of local anesthetics: Review of the literature and recommendations. *Anesth Analg* 85:1346, 1997.

45. Lyons G, Columb M, Wilson RC, et al. Epidural pain relief in labour: Potencies of levobupivacaine and racemic bupivacaine. *Br J Anaesth* 81:899, 1998.

46. Polley LS, Columb MO, Naughton NN, et al. Relative analgesic potencies of ropivacaine and bupivacaine for epidural anesthesia in labor: Implications for therapeutic indexes. *Anesthesiology* 90(4):944, 1999.

47. Casati A, Santorsola R, Aldegheri G, et al. Intraoperative epidural anesthesia and postoperative analgesia with levobupivacaine for major orthopedic surgery: A double blind, randomized comparison of racemic bupivacaine and ropivacaine. *J Clin Anesth* 15:126, 2003.

48. Murdoch JA, Dickson UK, Wilson PA, et al. The efficacy and safety of three concentrations of levobupivacaine administered as a continuous epidural infusion in patients undergoing orthopedic surgery. *Anesth Analg* 94:438, 2002.

49. Auroy Y, Narchi P, Messiah A, et al. Serious complications related to regional anesthesia. *Anesthesiology* 87:479, 1997.

50. Auroy Y, Benhamou D, Bargues L, et al. Major complications of regional anesthesia in France: The SOS regional anesthesia hot line service. *Anesthesiology* 97:1274, 2002.

51. Pollard JB. Can we explain the high incidence of cardiac arrest during spinal anesthesia for hip surgery? *Anesthesiology* 99:754, 2003.

52. Greene NM. Distribution of local anesthetic solutions within the subarachnoid space. *Anesth Analg* 64:715, 1985.

53. Carpenter RL, Hogan QH, Liu SS, et al. Lumbosacral cerebrospinal fluid volume is the primary determinant of sensory block extent and duration during spinal anesthesia. *Anesthesiology* 89:24, 1998.

54. Taivainen T, Tuominen M, Rosenberg PH. Spread of spinal anesthesia using various doses of plain 0.5% bupivacaine injected at the L IV-V interspace. *Acta Anaesthesiol Scand* 33:652, 1989.

55. Taivainen T, Tuominen M, Rosenberg PH. Influence of obesity on the spread of spinal analgesia after injection of plain 0.5% bupivacaine at the L3-4 or L4-5 interspace. *Br J Anaesth* 64:542, 1990.

56. Atchison SR, Wedal DJ, Wilson PR. Effect of injection rate on level and duration of hypobaric spinal anesthesia. *Anesth Analg* 69:496, 1989.

57. Horlocker TT, Wedel DJ, Wilson PR. Effect of injection rate on sensory level and duration of hypobaric bupivacaine spinal anesthesia for total hip arthroplasty. *Anesth Analg* 79:773, 1994.

58. Faust A, Fournier R, Van Gessel EV, et al. Isobaric versus hypobaric spinal bupivacaine for total hip arthroplasty in the lateral position. *Anesth Analg* 97:589, 2003.

59. Tuominen M, Kalso E, Rosenberg PH. The effects of posture in the spread of spinal anesthesia with isobaric 0.75% or 0.5% bupivacaine. *Br J Anaesth* 54:313, 1982.

60. Frey K, Holman S, Mikat-Stevens M, et al. The recovery profile of hyperbaric spinal anesthesia with lidocaine, tetracaine, and bupivacaine. *Reg Anesth Pain Med* 23:159, 1998.

61. Bridenbaugh PO, Greene NM, Brull SJ. Spinal (subarachnoid) neural blockade. In: Cousins MJ, Bridenbaugh PO, eds, *Neural Blockade in Clinical Anesthesia and Pain Management*, 3rd ed. Philadelphia, PA: Lippincott-Raven, 1998, p. 203.

62. Chambers WA, Littlewood DG, Scott DB. Spinal anesthesia with hyperbaric bupivacaine: Effect of added vasoconstrictors. *Anesth Analg* 61:49, 1982.

63. Racle JP, Benkhadra A, Poy JY, et al. Effect of increasing amounts of epinephrine during isobaric bupivacaine spinal anesthesia in elderly patients. *Anesth Analg* 66:882, 1987.

64. Ben-David B, Frankel R, Arzumonou T. Minidose bupivacaine-fentanyl spinal anesthesia for surgical repair of hip fracture in the aged. *Anesthesiology* 92:6, 2000.

65. Klimscha W, Chiari A, Krafft P, et al. Hemodynamic and analgesic effects of clonidine added repetitively to continuous epidural and spinal blocks. *Anesth Analg* 80:322, 1995.

66. Favarel-Garrigues JF, Sztark F, Petitjean ME, et al. Hemodynamic effects of spinal anesthesia in the elderly: Single dose versus titration through a catheter. *Anesth Analg* 82:312, 1996.

67. Collard C, Eappen S, Lynch E, et al. Continuous spinal anesthesia with invasive hemodynamic monitoring for surgical repair of the hip in two patients with severe aortic stenosis. *Anesth Analg* 81:195, 1995.

68. Van Gessel EV, Forster A, Gamulin Z. A prospective study of the feasibility of continuous spinal anesthesia in a university hospital. *Anesth Analg* 80:880, 1995.

69. Horlocker TT, McGregor DG, Matssushige DK, et al. Neurologic complications of 603 consecutive continuous spinal anesthetics using macrocatheter and microcatheter techniques. *Anesth Analg* 84:1063, 1997.

70. Horlocker TT, McGregor DG, Matsushige DK, et al. A retrospective review of 4767 consecutive spinal anesthetics: Central nervous systems complications. *Anesth Analg* 84:578, 1997.

71. Ilias WK, Klimscha W, Skrbensky G, et al. Continuous microspinal anesthesia: Another perspective on mechanisms inducing cauda equina syndrome. *Anaesthesia* 53:618, 1998.

72. Biboulet P, Capdevila X, Aubas P, et al. Causes and prediction of maldistribution during continuous spinal anesthesia with isobaric or hyperbaric bupivacaine. *Anesthesiology* 88:1487, 1998.

73. Cook TM. Combined spinal–epidural techniques. *Anaesthesia* 55:42, 2000.

74. Hoffmann VLH, Vercauteren MP, Buczkowski PW, et al. A new combined spinal epidural apparatus: Measurement of the distance to the epidural and subarachnoid spaces. *Anaesthesia* 52:350, 1997.

75. Ready BL. Acute pain: Lessons learned from 25,000 patients. *Reg Anesth Pain Med* 24:499, 1999.

76. Westbrook JL, Donald F, Carrie LES. An evaluation of a combined spinal/epidural needle set utilizing a 26-gauge, pencil point spinal needle for cesarean section. *Anaesthesia* 47:990, 1992.

77. Eappen S, Blinn A, Segal S. Incidence of epidural catheter replacement in parturients: A retrospective chart review. *Int J Obstet Anesth* 7:220, 1998.

78. Holmstrom B, Rawal N, Axelsson K, et al. Risk of catheter migration during combined spinal epidural block: Percutaneous epiduroscopy study. *Anesth Analg* 80:747, 1995.

79. Rawal N, Zundert AV, Holmstrom B, et al. Combined spinal-epidural technique. *Reg Anesth* 22:406, 1997.

80. Bernards CM, Kopacz DJ, Michel MZ. Effect of needle puncture on morphine and lidocaine flux through the spinal meninges of the monkey in vitro. Implications for combined spinal–epidural anesthesia. *Anesthesiology* 80:853, 1994.

81. Goy RWL, Sia ATH. Sensorimotor anesthesia and hypotension after subarachnoid block: Combined spinal–epidural versus single shot spinal technique. *Anesth Analg* 98:491, 2004.

82. Klasen J, Junger A, Hartmann B, et al. Differing incidences of relevant hypotension with combined spinal-epidural anesthesia and spinal anesthesia. *Anesth Analg* 96:1491, 2003.

83. Rawal N, Schollin J, Wesstrom G. Epidural versus spinal epidural block for cesarean section. *Acta Anesthesiol Scand* 32:61, 1988.

84. Stienstra R, Dahan A, Alhadi BZR, et al. Mechanism of action of an epidural top-up in combined spinal epidural anesthesia. *Anesth Analg* 83:382, 1996.

85. Stienstra R, Alhadi BZR, Dahan A, et al. The epidural "top-up" in combined spinal-epidural anesthesia: The effect of volume versus dose. *Anesth Analg* 88:810, 1999.

86. Takiguchi T, Okano T, Egawa H. The effect of epidural saline injection on analgesic level during combined spinal-epidural anesthesia assessed clinically and myelographically. *Anesth Analg* 85:1097, 1997.

87. Leeda M, Stienstra R, Arbous S, et al. The epidural "top-up": Predictors of increase of sensory blockade. *Anesthesiology* 96:1310, 2002.

88. Tetzlaff JE, Yoon HJ, Walsh M. Regional anesthetic technique and the incidence of tourniquet pain. *Can J Anaesth* 40:591, 1993.

89. Concepcion MA, Lambert DH, Welch KA, et al. Tourniquet pain during spinal anesthesia: A comparison of plain solutions of tetracaine and bupivacaine. *Anesth Analg* 67:828, 1988.

90. Bonnet F, Zozime JP, Marcandoro J, et al. Tourniquet pain during spinal anesthesia: Hyperbaric versus isobaric tetracaine *Reg Anesth* 13:29, 1988.

91. Bridenbaugh PO, Hagenouw R, Gielen MJ, et al. Addition of glucose to bupivacaine in spinal anesthesia increases incidence of tourniquet pain. *Anesth Analg* 65:1181, 1986.

92. Stewart A, Lambert DH, Concepcion MA, et al. Decreased incidence of tourniquet pain during spinal anesthesia with bupivacaine. *Anesth Analg* 67:833, 1988.

93. Gissen AJ, Covino BG, Gregus J. Differential sensitivities of mammalian nerve fibers to local anesthetic agents. *Anesthesiology* 53:467, 1980.

94. Cherng CH, Wong CS, Chang FL, et al. Epidural morphine delays the onset of tourniquet pain during epidural lidocaine anesthesia. *Anesth Analg* 94:1614, 2002.

95. Tuominen M, Valli H, Kalso E, et al. Efficacy of 0.3 mg morphine intrathecally in preventing tourniquet pain during spinal anesthesia with hyperbaric bupivacaine. *Acta Anesthesiol Scand* 32:113, 1988.

96. Bierbaum BE, Callaghan JJ, Galante JO, et al. An analysis of blood management in patients having a total hip or knee arthroplasty. *J Bone Joint Surg* 81:2, 1999.

97. Spahn DR, Casutt M. Eliminating blood transfusion. New aspects and perspectives. *Anesthesiology* 93:242, 2000.

98. Etchason J, Petz L, Keeler E, et al. The cost effectiveness of preoperative autologous blood donations. *N Engl J Med* 332:719, 1995.

99. Birkmeyer JD, Goodnough LT, AuBuchon JP, et al. The cost-effectiveness of preoperative autologous blood donations for total hip and knee replacement. *Transfusion* 33:544, 1993.

100. Couvert C, Laffon M, Baud A, et al. A restrictive use of both autologous donation and recombinant human erythropoietin is an efficient policy for primary total hip or knee arthroplasty. *Anesth Analg* 99:262, 2004.

101. Halpern NA, Alicea M, Seabrook B, et al. Cell Saver autologous transfusion: Metabolic consequences of washing blood with normal saline. *J Trauma* 41:407, 1996.

102. Murkin JM, Shannon NA, Bourne RB, et al. Aprotinin decreases blood loss in patients undergoing revision or bilateral total hip arthroplasty. *Anesth Analg* 80:343, 1995.

103. Schmied H, Kurz A, Sessler DI, et al. Mild hypothermia increases blood loss and transfusion requirements during total hip arthroplasty. *Lancet* 347:289, 1996.

104. Hartmann B, Junger A, Klasen J, et al. The incidence and risk factors for hypotension after spinal anesthesia induction: An analysis with automated data collection. *Anesth Analg* 94:1521, 2002.

105. Tarkkila P, Isola J. A regression model for identifying patients at high risk of hypotension, bradycardia and nausea during spinal anesthesia. *Acta Anesthesiol Scand* 36:554, 1992.

106. Carpenter RL, Caplan RA, Brown DL, et al. Incidence and risk factors for side effects of spinal anesthesia. *Anesthesiology* 76:906, 1992.

107. Critchley LA, Stuart JC, Short TG, et al. Hemodynamic effects of subarachnoid block in elderly patients. *Br J Anaesth* 73:464, 1994.

108. Buggy DJ, Power CK, Meeke R, et al. Prevention of spinal anesthesia-induced hypotension in elderly: I.M. methoxamine or combined hetastarch and crystalloid. *Br J Anaesth* 80:199, 1998.

109. Buggy D, Higgins P, Moran C, et al. Prevention of spinal anesthesia induced hypotension in the elderly: Comparison between preanesthetic administration of crystalloids, colloid and no prehydration. *Anesth Analg* 84:106, 1997.

110. Critchley LAH, Conway F. Hypotension during subarachnoid anesthesia: Hemodynamic effects of colloid and metaraminol. *Br J Anaesth* 76:734, 1996.

111. Nishikawa K, Yamakage M, Omote K, et al. Prophylactic IM small—dose phenylephrine blunts spinal anesthesia induced hypotensive response during surgical repair of hip fracture in the elderly. *Anesth Analg* 95:751, 2002.

112. Orsini, EC, Byrick RJ, Mullen BM, et al. Cardiopulmonary function and pulmonary emboli during arthroplasty using cemented or non-cemented components. The role of intramedullary pressure. *J Bone Joint Surg* 69:822, 1987.

113. Wenda K, Degreif J, Runkel M, et al. Pathogenesis and prophylaxis of circulatory reactions during total hip replacement. *Arch Orthop Trauma Surg* 112:260, 1993.

114. Ereth MH, Weber JG, Abel MD, et al. Cemented versus non-cemented total hip arthroplasty: Embolism, hemodynamics, and intrapulmonary shunting. *Mayo Clin Proc* 67:1066, 1992.

115. Patterson BM, Healey JH, Cornell CN, et al. Cardiac arrest during hip arthroplasty with a cemented long-stem component. *J Bone Joint Surg* 73:271, 1991.

116. Pitto RP, Hamer H, Fabiani R, et al. Prophylaxis against fat and bone-marrow embolism during total hip arthroplasty reduces the incidence of post-operative deep-vein thrombosis: A controlled clinical trial. *J Bone Joint Surg* 84:39, 2002.

117. Pitto RP, Koessler M, Kuehle JW. Comparison of fixation of the femoral component without cement and fixation with use of a bone vacuum cementing technique for the prevention of fat embolism during total hip arthroplasty: A prospective randomized clinical trial. *J Bone Joint Surg* 81:831, 1999.

118. Pitto RP, Koessler M, Klaus D. Prophylaxis of fat and bone marrow embolism in cemented total hip arthroplasty. *Clin Orthop Relate Res* 355:23, 1998.

119. Singelyn FJ, Deyart M, Joris D, et al. Effects of intravenous patient controlled analgesia with morphine, continuous epidural analgesia, and continuous three-in-one block on postoperative pain and knee rehabilitation after unilateral total knee arthroplasty. *Anesth Analg* 87:88, 1998.

120. Souron V, Delaunay L, Schifrine P. Intrathecal morphine provides better postoperative analgesia than psoas compartment block after primary hip arthroplasty. *Can J Anaesth* 50:574, 2003.

121. Slappendel R, Weber EWG, Dirksen R, et al. Optimization of the dose of intrathecal morphine in total hip surgery: A dose finding study. *Anesth Analg* 88:822, 1999.

122. Whitesides TE, Heckman MM. Acute compartment syndrome: Update on diagnosis and treatment. *J Am Acad Orthop Surg* 4(4):209, 1996.

123. Iaquinto JM, Pienkowski D, Thornsberry R, et al. Increased neurologic complications associated with postoperative epidural analgesia after tibial fracture fixation. *Am J Orthop* 604, 1997.

124. Badner NH, Reid D, Sullivan P, et al. Continuous epidural infusion of ropivacaine for the prevention of postoperative pain after major orthopaedic surgery: A dose finding study. *Can J Anaesth* 43:17, 1996.

125. Bertini L, Mancini S, Di Benedetto P, et al. Postoperative analgesia by combined continuous infusion and patient-controlled epidural analgesia (PCEA) following hip replacement: Ropivacaine versus bupivacaine. *Acta Anesthesiol Scand* 45:782, 2001.

126. Rathmell JP, Pino CA, Taylor R, et al. Intrathecal morphine for postoperative analgesia: A randomized, controlled, dose-ranging study after hip and knee arthroplasty. *Anesth Analg* 97:1452, 2003.

127. Murphy PM, Stack D, Kinirons B, et al. Optimizing the dose of intrathecal morphine in older patients undergoing hip arthroplasty. *Anesth Analg* 97:1709, 2003.

128. Jacobson L, Chabal C, Brody MC. A dose-response study of intrathecal morphine: Efficacy, duration, optimal dose, and side effects. *Anesth Analg* 67:1082, 1988.

129. Viscusi ER, Martin G, Hartrick CT, et al. Postoperative pain relief following hip arthroplasty with epidural sustained-release morphine (SKY0401). *Anesthesiology* 99:A1120, 2003.

130. Moen V, Dahlgren N, Irestedt L. Severe neurologic complications after central neuraxial blockades in Sweden 1990–1999. *Anesthesiology* 101:950, 2004.

131. Schmalzried TP, Noordin S, Amstutz H. Update on nerve palsy associated with total hip replacement. *Clin Orthop Relat Res* 344:188, 1997.

132. Edward BH, Tullos HS, Noble PC. Contributory factors and etiology of sciatic nerve palsy in total hip arthroplasty. *Clin Orthop* 218:136, 1987.

133. Rigler ML, Drasner K, Krejcie TC, et al. Cauda equina syndrome after continuous spinal anesthesia. *Anesth Analg* 72:275, 1991.

134. Reisner LS, Hochman BN, Plumer MH. Persistent neurologic deficit and adhesive arachnoiditis following intrathecal 2-chloroprocaine injection. *Anesth Analg* 59:452, 1980.

135. Reynolds F. Damage to conus medullaris following spinal anesthesia. *Anaesthesia* 56:235, 2001.

136. Holloway J, Seed PT, O'Sullivan G, et al. Paresthesia and nerve damage following combined spinal epidural and spinal anesthesia: A pilot survey. *Int J Obstet Anesth* 9:151, 2000.

137. Saifuddin A, Burnett SJD, White J. The variation of position of the conus medullaris in an adult population. *Spine* 23:1452, 1998.

138. Broadbent CR, Maxwell WB, Ferrie R, et al. Ability of anesthetists to identify a marked lumbar interspace. *Anaesthesia* 50:1106, 2000.

Neuraxial Anesthesia for Cardiac, Thoracic, and Vascular Surgery

CHAPTER 8

Hak Yui Wong

INTRODUCTION

The unique value of neuraxial anesthesia and the rationale for employing the various neuraxial anesthetic techniques (spinal, epidural, and combined spinal-epidural [CSE]) are predicated on two premises. First, neuraxial anesthesia makes it possible to avoid anesthetizing the brain and disabling most brain functions. It is assumed that by not "tampering with" the brain, potential central nervous system complications can be avoided. Preservation of the neural drive for spontaneous respiration and airway protective reflexes may obviate the need for respiratory interventions and accompanying morbidities. Second, complete sensory-motor nerve blockade (deafferentation) of the surgical site by neuraxial anesthesia not only provides superior analgesia, but may also mitigate or eliminate the systemic stress response. These two premises are better met when the site of surgery is located in more peripheral parts of the body (relative to the head and the thorax), hence the feasibility, widespread utility, and demonstrated benefits of neuraxial anesthesia for surgery on the limbs.

The case for neuraxial anesthesia becomes less clear the more central the site of the surgical procedure, as in cardiac, thoracic, and major vascular surgery. These surgical procedures, by virtue of their anatomic locations, are likely to encroach upon and compromise the respiratory system, often necessitating measures that counteract these adverse effects. In fact, some of these central procedures directly interrupt the workings of the lungs and ventilation, making control of patient's airway and mechanical ventilation mandatory. In this case, neuraxial anesthesia cannot eliminate the need for respiratory system intervention.

The positive impact of neuraxial anesthesia, in terms of deafferentation and reduction in systemic stress response, is less easy to demonstrate for patients who are undergoing cardiac, thoracic, or major vascular surgery, compared to patients undergoing more peripheral procedures. Complete deafferentation of the thoracic and abdominal wall and viscera is difficult to accomplish due to the complex innervation of these organs. Other triggering mechanisms of the stress response are also more likely with these invasive operations. For example, during cardiac surgery the process of cardiopulmonary bypass itself is a major provocateur of the systemic stress and inflammatory responses. Deafferentation by neuraxial anesthesia would therefore appear to have a much less pivotal role in stress response reduction, weakening the argument for its use in these types of surgical procedures.

The benefit(s) of neuraxial anesthesia also need(s) to be weighed against the risks in the context of these specific surgical procedures. Initiating neuraxial anesthesia carries an inherent risk of bleeding in tissues both external and internal to the spinal canal. The safety of neuraxial anesthesia for peripheral procedures, and the rarity with which spinal cord or nerve compression occurs after spinal or epidural technique, are contingent on a functioning coagulation system (see Chaps. 5 and 6). In the context of cardiac and vascular surgery, this assumption of safety may be invalidated by iatrogenic anticoagulation. Many of these procedures require initiation of an anticoagulated state (albeit temporary or low level), many of the patients presenting for these procedures are receiving preoperative anticoagulant or antiplatelet therapy, and many patients will require initiation or continuation of anticlotting therapy at the end of the procedure.

Questions remain as to the risk of initiating anticoagulation soon after subarachnoid puncture or epidural catheter insertion. Specific questions include: what is the minimum time interval between the performance of a neuraxial technique and anticoagulation; what is the difference in risk imposed by different size needles; and what is the appropriate action in the event of frank blood return via the needle or catheter (indicating direct trauma or cannulation of a blood vessel) during the performance of the neuraxial technique?

Various strategies have been devised to address these issues, but there are no data from controlled studies that can help define a zero-risk course of action. For example, many practitioners adhere to an interval of 1 h or more between a neuraxial procedure and initiating anticoagulation, under the assumption that bleeding induced by the spinal or epidural needle trauma will have stopped after 30 min, and heparin does not dissolve preexisitng clot. For patients who will require full heparin anticoagulation for cardiac surgery, placement of epidural catheter 24 h prior to the surgery has been advocated. Some practitioners advocate canceling the planned surgical procedure in the event frank blood is visualized in the epidural needle or catheter, and keeping the patient under surveillance for 24 h. Postoperative manipulation or discontinuation of epidural catheter is timed to coincide with the trough of anticoagulant level. To enable monitoring of the neurologic status at the end of the procedure, the concentration of local anesthetics, especially those administered for postoperative analgesia, is minimized to the lowest effective analgesic concentration.

A useful consensus statement on risk and the use of neuraxial anesthesia techniques in patients with compromised coagulation systems has been issued by the American Society of Regional Anesthesia and Pain Medicine.[1] However, the clinical decision to use neuraxial anesthesia is ultimately dependent on a risk-benefit analysis for individual patients and operations.

The goal of this chapter is to consider the utility of neuraxial anesthesia in cardiac, thoracic, and vascular surgery. Given that the use of neuraxial anesthesia has not been widespread in this arena, relatively little can be said about the standard of practice for these procedures. Instead, this chapter will discuss in broad terms the advantages and disadvantages of neuraxial techniques, as well as other issues that demand attention whenever neuraxial anesthesia is considered for cardiac, thoracic, and vascular surgery.

CARDIAC SURGERY

▶ Cardiac Surgery with Cardiopulmonary Bypass

Cardiac surgery performed with the aid of cardiopulmonary bypass presents several formidable challenges to the design and delivery of anesthetic care. The major surgical site is close to the head and full sternotomy is performed. Yet the origin of surgical pain can also be scattered across the body, and may involve the neck and the lower limbs (from harvest of saphenous veins), as well as the external thoracic cage and thoracic viscera. The pleural spaces may be breached and the resultant pneumothoraces will render intraoperative spontaneous ventilation and gas exchange difficult, if not impossible. Cardiopulmonary bypass creates a very artificial environment. Nonpulsatile blood flow, propelled by the heart-lung machine, courses through the body, often at a lower mean blood pressure than the patient's baseline. The effects of artificial perfusion and the induction of systemic hypothermia on (awake) cerebral function, consciousness, and respiratory control mechanisms are profound, but have not been systematically studied.

Given these considerations, and notwithstanding rare isolated case reports, neuraxial anesthesia has no role as the sole anesthetic for cardiac surgery with cardiopulmonary bypass. However, there may be advantages to including neuraxial anesthetic techniques as an adjuvant to general anesthesia for cardiac surgery. Purported benefits include sympatholysis of the heart, provision of postoperative analgesia, and reduction of the stress response and postoperative complications.[2,3]

Sympatholysis of the heart, as provided by high thoracic epidural anesthesia (TEA), may be beneficial in the context of myocardial ischemia. TEA, induced by bupivacaine, spanning the dermatomes of T1 to T6, has been shown to increase the diameter of stenotic segments of epicardial coronary arteries and relieve ischemia,[4] in addition to facilitating control of hemodynamics and maintaining myocardial oxygen supply/demand balance.[5]

Both continuous epidural infusion of an opioid/local anesthetic and single-shot intrathecal injection of long-acting opioids have been studied in terms of postcardiac surgery analgesic efficacy. To date, the data on the efficacy or advantages of epidural analgesia compared to intravenous analgesia are not conclusive.[5] The single bolus intrathecal administration of morphine prior to cardiac surgery has received the most attention. Intrathecal morphine 10 μg/kg can provide superior analgesia but at the expense of prolonged respiratory depression. Lower dosages such as 4 μg/kg may be effective but as a sole anesthetic agent does not appear to be advantageous over placebo or intravenous morphine.[6]

Reduction in postoperative cardiac, pulmonary, and renal complications has been shown with combined general anesthesia-TEA, although the evidence is not conclusive.[2,3,7] In a randomized study of coronary artery bypass surgery patients, TEA maintained with a continuous infusion of bupivacaine 0.125% and clonidine 0.0006% at 10 mL/h for 96 h was associated with a lower incidence of postoperative supraventricular dysrhythmias, respiratory infections, renal failure, and acute confusion (Table 8-1). In another study, TEA (as a supplement to general anesthesia and continued postoperatively) was associated with attenuation of the rise in heart rate and plasma epinephrine levels, release of troponin T, and a lower incidence of new ST-segment changes on the electrocardiogram (ECG).[3]

A major obstacle to the use of neuraxial anesthesia techniques as an adjuvant in cardiac surgery is extracorporeal

Table 8-1

Beneficial Effects of TEA and Analgesia in Addition to General Anesthesia for Postoperative Outcomes after Coronary Artery Bypass Graft Surgery

Complication	General Anesthesia* Combined with TEA (N = 206)	General Anesthesia* (N = 202)	Adjusted Odds Ratio (95% CI)
Supraventricular arrhythmias	21 (10.2%)	45 (22.3%)	2.56 (1.41–4.66)
Lower respiratory tract infection	31 (15.3%)	59 (29.2%)	2.06 (1.22–3.47)
Renal failure	4 (2%)	14 (6.9%)	
Acute confusion	3 (1.5%)	11 (5.5%)	
Significant bleeding	35 (17%)	23 (11%)	0.52 (0.28–0.96)
Any complications	84 (41%)	108 (53%)	1.44 (0.95–2.19)

*Values are number of patients (%).
Data from Ref. 2.

circulation or cardiopulmonary bypass, which mandates that the patient be profoundly anticoagulated, usually with high-dose heparin. This pharmacologically induced anticoagulated state may in turn be compounded by a complex picture of disordered hemostasis caused by cardiopulmonary bypass itself. The safety of performing neuraxial blockade in this context remains an unsettled question, even as the rarity of reported neurologic complication from spinal hematoma is acknowledged.[8] Using available data before 2000, Ho et al. estimated the 99% confidence interval (CI) of the risk of spinal-epidural hematoma in patients undergoing cardiac surgery to be 1:1000 to 1:150,000 after epidural anesthesia. After spinal anesthesia/analgesia the estimated risk was 1:2400 to 1:220,000.[8]

Various strategies to circumvent this ill-defined risk have been advocated, all of which are based on the assumption that the risk of intraspinal hematoma formation can be reduced by lengthening the time interval between the performance of the block (when trauma leading to bleeding occurs and clotting is triggered) and initiating pharmacologic anticoagulation. The reported time intervals range from 12 to 16 h (block performed in the evening prior to day of surgery) to 1 h. The short end of this range, 1 h, was deemed adequate in two large series of patients undergoing conventional coronary artery bypass surgery and valvular replacement surgery (total N > 1000).[9,10] Most of the other, smaller series have subscribed to a longer interval of up to 16 h, implying an extra day of inpatient care before the surgery.

The difficulty in defining and quantifying the risk of neuraxial blockade and neurologic complications should be compared with the relative safety and facility of modern general anesthesia and the availability of different, newer systemic sympatholytic and anticlotting therapies. Absent convincing data that show improved outcome when combining neuraxial and general anesthesia for cardiac surgery, compared to general anesthesia alone, the use of neuraxial anesthesia as adjunct to general anesthesia for cardiac surgery will remain a very select technique to be employed only after careful evaluation of individual risks and benefits, and for compelling reasons.

▶ Cardiac Surgery without Cardiopulmonary Bypass

Representative of the trend to reduce invasiveness of surgical procedures and the associated systemic response, surgical techniques, and instrumentation have evolved to allow coronary artery revascularization to be performed on the beating heart, without the use of cardiopulmonary bypass or aortic cross-clamping. The surgical approach for off-pump coronary artery bypass (OPCAB) surgery may be via full-length or partial median sternotomy, or via a small anterior thoracotomy if only the internal mammary artery is used as a conduit. Since cardiopulmonary bypass and systemic hypothermia are not used, physiologic trespass and anesthetic techniques of OPCAB surgery resembles more closely that of a thoracic procedure: the anterior mediastinum and the hemithoraces are breached, creating open-chest conditions that compromise the effectiveness of spontaneous ventilation, while at the same time lung inflation may obstruct the view of the operating site. Unique to OPCAB surgery is the intermittent and possibly extreme surgical "manhandling" of the heart itself that may cause sudden and profound fluctuation of hemodynamic status, and may necessitate rapid changes in patient position to compensate for the changes in venous return. In addition, the possibility always exists of converting to a conventional operation with cardiopulmonary bypass support. Systemic anticoagulation with heparin is required, although there is a trend to target a lower level of anticoagulation compared to that necessary for cardiopulmonary bypass. Because of all these factors, general anesthesia with endotracheal intubation and mechanical ventilation (with or without selective one-lung ventilation) is the preferred method of anesthesia for OPCAB surgery.

The perception, however, that OPCAB surgery is less invasive and provokes less systemic response does engender efforts to make the whole process of OPCAB surgery and recovery as minimally invasive as possible. Neuraxial anesthesia, specifically TEA may offer some advantages in this regard by reducing postoperative pain and the adverse effects of parenteral analgesic medications in the postoperative period. Theoretically, it can also obviate the perceived risk of general anesthesia and patient fear of various invasive interventions, such as the endotracheal tube. High TEA has been successfully employed as the sole anesthetic for OPCAB surgery in several small series.[11-14] In one series, the epidural catheter was inserted in the evening prior to the day of surgery. The intraoperative target level of sensory blockade, using 0.5% ropivacaine and sufentanil, was C7 to T9.[11] To date the problems of compromised ventilation during thoracotomy, risks posed by anticoagulation, and the necessary level of sedation have not been addressed or resolved. Pending definitive outcome data from controlled trials, the indication(s) for using neuraxial anesthesia in OPCAB surgery remains empiric.[6,15,16]

THORACIC SURGERY

The field of thoracic surgery encompasses many surgical procedures that present a wide variety of challenges to the perioperative care of these patients. For the purpose of planning the appropriate anesthetic strategy, thoracic surgical procedures may be classified into several working categories (Box 8-1).

Central to considering the role of neuraxial anesthesia is the organization of the nerve supply of the thorax and its content. Much to the inconvenience of design of neuraxial anesthesia, the thorax and the thoracic viscera receive innervation from diverse, noncontiguous origins. The upper airway is largely subserved by cranial nerves V, IX, and X. The thoracic cage is supplied by somatic nerves originating at the C4 level (supraclavicular nerves) and the thoracic spinal cord (intercostal nerves). The vagal and phrenic nerves constitute the main nerve supply of thoracic viscera and the diaphragm. Sympathetic nerve fibers from the thoracic spinal cord also innervate the thoracic viscera, including the heart (via the cardiac accelerator nerves).

Box 8-1
Categories of Thoracic Procedures
Upper airway, gastrointestinal endoscopy, and cervical mediastinoscopy
Tracheal and large intrathoracic airway
Supraclavicular region and extrapleural chest wall
Anterior mediastinum via a median sternotomy (e.g., thymoma resection)
Intrathoracic pulmonary (e.g., lung resections)
Posterior mediastinum (e.g., esophagus and descending thoracic aorta)
Minimally invasive procedures (e.g., video-assisted thoracoscopic surgery [VATS])

▶ Surgical Procedures Outside the Thoracic Cavity

Due to the complex and cranial origin of innervation of the large airways, as well as the tenuous state of the upper airway as a result of airway instrumentation, neuraxial anesthesia is neither optimal nor appropriate for endoscopies and surgical procedures in the large airways.

Cervical mediastinoscopy requires only a supramanubrial incision, which can be easily anesthetized with local anesthetic infiltration or a cervical epidural anesthetic. However, the procedure requires the patient to assume an uncomfortable posture, often entails extensive mechanical pressure on the trachea (which may provoke the cough reflex), as well as compression of the innominate artery anteriorly against the manubrium. Neuraxial anesthesia is therefore an inadequate form of anesthesia for this procedure.

For surgical procedures involving the supraclavicular region, extrapleural chest wall, or the anterior mediastinum (via either median sternotomy or anterior thoracotomy), neuraxial anesthesia is a feasible option.[17] Since the possible site of subarachnoid injection is limited anatomically to the lumbar region, a subarachnoid anesthetic for the thoracic region will necessitate extensive (and less than desirable) sensory-motor blockade, including blockade of the abdomen and lower extremities. TEA is the only appropriate neuraxial technique for the thoracic torso. An epidural catheter introduced through the midpoint of the thoracic spine is most likely to achieve segmental blockade of the thoracic dermatomes. For example, Groeben et al. described the use of TEA for mastectomies in patients with severe obstructive lung disease. They introduced epidural catheters at T2 to T4. The mean (± SD) volume of bupivacaine or ropivacaine

0.75% was 6.6 ± 0.5 mL. Sensory blockade extended from approximately C4 to T9.[17]

Several clinical issues will require special attention when TEA is used for surgical procedures on the supraclavicular area or the upper torso. Firstly, the proximity of the operative site to the patient's head and face may be psychologically unacceptable to the patient. This proximity may also compromise the patient's airway and ventilation. Secondly, a high, and sufficiently dense, thoracic epidural blockade may compromise the working of the diaphragm (due to blockade of the phrenic nerves), as well as the muscles that maintain airway patency and swallowing ability. Thirdly, extensive or complete blockade of thoracic sympathetic outflow, including the sympathetic nerves to the heart, may unmask dominant vagal tone and lead to profound bradycardia or heart conduction block, and hypotension. This is especially hazardous in the presence of a large anterior mediastinal mass, which may by itself pose a threat to cardiovascular homeostasis.

Surgical Procedures within the Thoracic Cavity

Surgical procedures within the thoracic cavity include operative procedures on the lungs, as well as procedures on structures in the posterior mediastinum; for example, esophageal procedures. Achieving optimal operating conditions for these procedures involves meeting a common set of prerequisites and compensating for the sequelae of the manipulated environment (Box 8-2). One of the hemithoraces is entered into surgically, creating an open pneumothorax and one of the two lungs is made quiescent and deflated. The quiescent/deflated lung becomes a significant right-to-left intrapulmonary shunt, which may result in severe hypoxemia. The contralateral (undeflated) lung must function optimally (for gas exchange): adequate expansion, adequate alveolar oxygen tension, and protection from secretions or contamination from the operative side. The patient is most often placed in a lateral decubitus position, and this along with the open thorax and unilateral lung deflation, contributes to changes in the dynamics of the mediastinal structures and potential for hemodynamic perturbations.

The creation of an open pneumothorax and the requirement for lung isolation during these procedures dictate the necessity of introducing specialized airway tubes and mechanical (positive pressure) ventilation of the nondeflated lung. Parenthetically, the development and availability of dependable, safe intubation techniques and mechanical ventilation arguably has played a "permissive" role in the development and advancement of modern thoracic surgical operations, in particular those on the lungs.

If neuraxial anesthesia cannot suffice as the sole anesthetic for intrathoracic procedures due to airway and ventilation considerations, it may yet, if administered along with general anesthesia, confer benefits of reduced stress response, enhanced postoperative analgesia, and improved postoperative respiratory function by virtue of its sympatholytic and deafferentation effects.[18] Segmental epidural blockade of the thoracic dermatomes (T1 to T10 level) affords sensory blockade of the thoracotomy incision, as well as chest tube insertion site. Neuraxial surgical anesthesia/analgesia may serve as a segue into postoperative analgesia, a crucial component of the perioperative care of these patients. In practice, however, complete deafferentation of body areas that are affected by thoracic operations may prove to be impossible to attain (see "Potential Disadvantages of Neuraxial Anesthesia as a Supplement," later). Furthermore, although certain beneficial effects on postoperative outcome are associated with the use of neuraxial anesthetic techniques, it is not known whether these beneficial effects are contingent on the neuraxial blockade being established during the intraoperative period, or if an equivalent effect can occur if the neuraxial blockade is administered only in the postoperative period. The answer to this question has significant implications because the concurrent administration of high TEA and general anesthesia is not without hazard (Box 8-3).

Box 8-2

Requirements and Challenges of Intrathoracic Surgery

Creation of unilateral open pneumothorax

Deflation and quiescence of one lung

Creation of right-to-left intrapulmonary shunt

Total dependence on contralateral lung function

Lateral decubitus patient position

Potential for mediastinal shift

Box 8-3

Potential Sequelae of Thoracic Denervation and Sympatholysis

Cardiac sympathectomy: bradycardia, AV conduction block, inadequate cardiac output

Peripheral and splanchnic vasodilation: hypotension

Possible bronchoconstriction

Possible inhibition of HPV

▶ Potential Disadvantages of Neuraxial Anesthesia as a Supplement

The initiation of TEA in order to achieve the desired deafferentation effect for intrathoracic procedures may bring about several potential complications. The source of innervation of the thoracic wall and viscera is diverse and widespread and includes the intercostal nerves, the thoracic sympathetic nerves (from T1 to T5 levels of spinal cord, via the cervical sympathetic ganglion), the phrenic nerves, and the vagal nerves. It is theoretically feasible, but clinically impractical, to provide neuraxial blockade that covers all these sources of innervation simultaneously: to block the vagal nerves would require blockade of the brainstem. Even epidural blockade limited only to the thoracic dermatomes is liable to cause complete sympathectomy, including cardiac sympathetic denervation. The ensuing vasodilation and bradycardia lead to hypotension, poor tolerance of mechanical interference with the heart, and inability to respond to acute changes in intravascular volume or body position. This symptom complex is especially troublesome to manage during intrathoracic operations when avoidance of hypervolemia is emphasized.

Thoracic sympathectomy has two other potential consequences: effect on bronchomotor tone and effect on oxygenation. The neural pathway that controls bronchomotor tone and airway resistance in humans is complex: adrenergic (sympathetic) nerve endings are sparsely located in the bronchial smooth muscles, and the vagal nerves appear to be predominant directly or indirectly via neurohumoral mechanisms. The effect of total thoracic sympathectomy on bronchial tone and airway resistance in humans has not been studied in detail. However, the possibility that airway resistance may change as a result of thoracic sympathectomy should be taken into consideration in patients whose chronic obstructive airway disease has an active bronchospastic component.

During intrathoracic procedures using one-lung ventilation, a right-to-left intrapulmonary shunt is intentionally created (in the form of the nonventilated lung). The ensuing arterial oxygen tension (PaO_2) is determined by a complex interaction involving cardiac output, mixed venous oxygen tension, the status of the ventilated lung, size of the shunt, and most significantly, hypoxic pulmonary vasoconstriction (HPV).

HPV diverts pulmonary blood flow away from the shunt by vasoconstriction in the nonventilated lung, and is the principal adaptive defense mechanism against arterial hypoxemia during one-lung ventilation. The cellular mechanism and regulation of HPV, and the possible role of the autonomic nervous system, are not completely understood. The effect of thoracic sympathectomy on HPV is even less well understood.[19,20] Since potent vasodilators such as nitroprusside antagonize HPV-induced vasoconstriction and lower the arterial oxygen tension, it is reasonable to assume that HPV will become less effective with thoracic sympathectomy. Clinical studies have produced conflicting conclusions, most probably because direct measurement of HPV is not possible in human studies, and the surrogate endpoint examined, PaO_2, is determined not only by HPV, but also by a host of interacting factors, some of which may be affected by the sympathectomy and cannot be held constant.[18,21,22] In summary, a full-fledged thoracic epidural anesthetic during one-lung ventilation may be neutral on arterial oxygenation, but the added thoracic sympathectomy may cause deterioration of oxygenation in patients who have borderline oxygen tension and who develop hypotension and low cardiac output from the sympatholysis.

▶ Minimally Invasive/Video-Assisted Thoracoscopic Surgery

Minimally invasive/video-assisted thoracoscopic surgical procedures are performed using long, thin instruments under the guidance of an image obtained via a miniature video camera (videoscope), all introduced through small incisions into the thoracic cavity. A pneumothorax must be created to provide room for visualization of anatomic structures and maneuvering of the instrument(s).

For procedures performed on superficial structures, a small pneumothorax, allowing the lung to fall just a small way away from the parietal pleura, may be sufficient. Examples are pleural biopsy, thoracentesis, pleurodesis, or drainage of empyema. Due to the small size of the pneumothorax and nonobtrusiveness of lung movement to the surgical procedure, neuraxial anesthesia, specifically TEA, has been used in this setting.[23-25] Potential pitfalls of using TEA for these procedures include the inability of the patient to tolerate the required positioning, patient coughing (due to preexisting disease or secondary to stimulation of the trachea and carina by the instruments), and discomfort when the diaphragm or hilum of the lung is stimulated (due to the cervical and cranial innervation of these structures).

The vast majority of modern thoracoscopic surgical procedures are now performed on structures hidden deeper in lung parenchyma or located posteriorly close to the spinal column. Examples of the former are wedge resection of lung lesions and complete lobectomy, and of the latter, thoracic sympathectomy. This form of thoracoscopic surgery requires a large pneumothorax and complete deflation of the lung, and the anesthetic consideration for this procedure is the same as that for open intrathoracic operations: general anesthesia with provision for one-lung ventilation. Since postoperative pain is often reported to be much less intense than after open thoracotomy, the indication for supplementary epidural anesthetic is less clear-cut. It may be selectively indicated for patients who are at high risk of developing respiratory failure from any new decrease in their reserve, and for patients who cannot tolerate oral and parenteral analgesics.

VASCULAR SURGERY

The overwhelming majority of vascular surgical procedures are performed for atherosclerosis-related vascular disorders. Therefore, more often than not, vascular surgery patients present with a complex litany of medical problems, including other atherosclerosis-related diseases, as well as the sequelae of diabetes mellitus, tobacco abuse, and chronic hypertension. Much progress has been made in the medical therapy of atherosclerotic disease, such as the advent of powerful antiplatelet and newer anticoagulant drugs. Percutaneous interventional procedures such as thrombolytic therapy, balloon angioplasty, and stent placement are being performed frequently. As a result, vascular surgery patients who present to the operating room today often represent the more complicated and difficult end of the spectrum and also have a high probability of having received some form of antiplatelet or anticoagulant therapy. Indeed, continual and rapid evolution of medical and interventional therapies as first-line treatments before surgical intervention will most likely alter the context in which neuraxial anesthesia is an option for vascular surgery in the near future.

In addition to the presence of presurgical anticoagulant and antiplatelet therapy, a low level of systemic anticoagulation is normally initiated during the course of vascular surgery, when temporary occlusion of blood vessel(s) is performed, or when a large catheter is inserted and left to dwell in a blood vessel. Depending on the immediate result of the surgical procedure and the condition of the blood vessel, the level of anticoagulation may have to be escalated or maintained well into the postoperative period. Antiplatelet drugs may also be added. An additional consideration is the hypercoagulability seen during and after vascular surgery procedures and the need to counter this with an anticoagulating modality.

The decision to use neuraxial anesthesia/analgesia in vascular surgery should be made after weighing the risk of neurologic complication from intraspinal bleeding and hematoma formation against the various benefits that can be expected from the neuraxial technique. This risk-benefit analysis will vary according to the type of vascular surgical procedures. For this purpose, vascular surgical procedures, which encompass a large group of operations that vary greatly in characteristics, degree of trauma to patients, and anesthetic requirements, can be classified into four working categories: infrainguinal vascular bypasses and other infrainguinal procedures, suprainguinal or abdominal procedures, endovascular procedures, and thoracic vascular procedures.

▶ Infrainguinal Vascular Bypasses and Other Infrainguinal Procedures

Infrainguinal vascular bypass procedures include various lower extremity revascularization operations, such as arterial bypasses using saphenous vein or synthetic graft, embolectomy, and thrombectomy. In addition to other significant atherosclerosis-related comorbidities, patients who undergo these procedures are very likely to suffer from chronic illnesses such as chronic renal insufficiency, diabetes mellitus, and other metabolic disturbances. Although there is less cardiac and pulmonary system surgical trespass compared to intra-abdominal vascular procedures, patients who undergo this group of operations are at high risk of developing postoperative cardiovascular, pulmonary, and renal complications. In addition, vascular surgery is associated with increased activation of clotting factors and decreased fibrinolysis, resulting in a hypercoagulable state in the postoperative period. Not surprisingly, it is for this group of patients that neuraxial anesthesia has held special interest.

The appeal of neuraxial anesthesia/analgesia for this high-risk group of patients and procedures lies in the avoidance of general anesthesia, reduction of stress response to surgery, and increased blood flow to the lower extremities, which may translate into improved outcomes such as reduction of postoperative cardiopulmonary morbidities and mortality, reduction of thromboembolic complications, and enhancement of graft patency rate. Multiple clinical studies, however, have yet to demonstrate definitive reduction of perioperative cardiovascular or pulmonary morbidity or mortality by the intraoperative use of neuraxial anesthesia (Table 8-2).[26,27] Two prospective studies suggest that neuraxial anesthesia extended into the postoperative period may be associated with a lower rate of graft occlusion and need for reoperation,[27,28] but there is also evidence to the contrary.[26] It is not known if these results can be emulated by more aggressive and detailed postsurgical management of the coagulation system using the large variety of new drugs that has become available in the last decade.

The choice of neuraxial anesthesia techniques is limited by the fact that many of these procedures are technically tedious and of long duration, making single-shot subarachnoid anesthesia an impractical choice, even with long-acting local anesthetic agents. Addition of epinephrine to the local anesthetic should be avoided in this group of patients, due to concern about the additional vasoconstrictive effect of epinephrine on the sometimes already tenuous blood supply to the spinal cord. A CSE or simple lumbar epidural technique is a more dependable option, although the use of epidural catheters may theoretically incur a higher risk for intraspinal hematoma. A commonly used CSE technique involves administering intrathecal hyperbaric bupivacaine 7.5–9 mg, followed by an infusion of 0.5% bupivacaine

Table 8-2

Prospective, Randomized Trials of Anesthesia and Lower Extremity Vascular Bypass

Study	Technique	N	Anesthetic	Mortality	Nonfatal MI	Morbidity Unstable angina	Infection	Renal failure	Reoperation
Christopherson et al. (1992)[27]	GA	51	Thiamylal, fentanyl, enflurane, N$_2$O, PCA	3/51	2/51	2/51	2/51	3/51	36%
	Regional	49	Epidural: bupivacaine	4/49	2/49	0/49	1/49	3/49	12%
Bode et al. (1996)[26]	GA	112	Thiopental, fentanyl, isoflurane, or enflurane N$_2$O	3/112	4/112	7/112			n.d.
	Regional	96	Epidural: lidocaine + bupivacaine	3/96	6/96	10/96			n.d.
		107	Spinal: tetracaine	0/107	4/107	7/107			n.d.

Abbreviations: n.d. = no difference between the GA and regional groups in reoperation rates, PCA = patient-controlled analgesia, MI = myocardial infarction.

(4–6 mL/h) via the epidural catheter (Box 8-4). The duration of bupivacaine infusion should be timed to allow motor blockade to dissipate in time for postprocedure

Box 8-4

CSE Technique for Intrainguinal Vascular Procedures

Intrathecal hyperbaric bupivacaine 7.5–9 mg

Continuous intraoperative epidural infusion: 0.5% bupivacaine 4–6 mL/h

Discontinue infusion approximately 1 h before the end of surgical procedure

Perform postoperative neurologic examination at the end of surgical procedure

Initiate postoperative epidural analgesia: 0.25% bupivacaine infusion

Consider anticoagulation status before discontinuing epidural catheter

evaluation of motor function. In general, the infusion should be stopped 1 h prior to the anticipated end of surgery. After the patient has demonstrated return of muscle function, infusion of a lower concentration of bupivacaine can be reinstituted to provide postoperative analgesia. The duration of postoperative epidural analgesia will depend on the timing of patient ambulation, time to patient's tolerance of oral analgesics, and initiation of oral antiplatelet drug and anticoagulant. Removal of the epidural catheter will need to be timed to occur when heparin effect is at its trough, and before oral anticoagulation (from Warfarin) has taken hold (see Chap. 7)

Perioperative monitoring should be instituted based on the usual and customary criteria and clinical findings of the patient. Neuraxial anesthesia does not preclude or obviate indicated invasive monitors such as intra-arterial blood pressure and central venous pressure monitoring. One disadvantage associated with neuraxial anesthesia is that transesophageal echocardiography, which may be very useful for patients with certain cardiopulmonary conditions, is not feasible. Perhaps transthoracic echocardiography may find increasing use by the anesthesiologist in this situation.

Another clinical problem with use of neuraxial anesthesia is the difficulty in maintaining patient immobility and physical comfort for prolonged periods, particularly in patients who have positional dyspnea, arthritis, or psychologic problems associated with chronic illness. Supplemental sedation or even "light" general anesthesia may be required, and in the case of the latter, may negate some of the theoretical benefits of avoiding a general anesthetic. Finally, the sympathectomy and peripheral vasodilation resulting from neuraxial anesthesia may make maintenance of normothermia more difficult in these patients who are prone to intraoperative hypothermia due to the large area of body surface exposed to room air.

Suprainguinal Abdominal Vascular Procedures

Suprainguinal vascular procedures include operations on the abdominal aorta and its larger branches, such as aortofemoral bypass, renal artery bypass, mesenteric artery bypass, and repair of abdominal aortic aneurysms. Surgery that involves the abdominal aorta necessitates trespass into the peritoneal cavity. Surgical retractors and abdominal packing under the diaphragm are liable to compromise the compliance of the thoracic cavity. Although the abdominal aorta is usually approached transperitoneally via a midline incision, under certain situations it can be approached retroperitoneally via a left thoracolumbar incision, in which case the patient will be in a physically stressful right lateral decubitus position with the torso flexed acutely toward the right (in the direction toward the floor). Obligatory temporary occlusion of the aorta is associated with major hemodynamic disturbances, such as marked and acute increases and decreases of blood pressure, myocardial ischemia, or frank heart failure. These changes, as well as the often vigorous resuscitative measures needed to counter sudden massive blood loss, may be associated with untoward symptoms in the awake patient. Application of the cross-clamp to the aorta, especially when applied cephalad to the renal arteries, carries a finite risk of spinal cord ischemia. Hence, the anesthesia plan must take into account the need for prompt neurologic evaluation of the lower extremities at conclusion of the surgical procedure.

Because of the aforementioned issues and concerns, neuraxial anesthesia is neither practical nor desirable as the sole anesthetic technique for the patient undergoing surgery involving the abdominal aorta. At least some elements of general anesthesia and positive pressure ventilation are needed to maintain respiratory homeostasis and patient comfort. Advocates of neuraxial anesthesia would maintain that some benefits may accrue from neuraxial anesthesia even if combination with general anesthesia is necessary.

Deafferentation or "sensory blockade" of the entire anatomic region involved in the surgery, in this instance the entire abdomen and the diaphragm, may blunt the acute neuroendocrine stress response and stress to the cardiovascular system. Empirically, superior pain control afforded by continuation of neuraxial anesthesia into the early postoperative period is not only humane, but also appears to facilitate early extubation of the trachea, improve postoperative respiratory mechanics, facilitate functional recovery, permit early ambulation, and decrease the incidence of thromboembolism. It is not known, however, if these salutary effects of neuraxial anesthesia result from intraoperative neuraxial blockade, extension of the blockade into the postoperative period, or both. It also appears that benefit on cardiovascular stress response and mortality is only obtained when the blockade is extensive enough to provide sympathetic denervation of the heart (T1 to T4 spinal segments).[29] To date, the question of whether neuraxial anesthesia independently improves outcome after abdominal vascular surgery has not been definitively answered.

Using neuraxial anesthesia as a supplement to general anesthesia for abdominal aortic surgery raises several practical issues. To achieve the desired denervation of the surgical site, sensory blockade of the extensive abdominal incision (T6 to T12 dermatomes) and the viscera (T4 to T12) is needed. Single-shot subarachnoid anesthetic has limited duration of action, and the larger dose necessary to achieve extensive sensory blockade will likely cause high levels of sympathetic blockade, resulting in extreme hypotension and bradycardia. TEA is a more logical route to provide blockade of thoracic dermatomes, but can be technically challenging to accomplish in the older patient population with a higher incidence of spinal deformity and ossification.

A common method of establishing epidural anesthesia as a supplement to general anesthesia consists of the following: inserting an epidural catheter in the upper midthoracic level (and administering the appropriate test dose) before induction of general anesthesia, injecting an induction dose of about 5 mL of 0.5% bupivacaine on stabilization of the vital signs after general anesthesia induction, and beginning a continuous infusion of 0.5% bupivacaine at 5 mL/h. With attainment of a high thoracic epidural blockade, extensive sympathectomy is unavoidable and this may complicate the management of hemodynamic and blood volume perturbations that accompany aortic cross-clamping and unclamping. The choice of local anesthetic and timing of infusion should take into consideration that prompt return of sensory and motor functions in the lower extremities at the end of the procedure is desirable. The risks of intraspinal hematoma posed by low level of perioperative anticoagulation or an incompetent coagulation system are similar to those faced by patients undergoing an infrainguinal vascular procedure, with the exception that the consequences of a thoracic epidural hematoma would be more devastating than those from a lumbar epidural hematoma.

Endovascular Procedures

Endovascular procedures include intraluminal balloon dilation of segmental arterial stenosis or occlusion, followed by placement of stents to prevent redevelopment of occlusion. Placement of intraluminal tubular grafts to exclude blood flow from the wall of aneurysms makes up the remainder of this category. As innovation and development of devices and technology continue, and as physicians continue to refine their techniques, the range of blood vessels and pathologies amenable to this form of treatment is expanding. Although the long-term outcome of these procedures as compared with surgical treatment is still being studied, this treatment modality is rapidly gaining popularity due to the perception of minimal trespass on the body and associated rapid recovery. It is particularly attractive for medically compromised or elderly patients who are at high risk for developing life-threatening complications in the postoperative period.

With rare exceptions, entry into the intravascular compartment is by surgical cut-down or percutaneous puncture of one or both of the femoral arteries. Noxious surgical stimuli arise from insertion of large (12–16 French) catheters into the femoral arteries, the manual pressure applied to the groin to stabilize these catheters, and prolonged localized pressure applied to the arterial puncture sites after removal of these catheters. Otherwise, besides the feeling of warmth or flushing as contrast agents are injected during angiography, the procedure is usually pain free. Low-level systemic anticoagulation using heparin is usually required.

Potential immediate risks include localized dissection of the femoral or iliac arteries that may require open surgical repair, blood loss from the arterial puncture or via the access catheters, fluid overload (from flushing of the catheters), and hypothermia. A fairly long period of immobility in the supine position on the operating/angiographic table is required of the patient, and this may be difficult for elderly patients, or those with musculoskeletal or other medical conditions that make maintaining this posture difficult. Therefore, although local anesthesia and intravenous sedation is technically sufficient from a procedure standpoint, general anesthesia or regional anesthesia is often necessary for safe patient management. A single-shot subarachnoid anesthetic aiming for a T10 sensory level is eminently suitable for this purpose. The single-shot technique, as opposed to an epidural catheter, minimizes the risk of spinal blood vessel trauma and hematoma formation. A sensory blockade up to the T10 level will cover the entire region subjected to painful stimuli without causing significant hypotension, anesthetize the lower extremities to reduce position-induced

discomfort, and enable the patient to be minimally sedated for monitoring of cerebral function, which is an important consideration for procedures involving the carotid or vertebral arteries. This level of subarachnoid anesthesia can easily be obtained by a single intrathecal injection of hyperbaric bupivacaine 9–12 mg combined with fentanyl 15–20 μg.

Thoracic Vascular Procedures

Procedures of the descending thoracic aorta represents some of the most stressful and challenging surgical operations. The list of acute challenges posed by these surgical procedures includes thoracotomy with its myriad implications on ventilation and gas exchange, patient positioning, dramatic hemodynamic changes induced by high aortic cross-clamping and unclamping, potential for massive blood loss, hypoperfusion of the spinal cord and paralysis, complex coagulopathy, and hypothermia. Some surgical teams use aortoaortic bypass or left atrial-aortic bypass to mitigate hemodynamic perturbations, in which case moderate-dose heparin anticoagulation is necessary. Because of these issues, neuraxial anesthesia has a very limited role, and there are no data pertaining to its use either as supplement to general anesthesia or as postoperative analgesia on outcome.

REFERENCES

1. Horlocker TT, Wedel DJ, Benzon H, et al. Regional anesthesia in the anticoagulated patient: Defining the risks (the second ASRA Consensus Conference on Neuraxial Anesthesia and Anticoagulation). *Reg Anesth Pain Med* 28(3):172, 2003.
2. Scott N, Turfrey D, Ray D, et al. A prospective randomized study of the potential benefits of thoracic epidural anesthesia and analgesia in patients undergoing CABG. *Anesth Analg.* 93:528, 2001.
3. Loick HM, Schmidt C, van Aken H, et al. High thoracic epidural anesthesia, but not clonidine, attenuates the perioperative stress response via sympatholysis and reduces the release of troponin T in patients undergoing coronary artery bypass grafting. *Anesth Analg* 88:701, 1999.
4. Blomberg SG, Emanuelson H, Kvist H, et al. Effects of thoracic epidural anesthesia on coronary arteries and arterioles in patients with coronary artery disease. *Anesthesiology* 73:840, 1990.
5. Blomberg SG, Emanuelson H, Ricksten SE. Thoracic epidural anesthesia and central hemodynamics in patients with unstable angina pectoris. *Anesth Analg* 69:558, 1989.
6. Cheng DCH. Regional analgesia and ultra-fast-track cardiac anesthesia. *Can J Anesth* 52:12, 2005.
7. Fillinger MP, Yeager MP, Dodds TM. Epidural anesthesia and analgesia: Effects on recovery from cardiac surgery. *J Cardiothorac Vasc Anesth* 16:15, 2000.
8. Ho AM, Chung DC, Joynt GM. Neuraxial blockade and hematoma in cardiac surgery: Estimating the risk of a rare adverse event that has not (yet) occurred. *Chest* 117:551, 2000.
9. Pastor MC, Sánchez MJ, Casas MA, et al. Thoracic epidural analgesia in coronary artery bypass graft surgery: Seven years' experience. *J Cardiothorac Vasc Anesth* 17:154, 2003.

10. Pastor MC, Casas MA, Sánchez MJ, et al. Thoracic epidurals in heart valve surgery: Neurologic risk evaluation. *J Cardiothorac Vasc Anesth* 16:723, 2002.

11. Aybek T, Kessler P, Khan MF, et al. Operative techniques in awake coronary artery bypass grafting. *J Thorac Cardiovasc Surg* 125:1394, 2003.

12. Karagoz HY, Kurtoglu M, Bakkaloglu B, et al. Coronary artery bypass grafting in the awake patient: Three years' experience in 137 cases. *J Thorac Cardiovasc Surg* 125:1401, 2003.

13. Chakravarthy M, Jawali V, Patil TA, et al. High thoracic epidural anesthesia as the sole anesthetic for performing multiple grafts in off-pump coronary artery bypass surgery. *J Cardiothorac Vasc Anesth* 17:160, 2003.

14. Chakravarthy M, Jawali V, Patil TA, et al. High thoracic epidural anesthesia as the sole anesthetic for redo off-pump coronary artery bypass surgery. *J Cardiothorac Vasc Anesth* 17:84, 2003.

15. Mangano CM. Risky business. *J Thorac Cardiovasc Surg* 125:1204, 2003.

16. Gravelee GP. Epidural analgesia and coronary artery bypass grafting: The controversy continues. *J Cardiothorac Vasc Anesth* 17:151, 2003.

17. Groeben H, Schafer B, Pavlakovic G, et al. Lung function under high thoracic segmental epidural anesthesia with ropivacaine or bupivacaine in patients with severe obstructive pulmonary disease undergoing breast surgery. *Anesthesiology* 96:536, 2002.

18. Von Dossow V, Welte M, Zaune U, et al. Thoracic epidural anesthesia combined with general anesthesia: The preferred anesthetic technique for thoracic surgery. *Anesth Analg* 92:848, 2001.

19. Ishibe Y, Shiokawa Y, Umeda T, et al. The effect of thoracic epidural anesthesia on hypoxic pulmonary vasoconstriction in dogs: An analysis of the pressure-flow curve. *Anesth Analg* 82:1049, 1996.

20. Brimioulle S, Vachiéry JL, Brichant JF, et al. Sympathetic modulation of hypoxic pulmonary vasoconstriction in intact dogs. *Cardiovasc Res* 34:384, 1997.

21. Garutti I, Quintana B, Olmedilla L, et al. Arterial oxygenation during one-lung ventilation: Combined versus general anesthesia. *Anesth Analg* 88:494, 1999.

22. Chow MY, Goh MH, Boey SK, et al. The effects of remifentanil and thoracic epidural on oxygenation and pulmonary shunt fraction during one-lung ventilation. *J Cardiothorac Vasc Anesth* 17:69, 2003.

23. Kempen PM. Complete analgesia during pleurodesis under thoracic epidural anesthesia. *Am Surg* 64:755, 1998.

24. Mukaida T, Andou A, Date H, et al. Thoracoscopic operation for secondary pneumothorax under local and epidural anesthesia in high-risk patients. *Ann Thorac Surg* 65:924, 1998.

25. Plummer S, Hartley M, Vaughan RS. Anaesthesia for telescopic procedures in the thorax. *Br J Anaesth* 80:223, 1998.

26. Bode RH, Lewis KP, Zarich SW, et al. Cardiac outcome after peripheral vascular surgery. Comparision of general and regional anesthesia. *Anesthesiology* 84:3, 1996.

27. Christopherson R, Beattie C, Frank SM. Perioperative morbidity in patients randomized to epidural or general anesthesia for lower extremity vascular surgery. *Anesthesiology* 79:422, 1993.

28. Tuman KJ, McCarthy RJ, March RJ, et al. Effects of epidural anesthesia and analgesia on coagulation and outcome after major vascular surgery. *Anesth Analg* 73:696, 1991.

29. Rodgers A, Walder N, Schug S, et al. Reduction of postoperative mortality and morbidity with epidural or spinal anaesthesia: Results from overview of randomized trials. *BMJ* 321:1493, 2000.

Neuraxial Anesthesia for General Surgery

CHAPTER 9

Nathaniel Diaz
Cynthia A. Wong

INTRODUCTION

Neuraxial anesthesia may be used as the primary anesthetic for outpatient general surgical procedures, such as inguinal hernia repair or anal surgery. Neuraxial ambulatory anesthesia is discussed in detail in Chap. 11. Cervical or thoracic epidural anesthesia (TEA) is appropriate for breast or chest wall procedures. Neuraxial anesthesia is also appropriate for lower abdominal procedures, including low anterior resection of the colon and sigmoid colectomy. More often neuraxial anesthesia is used as an adjunct to general anesthesia and for postoperative analgesia in patients undergoing major general surgical procedures, including upper and lower abdominal procedures. Neuraxial anesthesia/analgesia for breast and gastrointestinal procedures is the focus of this chapter. Epidural anesthesia as an adjunct to esophageal procedures requiring a thoracotomy is discussed in Chap. 8. Laparoscopic procedures usually require pneumoperitoneum and this may be an obstacle to using neuraxial anesthesia. Spinal or epidural anesthesia may be appropriate for some laparoscopic procedures, however, and this is discussed in Chap. 12. Finally, a limited number of studies have described the use of neuraxial anesthesia/analgesia for renal transplant surgery, donor hepatectomy, and major liver surgery. These indications require further study.

Denervation of the abdomen and its viscera requires blockade of spinal nerve roots from T1 through S4. The anatomic details are discussed in Chap. 1. This degree of blockade is accompanied by significant physiologic effects and these are discussed in Chap. 4. In contrast to the limbs, abdominal viscera and peritoneum are multiply innervated by segmental and heterosegmental (the phrenic and vagus nerves) nerves.[1] Briefly, parasympathetic innervation of abdominal viscera is via cranial (vagus nerve) and sacral (inferior hypogastric plexus and pelvic splanchnic nerves) components of the parasympathetic nervous system

(Fig. 1-19). The vagus nerve innervates the parts of the digestive system supplied by the celiac and superior mesenteric arteries (including the proximal gut up to the descending colon). Sacral parasympathetic efferents innervate the pelvic viscera, including the descending and sigmoid colon and the rectum. Because TEA blocks sympathetic, but not parasympathetic outflow, it is associated with increased gastrointestinal motility. Mid- to low-thoracic sympathetic blockade is associated with a dilation of splanchnic vascular beds and a marked decrease in preload to the right heart.

Surgical procedures of pelvic organs usually require blockade from T6 to S4. Surgical procedures of the upper abdomen require blockade to T1.

BREAST SURGERY

Thoracic epidural anesthesia and analgesia have been described for modified radical mastectomies,[2] breast augmentation,[3] and mastectomy with immediate transverse rectus abdominis musculocutaneous (TRAM) flap reconstruction.[4] Several studies randomizing patients to TEA or general anesthesia/systemic opioid analgesia have demonstrated that postoperative analgesia is superior, the incidence of nausea and vomiting is lower, patient satisfaction is higher, and hospital stays are shorter in the TEA compared to general anesthesia groups (Fig. 9-1).[2,4,5] Epidural anesthesia for breast procedures is usually initiated at the T3-T4 interspace (Table 9-1). A midline approach is possible at this level (see Chap. 2). The extent of sensory blockade depends on the specific procedure. Procedures limited to breast tissue (e.g., augmentation) require blockade from T1 to T7. Procedures which include the anterior chest wall (e.g., modified radical mastectomy) require blockade of the lateral and medical pectoral nerves (up to C5). Finally, mastectomies with TRAM flap reconstruction require more extensive

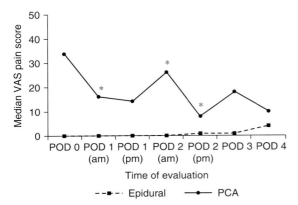

FIGURE 9-1. Pain scores (visual analog scale; VAS) in women randomized to thoracic epidural catheter (T8 to T10) or PCA (intravenous morphine) for postoperative analgesia (unilateral mastectomy with immediate TRAM flap reconstruction). POD = postoperative day, PCA = patient-controlled (intravenous) analgesia. *$P < 0.05$ PCA vs. epidural analgesia. *Used with permission from Correll DJ. Epidural analgesia compared with intravenous morphine patient-controlled analgesia: Postoperative outcome measures after mastectomy with immediate TRAM flap breast reconstruction. Reg Anesth Pain Med 26:444, 2001.*

abdominal wall blockade (C5 to L1). For these procedures the catheter is usually sited between T8 and T10.

Serious complications have not been reported in any study. Transient shivering, nasal congestion, and Horner syndrome have been observed. Some patients complained of subjective shortness of breath. The phrenic nerve, however, was not blocked and minute volume was unchanged.[3] Hypotension occurs in less than 10% of patients.[4]

Breast surgery patients randomized to preemptive epidural morphine analgesia had lower pain scores and required a significantly lower dose of morphine for postoperative analgesia compared to patients who received epidural saline.[1] In contrast, a preemptive effect of preoperative epidural morphine was not observed in patients who underwent gastrectomy or hysterectomy. The authors hypothesized that preemptive analgesia was effective for breast and limb, but not for intra-abdominal surgery because vagal input to abdominal viscera is not blocked by thoracic analgesia.

INTRA-ABDOMINAL PROCEDURES

Some general surgical procedures may be appropriate for central neuraxial blockade as the primary anesthetic, including inguinal hernia repair, appendectomy, low anterior resection of the colon, and sigmoid colectomy. Combined neuraxial/general anesthesia may be appropriate for other intra-abdominal procedures, including radical gastrectomy, vertical banded gastroplasty, upper abdominal surgery, esophageal surgery, and hepatic surgery.

▶ Outcomes

Benefits of neuraxial *anesthesia* include decreased physiologic stress response, decreased exposure to volatile inhaled agents, decreased muscle relaxant use, and decreased intraoperative opioid requirements. There is currently no evidence, however, to suggest that *anesthetic* technique influences overall outcome.[6] Benefits of epidural *analgesia* compared to systemic opioid analgesia include decreased duration of postoperative ileus, decreased incidence of postoperative nausea and vomiting and pulmonary complications, improved postoperative pain control, and improved short-term quality of life.[6,7] In particular, an intensive multimodal rehabilitation program that includes early feeding, epidural analgesia, and early ambulation has been shown to shorten hospital stays after gastrointestinal surgery.[8,9] Outcomes after neuraxial compared to systemic postoperative analgesia for mixed surgical procedures are discussed in detail in Chap. 16.

Duration of Ileus

Mechanisms of postoperative ileus include handling of the bowel, electrolyte imbalance, and opioid administration. In addition, abdominal pain and the stress response to surgery induce sympathetic activity which further inhibits bowel activity. Immobility secondary to pain and lack of enteral feedings also contribute to postoperative ileus. Epidural analgesia with local anesthetics may promote bowel activity by directly blocking thoracolumbar sympathetic outflow, by

Table 9-1

Epidural Anesthesia for Breast Surgery

	Procedures Limited to Breast Tissue	Procedures of Breast Tissue and Chest Wall	Procedures Including TRAM Flap Reconstruction
Extent of blockade	T1 to T7	C5 to T7	C5 to L1
Catheter insertion site	T3 to T4	T3 to T4	T8 to T10
Local anesthetic volume	8–15 mL	12–15 mL	20 mL

Review: Epidural local anaesthetics versus opioid-based analgesic regimens for postoperative gastrointestinal paralysis, PONV and pain after abdominal surgery
Comparison: 01 Epidural local anaesthetic (LA) vs opioid based regimens
Outcome: 03 Effect on time (h) to return of gastrointestinal function (flatus or stool)-subgroups

Study	Epidural LAN	Mean (SD)	Opioid based analg N	Mean (SD)	Weighted mean difference (Random) 95% CI	Weight (%)	Weighted mean difference (Random) 95% CI
01 Epi LA vs systemic opioid							
Ahn 1988	16	48.00 (10.00)	14	128.00 (21.00)		14.5	−80.00 [−92.04, −67.96]
Bredtmann 1990	57	71.00 (36.00)	59	96.00 (29.00)		14.5	−25.00 [−36.92, −13.08]
Liu 1995	14	40.00 (7.50)	12	81.00 (10.00)		15.1	−41.00 [−47.89, −34.11]
Riwar 1992	25	18.00 (12.00)	25	81.00 (18.00)		14.9	−63.00 [−71.48, −54.52]
Scheinin 1987	15	66.00 (28.00)	15	91.00 (35.00)		12.5	−25.00 [−47.68, −2.32]
Wallin 1988	12	43.00 (20.00)	15	39.00 (18.00)		14.1	4.00 [−10.53, 18.53]
Wattwill 1989	20	31.00 (22.00)	20	58.00 (14.00)		14.5	−27.00 [−38.43, −15.57]
Subtotal (95% CI)	159		160			100.0	−37.24 [−55.67, −18.82]

Test for heterogeneity chi-square = 116.86 df = 6 p < 0.00001
Test for overall effect = −3.96 p = 0.0001

02 Epi LA vs epi opioid							
Asantila 1991	20	46.00 (12.00)	20	55.00 (7.00)		29.1	−9.00 [−15.09, −2.91]
Liu 1995	14	40.00 (7.50)	14	71.00 (15.00)		27.5	−31.00 [−39.78, −22.22]
Scheinin 1987	15	66.00 (28.00)	30	93.00 (28.00)		21.2	−27.00 [−44.35, −9.65]
Thorén 1989	11	22.00 (16.00)	11	56.00 (22.00)		22.2	−34.00 [−50.08, −17.92]
Subtotal (95% CI)	60		75			100.0	−24.42 [−38.81, −10.03]

Test for heterogeneity chi-square = 21.62 df = 3 p = 0.0001
Test for overall effect = −3.33 p = 0.0009

03 Epi LA vs epi LA/opioid							
Asantila 1991	20	46.00 (12.00)	20	62.00 (19.00)		48.6	−16.00 [−25.85, −6.15]
Liu 1995	14	40.00 (7.50)	12	43.00 (14.00)		51.4	−3.00 [−11.84, 5.84]
Subtotal (95% CI)	34		32			100.0	−9.31 [−22.05, 3.42]

Test for heterogeneity chi-square = 3.71 df = 1 p = 0.0542
Test for overall effect = −1.43 p = 0.15

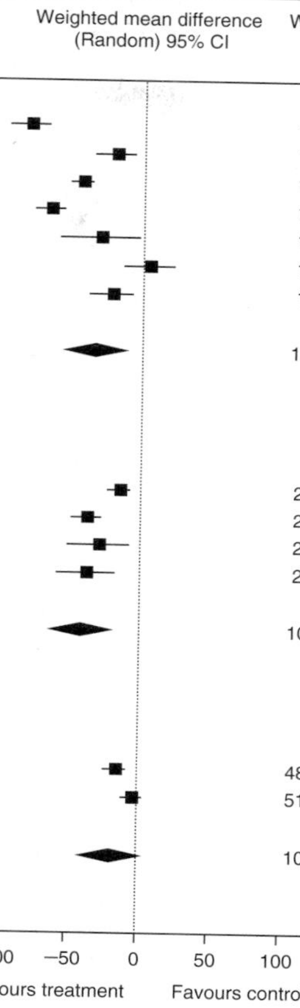

```
          −100    −50     0      50    100
            Favours treatment   Favours control
```

FIGURE 9-2. Meta-analysis of studies comparing epidural local anesthetic to systemic opioid analgesia, epidural local anesthetic to epidural opioid analgesia, and epidural local anesthetic analgesia with and without epidural opioids for duration of postoperative ileus as assessed by first flatus or stool. Epidural local anesthetic analgesia shortened duration to flatus by 24–48 h compared to both systemic and epidural opioid analgesia. The two studies comparing epidural local anesthetic analgesia with and without opioid have conflicting results. *Used with permission from Jorgensen H, Wetterslev J, Moiniche S, et al. Epidural local anaesthetics versus opioid-based analgesic regimens on postoperative gastrointestinal paralysis, PONV and pain after abdominal surgery.* Cochrane Database Syst Rev *CD001893, 2000.*

blocking nociceptive afferent nerves that contribute to sympathetic nervous system activation, and indirectly by controlling pain and allowing for earlier ambulation.[6,7] A meta-analysis of studies comparing local anesthetic epidural analgesia with systemic or epidural opioid analgesia in patients undergoing mixed abdominal procedures found that epidural analgesia with local anesthetics shortens the duration of postoperative ileus by 24–48 h (Fig. 9-2).[10] Thoracic epidural blockade is more effective than lumbar blockade in reducing the duration of ileus.[11,12] Two studies comparing epidural local anesthetic analgesia with and without opioid have conflicting results.[10] Duration of analgesia was shorter in one study, but not in the other, although

the addition of opioid improved analgesia. In a retrospective study of proctocolectomy patients, thoracic analgesia, but not lumbar analgesia, was associated with a shorter duration of ileus compared to intravenous opioid analgesia.[12]

Anastomotic Leakage

Theoretically, epidural anesthesia/analgesia with local anesthetics may alter the risk of anastomotic breakdown. Epidural anesthesia/analgesia might improve splanchnic blood flow, and thereby aid healing and reduce leakage. Alternatively, epidural anesthesia/analgesia might increase the risk of anastomotic breakdown because of sympathetic blockade and parasympathetic dominance, resulting in gut hypermotility. A meta-analysis of randomized-controlled trials in colorectal procedures found no evidence of increased anastomotic leakage in patients who received epidural anesthesia/analgesia with local anesthetics.[13] The authors concluded, however, that a larger trial is needed to adequately address this question.

Postoperative Analgesia

Without question, epidural compared to systemic opioid analgesia results in superior postoperative analgesia. In a meta-analysis of 29 trials in abdominal surgery patients, epidural analgesia, regardless of agents (local anesthetic with and without opioid or opioid only) and epidural catheter site (thoracic or lumbar), resulted in lower visual analog scores compared to parenteral opioid analgesia (Fig. 9-2).[14] Other meta-analyses of trials comparing epidural to patient-controlled (intravenous) analgesia (PCA) reached the same conclusion.[15,16] Patients undergoing colonic surgery under general anesthesia were randomized to epidural bupivacaine/morphine analgesia initiated 40 min before skin incision or at wound closure.[17] There were no differences in postoperative pain scores or supplemental morphine consumption between groups, suggesting timing of initiation of epidural analgesia does not play a role in its efficacy.

Epidural opioids work synergistically with local anesthetics (see Chap. 3). A systematic review of mixed surgical procedure studies supports the notion that epidural analgesia with a local anesthetic combined with opioid provides better analgesia than either type of medication administered alone.[18] The addition of opioid to local anesthetics allows for a lower dose of local anesthetic, thus minimizing the incidence of hypotension and motor blockade. The addition of local anesthetic to opioid, however, did not decrease the incidence of opioid-related side effects (e.g., pruritus, nausea, vomiting, and sedation).

Postoperative Pulmonary Complications

Pulmonary complications of abdominal surgery include hypoxemia, infection, and prolonged mechanical ventilation. The incidence of pulmonary complications depends on the extent and type of surgery (e.g., laparotomy vs. laparoscopy and upper vs. lower abdominal surgery), preexisting pulmonary disease, body habitus, and patient age.[7] The mechanisms of postoperative pulmonary complications are multifactorial and include pain, immobility, and dysfunction of the diaphragm, intercostal, and abdominal muscles. Functional residual capacity (FRC), vital capacity (VC), forced expiratory volume in 1 s (FEV1), peak expiratory flow rate, and oxygen saturation are all decreased after abdominal surgery.[7] Epidural analgesia may improve postoperative lung function by improving pain control. This allows the patient to breath deeply, cough, and ambulate. In addition, epidural analgesia that includes cervical dermatomes may block reflex inhibition of the phrenic nerve and prevent diaphragmatic dysfunction.

Several meta-analyses have addressed the incidence of pulmonary complications in patients randomized to neuraxial anesthesia/analgesia compared to general anesthesia/systemic analgesia.[19,20] No randomized-controlled trial or systemic review has addressed this issue specifically in patients undergoing gastrointestinal procedures. Compared with systematic opioid analgesia, epidural opioid analgesia decreased the incidence of pulmonary atelectasis and had a weak tendency to reduce the incidence of pulmonary infections, and overall pulmonary complications. Epidural local anesthetics were associated with an increased PaO_2 and a decreased incidence of pulmonary infections and overall pulmonary complications compared with systemic opioid analgesia.[19]

Other Outcomes

Epidural analgesia does not appear to be associated with decreased mortality after abdominal surgery. A systematic review found no difference in mortality in patients who received neuraxial anesthesia/analgesia compared to general anesthesia/systemic analgesia for abdominal procedures.[20] A secondary analysis of a subset of high-risk patients in a large multicenter randomized-controlled study of epidural compared to systemic analgesia for abdominal surgery found no difference in mortality between the two groups.[21]

TEA does not appear to influence postoperative cardiac outcome. Most postoperative myocardial ischemia, however, develops on postoperative day 2–3. Many studies of epidural analgesia do not continue this long; therefore, a large study with prolonged epidural analgesia (3 days) is required to definitively answer this question.[7]

Neuraxial anesthesia is associated with decreased intraoperative blood loss after orthopedic procedures. Studies in gastrointestinal surgery patients have not found a difference in blood loss or transfusion requirements.[7] Similarly, although neuraxial anesthesia is associated with a decreased incidence of deep venous thrombosis and pulmonary embolus in orthopedic patients, this has not been demonstrated in bowel surgery patients.

TEA and postoperative analgesia block the stress response to intra-abdominal surgery (see Chap. 4). The intraoperative response was more profoundly inhibited by sensory blockade to high cervical levels (C3 to C4) compared to low cervical-high thoracic (T2 to C8) levels in patients undergoing upper abdominal surgery.[22] This suggests that the phrenic nerve may also play a role in the stress response to upper abdominal surgery.[22]

Clinical pathways that include early feeding, epidural analgesia, and early ambulation have been shown to shorten hospital stays after gastrointestinal surgery.[8,9] Early feeding has been shown in a randomized-controlled trial in colorectal surgery patients to be associated with shorter duration of ileus and shorter hospital stay.[23] Although randomized trials of epidural compared to systemic analgesia have demonstrated better analgesia and shorter duration of ileus, they have failed to find a shorter duration of hospital stay after colon surgery.[6] These results suggest that aggressive rehabilitation that includes early feeding and excellent analgesia should be part of a fast-track clinical pathway in these patients.

Combined neuraxial/general anesthesia may be associated with less pain, less sedation, and improved psychomotor function in the immediate postoperative period.[7] Epidural *analgesia* for colon surgery may allow earlier resumption of daily activities and improved quality of life after hospital discharge. Patients who participated in a fast-track clinical pathway were randomized to intravenous morphine or thoracic epidural bupivacaine/fentanyl analgesia.[24] Although hospital duration of stay was not different between the two groups, functional exercise capacity and quality of life scores were significantly better at 3 and 6 weeks after discharge in the epidural group. Epidural blockade may block the catabolic response to surgery, and this combined with excellent postoperative nutrition may better preserve muscle mass and decrease deconditioning.[25,26]

▶ Management of Epidural Anesthesia/Analgesia

There are many "recipes" for postoperative epidural analgesia after abdominal surgery. Specific drugs and drug doses are discussed in Chap. 16. In general, an epidural catheter is sited in the awake patient in the immediate preoperative period. The patient may be lightly sedated, but should be awake enough to cooperate with positioning and to recognize and communicate the presence of paresthesias. The catheter should be sited at the vertebral interspace which corresponds to the middle of the surgical field (Box 9-1). The placement of an epidural catheter that is "incision congruent" results in a lower incidence of analgesic drug-induced side effects (e.g., pruritus, nausea, vomiting, hypotension, urinary retention, and lower extremity motor block).

The epidural catheter may be tested at the time of catheter placement or immediately before drug injection. The authors prefer to test the catheter at the time of insertion. This allows the replacement of a catheter that is malpositioned. The epidural test dose is more sensitive in an awake patient. The injection of a test dose containing

Box 9-1		
PCEA for Abdominal Surgery		
Site epidural catheter		Upper abdominal procedure: T5 to T8
		Lower abdominal procedure: T9 to T11
Basal infusion rate*		4–6 mL/h
Patient-activated bolus dose		2–4 mL
Lockout interval		15–20 min
Maximum dose per hour		20 mL/h

*Commonly used bupivacaine infusion concentrations vary from 0.0625 to 0.125% or an equipotent ropivacaine dose. Opioid infusion concentrations are listed in Table 16-3. If the patient experiences breakthrough pain, a bolus is administered (4 mL) and the basal infusion rate is increased by 1 mL/h. If the patient is > 65 years, initially settings are decreased by 25%. The infusion drug combination can be altered to treat or minimize the incidence of side effects (e.g., hypotension or sedation).

lidocaine 45 mg, allows the anesthesiologist to test for the presence of sensory blockade approximately 15 min after injection. Lack of blockade suggests that the catheter is not correctly positioned in the epidural space and that it should be replaced. It is much easier to replace a catheter in the preoperative compared to postoperative period.

The anesthesiologist may elect to proceed with epidural anesthesia (lower abdominal procedures), combined epidural/general anesthesia, or general anesthesia, all followed by epidural analgesia. If epidural anesthesia is initiated, it is a simple matter to convert to epidural analgesia at the end of the surgical procedure. If epidural anesthesia is not chosen, epidural analgesia is usually initiated at the time of wound closure with an epidural bolus of local anesthetic, opioid, or a combination of the two. This allows the patient to emerge from general anesthesia without pain. If analgesia is initiated at wound closure, the anesthesiologist will need to estimate the required drug dose. The titration of additional drug may be necessary on awakening if the extent of blockade is inadequate for analgesia. The dose should be titrated lower for the elderly.

Current evidence favors the use of local anesthetic only, or the combination of low-dose local anesthetic and an opioid. In a meta-analysis of mixed surgical procedures, epidural analgesia with either local anesthetic alone or combined local anesthesia/opioid provided superior analgesia

Table 9-2

Systematic Review: Pain Scores of Epidural Compared to Parenteral Opioid Analgesia

Site of Epidural	Epidural Infusion Drugs	N	VAS (mm)*			P-value
			Parenteral	Epidural	Weighted Mean Difference (95% CI)	
Thoracic	Local anesthesia with or without opioid	2591	28.0 (0.3)	17.1 (0.2)	10.9 (10.1–11.6)	<0.001
	Opioid alone	284	38.1 (1.1)	31.4 (0.9)	6.7 (3.4–9.6)	<0.001
Lumbar	Local anesthesia with or without opioid	342	33.9 (0.8)	16.0 (0.6)	17.8 (15.8–19.9)	<0.001
	Opioid alone	438	34.3 (0.8)	25.8 (0.8)	8.5 (6.2–10.8)	<0.001

Abbreviations: VAS = visual analog scale (0–100 mm, where 0 = no pain and 100 = worst pain imaginable), CI = confidence interval.
*VAS values are stated as mean (standard error of the mean).
Source: Data from Ref. 14.

compared to intravenous patient-controlled intravenous opioid, but epidural analgesia with a hydrophilic opioid did not.[16] Hydrophilic epidural opioid alone was inferior to lipophilic opioid alone.

The most common methods of maintaining analgesia are continuous epidural infusion or patient-controlled epidural analgesia (PCEA). PCEA is associated with lower local anesthetic consumption compared to a continuous technique. A meta-analysis in mixed surgical populations found that pain scores and the incidence of pruritus were lower, but total anesthetic dose was higher, as was the incidence of nausea and vomiting and motor blockade in patients randomized to receive a continuous infusion compared to PCEA (Table 9-2).[16] PCEA may be administered with or without a background infusion. A study in gastrectomy patients found that the nighttime institution of a background infusion resulted in less interrupted sleep and fewer patient-activated boluses compared to a control group.[27] Further study is required to assess the advantages and disadvantages between these two PCEA techniques. A suggested PCEA regimen for abdominal surgery is detailed in Box 9-1.

The optimal duration of epidural analgesia after abdominal surgery is unclear and may depend on type of surgery and patient risk factors. Most institutions discontinue analgesia between 24 and 72 h postoperatively. The effective maintenance of epidural analgesia is labor intensive and best accomplished by an acute pain service. In a retrospective audit, 13% of patients had catheter technical failure and 20% of patients had poor pain relief.[28] In a review of postoperative pain literature, the incidence of catheter dislodgement was 6%.[29]

SUMMARY

Breast surgery can be performed under epidural anesthesia or combined epidural/general anesthesia. Postoperative analgesia, incidence of nausea and vomiting, and duration of hospital stay may be shorter compared to general anesthesia/systemic analgesia.

The abdominal viscera have dual innervation (segmental spinal sympathetic and cranial/sacral parasympathetic). This results in a contracted gut during thoracic anesthesia/analgesia with local anesthetics. Mortality does not appear to be different for general compared to epidural anesthesia; however, epidural analgesia is associated with improved postoperative analgesia, shorter duration of ileus, a decreased incidence of pulmonary complication, and improved postdischarge quality of life. Thoracic epidural compared to lumbar epidural analgesia is associated with fewer side effects. Analgesic and gut motility outcomes are improved with epidural local anesthetic with or without opioid compared to epidural opioid alone.

REFERENCES

1. Aida S, Baba H, Yamakura T, et al. The effectiveness of preemptive analgesia varies according to the type of surgery: A randomized, double-blind study. *Anesth Analg* 89:711, 1999.
2. Sundarathiti P, Pasutharnchat K, Kongdan Y, et al. Thoracic epidural anesthesia (TEA) with 0.2% ropivacaine in combination with ipsilateral brachial plexus block (BPB) for modified radical mastectomy (MRM). *J Med Assoc Thai* 88:513, 2005.
3. Lai CS, Yip WH, Lin SD, et al. Continuous thoracic epidural anesthesia for breast augmentation. *Ann Plast Surg* 36:113, 1996.
4. Correll DJ, Viscusi ER, Grunwald Z, et al. Epidural analgesia compared with intravenous morphine patient-controlled

analgesia: Postoperative outcome measures after mastectomy with immediate TRAM flap breast reconstruction. *Reg Anesth Pain Med* 26:444, 2001.

5. Yeh CC, Yu JC, Wu CT, et al. Thoracic epidural anesthesia for pain relief and postoperation recovery with modified radical mastectomy. *World J Surg* 23:256, 1999.

6. Liu SS. Anesthesia and analgesia for colon surgery. *Reg Anesth Pain Med* 29:52, 2004.

7. Fotiadis RJ, Badvie S, Weston MD, et al. Epidural analgesia in gastrointestinal surgery. *Br J Surg* 91:828, 2004.

8. Bradshaw BG, Liu SS, Thirlby RC. Standardized perioperative care protocols and reduced length of stay after colon surgery. *J Am Coll Surg* 186:501, 1998.

9. Kehlet H, Mogensen T. Hospital stay of 2 days after open sigmoidectomy with a multimodal rehabilitation programme. *Br J Surg* 86:227, 1999.

10. Jorgensen H, Wetterslev J, Moiniche S, et al. Epidural local anaesthetics versus opioid-based analgesic regimens on postoperative gastrointestinal paralysis, PONV and pain after abdominal surgery. *Cochrane Database Syst Rev* CD001893, 2000.

11. Steinbrook RA. Epidural anesthesia and gastrointestinal motility. *Anesth Analg* 86:837, 1998.

12. Scott AM, Starling JR, Ruscher AE, et al. Thoracic versus lumbar epidural anesthesia's effect on pain control and ileus resolution after restorative proctocolectomy. *Surgery* 120:688, 1996.

13. Holte K, Kehlet H. Epidural analgesia and risk of anastomotic leakage. *Reg Anesth Pain Med* 26:111, 2001.

14. Block BM, Liu SS, Rowlingson AJ, et al. Efficacy of postoperative epidural analgesia: A meta-analysis. *JAMA* 290:2455, 2003.

15. Werawatganon T, Charuluxanun S. Patient controlled intravenous opioid analgesia versus continuous epidural analgesia for pain after intra-abdominal surgery. *Cochrane Database Syst Rev* CD004088, 2005.

16. Wu CL, Cohen SR, Richman JM, et al. Efficacy of postoperative patient-controlled and continuous infusion epidural analgesia versus intravenous patient-controlled analgesia with opioids: A meta-analysis. *Anesthesiology* 103:1079, 2005.

17. Dahl JB, Hansen BL, Hjortso NC, et al. Influence of timing on the effect of continuous extradural analgesia with bupivacaine and morphine after major abdominal surgery. *Br J Anaesth* 69:4, 1992.

18. Walker SM, Goudas LC, Cousins MJ, et al. Combination spinal analgesic chemotherapy: A systematic review. *Anesth Analg* 95:674, 2002.

19. Ballantyne JC, Carr DB, deFerranti S, et al. The comparative effects of postoperative analgesic therapies on pulmonary outcome: Cumulative meta-analyses of randomized, controlled trials. *Anesth Analg* 86:598, 1998.

20. Rodgers A, Walker N, Schug S, et al. Reduction of postoperative mortality and morbidity with epidural or spinal anaesthesia: Results from overview of randomised trials. *BMJ* 321:1493, 2000.

21. Peyton PJ, Myles PS, Silbert BS, et al. Perioperative epidural analgesia and outcome after major abdominal surgery in high-risk patients. *Anesth Analg* 96:548, 2003.

22. Segawa H, Mori K, Kasai K, et al. The role of the phrenic nerves in stress response in upper abdominal surgery. *Anesth Analg* 82:1215, 1996.

23. Stewart BT, Woods RJ, Collopy BT, et al. Early feeding after elective open colorectal resections: A prospective randomized trial. *Aust N Z J Surg* 68:125, 1998.

24. Carli F, Mayo N, Klubien K, et al. Epidural analgesia enhances functional exercise capacity and health-related quality of life after colonic surgery: Results of a randomized trial. *Anesthesiology* 97:540, 2002.

25. Carli F, Halliday D. Continuous epidural blockade arrests the postoperative decrease in muscle protein fractional synthetic rate in surgical patients. *Anesthesiology* 86:1033, 1997.

26. Schricker T, Wykes L, Eberhart L, et al. The anabolic effect of epidural blockade requires energy and substrate supply. *Anesthesiology* 97:943, 2002.

27. Komatsu H, Matsumoto S, Mitsuhata H. Comparison of patient-controlled epidural analgesia with and without nighttime infusion following gastrectomy. *Br J Anaesth* 87:633, 2001.

28. McLeod G, Davies H, Munnoch N, et al. Postoperative pain relief using thoracic epidural analgesia: Outstanding success and disappointing failures. *Anaesthesia* 56:75, 2001.

29. Dolin SJ, Cashman JN, Bland JM. Effectiveness of acute postoperative pain management: I. Evidence from published data. *Br J Anaesth* 89:409, 2002.

Neuraxial Anesthesia for Adult Genitourinary Procedures

Michele Sproviero

INTRODUCTION

Urologic procedures account for 10–20% of most anesthesia practices. The patient population that typically undergoes genitourinary procedures is elderly with multiple comorbidities. Neuraxial anesthesia is often an appropriate anesthetic option either as the primary anesthetic or as an adjunct to general anesthesia for postoperative pain control. The urologic procedures which are most amenable to neuraxial anesthesia include transurethral resection of the prostate, extracorporal shock wave lithotripsy (ESWL), radical retropubic prostatectomy, radical open nephrectomy, and cystectomy/ileoconduit bladder reconstruction. Indications for urologic laparoscopic surgery continue to develop. In general, as these procedures are lengthy and require steep Trendelenburg position with carbon dioxide insufflation, general anesthesia with controlled ventilation is indicated.

INNERVATION OF THE GENITOURINARY SYSTEM

The genitourinary system is innervated by both the sympathetic and parasympathetic nervous systems (Fig. 10-1 and Figs. 1-19 and 1-20). The kidney receives sympathetic innervation from the eighth thoracic through first lumbar spinal segments and parasympathetic innervation from the vagus nerve.[1] Pain is conducted via nerves to the T10 to L1 spinal levels. Sympathetic fibers to the ureter originate from the T10 to L2 segments. Parasympathetic input is from the S2 to S4 spinal segments.

Sympathetic nerves to the bladder and urethra originate from the T11 to L2 segments and supply the bladder through the right and left hypogastric nerves.[2] Parasympathetic innervation to the bladder originates from the S2 to S4 segments and from the pelvic and hypogastric plexuses.

There are more parasympathetic fibers supplying the bladder than sympathetic fibers. The afferents carrying sensations of stretch and fullness of the bladder accompany parasympathetic fibers, while sympathetic nerves carry the sensations of pain, touch, and temperature.

The prostate and the prostatic urethra receive both sympathetic and parasympathetic supply from the prostatic plexus arising from the pelvic parasympathetic plexus. The origin of this nerve supply is lumbrosacral.[2]

The dermatome blockade requirements for urologic surgical procedures are listed in Table 10-1.

TRANSURETHRAL RESECTION OF THE PROSTATE

Benign prostate hypertrophy is the most common benign tumor in men and can lead to symptomatic bladder outlet obstruction. Surgical management is often indicated in men who have failed conservative pharmacologic therapy. Approximately one-third of all males who live to the age of 80 require a prostatectomy.[3] Several procedures exist to remove the hypertrophied prostatic tissue but the most common and least invasive is a transurethral resection of the prostate (TURP). TURP involves urethral introduction of a resectoscope, an instrument which is capable of both cutting and coagulation, through a modified cystoscope. The protruding prostatic tissue is then resected from the prostatic urethra.

▶ TURP Syndrome

Continuous irrigation of the bladder and prostatic urethra is required to maintain visibility, distend the operative site, and remove tissue and blood.[4] The ideal irrigating fluid for TURP is isotonic, nonhemolytic, nonelectrolytic (in order

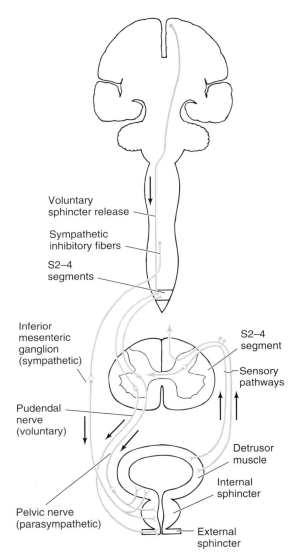

Voluntary sphincter release

Sympathetic inhibitory fibers

S2–4 segments

Inferior mesenteric ganglion (sympathetic)

Pudendal nerve (voluntary)

Pelvic nerve (parasympathetic)

S2–4 segment

Sensory pathways

Detrusor muscle

Internal sphincter

External sphincter

FIGURE 10-1. Innervation of the genitourinary system. *Used with permission from Waxman SG.* Clinical Neuroanatomy, *25th ed. New York: McGraw-Hill, 2003.*

Table 10-1	
Genitourinary Procedures and Required Sensory Level of Anesthesia	
Organ	Sensory blockade
Kidney	T8 to L1
Ureter	T10 to L2
Bladder	T11 to L2
Prostate	T11 to L2
Penis	L1 to L2
Testes	T10 to L2

potential to cause hypoosmolarity, hyponatremia, and fluid overload, a condition known as TURP syndrome.

TURP syndrome causes adverse effects in the cardiovascular, respiratory, and central nervous systems, in addition to metabolic changes (Box 10-1). These changes are primarily a result of hypervolemia, hypoosmolarity, and hyponatremia.

Box 10-1

TURP Syndrome

Cardiovascular and respiratory

Hypertension

Brady/tachyarrhythmia

Congestive heart failure

Pulmonary edema and hypoxemia

Myocardial infarction

Hypertension

Central nervous system

Agitation/confusion

Seizures

Coma

Visual disturbances (blindness)

Metabolic

Hyponatremia

Hyperglycemia

Hyperammonemia

Other

Hypoosmolarity

Hemolysis

to disperse electrical current), transparent (to allow clear visibility), nonmetabolized, nontoxic, rapidly excreted, and inexpensive.[5] Unfortunately, no such irrigation fluid exists. Initially, water was used for irrigation. However, since water has very low tonicity, water absorbed through open venous sinuses of the prostate caused massive intravascular hemolysis, hemoglobinemia, and rarely renal failure.[6] Consequently, less hypoosmolar substances have been employed including glycine, mannitol, and sorbitol. Since none of these substances are isotonic, they all have the

The syndrome occurs in approximately 10–15% of patients and has a mortality rate of 0.2–0.8%.

The classic triad of symptoms which has been described includes increases in systolic and diastolic blood pressure, bradycardia, and mental status changes.[5] TURP syndrome manifests initially with mental status changes, including restlessness, agitation, and confusion, and later with seizures, coma, and death. Central nervous system symptoms result from hyponatremia and water intoxication leading to cerebral edema. Cardiovascular effects include widening of the QRS complex, elevated ST segments, and finally ventricular tachycardia or fibrillation. In addition, fluid overload and pulmonary edema can develop, especially in patients who already have impaired cardiac function and a history of congestive heart failure.

In addition to TURP syndrome, irrigation fluids have a variety of other undesired metabolic side effects including transient blindness, hyperglycemia, and hyperammonemia. Other complications of TURP include bleeding and perforation of the prostatic capsule. Perforation occurs in 1–2% of patients[7] and can occur extraperitoneally resulting in suprapubic pain, or intraperitoneally resulting in referred shoulder pain. Bacteremia and deep venous thrombosis are postoperative complications of TURP syndrome.

Neuraxial Anesthesia for TURP

Neuraxial anesthesia has widely been considered the anesthetic of choice for TURP. There are several theoretical advantages to neuraxial compared to general anesthesia for TURP (Box 10-2). Since the patient is awake, mental status changes associated with TURP syndrome are more readily observed. This can aid in the early diagnosis and treatment of the syndrome. Also, if the prostatic capsule is perforated, breakthrough pain usually occurs, thus alerting the anesthesiologist

---

Box 10-2
Advantages of Spinal Anesthesia Compared to General Anesthesia for TURP
▸ Early detection of mental status changes
▸ Early detection of bladder perforation (patient will experience breakthrough pain)
▸ Decreased incidence of deep vein thrombosis
▸ Decreased incidence of fluid overload (secondary to increased venous capacitance)
▸ Decreased blood loss
▸ Improved immediate postoperative pain control

---

and surgeon to the perforation. Neuraxial anesthesia-associated sympathetic blockade increases venous capacitance and may decrease the risk of fluid overload. Bleeding may be decreased with neuraxial compared to general anesthesia. Finally, the postoperative risk of deep venous thrombosis is decreased[8] and immediate postoperative analgesia is better.

Although most anesthesiologists believe that spinal anesthesia is the anesthetic of choice for TURP, studies comparing spinal to general anesthesia have failed to find a difference in outcome. There was no difference in blood loss between regional and general anesthesia,[9,10] nor was there any difference in long-term cognitive function between the two techniques.[11] Morbidity, mortality, and the incidence of myocardial infarction also appear to be the same with both techniques.[12,13]

Either spinal or epidural anesthesia with a T10 sensory level is appropriate for TURP. Spinal is often preferred to epidural anesthesia because of better sacral coverage and denser sensory blockade. A T10 sensory level is necessary because of bladder distention; however, if there is minimal distention a lower sensory level is acceptable. The duration of the procedure is usually limited to less than 90 min, as the incidence of TURP syndrome increases with increased length of the procedure. Therefore, an intermediate or long-acting local anesthetic is appropriate. Intrathecal bupivacaine appears to be more potent than ropivacaine with similar motor and hemodynamic effects for TURP.[14] Several studies have shown that low-dose bupivacaine or tetracaine combined with fentanyl may be beneficial compared to higher-dose local anesthetic techniques.[15,16] Since many patients undergoing TURP are elderly and have coexisting cardiac or pulmonary disease, spinal anesthesia with low doses of local anesthetics may limit the distribution of the blockade, thus minimizing the side effects while still providing adequate anesthesia. The addition of opioid to the local anesthetic can create a denser sensory block without increasing hemodynamic side effects. A typical dose of bupivacaine without the addition of an opioid for TURP is 7.5–10 mg. With the addition of 15–20 µg of fentanyl, the dose of bupivacaine may be decreased to 5–7.5 mg.

EXTRACORPOREAL SHOCK WAVE LITHOTRIPSY

Extracorporal shock wave lithotripsy was introduced in the 1980s as a noninvasive technique for treating urolithiasis. All lithotriptors have an energy source, a focusing device, a coupling medium, and a stone localization system.[17] The energy source transmits shock waves, which exert a pressure on a focal point centered on the calculus. Water is used as a coupling medium, allowing the shock wave to pass into the body without dissipation because the impedance of the body tissue is close to that of water.[18]

The original lithotriptor was a Dornier HM-3, which delivers a high intensity shock wave of 18–22 kV. This corresponds to a pressure of approximately 900–1100 lbs/in.^{2} at the focal point.[19] Patients are immersed in a water bath, and usually require a general or regional anesthetic because of the high intensity of the shock waves, which is proportional to the pain the patient experiences. Water bath immersion is associated with significant changes in the cardiovascular and respiratory systems. This includes an increase in central blood volume, central venous pressure, and pulmonary blood flow, a decrease in vital capacity, functional residual capacity, and tidal volume, and an increase in respiratory rate.[20]

In contrast, the newer lithotriptors are coupled directly to the skin and do not require a water bath. These lithotriptors use a lower intensity shock wave and elicit less pain. Therefore, light analgesia-sedation is usually adequate.

▶ Neuraxial Anesthesia for Water Immersion ESWL

Neuraxial and general anesthesia, flank infiltration with and without intercostal nerve blocks, and intravenous analgesia-sedation have all been described for water immersion ESWL anesthesia/analgesia. Neuraxial anesthesia facilitates positioning and monitoring compared to general anesthesia. Profound analgesia can be provided without sedation and possible respiratory and airway compromise. Epidural or spinal anesthesia with a T6 to T12 sensory level may be used for ESWL. This is usually achieved best with an epidural catheter placed in the mid- to low-thoracic spine. Spinal anesthesia has the advantage of faster onset than epidural anesthesia, but has been associated with a higher incidence of intraoperative hypotension.[21] Since the hydrostatic forces of the water bath may partially compensate for the sympathetic blockade, hypotension may be more profound after the patient has been removed from the water.

Intrathecal opioid analgesia may provide adequate anesthesia for ESWL with less hemodynamic instability than that associated with local anesthetics.[22] Eaton et al. randomized patients to intrathecal sufentanil 12.5 µg or lidocaine 75 mg. The maximum mean decrease in mean arterial pressure was 12 mmHg in the sufentanil group compared to 26 mmHg in the lidocaine group. Time to void and discharge time was earlier in the female sufentanil patients, but there were no differences between groups for male patients. The most common side effect of intrathecal opioid analgesia is pruritus, which appears to be dose dependent.[23] Lau et al. compared sufentanil 12.5, 15, 17.5, and 20 µg, and concluded that doses between 15 and 17.5 µg provided the best analgesia with fewest side effects.

Epidural anesthesia has the advantages of less sympathetic blockade, greater control of the sensory level, and the provision of continuous anesthesia. Theoretically, as little air as possible should be used when placing an epidural with the loss-of-resistance to air technique since air in the epidural space can dissipate shock waves and promote injury to neural tissue. The epidural catheter and dressing should be secured to the flank opposite the procedure site, as dressings may block the shock path and absorb the shock wave energy.

A theoretical disadvantage of neuraxial compared to general anesthesia for ESWL is the inability to control ventilation and diaphragmatic movement. Large diaphragmatic excursion during spontaneous ventilation can move the calculus in and out of focus. Clinical experience, however, would suggest that stone movement with spontaneous respiration (with a neuraxial or intravenous analgesia-sedation technique) does not negatively impact ESWL success. Patients may recover more quickly from a general anesthetic than from a neuraxial technique.[24]

RADICAL RETROPUBIC PROSTATECTOMY

Cancer of the prostate is the most commonly diagnosed cancer in men. It may be managed surgically or medically depending on the stage of the cancer and the comorbidities and age of the patient. The most common surgical technique for prostate cancer is a radical retropubic prostatectomy. This procedure involves the en bloc surgical removal of the entire prostate gland, the seminal vesicles, the ejaculatory ducts, and a portion of the bladder neck. General, neuraxial, or combined epidural-general anesthesia may be used for the open procedure.

A T6 sensory level is necessary for neuraxial anesthesia. The length of the procedure can vary greatly depending on the patient's anatomy and pathology, therefore an epidural or combined spinal epidural anesthetic is preferred to a single-shot spinal technique if the anticipated duration of surgery is long or unknown. An epidural catheter placed in the midthoracic region provides the best coverage for the procedure. Potential advantages of a neuraxial technique are decreased blood loss and decreased incidence of postoperative thromboembolic complications, along with faster recovery of bowel function and hospital discharge, and improved postoperative analgesia. Potential disadvantages of neuraxial anesthesia are an unsecured airway and patient discomfort. Hemorrhage is the most common complication of a radical retropubic prostatectomy. Acute blood loss may be less well tolerated in an awake patient with neuraxial anesthesia. Radical retropubic prostatectomies can be lengthy procedures with the patient in the supine Trendelenburg position with back extension. Resulting airway edema can make intubation difficult, if required. Also, this position tends to be quite uncomfortable, so that patient often requires generous sedation in addition to a neuraxial technique.

A number of randomized-controlled trials have compared outcomes in patients randomized to general anesthesia, neuraxial anesthesia, or combined general-neuraxial anesthesia (Table 10-2).[25–30] Review of the data suggests that neuraxial analgesia, whether alone or combined with general anesthesia, is associated with decreased blood loss.[26,27,29] Shir et al. compared general anesthesia, epidural-general anesthesia with mechanical ventilation, and epidural anesthesia with spontaneous ventilation and found that blood loss and transfusion requirements were less in the epidural group compared to the other two groups (Fig. 10-2).[29] They suggested that an intraoperative factor common to both general and combined epidural-general anesthesia, for example, mechanical ventilation or effects of general anesthetic agents, were responsible for greater blood loss. Stevens et al. observed decreased blood loss in a group of patients randomized to epidural-general anesthesia with spontaneous ventilation compared to general anesthesia with mechanical ventilation.[27] Blood loss was less in patients randomized to spinal

compared to general anesthesia.[26] Taken together, these data suggest that mechanical ventilation increases blood loss and avoidance of mechanical ventilation with either a pure neuraxial technique, or a combined neuraxial-light general anesthesia technique results in less blood loss. Most studies were underpowered to determine if this resulted in fewer transfusions.

Most studies suggest that analgesia, at least in the immediate postoperative period, is improved with techniques incorporating neuraxial anesthesia/analgesia compared to general anesthesia/systemic analgesia.[25,26,28,30] Improved analgesia and level of activity was noted even 9 weeks postoperatively in one study.[30] Several studies found faster return of bowel function after neuraxial anesthesia.[26,27] Data are equivocal regarding differences in hospital discharge between neuraxial and general anesthesia.[25,27] At the current time it is not known whether overall outcome is influenced by anesthetic technique. Established clinical pathways appear to play an important role in length of stay and hospital cost.[31] Personal preference of the surgeon, anesthesiologist, and patient are the usual deciding factors as to anesthetic technique. More recently, we have seen the introduction of laparoscopic

Table 10-2

Outcomes After Neuraxial Anesthesia for Radical Prostatectomy

Study	N	Group	EBL	Analgesia	Return Bowel Function	Hospital Discharge
Shir Y[28]	96	EA EA/GA GA		EA > GA EA > EA/GA		
Shir Y[29]	100	EA EA/GA GA	EA < GA EA < EA/GA GA = EA/GA			
Gottschalk A[30]	100	EAB/GA EAF/GA GA		EAB/GA > GA EAF/GA > GA		
Stevens R[27]	40	EA/GA GA	EA/GA < GA	EA/GA = GA	EA/GA < GA	EA/GA = GA
Salonia A[26]	72	SA GA	SA < GA	SA > GA	SA < GA	
Brown DR[25]	100	SA/GA GA		SA/GA > GA		SA/GA < GA

Abbreviations: EA = epidural anesthesia, EA/GA = combined epidural-general anesthesia, GA = general anesthesia, EAB/GA = combined bupivacaine epidural-general anesthesia, EAF/GA = combined epidural fentanyl-general anesthesia, SA = spinal anesthesia, SA/GA = combined spinal-general anesthesia, EBL = estimated blood loss. EBL: < means less blood loss; analgesia: > means improved analgesia; return of bowel function: < means fewer days; hospital discharge: < means fewer days.

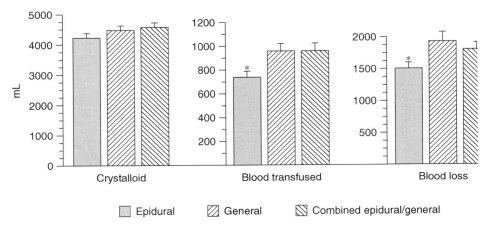

FIGURE 10-2. Intraoperative blood loss, intravenous crystalloid, and transfusion requirements in patients randomized to epidural, general, or combined epidural-general (with mechanical ventilation) anesthesia for radical prostatectomy. Blood loss and transfusion requirements were significantly less in the epidural group compared to the general and combined epidural-general groups, $P < 0.05$. *Used with permission from Shir Y, Raja SN, Frank SM, et al. Intraoperative blood loss during radical retropubic prostatectomy: Epidural versus general anesthesia. Urology 45:993, 1995.*

radical retropubic prostatectomy. Neuraxial anesthesia alone or general anesthesia with spontaneous ventilation may not be options for these procedures.

RADICAL CYSTECTOMY AND URINARY DIVERSION

Radical cystectomy is the current standard of care for the treatment of muscle-invasive bladder cancer. All anterior pelvic organs, including the bladder, prostate, and seminal vesicles, are removed in males, while the uterus, cervix, ovaries, and part of the anterior vaginal vault must be excised in females. This is usually done through a midline incision that extends from the pubis to the xiphoid process. Given the large incision, large fluid shifts, and the length of the procedure (usually 4–6 h), a general or combined general-epidural anesthetic is required. The addition of epidural anesthesia/analgesia has several potential benefits. First, it can aid in providing controlled hypotension, which is associated with decreased blood loss and improved surgical visualization during cystectomy.[32] Secondly, epidural analgesia may be used for postoperative pain control. A midthoracic epidural catheter with a T5 sensory level is appropriate. An infusion of local anesthetic with or without opioid may be used intraoperatively for analgesia in conjunction with a general anesthetic. Alternatively, the epidural analgesia may be initiated postoperatively for pain control. The advantage of administering intraoperative epidural analgesia is excellent anesthesia with minimal or no

intravenous opioid administration. This decreases the incidence of postoperative side effects associated with opioid administration and may facilitate quick and complete emergence at the end of the procedure. The disadvantage is that intraoperative epidural local anesthetic injection may cause hypotension, especially in the presence of large blood loss. The results of several small studies suggest decreased blood loss and improved analgesia with a combined epidural-general anesthesia and postoperative epidural analgesia technique,[33] particularly when combined with multimodal perioperative management.[34] These results remain to be confirmed with larger studies.

Urinary diversion is usually performed immediately following a cystectomy. Regardless of which urinary diversion procedure is used, the ureters are implanted in a segment of bowel which functions as a conduit or a reservoir. Neuraxial anesthesia may produce unopposed parasympathetic activity, which may result in a contracted, hyperactive bowel. This can make construction of a continent reservoir technically difficult. Papaverine (100–150 mg as a slow intravenous infusion over 2–3 h), an anticholinergic (glycopyrrolate 1 mg), or glucagon 1 mg may be administered to alleviate this problem.

RADICAL NEPHRECTOMY

Renal cell carcinoma accounts for approximately 3% of all adult malignancies. Radical nephrectomy is the definitive treatment. The operation may be carried out through several approaches, but the most common is with the patient in a flexed lateral decubitus position. General anesthesia or combined general-epidural anesthesia must be used because this position is very uncomfortable. Resection of tumor which extends into the inferior vena cava and right atrium may be accompanied by large blood losses and hemodynamic instability, exacerbating epidural local anesthetic-induced hypotension. Epidural analgesia with local anesthetics and/or opioids, however, is often very effective for postoperative pain management.

SUMMARY

Spinal anesthesia is considered the anesthetic of choice for TURP and may contribute to earlier recognition of TURP syndrome compared to general anesthesia. Spinal or epidural anesthesia is quite common for immersion extracorporeal shock wave lithotripter procedures, although these lithotripters are becoming obsolete. Epidural anesthesia is often used as an adjunct to general anesthesia for radical urologic cancer procedures. Particularly in combination with spontaneous ventilation, there is evidence for less blood loss compared to general anesthesia with mechanical ventilation, and improved postoperative analgesia.

REFERENCES

1. Kabalin J. Anatomy of the retroperitoneum and the kidney. In: Walsh PC, ed, *Campbell's Urology*, 8th ed. Philadelphia, PA: W.B. Saunders, 2002, p. 3.
2. Brooks J. Anatomy of the lower urinary tract and male genitalia. In: Walsh PC, ed, *Campbell's Urology,* 8th ed. Philadelphia, PA: W.B. Saunders, 2002, p. 41.
3. Riehmann M, Bruskewitz R. Evaluation of benign prostate hyperplasia. In: Bahnson RR, ed, *Management of Urologic Disorders*. London: Wolfe, 1994, p. 1A2.
4. Hatch PD. Surgical and anaesthetic considerations in transurethral resection of the prostate. *Anaesth Intensive Care* 15:203, 1987.
5. Jensen V. The TURP syndrome. *Can J Anaesth* 38:90, 1991.
6. Marx G. Complications associated with transurethal surgery. *Anesthesiology* 23:802, 1962.
7. Mebust WK, Holtgrewe HL, Cockett AT, et al. Transurethral prostatectomy: Immediate and postoperative complications. A cooperative study of 13 participating institutions evaluating 3,885 patients. 1989. *J Urol* 167:999, 2002.
8. Bernstein S, Malhotra V. Regional anesthesia for genitourinary surgery. In: Malhotra V, ed, *Anesthesia for Renal and Genitourinary Surgery*. New York: McGraw-Hill, 1996.
9. Abrams PH, Shah PJ, Bryning K, et al. Blood loss during transurethral resection of the prostate. *Anaesthesia* 37:71, 1982.
10. McGowan SW, Smith GF. Anaesthesia for transurethral prostatectomy. A comparison of spinal intradural analgesia with two methods of general anaesthesia. *Anaesthesia* 35:847, 1980.
11. Chung FF, Chung A, Meier RH, et al. Comparison of perioperative mental function after general anaesthesia and spinal anaesthesia with intravenous sedation. *Can J Anaesth* 36:382, 1989.
12. Hosking MP, Lobdell CM, Warner MA, et al. Anaesthesia for patients over 90 years of age. Outcomes after regional and general anaesthetic techniques for two common surgical procedures. *Anaesthesia* 44:142, 1989.
13. Edwards ND, Callaghan LC, White T, et al. Perioperative myocardial ischaemia in patients undergoing transurethral surgery: A pilot study comparing general with spinal anaesthesia. *Br J Anaesth* 74:368, 1995.
14. Malinovsky JM, Charles F, Kick O, et al. Intrathecal anesthesia: Ropivacaine versus bupivacaine. *Anesth Analg* 91:1457, 2000.
15. Kararmaz A, Kaya S, Turhanoglu S, et al. Low-dose bupivacaine-fentanyl spinal anaesthesia for transurethral prostatectomy. *Anaesthesia* 58:526, 2003.
16. Chen TY, Tseng CC, Wang LK, et al. The clinical use of small-dose tetracaine spinal anesthesia for transurethral prostatectomy. *Anesth Analg* 92:1020, 2001.
17. Preminger GM. Surgical management of calculus disease. In: Bahnson RR, ed, *Management of Urologic Disorders*. London: Wolfe, 1994, p. 14.2.
18. Eide TR. Anesthetic considerations for extracorporal shock wave lithotripsy. In: Lebowitz PW, ed, *Anesthesia for Urological Surgery*. Boston, MA: Little, Brown, 1993, p. 47.
19. Newman RC, Riehle RA. Principles of treatment. In: Newman RC, ed, *Principles of Extracorporal Shock Wave Lithotripsy*. New York: Churchill Livingstone, 1987, p. 79.
20. Weber W. Cardiocirculatory changes during anesthesia for extracorporal shock wave lithotripsy. *J Urol* 4:246A, 1984.
21. London RA, Kudlak T, Riehle RA. Immersion anesthesia for extracorporeal shock wave lithotripsy. Review of two hundred twenty treatments. *Urology* 28:86, 1986.
22. Eaton M, Chhibber AK, Green DR. Subarachnoid sufentanil versus lidocaine spinal anesthesia for extracorporal shock wave lithotripsy. *Reg Anesth* 22:515, 1997.
23. Lau WC, Green CR, Faerber GJ, et al. Determination of the effective therapeutic dose of intrathecal sufentanil for extracorporeal shock wave lithotripsy. *Anesth Analg* 89:889, 1999.
24. Richardson MG, Dooley JW. The effects of general versus epidural anesthesia for outpatient extracorporeal shock wave lithotripsy. *Anesth Analg* 86:1214, 1998.
25. Brown DR, Hofer RE, Patterson DE, et al. Intrathecal anesthesia and recovery from radical prostatectomy: A prospective, randomized, controlled trial. *Anesthesiology* 100:926, 2004.
26. Salonia A, Crescenti A, Suardi N, et al. General versus spinal anesthesia in patients undergoing radical retropubic prostatectomy: Results of a prospective, randomized study. *Urology* 64:95, 2004.
27. Stevens RA, Mikat-Stevens M, Flanigan R, et al. Does the choice of anesthetic technique affect the recovery of bowel function after radical prostatectomy? *Urology* 52:213, 1998.
28. Shir Y, Raja SN, Frank SM. The effect of epidural versus general anesthesia on postoperative pain and analgesic requirements in patients undergoing radical prostatectomy. *Anesthesiology* 80:49, 1994.
29. Shir Y, Raja SN, Frank SM, et al. Intraoperative blood loss during radical retropubic prostatectomy: Epidural versus general anesthesia. *Urology* 45:993, 1995.
30. Gottschalk A, Smith DS, Jobes DR, et al. Preemptive epidural analgesia and recovery from radical prostatectomy: A randomized controlled trial. *JAMA* 279:1076, 1998.

31. Worwag E, Chodak GW. Overnight hospitalization after radical prostatectomy: The impact of two clinical pathways on patient satisfaction, length of hospitalization, and morbidity. *Anesth Analg* 87:62, 1998.

32. Raj PP. Rational and choice for surgical procedures. In: Raj PP, ed, *Clinical Practice of Regional Anesthesia*. New York: Churchill Livingstone, 1991, p. 197.

33. Ozyuvaci E, Altan A, Karadeniz T, et al. General anesthesia versus epidural and general anesthesia in radical cystectomy. *Urol Int* 74:62, 2005.

34. Brodner G, Van Aken H, Hertle L, et al. Multimodal perioperative management—combining thoracic epidural analgesia, forced mobilization, and oral nutrition—reduces hormonal and metabolic stress and improves convalescence after major urologic surgery. *Anesth Analg* 92:1594, 2001.

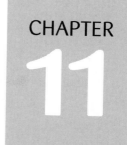
Spinal and Epidural Anesthesia for Ambulatory Surgery

Dominic Cottrell
Lynn Broadman

INTRODUCTION

Many anesthetic techniques have been used for minor surgery in the outpatient setting. Local anesthesia, local anesthesia with monitored anesthesia care (MAC), total intravenous anesthesia (TIVA), and general inhalational anesthesia have all been successfully employed for anal surgery, hernia repair, minor orthopedic, and other surgical procedures. Neuraxial anesthesia has also been used for many years for outpatient surgery.[1] Survey data demonstrate that increasing numbers of orthopedic surgeons are directing their patients to choose regional anesthesia techniques,[2] and spinal and epidural anesthesia can be highly effective for these procedures. Specific issues are important to consider when employing a neuraxial technique in the outpatient setting, including urinary retention, early ambulation and discharge, and postoperative analgesia. The best anesthetic for individual patients ultimately depends on the expectations of the patient and the surgeon expectations, cost considerations, and postoperative nursing management.[3] Patient satisfaction with an outpatient anesthetic depends on providing a short-acting anesthetic with few side effects that is tailored to the length of the surgical procedure. A fast and smooth recovery that produces a wide-awake, fully functional, and pain-free patient is also essential.

ADVANTAGES AND DISADVANTAGES OF NEURAXIAL ANESTHESIA

▶ Advantages

There are advantages and disadvantages, and benefits and risks to ambulatory neuraxial anesthesia (Box 11-1). Patients who undergo spinal or epidural anesthesia for outpatient surgery may be more alert and more comfortable in the immediate postoperative period than surgical patients who elect to have a general anesthetic for their procedures.[4–6] The success rate of neuraxial anesthesia is higher than that for peripheral nerve blocks. Moreover, reduced postoperative nausea and vomiting (PONV) may be a major advantage of neuraxial anesthesia for ambulatory surgery,[4] although data to support this claim are limited.[7,8] In relatively lengthy prothrombogenic procedures, such as total hip arthroplasty, spinal anesthesia has been shown to reduce the incidence of deep vein thrombosis (DVT), thromboembolic disease, and blood loss.[9] From a technical standpoint, neuraxial blockade is simple to perform. With proper local anesthetic agent selection these blocks offer rapid onset and quick recovery.[4] Many patients wish to be awake for their surgical procedure. Neuraxial anesthesia has a high success rate, and provides both profound operative anesthesia and postoperative analgesia without the use of sedative-hypnotic agents.

▶ Disadvantages

Discharge Readiness

The availability of newer, short-acting general anesthetic agents such as propofol, sevoflurane, and desflurane has made recovery from general anesthesia faster. Local anesthesia

---

Box 11-1

Advantages and Disadvantages to Ambulatory Neuraxial Anesthesia

Advantages	Disadvantages
Simple to perform	Discharge readiness
Rapid onset	PDPH
Quick recovery of alertness	Back pain/TNS
Reduced incidence of PONV	Urinary retention

supplemented with short-acting sedative agents is also an option for many ambulatory surgical procedures. Time to discharge was shorter after local anesthesia with sedation compared to spinal and general anesthesia for herniorrhaphy (spinal bupivacaine 9–11 mg with fentanyl)[10] and anorectal surgery (spinal lidocaine 30 mg with fentanyl).[11] In contrast, other investigators found no difference in discharge time in patients randomized to spinal lidocaine 50 mg compared to propofol-fentanyl-isoflurane general anesthesia with a laryngeal mask airway.[6] Discharge time after spinal anesthesia can be reduced by strict attention to medications and dose, as well as patient selection. In addition, discharge time can be reduced in low-risk patients by modifying discharge criteria (see "Discharge Concerns," later).

Postdural Puncture Headache

While postdural puncture headache (PDPH) can occur following spinal or epidural anesthesia, the incidence with small-gauge, pencil-point needles is very low, particularly in the elderly (see Chaps. 2 and 6). This is especially important in the outpatient setting where patients and surgeons anticipate a speedy discharge after surgery. More importantly, many patients may have to travel a considerable distance for follow-up care should a PDPH develop.

Pittoni et al. compared 22- and 25-gauge Sprotte needles in 234 patients undergoing elective outpatient arthroscopy of the knee joint.[12] The incidence of PDPH was 0.9% (1 of 117 patients) in the 22-gauge needle group and 0% in the 25-gauge needle group. Another group of investigators described the use of 27-gauge Sprotte needles in 116 patients undergoing ambulatory arthroscopic knee surgery.[13] The incidence of PDPH was 0.9% (1/116).

Back Pain and Transient Neurologic Symptoms

Back pain and transient neurologic symptoms (TNS) are the most troublesome side effects associated with neuraxial blockade for ambulatory surgery. Focal back pain may occur at the skin site, and this must be differentiated from TNS. TNS are discussed in detail in Chap. 6 and have been reviewed elsewhere.[14] Our readers are urged to review the aforementioned material because there are many important TNS features which are germane to ambulatory surgery and anesthesia. The incidence of back pain and other forms of TNS following spinal anesthesia depends on a number of factors (Box 11-2); however, it appears that the most important single factor may be the selection of the intrathecal local anesthetic.[15] Lidocaine is most commonly implicated in TNS, and because of its short duration of action, it is also the local anesthetic agent most suitable for use during ambulatory surgical procedures. The risk of TNS was five times

---

Box 11-2

Risk Factors for TNS

Intrathecal lidocaine
Lithotomy position
Arthroscopic knee surgery
Obesity
Ambulatory surgery (unclear)

---

higher after lidocaine spinal anesthesia compared to bupivacaine and tetracaine.[16] There was an increased incidence of TNS following knee arthroscopies compared to hernia repair.[17] In addition, lithotomy position for surgery was related to a higher incidence of TNS following lidocaine spinal anesthesia.[16] A prospective survey involving over 1800 patients identified ambulatory surgery as a risk factor for TNS.[16] In contrast, Swedish investigators randomized patients undergoing lidocaine spinal anesthesia to two groups: early ambulation (immediately after block regression) or delayed ambulation (after 12 h bedrest). This study found no difference in the incidence of TNS between the two groups.[18] Factors that do not increase the risk of TNS include needle size and other technical aspects of the spinal procedure, such as concentration of the local anesthetic solution, or the addition of opioids or dextrose to the intrathecal local anesthetic solution. Pollock et al. clearly demonstrated in a prospective, double-blind study that epinephrine added to lidocaine did not cause an increased incidence of back pain or TNS.[17]

Diagnosis and Treatment of TNS. Treatment options for TNS have been well documented in a recent review article.[14] Many patients with this syndrome complain about being troubled by bilateral thigh pain. The pain is further described as achy, burning, or crampy. In addition, the pain may radiate from the site of origin, usually to the anterior or posterior thighs. A very important pertinent negative finding is that no patient has ever been reported with TNS and a concomitant objective neurologic deficit. This establishes the importance of ruling out epidural hematoma or nerve root damage in patients with positive neurologic deficits.

TNS usually responds to conservative therapy and symptoms frequently resolve within 1–4 days. Nonsteriodal anti-inflammatory drugs (NSAIDs) and warm compresses, along with comfortable positioning are the most simple and efficacious treatment options for the management of TNS. Oral opioids, muscle relaxants, physical therapy, and transcutaneous electrical nerve stimulation (TENS) are alternative treatment modalities. Advanced treatment paradigms for the patient with TNS include trigger point injections.[14]

Urinary Retention

Voiding difficulties occur with some regularity after spinal and epidural anesthesia. There appears to be an increased risk with anorectal surgery and inguinal hernia repairs, primarily due to concurrent surgical issues. A volunteer crossover study revealed that the addition of epinephrine to lidocaine significantly increased the time to void by over an hour.[19] Studies differ as to the risk factors for postoperative urinary retention. Age and male sex have been identified as risk factors in some studies,[20–23] but not in others.[24,25] Prospective observational studies on inpatients have identified spinal compared to general anesthesia as a risk factor for urinary retention.[20,23] However, in a prospective study of low-risk ambulatory patients, only 3 of 201 patients who received short-acting, low-dose spinal or epidural anesthesia required bladder catheterization before discharge.[26] This incidence is similar to that observed in other studies in patients undergoing general anesthesia.

Short-acting neuraxial local anesthetics decrease the risk of urinary retention. The addition of fentanyl 20 µg to intrathecal lidocaine did not prolong time to first void.[27] Mulroy et al. demonstrated that there was no reason to delay discharge due to inability to void after outpatient spinal or epidural anesthesia with short-acting anesthetic agents in patients undergoing low-risk (for urinary retention) procedures.[26]

Bleeding and Infection

The potential for neuraxial hematoma formation or infection exists following spinal or epidural anesthesia (see Chap. 6). However, spinal-epidural hematoma and infection are rare complications, especially in the outpatient setting following either spinal or epidural anesthesia. There is at least one case report, however, describing an otherwise healthy patient who developed an epidural hematoma following epidural anesthesia for outpatient knee arthroscopy.[28] An additional case report describes transient paraparesis from a spinal hematoma in a patient who received postoperative ketorolac.[29] The risk of epidural hematoma formation appears to be dependent on the patient and the presence of medications that alter the coagulation cascade or platelet function. Increasing numbers of ambulatory patients are being treated with warfarin, low molecular weight heparin, NSAIDs, and platelet inhibitors, such as clopidogrel. A consensus statement from the American Society of Regional Anesthesia and Pain Medicine is available to help practitioners make appropriate decisions regarding the placement of neuraxial

blocks in the aforementioned patient populations (see Chap. 5).[30] Aspirin and other nonsteroidal anti-inflammatory agents and prophylactic subcutaneous unfractionated heparin, in the absence of other anticoagulants or a prior history of bleeding, are not a contraindication to neuraxial anesthesia. Therapeutic heparin and other anticoagulants require special consideration when neuraxial anesthesia is planned.

SPINAL ANESTHESIA

Subarachnoid block with short-acting local anesthetics is a useful technique in the outpatient setting; however, because spinal anesthetic blockade can potentially result in a prolonged discharge time, the duration of blockade must be tailored to the duration of the procedure. Lidocaine or lidocaine with fentanyl are currently the most widely used agents for spinal anesthesia in the ambulatory surgery setting. Recent research from a single institution has focused on intrathecal 2-chloroprocaine (2-CP) for spinal anesthesia (see "2-Chloroprocaine," later).

▶ ## Local Anesthetics

Lidocaine

Lidocaine is an ideal local anesthetic for spinal anesthesia in the ambulatory setting because it provides rapid onset and short duration of action. The addition of fentanyl appears to prolong the duration of surgical anesthesia, but not the time to recovery.[27] Epinephrine, however, prolongs both the duration of blockade, and the length of recovery (as measured by time to first void) when added to lidocaine.[19]

The selection of an appropriate lidocaine dose is a function of matching the dose with the anticipated surgical time (Table 11-1). Ben-David et al. reported the successful use of intrathecal hyperbaric 0.5% lidocaine 20 mg, combined with fentanyl 20 µg for knee arthroscopy.[31] Lennox et al.

Table 11-1

Lidocaine for Ambulatory Spinal Anesthetic Blockade: Dose, Adjuvant, Duration

Agent	Dose (mg)	Adjunct	Dose (µg)	Duration (min)
Lidocaine	25–35	–	–	30
Lidocaine	25–40	Fentanyl	25–40	60–90
Lidocaine	50	Fentanyl	50	>90

have used as little as lidocaine 10 mg (1%) combined with sufentanil 10 μg for very short outpatient laparoscopic procedures and similar short duration procedures.[32,33] Hyperbaric lidocaine (5%) was clinically indistinguishable from hyperbaric lidocaine (1.5%).[34]

The authors use lidocaine or lidocaine with fentanyl for almost all spinal anesthetics for ambulatory procedures. These agents are particularly useful for urologic and gynecologic procedures, as well as inguinal hernia, knee arthroscopy, and anorectal surgery.

Bupivacaine

The use of spinal-epidural bupivacaine for ambulatory surgical cases is quite limited due to its long duration of action.[35] Recovery time is generally too long for the ambulatory setting. Hypobaric bupivacaine 5 mg, administered in a concentration of 0.1% in the jackknife position was shown to be effective for outpatient anorectal surgery.[36] Postoperative analgesia was excellent without motor blockade. The addition of fentanyl (25 μg) to bupivacaine (12 mg) resulted in prolonged postoperative analgesia, but onset time and duration of the block were not affected.[37] Ben-David et al. compared two "low-dose" bupivacaine techniques for knee arthroscopy: hyperbaric bupivacaine (5 mg) with and without fentanyl (10 μg).[38] The mean time to S2 block regression was prolonged in the fentanyl group (120 min vs. 146 min, $P < 0.05$), however, there was no difference in the discharge time between groups (187 min vs. 195 min). Unfortunately, three hours is a long time for patients to linger in a busy ambulatory surgery center and it is the opinion of your authors that the duration of bupivacaine blockade is too long to make the drug useful for most ambulatory procedures. Moreover, hypobaric and hyperbaric bupivacaine have different pharmacokinetic profiles, and this must be considered when this agent is used to perform ambulatory spinal anesthesia.

Ropivacaine

Ropivacaine is a relatively new local anesthetic. When used for spinal anesthesia, it appears to have no advantage over bupivacaine. It is currently not approved for intrathecal use in the United States.

2-Chloroprocaine

Investigators have recently revisited 2-CP for subarachnoid anesthesia. Kouri and Kopacz compared this agent to lidocaine in a small, double-blinded crossover study in volunteers.[39] They found that 40 mg of 2% preservative-free 2-CP was as effective as 40 mg of 2% lidocaine for both sensory and motor blockade. Median block height was T8. Resolution

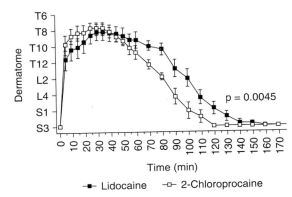

FIGURE 11-1. Resolution of sensory block determined by pinprick anesthesia, 2-CP (40 mg preservative-free 2% 2-CP) vs. lidocaine (40 mg preservative-free 2% lidocaine). *Used with permission from Kouri ME, Kopacz DJ. Spinal 2-chloroprocaine: A comparison with lidocaine in volunteers. Anesth Analg 98:75, 2004.*

of sensory blockade was shorter after 2-CP (103 min vs. 126 min; Fig. 11-1), as was time to simulated discharge (104 min vs. 134 min).

The investigators also studied the addition of adjuncts to 2-CP in another dose-ranging study. Epinephrine combined with 2-CP resulted in flu-like symptoms being reported by the study participants. Recovery times were prolonged when epinephrine was added to low-dose 2-CP (30 mg).[40] The investigators recommended against the use of 2-CP combined with epinephrine because of these side effects. Fentanyl (20 μg) mildly prolonged block duration and duration of tourniquet tolerance when combined with 2-CP (40 mg).[41] Clonidine (15 μg) combined with 2-CP (30 mg) prolonged duration to simulated discharge (99 min vs. 131 min), but did not increase side effects.[42] The addition of dextrose to 2-CP did not significantly alter block characteristics.[43] TNS was not reported in any volunteer in any of these studies.

Finally, this group of investigators studied the clinical use of spinal 2-CP in 121 patients undergoing short outpatient procedures. 2-CP (30–40 mg) with or without fentanyl (10–20 μg) resulted in mean block height between T6 and T8. Time to discharge was 155 min (plain) to 208 min (with fentanyl).[44]

The above reports are from a single institution. As more information becomes available on the use of 2-CP for ambulatory surgery, anesthesia providers will be able to make important patient care decisions about its use compared to lidocaine in the outpatient setting. One must be aware that local anesthetic preparations containing preservatives can cause irreversible neurologic injury when injected into the subarachnoid space. The use of such preparations must be avoided for spinal axis anesthetics. 2-CP is currently not approved for intrathecal injection in the United States and therefore, intrathecal injection is considered an "off-label" use of this drug.[45]

Opioids and Other Adjuncts to Spinal Anesthesia

The risk of delayed respiratory depression limits neuraxial opioid use in ambulatory patients to the short-acting, lipid-soluble opioids. Respiratory drive may become compromised due to the rostral spread of hydrophilic opioids and inhibition of the respiratory centers in the brainstem (see Chap. 6). This may occur many hours after intrathecal administration. Lipid-soluble opioids, however, are excellent adjuncts for ambulatory spinal and epidural anesthesia. The authors recommend that only short-acting opioids, such as fentanyl, be used on day surgery patients.

Fentanyl

Opioids are often combined with intrathecal local anesthetics. The addition of fentanyl produces a more dense motor and sensory block, and it also increases the block duration. In addition, the addition of fentanyl produces profound postoperative analgesia which may last as long as 4 h after all signs of motor block have resolved. Finally, the addition of fentanyl allows one to use a decreased dose of local anesthetic and thus decrease the incidence and severity of local anesthetic-related adverse side effects (see Chap. 3).

Face, neck, and chest pruritus is a common side effect of all neuraxial opioids, and is likely due to the cephalad spread of the drug in the cerebrospinal fluid. Pruritus is less common with lipid-soluble opioids and is effectively treated with a small systemic dose of an opioid agonist-antagonist agent (see Chap. 6). Antihistamines (H_1-blocking agents) may be an effective treatment because of their sedating effects, although the mechanism of pruritus is not histamine related.

The incidence of urinary retention may also be increased by the addition of neuraxial opioids. This effect is thought to be due to receptor-mediated drug effects in the sacral spinal cord that result in bladder muscle relaxation and increased bladder volume capacity (see Chap. 6).

Fentanyl 20–25 µg may be combined with any intrathecal local anesthetic to prolong its duration (Fig. 11-2). Tolerance to tourniquet pain was prolonged an average of 48% when fentanyl 20 µg was combined with lidocaine 50 mg.[27] It is especially effective when mixed in equal volumes of hyperbaric lidocaine (e.g., lidocaine 0.8 mL, 5% hyperbaric lidocaine [40 mg] and fentanyl 0.8 mL, 50 µg/mL [40 µg]). This mixture provides 60–90 min of anesthesia and 3–4 h of profound postoperative analgesia and is particularly useful

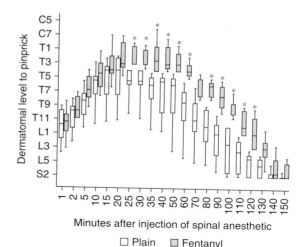

FIGURE 11-2. Regression of sensory analgesia to pinprick after lidocaine (50 mg 5% hyperbaric lidocaine) with and without fentanyl 20 µg. Box plot displays median and 10th and 90th percentiles. *Different from lidocaine without fentanyl, $P < 0.05$. *Used with permission from Liu S, Chiu AA, Carpenter RL, et al. Fentanyl prolongs lidocaine spinal anesthesia without prolonging recovery. Anesth Analg 80:730, 1995.*

and effective for inguinal hernia, knee arthroscopy, and anorectal surgery.

Meperidine

Meperidine is the only opioid that also possesses local anesthetic properties (see Chap. 3). Its use as the sole intrathecal agent for outpatient spinal anesthesia for perianal or inguinal procedures has been described.[46] Patients demonstrated prolonged postoperative analgesia. Side effects included nausea and vomiting, hypotension, pruritus, and urinary retention. Motor block is often poor or absent. In addition, respiratory depression can occur with neuraxial meperidine. For this reason, the authors of this chapter recommend that meperidine and all other long-acting opioids *not* be used for spinal anesthesia, or as an adjunct to spinal anesthesia, in the ambulatory surgery patient.

Clonidine

Intrathecal clonidine has been used as an adjunct to spinal anesthesia. In a randomized double-blinded study, investigators combined clonidine (0, 15 or 30 µg) with bupivacaine (6 mg) for inguinal hernia surgery.[47] All patients who received clonidine had satisfactory surgical anesthesia, whereas this was not true for some patients in the plain bupivacaine group. Although mean arterial blood pressures were lower in patients who received clonidine, no one required treatment.

Time to first void, however, was approximately 360 min in all groups.

In a study of knee arthroscopy patients, clonidine 0, 15, 45, or 75 μg was added to intrathecal ropivacaine 8 mg.[48] Clonidine 15 μg improved surgical anesthesia without prolonging time to first void (approximately 180 min). Higher doses of clonidine were associated with a longer recovery period, lower blood pressure, and clinical sedation. Adequate dose response studies for intrathecal lidocaine and clonidine are currently lacking.

Epinephrine

The addition of epinephrine to intrathecally administered local anesthetic agents prolongs surgical blockade, as well as recovery time. In a recent crossover study involving 12 volunteers, Moore et al. showed that the addition of epinephrine (200 μg) to bupivacaine (7.5 mg) increased tolerance to tourniquet pain by an average of 30 min, but prolonged simulated discharge time by 48 min.[49]

▶ Bilateral Compared to Unilateral Blockade

A unilateral spinal anesthetic block may be a suitable anesthetic option for some patients in the ambulatory setting (see Chap. 2). Unilateral blockade can provide a profound and long-lasting block in the operative limb, with similar discharge times when compared to bilateral blockade.[50] This approach is usually carried out by initiating the spinal anesthetic with the patient in the lateral decubitus position. Hyperbaric local anesthetic solution is preferentially distrib-uted to the dependent portion of the subarachnoid space, thus the operative side is placed down. If a hypobaric local anesthetic solution is used, the operative limb is placed in the nondependent position (up). Most practitioners keep the patient in the lateral position for 10–15 min after the intrathecal injection. Each anesthesia provider will have to decide whether this delay is cost-effective in his or her particular setting.

Valanne et al. studied low-dose hyperbaric bupivacaine (4 and 6 mg) for unilateral spinal block for outpatient knee arthroscopy.[51] Bupivacaine was injected slowly (over 2 min) toward the dependent side and patients were maintained in the lateral decubitus position for at least 10 min. Surgical anesthesia was obtained in most patients (Table 11-2) and discharge readiness was faster than usually described following bilateral bupivacaine spinal anesthesia.

Similar results were reported by Borghi.[52] Patients were maintained in the lateral position for 15 min after intrathecal injection. Kiran and Upma have described the successful use of doses as small as 3 mg of hyperbaric bupivacaine in outpatient knee arthroscopy.[53] Duration of motor blockade averaged 75 min, and time to first void was 200 min in their study of 40 adult patients. Studies of unilateral spinal anesthesia with lidocaine have not been reported.

EPIDURAL ANESTHESIA

Epidural anesthesia can be used in many procedures, but may not be ideal for procedures of short duration. Onset of blockade is slower after epidural compared to spinal anesthesia and the failure rate is also higher. The PDPH rate is similar.

Table 11-2

Unilateral Bupivacaine Spinal Anesthesia for Knee Arthroscopy

Block Characteristic	Bupivacaine Dose*		
	4 mg	6 mg	8 mg
Valanne et al. ($n = 99$)			
Inadequate anesthesia (n)	3/48	1/51	–
Time to void (min)	172 (115, 319)	203 (122, 377)[†]	–
Home readiness (min)	181 (115, 319)	209 (147, 377)	–
Borghi ($n = 90$)			
Inadequate anesthesia (n)	0/30	0/30	0/30
Home readiness (min)	104[‡]	148	161

*Data are presented as number/total, median (range), or mean.
[†]Different from 4 mg, $P < 0.05$.
[‡]Different from 6 and 8 mg, $P < 0.05$. Patients were not required to void before home discharge in the Borghi study.
Source: Data from Refs. 51, 52.

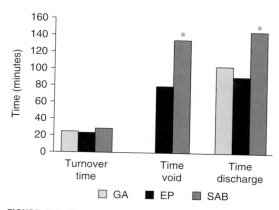

FIGURE 11-3. Comparison of operating room turnover time, time to void, and time to discharge for general anesthesia (GA) (propofol-nitrous oxide), epidural anesthesia (EP) (3% 2-CP), and spinal anesthesia (SAB) (procaine 75 mg with fentanyl 20 μg) for outpatient knee arthroscopy. GA patients were not required to void prior to discharge. *$P < 0.05$. Data are from Ref. 56. *Used with permission from Mulroy MF, Larkin KL, Hodgson PS, et al. A comparison of spinal, epidural, and general anesthesia for outpatient knee arthroscopy. Anesth Analg 91:860, 2000.*

Box 11-3

Order of Return of Neurologic Function after Spinal Anesthesia and Suggested Discharge Criteria after Spinal Anesthesia

Reversal of sympathetic block

    Spontaneous increase in mean arterial pressure

    Spontaneous increase in pulse rate

Return of pinprick sensation

    S4 to S5 dermatomes = perianal area

Return of motor function

    Plantar flexion of foot in supine position, at motor strength equivalent to preanesthetic levels

Adequate proprioception (feet)

    Position changes in great toe

Data from Ref. 56.

Theoretical advantages of epidural compared to spinal anesthesia include ability to titrate (one can use a short-acting drug followed by reinjection as necessary) and decreased risk of TNS.

Mulroy et al. compared general (propofol-nitrous oxide), spinal (procaine-fentanyl), and epidural (3%, 2-CP) anesthesia for outpatient knee arthroscopy.[54] Twenty-five percent of patients with epidural anesthesia required a second bolus dose of 2-CP. Operating room turnover time and patient satisfaction were similar among groups. Time to discharge was longer after spinal anesthesia compared to general and epidural anesthesia. This may have been due to the fact that patients were required to void before discharge after both neuraxial techniques, and not after general anesthesia (Fig. 11-3). In another study of epidural anesthesia for outpatient knee arthroscopy, discharge time was significantly longer following lidocaine compared to 2-CP epidural anesthesia.[55]

Although epidural anesthesia with a short-acting local anesthetic is theoretically clinically effective for outpatient surgery, the authors perceive no real advantage for the routine use of 2-CP epidural anesthesia compared to spinal anesthesia with a short-acting agent such as lidocaine for most ambulatory surgical procedures.

DISCHARGE CONCERNS

Establishment of criteria for safe and successful patient discharge, either to home or to another hospital care area, must be based on physiologic parameters. The Bromage scale for

regression of motor blockade have been used in many institutions. Many institutions require full regression of spinal blockade (sensory, motor, sympathetic, and proprioception), although this has not been well studied in the ambulatory setting. Pflug et al. studied the return of neurologic function during resolution of tetracaine spinal anesthesia.[56] Sympathetic nervous systemic activity returned first, followed by sensation to pinprick, somatic motor function, and finally proprioception in the feet. The Pflug et al. criteria for discharge following spinal anesthesia are outlined in Box 11-3.[56] The ability of patients to urinate was not assessed by Pflug et al.

The authors of this chapter use the following simple test to determine if patients are suitable for discharge following spinal anesthesia in the outpatient setting. Two strong people support the patient under each armpit and the patient is asked to perform a deep knee bend. If the patient is able to resume an erect posture without any help, she can go home.

Mulroy's group addressed the issue of required voiding prior to discharge. They studied patients undergoing ambulatory surgery, but excluded patients undergoing hernia, rectal, or urologic procedures. In addition, only patients younger than 70 years were enrolled. This study in low-risk patients found that patients could be discharged home safely without voiding spontaneously. However, those patients who did not void spontaneously within 2 h received a single urinary catheterization if the presence of bladder volumes of 400 mL or more was diagnosed by ultrasound.[26]

SUMMARY

Neuraxial anesthesia is appropriate for selected ambulatory procedures. Advantages include postoperative analgesia and minimal need for sedative-hypnotic administration. The anesthetic must be tailored to the length of the surgical procedure and steps should be taken to minimize the incidence of side effects that prolong discharge times, for example, urinary retention. Spinal anesthesia with low-dose lidocaine combined with fentanyl is currently the most frequently used technique in the ambulatory setting, but transient neurologic symptoms remain an issue.

REFERENCES

1. Louthan BW, Jones JR, Henschel EO, et al. Isobaric spinal anesthesia for anorectal surgery. *Anesth Analg* 44:742, 1965.
2. Oldman M, McCartney CJ, Leung A, et al. A survey of orthopedic surgeons' attitudes and knowledge regarding regional anesthesia. *Anesth Analg* 98:1486, 2004.
3. Horlocker TT, Hebl JR. Anesthesia for outpatient knee arthroscopy: Is there an optimal technique? *Reg Anesth Pain Med* 28:58, 2003.
4. Mulroy MF, McDonald SB. Regional anesthesia for outpatient surgery. *Anesthesiol Clin North America* 21:289, 2003.
5. Erhan E, Ugur G, Anadolu O, et al. General anaesthesia or spinal anaesthesia for outpatient urological surgery. *Eur J Anaesthesiol* 20:647, 2003.
6. Wong J, Marshall S, Chung F, et al. Spinal anesthesia improves the early recovery profile of patients undergoing ambulatory knee arthroscopy. *Can J Anaesth* 48:369, 2001.
7. Urmey WF. Spinal anaesthesia for outpatient surgery. *Best Pract Res Clin Anaesthesiol* 17:335, 2003.
8. Carpenter RL, Caplan RA, Brown DL, et al. Incidence and risk factors for side effects of spinal anesthesia. *Anesthesiology* 76:906, 1992.
9. Geerts WH, Heit JA, Clagett GP, et al. Prevention of venous thromboembolism. *Chest* 119:132S, 2001.
10. Song D, Greilich NB, White PF, et al. Recovery profiles and costs of anesthesia for outpatient unilateral inguinal herniorrhaphy. *Anesth Analg* 91:876, 2000.
11. Li S, Coloma M, White PF, et al. Comparison of the costs and recovery profiles of three anesthetic techniques for ambulatory anorectal surgery. *Anesthesiology* 93:1225, 2000.
12. Pittoni G, Toffoletto F, Calcarella G, et al. Spinal anesthesia in outpatient knee surgery: 22-gauge versus 25-gauge Sprotte needle. *Anesth Analg* 81:73, 1995.
13. Garcia F, Bustos A, Sariego M, et al. Intradural anesthesia with a 27-gauge Sprotte needle for arthroscopic knee surgery in ambulatory patients under 40 years of age. *Rev Esp Anestesiol Reanim* 45:263, 1998.
14. Pollock JE. Transient neurologic symptoms: Etiology, risk factors, and management. *Reg Anesth Pain Med* 27:581, 2002.
15. Hodgson PS, Neal JM, Pollock JE, et al. The neurotoxicity of drugs given intrathecally (spinal). *Anesth Analg* 88:797, 1999.
16. Freedman JM, Li DK, Drasner K, et al. Transient neurologic symptoms after spinal anesthesia: An epidemiologic study of 1,863 patients. *Anesthesiology* 89:633, 1998.
17. Pollock JE, Neal JM, Stephenson CA, et al. Prospective study of the incidence of transient radicular irritation in patients undergoing spinal anesthesia. *Anesthesiology* 84:1361, 1996.
18. Lindh A, Andersson AS, Westman L. Is transient lumbar pain after spinal anaesthesia with lidocaine influenced by early mobilisation? *Acta Anaesthesiol Scand* 45:290, 2001.
19. Chiu AA, Liu S, Carpenter RL, et al. The effects of epinephrine on lidocaine spinal anesthesia: A cross-over study. *Anesth Analg* 80:735, 1995.
20. Lau H, Lam B. Management of postoperative urinary retention: A randomized trial of in-out versus overnight catheterization. *Aust N Z J Surg* 74:658, 2004.
21. Tammela T. Postoperative urinary retention: Why the patient cannot void. *Scand J Urol Nephrol Suppl* 175:75, 1995.
22. Petros JG, Rimm EB, Robillard RJ, et al. Factors influencing postoperative urinary retention in patients undergoing elective inguinal herniorrhaphy. *Am J Surg* 161:431, 1991.
23. Lamonerie L, Marret E, Deleuze A, et al. Prevalence of postoperative bladder distension and urinary retention detected by ultrasound measurement. *Br J Anaesth* 92:544, 2004.
24. Stallard S, Prescott S. Postoperative urinary retention in general surgical patients. *Br J Surg* 75:1141, 1988.
25. Haskell DL, Sunshine B, Heifetz CJ. A study of bladder catheterization with inguinal hernia operations. *Arch Surg* 109:378, 1974.
26. Mulroy MF, Salinas FV, Larkin KL, et al. Ambulatory surgery patients may be discharged before voiding after short-acting spinal and epidural anesthesia. *Anesthesiology* 97:315, 2002.
27. Liu S, Chiu AA, Carpenter RL, et al. Fentanyl prolongs lidocaine spinal anesthesia without prolonging recovery. *Anesth Analg* 80:730, 1995.
28. Gilbert A, Owens BD, Mulroy MF. Epidural hematoma after outpatient epidural anesthesia. *Anesth Analg* 94:77, 2002.
29. Gerancher JC, Waterer R, Middleton J. Transient paraparesis after postdural puncture spinal hematoma in a patient receiving ketorolac. *Anesthesiology* 86:490, 1997.
30. Horlocker TT, Wedel DJ, Benzon H, et al. Regional anesthesia in the anticoagulated patient: Defining the risks (the second ASRA Consensus Conference on Neuraxial Anesthesia and Anticoagulation). *Reg Anesth Pain Med* 28:172, 2003.
31. Ben-David B, DeMeo PJ, Lucyk C, et al. A comparison of minidose lidocaine-fentanyl spinal anesthesia and local anesthesia/propofol infusion for outpatient knee arthroscopy. *Anesth Analg* 93:319, 2001.
32. Lennox PH, Chilvers C, Vaghadia H. Selective spinal anesthesia versus desflurane anesthesia in short duration outpatient gynecological laparoscopy: A pharmacoeconomic comparison. *Anesth Analg* 94:565, 2002.
33. Lennox PH, Vaghadia H, Henderson C, et al. Small-dose selective spinal anesthesia for short-duration outpatient laparoscopy: Recovery characteristics compared with desflurane anesthesia. *Anesth Analg* 94:346, 2002.
34. Markey JR, Montiague R, Winnie AP. A comparative efficacy study of hyperbaric 5% lidocaine and 1.5% lidocaine for spinal anesthesia. *Anesth Analg* 85:1105, 1997.
35. Liu SS, Ware PD, Allen HW, et al. Dose-response characteristics of spinal bupivacaine in volunteers. Clinical implications for ambulatory anesthesia. *Anesthesiology* 85:729, 1996.
36. Maroof M, Khan RM, Siddique M, et al. Hypobaric spinal anaesthesia with bupivacaine (0.1%) gives selective sensory block for ano-rectal surgery. *Can J Anaesth* 42:691, 1995.

37. Roussel JR, Heindel L. Effects of intrathecal fentanyl on duration of bupivacaine spinal blockade for outpatient knee arthroscopy. *AANA J* 67:337, 1999.

38. Ben-David B, Solomon E, Levin H, et al. Intrathecal fentanyl with small-dose dilute bupivacaine: Better anesthesia without prolonging recovery. *Anesth Analg* 85:560, 1997.

39. Kouri ME, Kopacz DJ. Spinal 2-chloroprocaine: A comparison with lidocaine in volunteers. *Anesth Analg* 98:75, 2004.

40. Smith KN, Kopacz DJ, McDonald SB. Spinal 2-chloroprocaine: A dose-ranging study and the effect of added epinephrine. *Anesth Analg* 98:81, 2004.

41. Vath JS, Kopacz DJ. Spinal 2-chloroprocaine: The effect of added fentanyl. *Anesth Analg* 98:89, 2004.

42. Davis BR, Kopacz DJ. Spinal 2-chloroprocaine: The effect of added clonidine. *Anesth Analg* 100:559, 2005.

43. Warren DT, Kopacz DJ. Spinal 2-chloroprocaine: The effect of added dextrose. *Anesth Analg* 98:95, 2004.

44. Yoos JR, Kopacz DJ. Spinal 2-chloroprocaine for surgery: An initial 10-month experience. *Anesth Analg* 100:553, 2005.

45. Drasner K. Chloroprocaine spinal anesthesia: Back to the future? *Anesth Analg* 100:549, 2005.

46. Famewo CE, Naguib M. Spinal anaesthesia with meperidine as the sole agent. *Can Anaesth Soc J* 32:533, 1985.

47. Dobrydnjov I, Axelsson K, Thorn SE, et al. Clonidine combined with small-dose bupivacaine during spinal anesthesia for inguinal herniorrhaphy: A randomized double-blinded study. *Anesth Analg* 96:1496, 2003.

48. De Kock M, Gautier P, Fanard L, et al. Intrathecal ropivacaine and clonidine for ambulatory knee arthroscopy: A dose-response study. *Anesthesiology* 94:574, 2001.

49. Moore JM, Liu SS, Pollock JE, et al. The effect of epinephrine on small-dose hyperbaric bupivacaine spinal anesthesia: Clinical implications for ambulatory surgery. *Anesth Analg* 86:973, 1998.

50. Fanelli G, Borghi B, Casati A, et al. Unilateral bupivacaine spinal anesthesia for outpatient knee arthroscopy. Italian Study Group on Unilateral Spinal Anesthesia. *Can J Anaesth* 47:746, 2000.

51. Valanne JV, Korhonen AM, Jokela RM, et al. Selective spinal anesthesia: A comparison of hyperbaric bupivacaine 4 mg versus 6 mg for outpatient knee arthroscopy. *Anesth Analg* 93:1377, 2001.

52. Borghi B. Unilateral spinal block for outpatient knee arthroscopy: A dose-finding study. *J Clin Anesth* 15:351, 2003.

53. Kiran S, Upma B. Use of small-dose bupivacaine (3 mg vs 4 mg) for unilateral spinal anesthesia in the outpatient setting. *Anesth Analg* 99:302, 2004.

54. Mulroy MF, Larkin KL, Hodgson PS, et al. A comparison of spinal, epidural, and general anesthesia for outpatient knee arthroscopy. *Anesth Analg* 91:860, 2000.

55. Neal JM, Deck JJ, Kopacz DJ, et al. Hospital discharge after ambulatory knee arthroscopy: A comparison of epidural 2-chloroprocaine versus lidocaine. *Reg Anesth Pain Med* 26:35, 2001.

56. Pflug AE, Aasheim GM, Foster C. Sequence of return of neurological function and criteria for safe ambulation following subarachnoid block (spinal anaesthetic). *Can Anaesth Soc J* 25:133, 1978.

Spinal and Epidural Blockade for Gynecologic Surgery

Klaus Kjaer
Joon Kim

INTRODUCTION

Gynecologic surgery includes a wide variety of procedures, many of which are performed in the ambulatory setting. Procedures range from the relatively simple dilation and curettage (D&C) to the more complex staging laparotomy for advanced gynecologic cancer. Pain pathways from pelvic structures are transmitted via sacral, lumbar, and thoracic nerve roots up to T10. Peritoneal irritation may involve nerve roots as high as T4. While a T4 block is not difficult to establish, general anesthesia is frequently chosen for a variety of reasons, particularly for procedures where blockade of thoracic dermatomes is necessary.[1]

Provider perceptions of time inefficiency in the operating room (OR) and the postanesthesia care unit (PACU) may be real or perceived. Efficiency can be increased by OR systems designed to take maximal advantage of neuraxial anesthesia, or by using newer low-dose techniques. Patient concerns can be effectively alleviated by preoperative education and reassurance from the anesthesiologist. Administration of intravenous opioids prior to block placement and intravenous anxiolytics during surgery can significantly increase patient comfort during a regional anesthetic. When administered skillfully, patient satisfaction with neuraxial blockade is very high (greater than 90%).[2]

This chapter will review the advantages, disadvantages, and unique considerations for applying neuraxial blocks for commonly performed gynecologic procedures.

GYNECOLOGIC LAPAROTOMY

Intraoperative Management

Laparotomy inevitably involves manipulation of bowel and peritoneum. Visceral pain from such manipulation can be difficult to control with neuraxial blockade, and a T4 thoracic

sensory block is required. Consequently, general anesthesia is preferred by many clinicians. When used, neuraxial anesthesia is often combined with heavy sedation or light general anesthesia.

Visceral pain from bowel and peritoneal manipulation is not well understood. Recent studies have implicated the dorsal column pathway as an important mediator of visceral pain.[3] It is clear that there is less visceral pain when the level of neuraxial blockade is higher. In a series of 200 patients who underwent abdominal hysterectomy under neuraxial anesthesia, those with sensory blockade higher than T3 required less rescue intravenous medications, and fewer needed to be converted to general anesthesia.[4] In addition, neuraxial opioids reduce visceral pain. This has been demonstrated in patients undergoing abdominal hysterectomy and laparoscopy.[5]

Spinal Anesthesia

Spinal anesthesia has the advantage of providing a fast, dense, and reliable block with a low dose of local anesthetic. The choice of local anesthetic drug should be individualized to the patient and the expected duration of laparotomy. Bupivacaine is popular due to its reliable sensory block, long duration at higher dosages, and low incidence of transient neurologic symptoms.[6,7] Hyperbaric preparations permit greater control of block height, as cephalad spread of local anesthetic can be regulated via patient positioning.[8]

A variety of adjuvants can be added to enhance the quality of a spinal block (Table 12-1).[9,10] For laparotomy, opioids in particular are beneficial because they prolong the duration of sensory analgesia and reduce visceral pain.[1] α-Adrenergic agents are also useful adjuncts for laparotomy. In a series of 73 patients undergoing mostly abdominal hysterectomies, adding 15–30 μg of clonidine to intrathecal bupivacaine 15 mg prolonged the duration of motor block, increased the cephalad extent of sensory block, and lengthened the

Table 12-1

Adjuvants to Spinal Anesthesia

Drug	Dose	Effect
Sufentanil	10 µg IT	Prolongs sensory analgesia by 60 min
		Reduces block failure at low bupivacaine doses[1]
Fentanyl	25 µg IT	Equivalent to sufentanil 10 µg
		Reduces shoulder pain from laparoscopy from 68 to 28%[5]
Meperidine	10 mg IT	Equivalent to sufentanil 5 µg
		Provides 60–90 min of additional analgesia
		Side effects: nausea, respiratory depression[9]
Epinephrine	0.2 mg IT	Prolongs sensory analgesia by 30 min
		Prolongs time to void by 80 min[12–14]
Clonidine	0.2 mg PO	Prolongs motor and sensory block with lidocaine by 30 min when given 1.5 h before block initiation
		Side effects: sedation, bradycardia[10]
	15–30 µg IT	Expanded sensory block, prolonged duration of motor block, and prolonged analgesia[11]
Neostigmine	1–5 µg IT	Combined with IT morphine 100 µg, time to first rescue analgesic doubles from 3 to 6 h and 24 h analgesic consumption decreases[25]
Nitrous oxide	50%	Increases sensory level by 2 cm after 10 min[1]

Abbreviations: IT = intrathecal, PO = oral.

duration of postoperative analgesia without additional side effects.[11]

Intrathecal epinephrine 200 µg prolongs surgical anesthesia by approximately 30 min, while 50 µg provides no additional benefit in terms of intraoperative analgesia or operating conditions.[12] Drawbacks to the use of epinephrine are prolonged motor block and delayed time to void by up to 80 min.[13,14] These drawbacks are less likely to be issues for laparotomy patients, who most often are admitted to the hospital after surgery with urinary catheters.

▶ Epidural Anesthesia

Epidural compared to spinal anesthesia has the advantage of being a continuous technique and allows the patient to receive epidural analgesia following surgery. However, sacral blockade is less reliable with an epidural technique and this is a significant drawback for procedures involving significant perineal pain. There is a growing interest in combined spinal-epidural anesthesia (CSE), as it combines some of the favorable elements of each technique while minimizing their respective disadvantages.

▶ Postoperative Analgesia

Improved postoperative pain control is a generally accepted benefit of neuraxial blockade and has been confirmed in gynecologic surgical populations. Compared to general anesthesia alone, neuraxial blockade either alone or in combination with general anesthesia was associated with reduced postoperative pain after uterine surgery.[15,16] The concept of preemptive analgesia has been proposed from observations that postoperative analgesia sometimes outlasts the known pharmacologic duration of the given analgesic. It has been hypothesized that neuraxial blockade limits neural afferent stimulation, which prevents a state of hyperexcitability, whereby subsequent stimuli further potentiate neural impulses and intensify pain. However, preincisional as opposed to preemergence epidural bupivacaine and fentanyl did not reduce 48-h postoperative morphine requirements after abdominal hysterectomy.[17] This was consistent with other hysterectomy studies in which preincisional as opposed to postincisional epidural bupivacaine administration, and preinduction as opposed to postextubation spinal bupivacaine administration, did not produce any preemptive analgesic effect.[18,19] Therefore, current evidence suggests that while neuraxial blockade improves postoperative analgesia, it does so without a preemptive analgesia effect.

Intrathecal morphine is a widely used adjuvant for postoperative analgesia. Drawbacks include nausea, pruritus, and the need for close surveillance for delayed respiratory depression. In 80 patients undergoing abdominal hysterectomy, patients were randomized to receive 0, 0.1, 0.3, and 0.5 mg intrathecal morphine.[20] Analgesia was deemed inadequate after morphine 0 and 0.1 mg, while the 0.5 mg dose was associated with an unacceptably high incidence of side effects. Therefore, the authors concluded that 0.3 mg was the optimal intrathecal morphine dose. No respiratory depression was observed with any dose. Another group of investigators randomized 343 gynecologic surgery patients to intrathecal morphine 0.2, 0.25, or 0.3 mg.[21] The authors concluded that the optimum dose was 0.2 mg, as higher doses did not provide better analgesia but resulted in more side effects. Combining the results of these studies suggests that 0.2 mg intrathecal morphine is the best analgesic dose for uterine procedures.

Other adjuvants are synergistic with intrathecal morphine as they enhance and prolong analgesia. Epinephrine 120 µg added to intrathecal tetracaine and morphine 0.2 mg enhanced the quality and duration of postoperative pain control after abdominal hysterectomy and oophorectomy without increasing the incidence of side effects, when compared to intrathecal morphine alone, or epinephrine alone (Fig. 12-1).[22] Use of neostigmine is more controversial. Intrathecal neostigmine 100 µg, in combination with bupivacaine, but without opioid, did not result in effective postabdominal hysterectomy analgesia. It was also associated with a high incidence of postoperative nausea and vomiting (PONV).[23] A follow-up study in vaginal hysterectomy

patients with neostigmine 25 µg, in combination with fentanyl 25 µg and bupivacaine, prolonged time to first rescue medication to 338 min compared with 238 min for fentanyl and bupivacaine alone. There was a slightly higher incidence of PONV, but this was not statistically significant.[24] Very low-dose neostigmine, 1–5 µg, in combination with intrathecal morphine 0.1 mg, doubled the time to first rescue analgesic from 3 to 6 h and decreased total analgesic consumption over 24 h without an increase in side effects compared to saline control.[25] Although the study was underpowered to find a statistical difference, the data suggest that the addition of low-dose neostigmine to morphine improved analgesia compared to morphine alone.

Epidural morphine also improves postoperative pain control after abdominal hysterectomy (Fig. 12-2).[26] Doses

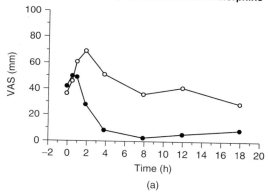

Extradural vs patient-controlled IV morphine

(a)

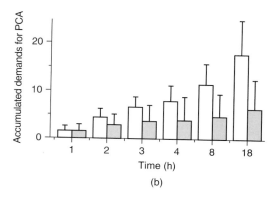

(b)

FIGURE 12-2. Comparison of epidural and patient-controlled intravenous morphine for postabdominal hysterectomy after standardized combined epidural-general anesthesia for abdominal hysterectomy. VAS = visual analog score, PCA = patient-controlled analgesia. Solid circles and bars are epidural morphine. Open circles and bars are intravenous morphine. There was a significant difference in pain scores ($P < 0.001$) (a) and accumulated PCA demands ($P < 0.001$) (b) between groups. *Used with permission from Eriksson-Mjoberg M, Svensson JO, Almkvist O, et al. Extradural morphine gives better pain relief than patient-controlled I.V. morphine after hysterectomy. Br J Anesth 78:10, 1997.*

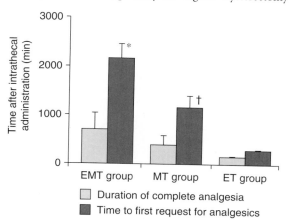

FIGURE 12-1. Duration of complete analgesia after tetracaine (T) spinal anesthesia for abdominal hysterectomy ($n = 31$) and oopherectomy ($n = 5$). Adjuvants studied were morphine (M) 0.2 mg and/or epinephrine (E) 0.12 mg. *$P < 0.05$ vs. MT and ET groups. †$P < 0.05$ vs. ET group. *Used with permission from Goyagi T, Nishikawa T. The addition of epinephrine enhances postoperative analgesia by intrathecal morphine. Anesth Analg 81: 508, 1995.*

between 2 and 4 mg were effective while minimizing adverse reactions.[27] Prophylactic intravenous dexamethasone 8 mg or ondansetron 4 mg reduced the incidence of PONV associated with epidural morphine 3 mg after abdominal hysterectomy.[28,29]

▶ Advantages of Neuraxial Anesthesia

Patients undergoing gynecologic surgery are at especially high risk for PONV, with a reported incidence of 50–93%.[30,31] While there are no data directly comparing regional and general anesthesia for gynecologic surgery with respect to PONV, recent studies of other surgical populations have shown that general anesthesia is associated with a higher incidence of PONV.[32]

Earlier return of bowel function is another potential benefit of epidural analgesia with local anesthetics and appears to be mostly secondary to a reduction in postoperative opioid requirements. Bowel function returned significantly earlier when patients were given epidural bupivacaine instead of parenteral opioids or epidural morphine after abdominal hysterectomy.[33] In a more recent study, use of postoperative epidural bupivacaine for 24 h accelerated time to first flatus, but not time to defecation when compared postoperative nonsteroidal anti-inflammatory drugs (NSAIDs) and acetaminophen, as both groups consumed similar amount of morphine 24–72 h after abdominal hysterectomy (Fig. 12-3).[34]

Another benefit of neuraxial blockade for laparotomy includes a reduction in the number of thromboembolic events after neuraxial compared to general anesthesia.[35] Patients who underwent hysterectomy with epidural anesthesia had lower factor VIII complex levels compared to those who had general anesthesia.[36] A decrease in the stress response was noted: plasma glucose and cortisol levels were lower in patients undergoing abdominal hysterectomy with neuraxial compared to general neuraxial anesthesia. The effect, however, was transient and correlated with regression of sensory analgesia.[37,38] Combining neuraxial and general anesthesia also limited the rise in plasma aldosterone levels.[39] The clinical implications of these findings are not known.

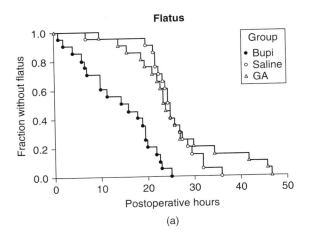

(a)

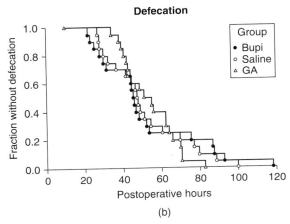

(b)

FIGURE 12-3. Fraction of patients with flatus (a) and defecation (b). ● = general anesthesia, intraoperative epidural lidocaine, and postoperative epidural bupivacaine; Δ = general anesthesia, postoperative epidural saline; and ○ = intraoperative epidural lidocaine and postoperative epidural saline. There was a significant difference in time to first flatus in the group that received postoperative bupivacaine compared to the other groups ($P = 0.009$), but no difference among groups in time to defecation. *Used with permission from Jorgensen H, Fomsgaard JS, Dirks J, et al. Effect of peri- and postoperative epidural anaesthesia on pain and gastrointestinal function after abdominal hysterectomy. Br J Anaesth 87: 577, 2001.*

VAGINAL HYSTERECTOMY

Vaginal hysterectomy eliminates the need for an abdominal incision and requires less muscle relaxation compared to abdominal hysterectomy. In addition, a lower dermatomal sensory blockade is needed due to decreased manipulation of the visceral structures. T10 sensory block should provide sufficient anesthesia. In a retrospective analysis of vaginal hysterectomies, there was no difference in OR time between spinal and general anesthesia. The spinal anesthesia group, however, remained in the PACU on average 27 min longer than patients who received general anesthesia secondary to prolonged motor block (168 min vs. 141 min).[40] Complete motor recovery was necessary for PACU discharge in this study population.

GYNECOLOGIC LAPAROSCOPY

Initially used for diagnoses of infertility and pelvic pain, laparoscopy is now used for a growing number of operative gynecologic procedures. Its advantages include less postoperative pain, decreased recovery time, decreased stress response, preserved immune function, fewer wound complications, and lower risk of adhesions.[41] The procedure entails inserting a Verres needle through the umbilicus by which CO_2 is insufflated into the peritoneal cavity. The Verres needle is then replaced by a large trocar. A camera with a fiberoptic light source is inserted through the trocar to visualize the peritoneum. One or more suprapubic incisions are made for additional trocars for forceps, cutting, coagulation, laser, suction, or irrigation. A uterine manipulator is often inserted vaginally as well.

CO_2 pneumoperitoneum creates extensive physiologic disturbances. Hemodynamic changes are summarized in Table 12-2. Increased intra-abdominal pressure and elevation of the diaphragm results in decreased functional residual capacity (FRC), increased dead space ventilation, increased ventilation-perfusion mismatch, decreased pulmonary compliance (47%), and increased peak airway pressures (50–81%). Absorption of insufflated CO_2 leads to acidosis and increased respiratory drive. Minute ventilation required to maintain constant $PaCO_2$ increases by up to 55%. Intracranial pressure increases regardless of $PaCO_2$ and is unresponsive to hyperventilation. Perfusion to splanchnic structures decreases due to mechanical compression of mesenteric vasculature. Urine output drops from reduced glomerular filtration rate and elevated serum levels of antidiuretic hormone (ADH). Many of these disturbances are further exacerbated by the Trendelenburg position.[41,42]

Table 12-2

Hemodynamic Changes During Laparoscopy

	Pneumoperitoneum	Gasless Laparoscopy
Heart rate	↔	↔
Systemic vascular resistance	↑	↑
Mean arterial pressure	↑	↑
Cardiac output	↓	↑
Central venous pressure	↑	↔
Pulmonary capillary wedge pressure	↑	↔

Respiratory compromise from pneumoperitoneum and the Trendelenburg position can be a significant obstacle to using neuraxial anesthesia. For lengthy operations or for those that require steep Trendelenburg position, general anesthesia with controlled ventilation has traditionally been the preferred technique. However, there is evidence that awake, spontaneously breathing patients can tolerate laparoscopy quite well. In one study of patients undergoing laparoscopy under epidural anesthesia with 20-degree Trendelenburg tilt, there was no increase in $PaCO_2$, as patients were able to autoregulate their minute ventilation.[43]

Laparoscopy is thought to increase the risk of gastroesophageal reflux due to increased intra-abdominal pressures and Trendelenburg (head-down) position. However, this fear appears to be unfounded as numerous studies have been unable to demonstrate a higher incidence of reflux or aspiration during laparoscopy. During pneumoperitoneum, it appears that the lower esophageal pressure increases to a greater degree than intragastric pressure which prevents regurgitation of gastric contents.[42]

Intraoperative referred shoulder pain, on the other hand, is a significant problem. It results from thermal, mechanical, and chemical irritation of diaphragm. As CO_2 expands during entry into the peritoneum, intraperitoneal temperatures can fall to as low as 27.7 degrees.[44] Intraperitoneal pH also decreases to 6.0 immediately after surgery and normalizes above 7.0 only by the second or third postoperative day.[45] Drying of peritoneal cells also results in cellular death.[46]

Using heated and humidified CO_2 can reduce patient discomfort. Fewer patients complained of shoulder pain (5% vs. 40%) and shivering (0% vs. 55%) when humidified CO_2 was used during awake microlaparoscopy.[47] For patients who experienced shoulder pain after their previous laparoscopy, using heated and humidified CO_2 resulted in better patient tolerance, decreased conversion to general anesthesia (10% vs. 50%), and shorter recovery times after awake laparoscopy. Fewer patients required sedation and more patients were able to tolerate insufflation of more than 1200 mL of CO_2 (65% vs. 20%).[46]

Laparoscopy can be performed without pneumoperitoneum. Also known as gasless laparoscopy, subcutaneous wires are used to lift the abdominal wall. Neuraxial anesthesia can be employed more easily for these operations since the physiologic disturbances and shoulder discomfort from CO_2 insufflation are mostly absent. In one study involving 279 gasless laparoscopic myomectomies, 57 were performed under epidural anesthesia by patient preference. No conversion to general anesthesia was necessary.[48] Another group reported 21 cases of gasless laparoscopy for gynecologic surgery, all under epidural anesthesia, without supplemental drugs.[49]

Intrathecal opioids reduce the incidence of shoulder and upper chest discomfort. In a double-blind prospective trial, addition of fentanyl 25 µg to lidocaine 20 mg reduced the

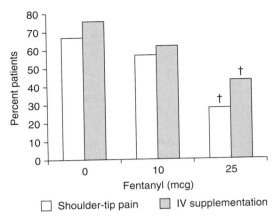

FIGURE 12-4. Decrease in shoulder-tip pain and need for intraoperative intravenous supplementation during lidocaine spinal anesthesia for laparoscopy with addition of intrathecal fentanyl 0, 10, and 25 µg. †$P < 0.05$ compared to fentanyl 0 µg. *Data from Ref. 5.*

occurrence of shoulder pain from 67 to 28% (Fig. 12-4). It also reduced the requirement for supplementation with IV analgesics intraoperatively, and prolonged time to first request for postoperative analgesia. Motor recovery and discharge times were similar.[5]

Other measures to maximize patient comfort include minimizing the degree of Trendelenburg tilt, minimizing insufflation pressures to below 15 mmHg, and limiting the total amount of insufflated CO_2.[50] Prophylactic glycopyrrolate is also useful to prevent vasovagal episodes that can occur with the combination of laparoscopy and spinal anesthesia.[51] A list of useful systemic pharmacologic adjuvants is provided in Table 12-3.

Table 12-3

Useful Local or Systemic Adjuvants to Neuraxial Anesthesia for Laparoscopy

Drug	Effect
Midazolam	Anxiolytic
Fentanyl	Analgesic
Infiltrate local anesthetic	Analgesic
Acetaminophen	Analgesic
NSAIDs	Analgesic/anti-inflammatory
5-HT$_3$ receptor antagonists	Antiemetic
Dexamethasone	Antiemetic
Perphenazine	Antiemetic
Glycopyrrolate	Vagolytic

Abbreviation: 5-HT$_3$ = serotonin 5-hydroxytryptamine 3.

In summary, despite potential problems, neuraxial anesthesia can play an important role in the care of patients undergoing laparoscopy. Neuraxial blockade is associated with improved postoperative pain and less PONV compared to general anesthesia. The ability to be awake and communicate with the surgeon can be an advantage, and even a prerequisite, for procedures such as pain mapping, and some patients prefer to be awake.[50]

▶ Selective Spinal Anesthesia

As many laparoscopies are performed on an outpatient basis, there has been a growing interest in using reduced doses of local anesthetics in order to minimize adverse effects such as hypotension, bladder distention, and prolonged recovery times. Opioids facilitate reduction in local anesthetic doses by prolonging sensory block, improving tolerance to visceral sensations such as bladder or bowel irritation and peritoneal stretch, without delaying time to void.

Short duration laparoscopies are successfully performed with intrathecal lidocaine 10–20 mg when an opioid (sufentanil 10 µg or fentanyl 25 µg) is added as an adjuvant.[52] This has been called selective spinal anesthesia (SSA), and results in anesthesia in which the nociceptive fibers are blocked with minimal doses of local anesthetics, but motor and dorsal column functions are preserved. The combination of lidocaine 10 mg and sufentanil 10 µg resulted in motor block of the shortest duration. While still in the OR, 80% of patients were able to perform deep knee bends at the end of a 15-min laparoscopy, and most were able to fulfill discharge criteria. There were no conversions to general anesthesia even though one procedure took 87 min. The incidence of shoulder pain was 60–100%, but this was successfully relieved with intravenous alfentanil. Since light touch and proprioception were preserved, patients required reassurance that they would be aware of stimuli such as preparation of the skin and perineum and insertion of instruments, but that they would not feel any pain during surgery.

SSA compares favorably to general anesthesia with respect to OR and PACU efficiency. In a study of 40 patients for outpatient gynecologic laparoscopy, SSA with lidocaine 10 mg and sufentanil 10 µg was compared to general anesthesia with propofol, mivacurium, fentanyl, and nitrous oxide. At the conclusion of surgery, both groups received perphenazine 1 mg IV, diclofenac 100 mg PR, and local infiltration of 0.25% bupivacaine at the incision sites. The times to leave the OR, perform straight leg raises, and perform deep knee bends, were all shorter with SSA. SSA patients spent more time in the PACU. This was due to discharge criteria requiring complete recovery of sensory function in spite of the ability to ambulate.[53]

The total economic cost was similar between SSA and general anesthesia with propofol.[49]

SSA also has a similar recovery profile to desflurane general anesthesia. Investigators compared SSA with lidocaine 10 mg and sufentanil 10 μg to general anesthesia with propofol and mivacurium induction, intratracheal lidocaine, and desflurane maintenance titrated to a bispectral index (BIS) between 45 and 65. All patients were given oral acetaminophen 975 mg 30 min preoperatively and diclofenac 100 mg rectal suppository, perphenazine 1 mg IV, and local infiltration with 0.25% bupivacaine at the incision sites. Patients in the SSA group exhibited faster emergence, better postoperative pain control, and a higher incidence of pruritus that resolved spontaneously without intervention. Again, although time to ambulation was shorter with SSA (3 min vs. 59 min), overall duration of PACU stay was similar in both groups because complete recovery of sensory block was required prior to discharge.[54] Allowing patients to ambulate in the presence of selective neuraxial block is an accepted practice in the obstetric setting; however, it remains controversial whether patients can be discharged with residual sensory block after ambulatory surgery.

As with lidocaine, addition of an opioid helps to establish effective blockade with low-dose bupivacaine. Hyperbaric bupivacaine 5.25 mg plus fentanyl 20 μg was found to have a similar profile to lidocaine 30 mg plus fentanyl 20 μg with respect to block height and time to T12 regression. The lidocaine group had longer duration of motor block (75 min vs. 56 min) but time to ambulation was the same (117 min). The bupivacaine group had a longer time to micturition (164 min vs. 133 min) and a lower incidence of transient neurologic symptoms (0% vs. 7%).[55]

Typical local anesthetic and opioid doses used for SSA for laparoscopic surgery are summarized in Table 12-4.

HYSTEROSCOPY

Hysteroscopy is used to visualize the intrauterine cavity in order to diagnose and treat causes of infertility and abnormal bleeding. After the cervix is dilated, the uterine cavity is distended with gas (CO_2), and a low viscosity fluid (normal saline, lactated Ringers, or glycine) or high viscosity fluid (dextran 70 or Hyskon). The hysteroscope is then introduced into the cervical canal and advanced into the uterine cavity under visual guidance. Other surgical instruments such as forceps, scissors, electrocautery, and laser are subsequently inserted for resection of submucous fibroids, polyps, or adhesions.

While operative hysteroscopy typically requires general or neuraxial anesthesia, diagnostic hysteroscopy can be performed under local anesthesia only.[56,57] However, endometrial ablation, which involves removal of the whole thickness of endometrium, requires either general or neuraxial anesthesia. A high viscosity fluid or glycine is typically used to distend the uterine cavity because its electroneutrality interferes less with electrocautery. However, absorption of hypotonic irrigation solution during resection of endometrium can result in dilutional hyponatremia, pulmonary edema, and cerebral edema. One study suggests that general anesthesia may offer an advantage over neuraxial anesthesia as less glycine was absorbed (380 mL vs. 648 mL).[58] The investigators hypothesized that sympathetic blockade from neuraxial anesthesia and subsequent vasodilation may have caused greater absorption of irrigation solution. Neuraxial anesthesia, however, allows the patient to report shortness of breath or mental status changes from significant absorption of hypotonic irrigation solution.

In a randomized trial of 40 women for hysteroscopic ablation of endometrial neoplasm, titration of short-acting intravenous anesthetic drugs such as propofol and remifentanil resulted in shorter preparation times, earlier discharge,

Table 12-4

SSA Drugs and Doses

	Time Until Regression to S3 Sensory Block* (min)	Duration of Full Motor Block (min)*
Lidocaine 20 mg + fentanyl 10 μg	87	34
Lidocaine 20 mg + fentanyl 25 μg	101	36
Lidocaine 20 mg + sufentanil 10 μg	135	34
Lidocaine 10 mg + sufentanil 10 μg	105	26

*Values are mean values.
Source: Data from Ref. 5, 52.

better patient acceptance, and no increased costs compared with spinal anesthesia with hyperbaric bupivacaine 10 mg. However, this is not surprising given the large dose of bupivacaine used.[59] It seems sensible to perform hysteroscopy under SSA, as has been done successfully for gynecologic laparoscopy.

DILATION AND CURETTAGE AND DILATION AND EVACUATION

A simple D&C may be performed for irregular, unusually heavy, or postmenopausal bleeding. A suction D&C is typically performed for removal of the products of conception prior to 12 weeks gestation. After 12 weeks gestation, this procedure is a second trimester termination and is referred to as a dilation and evacuation (D&E).

A simple D&C can be performed without difficulty under paracervical block, typically performed by the obstetrician. Systemic absorption of local anesthetic after a paracervical block is rapid, and this block has been associated with convulsions. However, plasma levels have been shown to remain below toxic levels if the lidocaine dose for paracervical blocks is limited to less than 100 mg.[60] Paracervical block has also been associated with higher levels of serum prolactin and cortisol, and a higher incidence of fever.[61] However, recent literature has established local anesthesia as safe and efficacious for suction D&C.[62]

On the other hand, general anesthesia with volatile agents has been associated with higher risk of cervical injury, uterine perforation, and hemorrhage.[63] Similarly, for D&E, local anesthesia was associated with fewer complications such as hemorrhage, unintended major surgery, and postoperative temperature greater than 38°C compared to general anesthesia.[64] These findings may be due in part to more aggressive surgical techniques when the patient is anesthetized with general anesthesia, and due in part to uterine relaxation caused by halogenated agents. When propofol is used instead of halogenated agents, the blood loss during D&C is significantly lower.[65,66]

Spinal anesthesia may be used when patients are at high risk for complications from general anesthesia, and would be expected to provide greater patient comfort than paracervical block. A T10 sensory blockade is sufficient to provide anesthesia for these procedures. Special attention needs to be paid when moving the patient from the supine to the lithotomy position, or the reverse, as this may blunt or exacerbate the hemodynamic changes associated with neuraxial anesthesia-induced sympathectomy.

Although it has not been specifically studied with these procedures, SSA is a reasonable technique for these outpatient procedures. Blood loss after spinal anesthesia has not been compared with blood loss after general anesthesia with propofol.

INFERTILITY PROCEDURES

Assisted reproductive technologies (ART) are now used to treat many etiologies of infertility including chronic fallopian tube disease, cervical abnormalities, endometriosis, ovulatory dysfunction, maternal antisperm antibodies, and male factor infertility. The four steps to ART are hormonal stimulation, oocyte retrieval, in vitro fertilization, and embryo transfer. The delivery rate is around 30% per oocyte retrieved.

Hormonal stimulation consists of down-regulation with gonadotropin-releasing hormone (GnRH), then hyperstimulation with human menopausal gonadotropin (hMG), followed by induced ovulation with human chorionic gonadotropin. Oocyte retrieval occurs 24–36 h later and typically takes 15–30 min for which brief deep anesthesia is usually required. Embryo transfer can by a transcervical or intrafallopian approach. The transcervical approach does not require anesthesia, while the intrafallopian approach does.

Anesthetic agents may impact the fertilization rate, early embryo division, and implantation. Anesthetic agents have been detected in follicular fluid in both animal and human studies. Some studies have found that various halogenated agents, N_2O, and propofol adversely affect fertilization and embryonic development, while other studies have found no difference.[67] In addition, NSAIDs administration should be avoided, as changes in prostaglandin production can affect embryo implantation.

Local anesthetics do not appear to interfere with ART. One investigation measured intrafollicular lidocaine levels after paracervical blocks with lidocaine 50 mg, and found no difference in lidocaine levels in fertilized and nonfertilized oocytes. Moreover, patients who did receive lidocaine exhibited no difference in fertilization, cleavage, and overall pregnancy rate compared to a control group of patients who did not receive lidocaine.[68]

Paracervical block may be insufficient for patient comfort during oocyte retrieval.[69] Spinal anesthesia with lidocaine 45 mg and fentanyl 10 µg has been used successfully.[70] Given concerns over transient neurologic syndrome (TNS) with lidocaine, attempts have been made to use low-dose bupivacaine. Bupivacaine 3.75 mg and fentanyl 25 µg resulted in no difference in time to onset and subsequent recovery of motor function compared to lidocaine 30 mg and fentanyl 25 µg. However, the bupivacaine group required more supplemental IV medications and had longer time to void and discharge (Table 12-5).[71]

Table 12-5

Bupivacaine Vs. Lidocaine Spinal Anesthesia for In Vitro Fertilization Procedures: Recovery Profile

	Bupivacaine + Fentanyl (n = 20)*	Lidocaine + Fentanyl (n = 20)†	P-value
	Time (min)‡		
Procedure duration	27 ± 9	29 ± 10	NS
Full motor recovery	53 ± 30	62 ± 21	NS
Full sensory recovery	93 ± 25	94 ± 28	NS
Ambulation	107 ± 37	103 ± 28	NS
Urination	159 ± 38	126 ± 38	<0.05
Hospital discharge	178 ± 41	144 ± 34	<0.05

*Bupivacaine group: hyperbaric bupivacaine 3.75 mg plus fentanyl 25 µg, †lidocaine group: hyperbaric lidocaine 30 mg plus fentanyl 25 µg.
‡Values are mean ± SD. NS = not significant.
Source: Data from Ref. 71.

PELVIC FLOOR PROCEDURES

▶ Urinary Incontinence Procedures

Laparoscopic Burch colposuspension and the tension-free vaginal tape (TVT) procedure are performed to correct stress incontinence. They are typically performed under local or neuraxial anesthesia in order to ensure the patient's ability to cooperate in demonstrating continence intraoperatively. With this approach, the bladder is filled with fluid, the patient is asked to cough, and the suspension is incrementally adjusted until the patient becomes continent under stress. This decreases the risk of postoperative voiding dysfunction.

Good surgical conditions for the TVT procedure can be achieved with local anesthetic infiltration and sedation.[72] Neuraxial anesthesia can also be used for this procedure, but results in relaxation of the pelvic floor and detrusor muscles. This can make assessment of incontinence more difficult.[73] In a prospective randomized comparison of local anesthetic infiltration and epidural anesthesia for the TVT procedure, there were no differences in pain, procedure duration, anxiety level, and blood loss. The local group had earlier voiding, smaller postvoid residuals, and shorter hospital stays. However, there were no differences in the long-term success rate of the procedure (Table 12-6).[74]

While general anesthesia precludes the ability to perform an intraoperative cough stress test, one study reported good results using intraoperative ultrasound instead of patient cooperation to ensure precise positioning of the vaginal tape.[75] A retrospective cohort study also showed that general anesthesia does not increase the risk of postoperative voiding dysfunction with TVT.[76]

Table 12-6

Local Compared to Epidural Anesthesia for TVT Procedures

	Local (n = 36)*	Epidural (n = 36)*	P-value
Peak pain score†	2.69 ± 0.62	2.75 ± 0.50	0.68
Postresidual void during hospitalization (mL)	98 ± 63	155 ± 16	<0.05
Hospital stay (days)	3.4 ± 1.4	5.5 ± 1.6	<0.05
Initial voiding > 6 h postoperatively, n (%)	2 (6)	10 (28)	<0.05
Objective success rate (%)			
Cure	86	86	1.0
Improved	6	3	0.56

*Local group: lidocaine 1%, 60 mL; epidural group: lidocaine 2%, 20 mL injected at L4-L5 interspace. Data are mean ± SD or as indicated.
†Pain assessed using the McGill Pain Questionnaire, adjective descriptor scale for present pain intensity.
Source: Data from Ref. 74.

▶ Anterior-Posterior Repair and Radical Vulvectomy

Anterior-posterior repair is an operation to correct prolapse of the pelvic organs, a condition associated with relaxation of the pelvic floor following vaginal delivery. The patient population presenting for this operation tends to be elderly, and neuraxial anesthesia is an excellent choice for these patients.[77] A saddle block performed by lumbar injection of hyperbaric local anesthetic while the patient maintains a sitting position for 3–5 min will provide excellent anesthesia for perineal areas while avoiding more cephalad spread.

BRACHYTHERAPY

Brachytherapy is an effective treatment for cervical cancer. It involves placement of radioactive seeds near the site of malignancy. Oxygenation status of cervical cancers is a significant prognostic factor for disease-free survival as tumor hypoxia can cause resistance to radiation therapy.[78] Spinal anesthesia has been found to have no influence on oxygenation status of cervical cancers. It should not interfere with the oncologist's ability to make reliable PO_2 measurements or affect oxygen-related efficacy of brachytherapy.[79]

Intrathecal ketamine has been used to supplement bupivacaine spinal anesthesia in order to reduce the dose of bupivacaine to facilitate faster recovery in patients receiving brachytherapy. Bupivacaine 7.5 mg with ketamine 25 mg was compared to bupivacaine 10 mg alone. Requirement for IV fluids and duration of motor block was lower in the ketamine group (116 min vs. 133 min) while analgesic duration was similar. However, the ketamine group had significantly more adverse events such as sedation, dizziness, nystagmus, "strange feelings," and PONV.[80] Ketamine is not approved for intrathecal use in the United States. SSA for brachytherapy has not been studied.

SUMMARY

Many factors which discourage the use of neuraxial blockade for gynecologic surgery can be overcome with appropriate techniques and adjuvant agents. Advantages of regional anesthesia for gynecologic surgery include better postoperative analgesia and less nausea. Gasless laparoscopy is an alternative to laparoscopy with pneumoperitoneum, and may be easier to perform under regional anesthesia. Intrathecal opioids permit very low doses of local anesthetic for spinal anesthesia, which can result in SSA. SSA has a highly favorable recovery profile. Finally, most gynecologic surgery performed via the vaginal approach can be performed under regional anesthesia.

REFERENCES

1. Vaghadia H. Spinal anesthesia for outpatients: Controversies and new techniques. *Can J Anaesth* 45:R64, 1998.
2. Vaghadia H, McLeod DH, Mitchell GW, et al. Small-dose hypobaric lidocaine-fentanyl spinal anesthesia for short duration outpatient laparoscopy. I. A randomized comparison with conventional dose hyperbaric lidocaine. *Anesth Analg* 84:59, 1997.
3. Palecek J. The role of dorsal columns pathway in visceral pain. *Physiol Res* 53:S125, 2004.
4. Mihic DN, Abram SE. Optimal regional anaesthesia for abdominal hysterectomy: Combined subarachnoid and epidural block compared with other regional techniques. *Eur J Anaesthesiol* 10:297, 1993.
5. Chilvers CR, Vaghadia H, Mitchell GW, et al. Small-dose hypobaric lidocaine-fentanyl spinal anesthesia for short duration outpatient laparoscopy. II. Optimal fentanyl dose. *Anesth Analg* 84:65, 1997.
6. Beilin Y, Zahn J, Abramovitz S, et al. Subarachnoid small-dose bupivacaine versus lidocaine for cervical cerclage. *Anesth Analg* 97:56, 2003.
7. Tsen LC, Schultz R, Martin R, et al. Intrathecal low-dose bupivacaine versus lidocaine for in vitro fertilization procedures. *Reg Anesth Pain Med* 26:52, 2001.
8. Chambers WA, Edstrom HH, Scott DB. Effect of baricity on spinal anaesthesia with bupivacaine. *Br J Anaesth* 53:279, 1981.
9. Ong B, Segstro R. Respiratory depression associated with meperidine spinal anaesthesia. *Can J Anaesth* 41:725, 1994.
10. Dobrydnjov I, Samarutel J. Enhancement of intrathecal lidocaine by addition of local and systemic clonidine. *Acta Anaesthesiol Scand* 43:556, 1999.
11. Juliao MC, Lauretti GR. Low-dose intrathecal clonidine combined with sufentanil as analgesic drugs in abdominal gynecological surgery. *J Clin Anesth* 12:357, 2000.
12. Vaghadia H, Solylo MA, Henderson CL, et al. Selective spinal anesthesia for outpatient laparoscopy. II. Epinephrine and spinal cord function. *Can J Anaesth* 48:261, 2001.
13. Moore JM, Liu SS, Pollock JE, et al. The effect of epinephrine on small-dose hyperbaric bupivacaine spinal anesthesia: Clinical implications for ambulatory surgery. *Anesth Analg* 86:973, 1998.
14. Chambers WA, Littlewood DG, Scott DB. Spinal anesthesia with hyperbaric bupivacaine: Effect of added vasoconstrictors. *Anesth Analg* 61:49, 1982.
15. Vaida SJ, Ben David B, Somri M, et al. The influence of pre-emptive spinal anesthesia on postoperative pain. *J Clin Anesth* 12:374, 2000.
16. Wang JJ, Ho ST, Liu HS, et al. The effect of spinal versus general anesthesia on postoperative pain and analgesic requirements in patients undergoing lower abdominal surgery. *Reg Anesth* 21:281, 1996.
17. Richards JT, Read JR, Chambers WA. Epidural anaesthesia as a method of pre-emptive analgesia for abdominal hysterectomy. *Anaesthesia* 53:296, 1998.
18. Espinet A, Henderson DJ, Faccenda KA, et al. Does pre-incisional thoracic extradural block combined with diclofenac reduce postoperative pain after abdominal hysterectomy? *Br J Anaesth* 76:209, 1996.
19. Dakin MJ, Osinubi OY, Carli F. Preoperative spinal bupivacaine does not reduce postoperative morphine requirement in women

undergoing total abdominal hysterectomy. *Reg Anesth* 21:99, 1996.

20. Sarma VJ, Bostrom UV. Intrathecal morphine for the relief of post-hysterectomy pain: A double-blind, dose-response study. *Acta Anaesthesiol Scand* 37:223, 1993.

21. Rodanant O, Sirichotewithayakorn P, Sriprajittichai P, et al. An optimal dose study of intrathecal morphine in gynecological patients. *J Med Assoc Thai* 86: S331, 2003.

22. Goyagi T, Nishikawa T. The addition of epinephrine enhances postoperative analgesia by intrathecal morphine. *Anesth Analg* 81:508, 1995.

23. Lauretti GR, Mattos AL, Gomes JM, et al. Postoperative analgesia and antiemetic efficacy after intrathecal neostigmine in patients undergoing abdominal hysterectomy during spinal anesthesia. *Reg Anesth* 22:527, 1997.

24. Lauretti GR, Hood DD, Eisenach JC, et al. A multi-center study of intrathecal neostigmine for analgesia following vaginal hysterectomy. *Anesthesiology* 89:913, 1998.

25. Almeida RA, Lauretti GR, Mattos AL. Antinociceptive effect of low-dose intrathecal neostigmine combined with intrathecal morphine following gynecologic surgery. *Anesthesiology* 98:495, 2003.

26. Eriksson-Mjoberg M, Svensson JO, Almkvist O, et al. Extradural morphine gives better pain relief than patient-controlled i.v. morphine after hysterectomy. *Br J Anaesth* 78:10, 1997.

27. Tanaka M, Watanabe S, Ashimura H, et al. Minimum effective combination dose of epidural morphine and fentanyl for posthysterectomy analgesia: A randomized, prospective, double-blind study. *Anesth Analg* 77:942, 1993.

28. Wang JJ, Ho ST, Liu YH, et al. Dexamethasone decreases epidural morphine-related nausea and vomiting. *Anesth Analg* 89:117, 1999.

29. Tzeng JI, Chu KS, Ho ST, et al. Prophylactic iv ondansetron reduces nausea, vomiting and pruritus following epidural morphine for postoperative pain control. *Can J Anaesth* 50:1023, 2003.

30. Suen TKL, Gin TA, Chen PP, et al. Ondansetron 4mgs for prevention of nausea and vomiting after minor gynaecological surgery. *Anaesth Intensive Care* 22:142, 1996.

31. Bodner M, White P. Antiemetic efficacy of ondansetron after outpatient laparoscopy. *Anesth Analg* 73:250, 1991.

32. Larsson S, Lundberg D. A prospective survey of postoperative nausea and vomiting with special regard to incidence and relations to patient characteristics, anesthetic routines and surgical procedures. *Acta Anaesthesiol Scand* 39:539, 1995.

33. Wattwil M, Thoren T, Hennerdal S, et al. Epidural analgesia with bupivacaine reduces postoperative paralytic ileus after hysterectomy. *Anesth Analg* 68:353, 1989.

34. Jorgensen H, Fomsgaard JS, Dirks J, et al. Effect of peri- and postoperative epidural anaesthesia on pain and gastrointestinal function after abdominal hysterectomy. *Br J Anaesth* 87:577, 2001.

35. Rodgers A, Walker N, Schug S, et al. Reduction of postoperative mortality and morbidity with epidural or spinal anaesthesia: Results from overview of randomised trials. *BMJ* 321:1493, 2000. Review.

36. Bredbacka S, Blomback M, Hagnevik K, et al. Per- and postoperative changes in coagulation and fibrinolytic variables during abdominal hysterectomy under epidural or general anaesthesia. *Acta Anaesthesiol Scand* 30:204, 1986.

37. Cowen MJ, Bullingham RE, Paterson GM, et al. A controlled comparison of the effects of extradural diamorphine and bupivacaine on plasma glucose and plasma cortisol in postoperative patients. *Anesth Analg* 61:15, 1982.

38. Moller IW, Hjortso E, Krantz T, et al. The modifying effect of spinal anaesthesia on intra- and postoperative adrenocortical and hyperglycaemic response to surgery. *Acta Anaesthesiol Scand* 28:266, 1984.

39. Petropoulos G, Vadalouca A, Siafaka I, et al. Renin-aldosterone system alterations during abdominal gynaecological operations under general or combined general and epidural anaesthesia. *Clin Exp Obstet Gynecol* 27:42, 2000.

40. Tessler MJ, Kardash K, Kleiman S, et al. A retrospective comparison of spinal and general anesthesia for vaginal hysterectomy: A time analysis. *Anesth Analg* 81:694, 1995.

41. O'Malley C, Cunningham AJ. Physiologic changes during laparoscopy. *Anesthesiol Clin North America* 19:1, 2001.

42. Smith I. Anesthesia for laparoscopy with emphasis on outpatient laparoscopy. *Anesthesiol Clin North America* 19:21, 2001.

43. Ciofolo MJ, Clergue F, Seebacher J, et al. Ventilatory effects of laparoscopy under epidural anesthesia. *Anesth Analg* 70:357, 1990.

44. Jacobs VR, Morrison JE Jr, Mettler L, et al. Measurement of CO(2) hypothermia during laparoscopy and pelviscopy: How cold it gets and how to prevent it. *J Am Assoc Gynecol Laparosc* 6:289, 1999.

45. Mouton WG, Bessell JR, Otten KT, et al. Pain after laparoscopy. *Surg Endosc* 13:445, 1999.

46. Demco L. Effect of heating and humidifying gas on patients undergoing awake laparoscopy. *J Am Assoc Gynecol Laparosc* 8:247, 2001.

47. Almeida OD Jr. Awake microlaparoscopy with the Insuflow device. *JSLS* 6:199, 2002.

48. Damiani A, Melgrati L, Marziali M, et al. Gasless laparoscopic myomectomy. Indications, surgical technique and advantages of a new procedure for removing uterine leiomyomas. *J Reprod Med* 48:792, 2003.

49. Li B, Hao J, Gao X, et al. Gynecological procedures under gasless laparoscopy. *Chin Med J (Engl)* 114:514, 2001.

50. Collins LM, Vaghadia H. Regional anesthesia for laparoscopy. *Anesthesiol Clin North America* 19:43, 2001. Review.

51. Chilvers CR, Goodwin A, Vaghadia H, et al. Selective spinal anesthesia for outpatient laparoscopy. V. Pharmacoeconomic comparison vs general anesthesia. *Can J Anaesth* 48:279, 2001.

52. Vaghadia H, Viskari D, Mitchell GW, et al. Selective spinal anesthesia for outpatient laparoscopy. I. Characteristics of three hypobaric solutions. *Can J Anaesth* 48:256, 2001.

53. Stewart AV, Vaghadi H, Collins L, et al. Small-dose selective spinal anaesthesia for short-duration outpatient gynaecological laparoscopy: Recovery characteristics compared with propofol anaesthesia. *Br J Anaesth* 86:570, 2001.

54. Lennox PH, Vaghadia H, Henderson C, et al. Small-dose selective spinal anesthesia for short-duration outpatient laparoscopy: Recovery characteristics compared with desflurane anesthesia. *Anesth Analg* 94:346, 2002.

55. Hampl KF, Heinzmann-Wiedmer S, Luginbuehl I, et al. Transient neurologic symptoms after spinal anesthesia: A lower incidence with prilocaine and bupivacaine than with lidocaine. *Anesthesiology* 88:629, 1998.

56. Soriano D, Ajaj S, Chuong T, et al. Lidocaine spray and outpatient hysteroscopy: Randomized placebo-controlled trial. *Obstet Gynecol* 96:661, 2000.

57. Zupi E, Luciano AA, Valli E, et al. The use of topical anesthesia in diagnostic hysteroscopy and endometrial biopsy. *Fertil Steril* 63:414, 1995.

58. Goldenberg M, Cohen SB, Etchin A, et al. A randomized prospective comparative study of general versus epidural anesthesia for transcervical hysteroscopic endometrial resection. *Am J Obstet Gynecol* 184:273, 2001.

59. Danelli G, Berti M, Casati A, et al. Spinal block or total intravenous anaesthesia with propofol and remifentanil for gynaecological outpatient procedures. *Eur J Anaesthesiol* 19:594, 2002.

60. Blanco LJ, Reid PR, King TM. Plasma lidocaine levels following paracervical infiltration for aspiration abortion. *Obstet Gynecol* 60:506, 1982.

61. Beksac MS, Beksac M, Kisnisci HA, et al. Stress-induced release of cortisol and prolactin during dilatation and curettage under general and local anesthesia. *Neuropsychobiology* 11:227, 1984.

62. Thonneau P, Fougeyrollas B, Ducot B, et al. Complications of abortion performed under local anesthesia. *Eur J Obstet Gynecol Reprod Biol* 81:59, 1998.

63. Grimes DA, Schulz KF, Cates W Jr, et al. Local versus general anesthesia: Which is safer for performing suction curettage abortions? *Am J Obstet Gynecol* 135:1030, 1979.

64. MacKay HT, Schulz KF, Grimes DA. Safety of local versus general anesthesia for second-trimester dilatation and evacuation abortion. *Obstet Gynecol* 66:661, 1985.

65. Kumarasinghe N, Harpin R, Stewart AW. Blood loss during suction termination of pregnancy with two different anaesthetic techniques. *Anaesth Intensive Care* 25:48, 1997.

66. Hall JE, Ng WS, Smith S. Blood loss during first trimester termination of pregnancy: Comparison of two anaesthetic techniques. *Br J Anaesth* 78:172, 1997.

67. Wilhelm W, Hammadeh ME, White PF, et al. General anesthesia versus monitored anesthesia care with remifentanil for assisted reproductive technologies: Effect on pregnancy rate. *J Clin Anesth* 14:1, 2002.

68. Wikland M, Evers H, Jakobsson AH, et al. The concentration of lidocaine in follicular fluid when used for paracervical block in a human IVF-ET programme. *Hum Reprod* 5:920, 1990.

69. Hammarberg K, Wikland M, Nilsson L, et al. Patients' experience of transvaginal follicle aspiration under local anesthesia. *Ann N Y Acad Sci* 541:134, 1988.

70. Martin R, Tsen LC, Tzeng G, et al. Anesthesia for in vitro fertilization: The addition of fentanyl to 1.5% lidocaine. *Anesth Analg* 88:523, 1999.

71. Tsen LC, Schultz R, Martin R, et al. Intrathecal low-dose bupivacaine versus lidocaine for in vitro fertilization procedures. *Reg Anesth Pain Med* 26:52, 2001.

72. Miklos JR, Sze EH, Karram MM. Vaginal correction of pelvic organ relaxation using local anesthesia. *Obstet Gynecol* 86:922, 1995.

73. Norris A, Scerri A, Powell M. Quality of anaesthesia for insertion of tension-free vaginal tape using local analgesia and sedation. *Eur J Anaesthesiol* 18:755, 2001.

74. Wang AC, Chen MC. Randomized comparison of local versus epidural anaesthesia for tension-free vaginal tape operation. *J Urol* 165:1177, 2001.

75. Lo TS, Huang HJ, Chang CL, et al. Use of intravenous anesthesia for tension-free vaginal tape therapy in elderly women with genuine stress incontinence. *Urology* 59:349, 2002.

76. Murphy M, Heit MH, Fouts L, et al. Effect of anesthesia on voiding function after tension-free vaginal tape procedure. *Obstet Gynecol* 101:666, 2003.

77. Heinonen PK. Transvaginal sacrospinous colpopexy for vaginal vault and complete genital prolapse in aged women. *Acta Obstet Gynecol Scand* 71:377, 1992.

78. Fyles AW, Milosevic M, Wong R, et al. Oxygenation predicts radiation response and survival in patients with cervix cancer. *Radiother Oncol* 48:149, 1998.

79. Weitmann HD, Gustorff B, Vaupel P, et al. Oxygenation status of cervical carcinomas before and during spinal anesthesia for application of brachytherapy. *Strahlenther Onkol* 179:633, 2003.

80. Kathirvel S, Sadhasivam S, Saxena A, et al. Effects of intrathecal ketamine added to bupivacaine for spinal anaesthesia. *Anaesthesia* 55:899, 2000.

Neuraxial Analgesia for Labor

David J. Birnbach
Marcelle Hernandez

Pain during childbirth was for many years seen as part of a natural and useful process, since it has the biologic function of indicating the beginning of labor to the parturient. As labor progresses, however, the "usefulness" of this pain diminishes. Labor pain is the experience that incorporates biologic mechanisms with the perception of pain, as well as the emotions and sensations that follow. Many obstetricians, therefore, believed that this natural experience should not be treated pharmacologically, but instead, handled with preparation and education of the parturient. As a result, until recent times, anesthesia for labor was considered unnatural and to some, even morally wrong. Many obstetricians and midwives believed that drugs administered to abolish pain were potentially dangerous to mother and infant and would alter uterine contractions, prolong the time to delivery, and increase the rate of operative deliveries.

As practiced today, however, properly administered neuraxial labor analgesia does not increase maternal or perinatal morbidity or mortality and is not associated with an increased risk of cesarean delivery.[1,2] The vast majority of anesthesia-related maternal deaths (ranked as the sixth most common cause of pregnancy-related deaths) occurred during general anesthesia and airway management for cesarean delivery.[3] The use of general anesthesia for cesarean deliveries has decreased from 41% (1984) to 16% (1992) and continues to further decrease today, as illustrated by the approximate 1% rate at the authors' institution. The number of neuraxial anesthesia-related deaths has likewise decreased since 1984, primarily because of improvements in technique and heightened awareness of local anesthetic toxicity.[3] In addition to its other advantages, it has been shown that parturients who receive neuraxial labor analgesia spend less time in delivery rooms and have a decreased incidence of postpartum depression.[4] This chapter will review the various methods available to safely treat the pain of childbirth, as illustrated in Fig. 13-1.

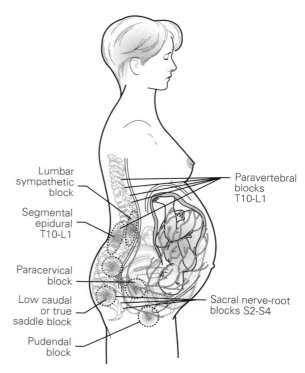

FIGURE 13-1. Pathways of labor pain. Labor pain has a visceral and somatic component. Uterine contractions may result in myometrial ischemia. In addition, stretching and distention of the lower uterine segment and cervix stimulate mechanoreceptors. The visceral noxious impulses follow sensory-nerve fibers that accompany sympathetic nerve endings, traveling through the paracervical region and the pelvic and hypogastric plexuses to enter the lumbar sympathetic chain. Signals pass through the white rami communicantes of the T10, T11, T12, and L1 spinal nerves to enter the dorsal horn of the spinal cord. Somatic impulses follow sacral nerves to enter the spinal cord at S2, S3, and S4. *Used with permission from Eltzschig HK, Lieberman ES, Camann WR. Regional anesthesia and analgesia for labor and delivery. N Engl J Med 348:319, 2003.*

MECHANISMS OF PAIN OF CHILDBIRTH

In order to fully understand the advantages and disadvantages of the various techniques used to provide labor analgesia, it is important to first appreciate the mechanisms of pain as labor progresses. One of the best estimations of the pain associated with labor is the McGill Pain Questionnaire (Fig. 13-2). Scores comparing the intensity and emotional impact of labor pain to other pain syndromes have illustrated that childbirth is one of the most painful experiences possible and most women categorized it as being severe or intolerable.[5,6] When compared to several pain syndromes such as cancer pain, postherpetic neuralgia, or phantom limb pain, labor pain has been found to be the most severe (Fig. 13-3).[5] While not every patient wants or needs labor analgesia, severe pain after commencement of labor may have harmful effects on mother and fetus and mothers who request analgesia for labor should receive it.

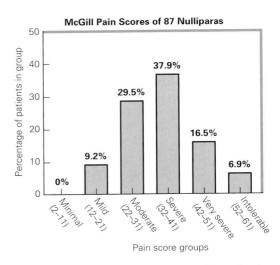

FIGURE 13-2. McGill pain scores in nulliparas. The severity of pain during labor as assessed by the McGill Pain Questionnaire for 87 nulliparous women. *Used with permission from Melzack R, Taenzer P, Feldman P, et al. Labour is still painful after prepared childbirth training. Can Med Assoc J 125:357, 1981.*

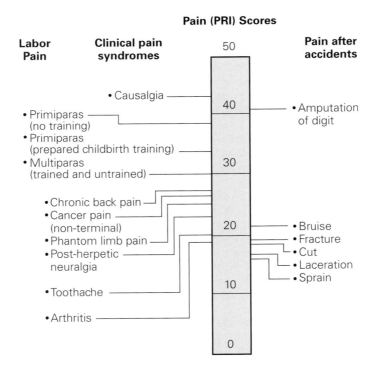

FIGURE 13-3. Comparison of pain scores, using the McGill Pain Questionnaire obtained from laboring women, general hospital, and emergency department patients. The pain-rating index (PRI) represents the sum of the rank values of all the words chosen from 20 sets of pain descriptors. *Used with permission from Melzack R. The myth of painless childbirth (The John J. Bonica Lecture). Pain 19:321, 1984.*

First Stage of Labor

Pain during the first stage of labor is visceral in nature, as it arises from afferents in the uterus and its adnexa during contractions. During this stage, there is dilation of the cervix and lower uterine segment, with subsequent distention and stretching.[7] Pain intensity is related to the strength of contractions and the pressure generated against a closed cervix and perineum.[8]

The uterine cervix has two different types of afferent innervation, and this is the basis for differences in sensory output and referred pain. The afferents which innervate the lower uterine segment and the endocervix have cell bodies in the thoracolumbar dorsal root ganglia.[9] The upper vagina and vaginal cervix have cell bodies in the sacral dorsal root ganglia. The thoracolumbar afferents are mostly C fibers, which enter the spinal cord through the dorsal root, ending in a loose network of synapses in the ventral horn and the superficial and deep dorsal horn. This anatomic composition explains the diffuse localization of visceral pain. Neurons at the dorsal horn transmit the signal to the contralateral ventral spinothalamic tract, stimulating the thalamus. Stimulation of the thalamus results in propagation of the message to the somatosensory cortex, where pain is perceived, and to other areas of the cortex that are responsible for the motor and emotional response, and memory of the event. This anatomic pathway suggests that in order to block the response to the release of inflammatory products that occurs during cervical ripening and labor (first stage of labor), analgesia in the T10 to L1 dermatome distribution is necessary.

Second Stage of Labor

The second stage of labor begins when full dilation of the cervix occurs. Contractions of the uterine body and distention of the lower uterine segments are predominantly responsible for nociceptive stimulation at this time. In addition, pressure of the fetal presenting part on pelvic structures gives rise to somatic pain which is transmitted principally via the pudendal nerves. The pudendal nerve supplies the motor fibers to the skeletal muscle of the pelvic floor and the perineum. The anterior perineum also receives fibers from the ilioinguinal nerve and the genital branch of the genitofemoral nerve. The lateral aspect of the perineum is also supplied by the posterior femoral cutaneous nerve.

During the second stage of labor the fascia and subcutaneous tissues of the lower birth canal begin to stretch and tear, the perineum distends, and pressure is applied to the perineal skeletal muscles. In contradistinction to the first stage of labor, this pain is sharply localized. This somatic pain is transmitted via C and A-delta fibers that enter the spinal cord through the dorsal roots at the sacral level and terminate in synapses in the ipsilateral superficial laminae of the dorsal horn. Therefore, in order to provide analgesia during the second stage of labor, the cephalad extent of blockade should extend to T10, and caudal extent must include the pudendal nerve, which is derived from the anterior primary divisions of S2 to S4 (Fig. 13-1).

During labor the visceral pain from the uterine contractions is diffuse and poorly localized, commonly referred to the lower back, abdomen, and rectum. These areas are supplied by spinal cord segments that also receive nociceptive input from the cervix and uterus. During the first stage of labor, as cervical dilation progresses to 3–4 cm and uterine contractions increase in intensity, blockade of the T10 to L1 dermatomes are key to pain relief. Referred pain via the dorsal rami of these nerve roots results in low back pain.[14] The differences between visceral and somatic pain are reviewed in Table 13-1.[10]

Table 13-1

Visceral Vs. Somatic Pain

	Somatic Pain	Visceral Pain
Site	Well-localized	Poorly localized
Radiation	May follow distribution of somatic nerve	Diffuse
Character	Sharp and definite	Dull and vague (may be colicky, cramping, squeezing)
Relation to stimulus	Hurts where the stimulus is associated with external factors	May be "referred" to another area, associated with internal factors
Temporal activity	Often constant	Often periodic and builds to peak (sometimes constant)
Associated symptoms	Nausea usually only with deep somatic pain owing to bone involvement	Often nausea, vomiting, sickening feeling

Data from Ref. 10.

Late during the first stage, and continuing during the second stage, the presenting fetal part begins descending in the birth canal, producing the sharp, well-localized somatic pain in the distribution of the pudendal nerve. This is consistent with the pain caused by stimulation of superficial somatic structures. Pain may be referred to the lower lumbar and sacral segments if there is pressure and traction occurring in the pelvic cavity and on its contents, including ligaments, fascia, muscles, uterine ligaments, tension of bladder, the urethra, and rectum.

▶ Other Labor Pain Factors

Perception of pain varies among individuals.[11] The degree of pain associated with labor and delivery is not only influenced by intensity, duration, and pattern of contractions, but also by physical, psychologic, ethnocultural, and neurohumoral factors.[11]

Physical Factors

The parturient's age, parity, and physical condition influence the course of labor. For example, there is an increased potential for severe and unrelieved pain of dysfunctional labor if the size of the infant is not proportionate to the size of the birth canal, the pelvis is contracted, or if the frequency of contractions or the speed and degree of cervical dilation are inadequate. In addition, while in labor, parturients may become fatigued and sleep deprived, and have exacerbations of preexisting medical conditions which may also affect their perception of pain.

Psychologic Factors

Parturients with anxiety, fear, expectations of pain, prior pain experiences, and lack of knowledge of the process of pregnancy and labor are more likely to perceive the nociceptive stimulus in a magnified way, increasing the risk of having a negative labor experience.[12] The presence of an expectant father with a positive attitude decreases parturients' apprehension, pain, and postpartum depression scores.[13] Women with antenatal education or a previous experience with labor, for example, multiparas, handle labor with more confidence, which decreases pain perception and analgesia use.[14]

Cultural Factors

Perception and expression of pain is affected by ethnicity, cultural background, level of education, and the socioeconomic status of the parturient.[11] Sheiner et al. performed a study in the southern part of Israel with parturients of two different ethnic groups (Jewish and Bedouin). They compared self-reported pain and exhibited pain (observed and interpreted by the attending obstetrician and midwife). The investigators also assessed whether the parturients' ethnic background, including different lifestyles, cultures, socioeconomic status, level of education, and parity, influenced the perception of pain. Despite differences in many of these variables, the self-assessment of pain intensity levels in the initial active phase of labor was similar in both groups, while the pain behavior was different between the Jewish and the Bedouin parturients.[15] The only variable found to inversely correlate to levels of self-evaluated pain in both ethnic groups was parity. Medical staff perceived that Bedouin women experienced less pain than Jewish women. This underestimation of pain in Bedouin parturients may have been related to the fact that the medical staff was of Jewish ethnicity, and may have been unable to recognize the presence of pain in parturients of a different culture.[15] Recognizing the existence of communication discrepancies is important for the diagnosis and treatment (e.g., epidural analgesia) of pain in the parturient.

Neurohumoral Factors

Neurohumoral changes in pregnancy may modify the response to pain.[16] Although substances released during labor have been identified and implicated in increasing the nociceptive threshold, the significance of these findings is not completely understood. Estrogen and progesterone modulate the mother's antinociceptive response.[17] Progesterone has been associated with increasing a parturient's sensitivity to analgesic agents and activating opioid receptors while decreasing the release of substance P.[18] Inhibitory neurotransmitters such as norepinephrine (NE) and acetylcholine (Ach) seem to play a role in antinociception.[19] Animal studies show that pain stimulates a surge of spinal cord NE, inducing Ach release and subsequent analgesia.[20] In addition, stimulation of afferent fibers in the hypogastric and pelvic nerves is thought to cause hypoalgesia via the spinal opioid system.

ANATOMY OF NEURAXIAL ANESTHESIA IN PREGNANCY

Knowledge of spinal anatomy is essential for successful performance of central neuraxial anesthesia in the obstetric patient (see Chap. 1). It is important to understand where to place the needle and how the injected agents will be distributed. The discussion here will concentrate on the

Table 13-2

Changes in Pregnancy that Affect Neuraxial Anesthesia

Anatomy	Change in Pregnancy	Consequences for Neuraxial Anesthesia/Analgesia
Weight	Increases	More difficult to palpate landmarks
Tuffier's line	More cephalad relative to L4 spinous process	Shorter distance (and one less interspace) between Tuffier's line and end of spinal cord
Vertebral column: Lumbar lordosis Thoracic kyphosis	Exaggerated, apex more caudad Reduced	Increased cephalad spread of hyperbaric spinal anesthetic solutions Reduced spinal anesthetic dose
Epidural space	Engorgement of epidural veins	Increased risk of inadvertent intravascular injection Decreased dose of epidural and spinal anesthetics
Hormones	Changes in levels	Decreased dose of epidural and spinal anesthetics
Autonomic nervous system Tone Receptors	Increased Down regulated	Increased dose of vasopressors necessary to treat hypotension Intravascular epidural test dose (epinephrine) less reliable

lumbar area of the spinal cord and how this differs during pregnancy (Table 13-2).

Tuffier's line is an imaginary line made by joining the top of the iliac crests. This landmark is often difficult to appreciate in the obstetric patient. In the nonpregnant individual the line crosses the spine at the level of the L4 spinous process. In the majority of adults, the spinal cord terminates at or above the L1-L2 intervertebral disk level. The frequency distribution of the vertebral level at which the spinal cord terminates and Tuffier's line crosses the vertebral column is shown in Fig. 13-4. Spinal anesthesia/analgesia is usually performed no more than two interspaces above Tuffier's line, to avoid possible cord trauma. In pregnant patients, however, the weight of the gravid uterus rotates the pelvis anteriorly and as lumbar spine lordosis increases, Tuffier's line moves more cephalad relative to the L4 spinous process. Therefore, caution should be exercised when performing spinal anesthesia more than one interspace above this landmark in obstetric patients. It has been reported that anesthesiologists actually identify an interspace one or more levels higher than they think 51% of the time, and they identify the correct interspace only 29% of the time.[21] This has serious implications in obstetric patients, in whom it may be difficult to appreciate landmarks due to weight gain.

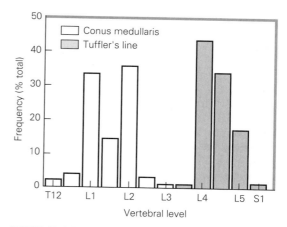

FIGURE 13-4. Frequency distribution of vertebral level where the spinal cord terminates and where Tuffier's line (between iliac crests) crosses the spine. Spaces between vertebral levels represent disk spaces. *Used with permission from Hogan QH. Tuffier's line: The normal distribution of anatomic parameters. Anesth Analg 78:194, 1994.*

In the supine position the human spine has four curvatures which affect the spread of spinal medications: cervical lordosis, lumbar lordosis, anterior concavity of the thoracic area, and anterior concavity of the sacrococcygeal area.

A

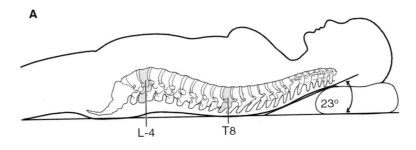

L-4   T8

B

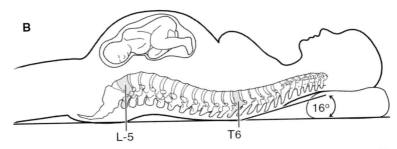

L-5   T6

FIGURE 13-5. Spinal configuration in the supine position in the nonpregnant female (top) and in late pregnancy (bottom). The apex of the lumbar lordosis is moved caudad and the thoracic kyphosis reduced in the parturient. Median high and low points of the two curves are shaded. Data are from reference 23.

These curves are increased in pregnancy as illustrated in Fig. 13-5. Parturients in the standing position have an exaggeration of the normal lumbar lordosis. Later, as pregnancy progresses and there is more weight from the uterus and increased laxity of spinal ligaments, there are changes in the lumbar lordosis and thoracic kyphosis when supine.[22] These changes are thought to contribute to the enhanced cephalad spread of hyperbaric local anesthetics during spinal anesthesia in pregnant patients.

Pregnancy alters other aspects of lumbar vertebral anatomy. The epidural space is a potential space which contains nerve roots (lateral), vessels, and fat. In pregnant patients, there is increased risk of intravascular injection due to engorgement of epidural veins, especially if the parturient lies in the supine position. The increase in intra-abdominal pressure and obstruction of the inferior vena cava due to the gravid uterus divert blood return from the legs and pelvic structures to the vertebral venous-azygous anastomotic system, and therefore causes significant engorgement of the extradural venous plexus.[23]

Young women are at increased risk for developing postdural puncture headache (PDPH) after dural puncture (see Chap. 6). To decrease its incidence, several changes to practice have been advocated. Noncutting, pencil-point (e.g., Whitacre, Sprotte, Gertie Marx, and Pencan) spinal needles are primarily used (see Chap. 2). When Quincke (cutting) tipped needles are

used, the needle should be inserted parallel to the dural fibers to decrease the risk of PDPH (see "Complications and Side Effects of Neuraxial Labor Analgesia," later).

▶ Epidural Space

The distance from the skin to the epidural space has been studied using MRI, sonography, and clinical experience.[24–26] When using a midline approach, on average a distance of 5 cm at the lumbar level has been found from skin to epidural space in both obstetric and nonobstetric patients. The distribution of skin to lumbar epidural space distance is illustrated in Fig. 13-6.[27,28] In obstetric patients, about 16% have a skin to epidural space distance of less than 4 cm, increasing the risk in those patients of inadvertent dural puncture.[27] The skin to epidural space distance may be increased in edematous patients. The ligamentum flavum-dura mater distance also varies, depending on spinal level and interspace. At the L3-L4 interspace, this distance averages 6–7 mm in the midline.[29]

Various studies have investigated the distance from the skin to the epidural space as it relates to mild scoliosis, age, weight, height, and position at the time of epidural puncture. Weight has been shown to have a direct relationship with the distance from skin to epidural space; the distance increased approximately 1 cm in patients with a high body mass index (BMI)[30] (greater than 30 kg/m^2). The second

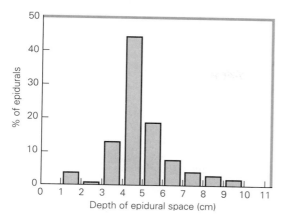

FIGURE 13-6. Distribution of skin to lumbar epidural space distance measured clinically in 4011 obstetric cases. Data are from references 27 and 28.

Box 13-1

Advantages of Epidural Labor Analgesia

More effective than parenteral analgesia

Improves uteroplacental blood flow

Blunts maternal hyperventilation-hypoventilation cycle

Ability to rapidly convert to epidural anesthesia for emergency cesarean delivery

factor is the patient's position at the time of epidural placement; the sitting position resulted in a shorter distance than the lateral position. The change in skin to epidural space depth associated with body position can cause epidural catheters to move in and out as body position changes (see "Epidural Analgesia Technique" below).

Epidural placement relies on indirect methods of identification of the epidural space such as loss-of-resistance (LOR) or the hanging-drop technique. In the cervicothoracic area, there is an ambient subatmospheric pressure that helps identify the space. In the lumbosacral area, however, the pressure of the epidural space reflects the resting abdominal pressure. Epidural pressure below the thoracic level tends to be more positive, especially with pregnancy and the sitting position.[31] An injection at the thoracic site would therefore have a more symmetric distribution. Solutions injected at the lumbar region, because of the epidural pressure gradient between lumbar and thoracic levels may spread more cephalad than caudad. Pregnancy has been associated with a decrease in dose requirements for central neuraxial blockade.[32] This effect has long been attributed to progesterone, with no proven mechanism.[33] Other possible explanations include physical changes of pregnancy due to the gravid uterus; for example, changes in spinal curvature favoring more cephalad spread and reduction of cerebrospinal fluid (CSF) volume by distention of epidural veins.

NEURAXIAL LABOR ANALGESIA TECHNIQUES

▶ Epidural Analgesia

Advances in the understanding of neural pathways and pain receptors, together with the diverse pharmacologic and technical supplies now available for epidural techniques,

have led to newer and safer ways to modify the pain of labor. Several advantages of epidural labor analgesia have been identified (Box 13-1). Studies that compared parenteral analgesia (e.g., intramuscular or intravenous meperidine) to epidural analgesia for relief of labor pain and discomfort universally found that epidural techniques are more effective.[34] Neuraxial analgesia for labor has been gaining popularity and its use may have several benefits in addition to better pain relief. Improved uteroplacental perfusion in conjunction with more effective uterine activity can result from the decrease in circulating maternal plasma catecholamines.[35] This may be particularly beneficial in pathologic conditions associated with decreased uteroplacental perfusion, for example, preeclampsia. In addition, effective epidural analgesia blunts the "hyperventilation-hypoventilation cycle" that accompanies painful uterine contractions. This prevents maternal respiratory alkalosis, which may cause a left shift of the oxyhemoglobin curve, potentially decreasing oxygen delivery to the fetus. An additional advantage is the ability to convert epidural analgesia to epidural anesthesia for urgent or emergency cesarean deliveries, thus avoiding the need and accompanying risk of general anesthesia.

Controversy exists regarding the appropriate time (in relation to cervical dilation) to initiate epidural analgesia during labor.[36] Recent data suggest that early epidural placement with lower doses of local anesthetics does not affect the incidence of cesarean or operative vaginal deliveries and may decrease the duration of labor or the incidence of operative vaginal deliveries.[37,38] A secondary analysis of a randomized study of active management of labor found that women who were managed with early initiation of epidural analgesia (less than equal to 4 cm cervical dilation) had decreased duration of labor when compared to those with late initiation.[37] In addition, the second stage of labor was not lengthened in the early versus late epidural initiation groups. Finally, a recent randomized prospective study of nulliparas in spontaneous labor found that women who were randomized to early (less than 4 cm cervical dilation) combined spinal-epidural (CSE) analgesia had no increase in cesarean or operative vaginal delivery rates, but shorter duration of the first stage of labor compared to women who received systemic opioid analgesia in early labor.[38]

Recently, the American College of Obstetricians and Gynecologists (ACOG) and the American Society of Anesthesiologists (ASA) have reiterated that "in the absence of a medical contraindication, maternal request is a sufficient medical indication for pain relief during labor" and that women should not be deprived of this service based on insurance or inadequate nursing participation with neuraxial analgesic modalities.[39] Of the various methods used for pain relief, ACOG describes neuraxial analgesia techniques (epidural, spinal, and CSE analgesia) as the most effective and least depressing to the central nervous system (CNS), allowing the mother to participate in the birth and enjoy an alert neonate. As relates to the timing of epidural analgesia initiation, ACOG suggests that decisions regarding analgesia "should be closely coordinated among the obstetrician, the anesthesiologist, the patient, and skilled support personnel."[40]

Informed consent should be obtained prior to proceeding with neuraxial analgesia. Several groups of investigators have reported that obstetrical patients find it very important to know the complications of epidural analgesia before consenting for it, regardless of the severity or risks.[41,42] Studies have shown that the discomfort from labor did not interfere with the ability of the parturient to comprehend information associated with the consent process.[41] Pattee et al. showed that the parturient's level of education cannot be used to judge who would want greater explanation of possible complications.[41]

After a preanesthetic evaluation and informed consent, assessment of maternal airway and back anatomy should be performed prior to initiation of the neuraxial block. Preanesthetic evaluation should also include a basic assessment of the fetus. Emergency airway equipment, oxygen, and drugs and supplies should be available in case serious complications arise. Monitoring maternal blood pressure and heart rate, the latter by electrocardiography or pulse oximetry, and fetal heart rate (FHR) is routine.[43] Many anesthesiologists administer a 500–1000 mL bolus of Ringer's lactate (or similar crystalloid solution without glucose) immediately prior to the procedure in an attempt to prevent hypotension secondary to sympathetic blockade, and maintain uteroplacental perfusion. This practice is controversial, as it may not decrease the incidence of hypotension, especially with newer neuraxial analgesia techniques. Avoidance of aortocaval compression is of the utmost importance, especially when using doses of medications that cause sympathetic blockade.

Technique

Initiation of epidural analgesia in the parturient is similar to the initiation of lumbar epidural anesthesia for the non-pregnant patient (see Chap. 2). Specific differences, and studies performed in obstetric patients are discussed later.

Epidural analgesia is usually initiated with the patient in the lateral decubitus or sitting position. Uteroplacental perfusion may be better in the lateral decubitus position.[44] In obese patients the sitting position has the advantage of easier identification of landmarks and better respiratory mechanics;[45] but the lateral recumbent head-down position may reduce the incidence of lumbar epidural venous puncture.[46] There is no "perfect" patient position and often the preference and experience of the anesthesiologist are the most important factors. For this reason, residents in the authors' program are encouraged to initiate analgesia with patients in both the sitting and lateral positions.

Aseptic precautions for epidural catheter placement have been an area of recent concern. The anesthesiologist should adhere to strict aseptic technique. Skin disinfection with povidone iodine (PI) or chlorhexidine is recommended. Unopened bottles or single-use packets of PI have proved to be more effective than previously opened bottles[47] and decrease the risk of contamination that may be associated with multi-use bottles.[48] Although in vitro studies favor iodine products, chlorhexidine continues to be evaluated and recent evidence suggests that chlorhexidine in alcohol solution is more efficient as an antimicrobial agent.[49] Although this agent has been extensively evaluated for use in placing central lines, it has not been thoroughly studied as relates to disinfection prior to epidural or spinal techniques. The use of face masks to prevent meningitis from the oropharyngeal flora of the anesthesiologist is also controversial.[50] Surveys among the United Kingdom obstetric anesthesiologists done in 1996 found that more than 50% did not wear face masks for either epidural or spinal procedures.[51] Reports of meningitis arising from bacteria in the nares of anesthesiologists, however, continue to be published[52] and have led infectious disease experts to recommend routine use of face masks.

After the lower back is prepared with the appropriate antiseptic solution and draped, the skin and subcutaneous tissue are anesthetized with local anesthesia. Clear plastic drapes offer the advantage of providing a sterile field while allowing better visualization of landmarks. The epidural needle is optimally inserted at the L3-L4 ± 1 vertebral interspace. There is controversy as to whether the LOR to saline technique or LOR to air technique is better (see Chap. 2). Some studies have assessed the quality of analgesia in women who have been randomized to either an air or saline LOR technique. Beilin et al. found a higher frequency of adequate analgesia when a saline-filled syringe was used in the LOR technique, whereas women in the air group requested additional medication more often after initial analgesia.[53] Air may cause mild pneumocephalus with resultant headache,[54] form air bubbles in the epidural space preventing effective spread of local anesthetic,[55] and may exert pressure on neural structures.[56] An advantage of LOR to air when performing the

CSE technique, however, is that there is no confusion between CSF and saline.

Since the duration of labor is indeterminate and emergency cesarean delivery may become necessary, most anesthesiologists insert an epidural catheter rather than performing a single-shot technique. Two types of epidural catheters are commonly used: single-orifice and multiorifice. A theoretical advantage of the single-orifice (open-end) catheters is that the anesthetic solution can be delivered only to a single anatomic site. Newly developed flexible-tip single-orifice catheters offer the advantage of decreased incidence of paresthesias and intravascular placement.[57] Multiorifice (closed-end) catheters, in theory, have the disadvantage of delivering anesthetic to more than one anatomic site, for example, simultaneous administration of drug to both the epidural and subarachnoid spaces. In a study by D'Angelo et al., these multiorifice catheters were not associated with multicompartment placement; and the incidence of intravenous cannulation and catheter dislodgement followed by replacement was similar for both the traditional (non-flexible-tip single-orifice) and multiorifice catheter types.[58] There is, however, clear evidence suggesting that multiorifice catheters are associated with a decreased frequency of inadequate analgesia and require less manipulation than traditional non-flexible-tip single-orifice catheters,[58] presumably due to a more even distribution of medication.[57] Since there are advantages and disadvantages to each type of catheter, the choice of which one to use is a matter of personal preference.

Some anesthesiologists inject 3–5 mL of saline through the epidural needle before threading the epidural catheter, expanding the epidural space, and possibly decreasing the likelihood of unintentional intravenous cannulation.[59] Multiorifice catheter insertion to a depth of 7 cm has been associated with the highest rate of insertion complications, while insertion to a depth of 5 cm has been associated with the highest incidence of satisfactory analgesia and minimal complications.[60] It should be noted that epidural catheters are not fixed in the epidural space and can move in or out, depending on the parturient's posture. If the patient's position is changed from the sitting to lateral recumbent position, the catheter may move 1–2.5 cm inward, resulting in a misplaced catheter and inadequate analgesia. To minimize the risk of catheter displacement, particularly in obese patients or those with an obese back, Hamilton et al.[61] recommended multiorifice catheter insertion to at least 4 cm into the epidural space and securing (taping) the catheter to the skin only after the patient has moved from the sitting to the lateral position.

The catheter is optimally inserted before therapeutic doses of local anesthetic are administered and a test dose may be used to confirm that spinal or intravenous placement has not occurred. Although somewhat controversial in laboring patients, the test dose is considered important by some anesthesiologists, as patients may subsequently require a large dose of concentrated local anesthetic for an emergency cesarean delivery.[62] If a continuous infusion has been administered for several hours and the parturient remains comfortable and has no signs of lower extremity weakness, the catheter can be considered to be appropriately sited in the epidural space. It is important to note that the test dose is used to determine if the epidural catheter is in the subarachnoid or intravenous space after insertion, not whether the epidural catheter is functioning.

Inadvertent intrathecal injection of the test dose, usually lidocaine 1.5% (45 mg) with epinephrine 1:200,000 (5 μg/mL), 3 mL,[63] will cause dense motor blockade within 2–4 min after administration. Intravascular injection of the same test dose results in tachycardia and less often, systemic symptoms of local anesthetic toxicity, such as lightheadedness and circumoral numbness or tingling, within 1 min of injection.[64] Since labor pain is associated with increased heart rate variability, the test dose should not be administered immediately before or during a uterine contraction. Aspiration of epidural catheters does not adequately identify all cases of intravascular or intrathecal catheter placement, especially if a single-orifice catheter is used.[65]

Local Anesthetics and Adjuvants

Bupivacaine. Bupivacaine is the local anesthetic most commonly administered for epidural labor analgesia (Table 13-3). Concentrations of 0.125% or less are usually injected or infused, as this provides adequate analgesia without a high degree of motor blockade. After bolus epidural administration of bupivacaine, pain relief is perceived within 10–15 min, but it may take approximately 20 min to achieve peak effect. Bupivacaine is highly protein bound (see Chap. 3) which limits placental transfer. The umbilical vein:maternal vein concentration ratio is 0.3.

The authors' practice is to use bolus solutions of bupivacaine 0.125%, 12 mL (three incremental injections of 4 mL) which is generally adequate during early labor, especially

Table 13-3		
Drugs for Epidural Labor Analgesia Initiation		
Drug	Concentration	Dose
Local anesthetic		
Bupivacaine	0.125%	10–15 mL
Ropivacaine	0.1–0.2%	10–15 mL
Lidocaine	0.75–1.5%	10–15 mL
Opioid		
Fentanyl		50–100 μg
Sufentanil		5–10 μg

Table 13-4

Drugs for Epidural Labor Analgesia Maintenance

Drug Solution	Local Anesthetic Concentration (%)	Opioid Concentration (µg/mL)	Infusion Rate (mL/h)*
Bupivacaine-fentanyl	0.0625–0.125	2–4	10–15
Bupivacaine-sufentanil	0.0625–0.125	0.2–0.33	10–15
Ropivacaine-fentanyl	0.08–0.15	2–4	10–15
Ropivacaine	0.2	–	10–15

*All or part of the total hourly infusion volume may be administered as part of a PCEA bolus. In case of epidural catheter malposition, patient-controlled bolus volumes should not contain a total mass of local anesthetic that exceeds the mass which could be safely injected into the subarachnoid space or into a blood vessel.

when combined with epidural fentanyl (see "Opioids," later). This produces excellent sensory analgesia with minimal motor blockade. If necessary, the concentration can be increased as labor progresses. For continuous epidural infusions (CEI), a solution of bupivacaine 0.0625–0.1% with the addition of fentanyl 2–4 µg/mL is commonly used (Table 13-4). Administering infusions of bupivacaine 0.125% maintains analgesia longer than 0.0625%, but with the disadvantage of causing more motor blockade.[65]

Ropivacaine. A homologue of bupivacaine and mepivacaine, ropivacaine is a local anesthetic formulated as a single levorotary enantiomer (see Chap. 3). Studies suggest less cardiodepressant and neurologic toxicity than bupivacaine. In addition, ropivacaine is cleared faster than bupivacaine after intravascular administration in sheep, suggesting a greater margin of safety after unintentional intravascular injection.

Recent investigations using the minimum local anesthetic concentration (MLAC) technique for determining local anesthetic potency have reported that ropivacaine is 40% less potent than bupivacaine when used as a bolus for initiation of epidural analgesia in early labor.[66,67] Controversy exists about the clinical application of these data. A study comparing both drugs showed less motor blockade with ropivacaine, but more sustained analgesia with bupivacaine.[68] Dilute ropivacaine (0.08%) with fentanyl (2 µg/mL) was used to initiate effective labor analgesia with preservation of spontaneous voiding and unassisted ambulation in parturients.[69] In a second study, bupivacaine and ropivacaine 0.075% were equally effective for labor analgesia using a patient-controlled epidural analgesia (PCEA) technique.[70] In conclusion, there appears to be no clear-cut advantage between ropivacaine and bupivacaine in either obstetric or neonatal outcome; however, a potential disadvantage of ropivacaine is its increased cost.

Levobupivacaine. The need for a long-acting local anesthetic with similar pharmacologic action to bupivacaine, but with less toxicity, led to the development of levobupivacaine. This purified levorotary enantiomer of racemic bupivacaine has less potential for cardiotoxicity and CNS toxicity (see Chap. 3).[71] Animal studies have demonstrated greater potency and longer duration of anesthesia with levobupivacaine when compared to bupivacaine, which may be related to its vasoconstrictor actions. In a study of epidural analgesia for labor, both drugs produced similar degrees of motor blockade and sensory analgesia, and reduction in visual analog pain scores.[70] In contrast, several other studies observed an absence of motor impairment in levobupivacaine-treated parturients compared to bupivacaine-treated parturients.[68,69,72] In addition, no difference was found in neonatal outcome after epidural administration of either of these two drugs for cesarean delivery.[73] Unfortunately, levobupivacaine is not available in the United States market at the present time.

Lidocaine. Lidocaine is an amide local anesthetic with a duration of action between that of bupivacaine and 2-chloroprocaine. While it is a superior agent for epidural anesthesia for cesarean delivery, it is not often used for labor analgesia. Solutions of lidocaine 0.75–1.5% provide satisfactory analgesia, but not comparable to that provided by bupivacaine,[74] and with less discrimination between motor and sensory block. At delivery, umbilical vein:maternal vein lidocaine concentration ratio is approximately twice that of bupivacaine. Studies comparing bupivacaine, 2-chloroprocaine, and lidocaine show similar neonatal outcomes with all three local anesthetics when used for epidural anesthesia for cesarean delivery (see Chap. 14).[75]

2-Chloroprocaine. 2-Chloroprocaine is an ester local anesthetic with a rapid onset, but short duration of action, which limits its usefulness for labor analgesia. Administration of 2-chloroprocaine, even in doses as low as those used as a test dose, may adversely affect the efficacy of subsequently administered bupivacaine and opioids.[76] Its metabolite, 4-amino-2-chlorobenzoic acid, has been found to stay in the nerve following recovery from neural blockade, potentially interfering with the subsequent action of bupivacaine.[77] For example, bupivacaine administered after 2-chloroprocaine may produce a blockade lasting 30–40 min instead of the anticipated 90–120 min. Although at high doses, 2-chloroprocaine has a binding affinity at mu and kappa opioid receptor sites, the decrease in analgesia of subsequently administered epidural fentanyl probably is not related to antagonist activity on these receptors.[78] Further investigation is needed to clarify these issues.

Chloroprocaine 3% is extremely useful for extending epidural blockade rapidly in the event of emergency cesarean or operative vaginal deliveries. Because of its short duration of action, it is not useful for routine maintenance of labor analgesia. In cases of "fetal distress," chloroprocaine is very attractive due to its maternal and fetal safety profile. It has a short half-life in maternal and fetal blood, thus minimizing potential impact on the fetus, as well as untoward responses to accidental intravascular injections. Placental transfer of 2-chloroprocaine is not increased by the presence of fetal acidosis and there are no reports of "ion trapping" (see Chap. 3) as with bupivacaine and lidocaine.[79] Although neurotoxicity was a concern with chloroprocaine in the 1980s (see Chap. 6), newer preservative-free preparations do not appear to be associated with neurotoxicity. Preservative containing formulations of 2-chloroprocaine and other local anesthetics are marketed in multiuse vials and anesthesiologists should take care that these solutions not be used for neuraxial anesthesia.[80]

Opioids. Opioids are frequently added to local anesthetics in the epidural space to provide analgesia during labor. Synergistic interactions occur between local anesthetics and opioids when given epidurally (see Chap. 3) and the addition of opioid shortens latency. Opioids treat visceral pain, but are less effective in treating somatic pain during the second stage of labor. Conversely, local anesthetics provide dense somatic analgesia, but not selective visceral analgesia. The combination of low concentration local anesthetic with a low-dose lipid-soluble opioid provides excellent analgesia while minimizing the side effects of both drugs. Advantages of an opioid added to a dilute solution of local anesthetic include decreased risk of systemic local anesthetic toxicity, decreased risk of high spinal anesthesia, decreased plasma concentrations of local anesthetic in the fetus, and decreased intensity of motor blockade. Adding local anesthetic to opioid decreases the opioid dose and therefore, decreases the risk of nausea and pruritus.

Morphine was one of the first opioids used to provide neuraxial labor analgesia. Because of its long latency (up to 60 min), side effect profile, and inconsistent analgesia, it has been replaced with more lipophilic agents such as fentanyl and sufentanil. Administration of 50–100 μg of fentanyl (Table 13-3) in the epidural space provides adequate analgesia for early labor that lasts for approximately 60 min.[81]

Higher doses are associated with increased systemic side effects. Typically, fentanyl is mixed with local anesthetic to initiate and maintain analgesia.

Epidural sufentanil, compared to fentanyl, has a larger volume of distribution when systemically absorbed, has greater potency (because of greater affinity to opioid receptors), and results in better penetration into the spinal cord (due to its greater lipid solubility). Because of its high solubility and high volume of distribution, only a small amount of drug is transferred across the placenta, resulting in low concentration of drug in the fetal circulation.

Meperidine is the only opioid to possess local anesthetic properties when administered at clinically useful doses. A 100 mg dose of epidural preservative-free meperidine provides analgesia similar to that provided by bupivacaine 0.25% with less motor block. However, more sedation, nausea, and pruritus are observed. This drug may be beneficial for use in the patient who is allergic to amide local anesthetics undergoing cesarean delivery, but is not routinely used for labor analgesia.

Epinephrine. The addition of epinephrine to epidural bupivacaine may speed up the onset of analgesia and increase the intensity of the motor blockade, with no effect on neonatal outcome or intervillous blood flow.[82,83] A small bupivacaine sparing effect is also seen, perhaps as the result of spinal cord α-adrenergic receptor stimulation. In obstetric patients, systemic absorption of epinephrine may increase maternal heart rate and may transiently decrease uterine activity as a result of β-adrenergic stimulation. The use of epinephrine in local anesthetic solutions is controversial in severely hypertensive parturients, since it may pose a significant risk for development of a dramatic hypertensive reaction.[84]

Epinephrine may also increase the efficacy of epidural opioids. Following injection of epinephrine, elimination of drugs in the epidural space is delayed because of vasoconstriction and decreased epidural blood flow. Since epinephrine is absorbed systemically, a slowing in labor may theoretically result from the stimulation of beta-2-uterine receptors. In summary, epinephrine may potentiate the analgesia provided by epidural administration of local anesthetics and opioids, but does not seem to play an important role in infusions.[85]

Maintenance of Epidural Analgesia

Since labor pain can last for many hours, a single epidural injection of local anesthetic with or without opioid does not last long enough to provide adequate analgesia for the duration of labor in most parturients. This problem is also encountered when administering single-shot spinal analgesia, as will be discussed later in this chapter. Unless the parturient is a multipara who presents late in labor, supplemental analgesic administration is usually required and often administered via continuous infusion, PCEA, or via intermittent bolus epidural analgesia.

Epidural Analgesia Technique and the Second Stage of Labor. Traditional epidural analgesia is associated with a longer second stage of labor. An advantage of low-dose local anesthetic neuraxial blockade is that motor blockade of the abdominal muscles is minimized. Maternal muscle strength is maintained and this may be important for pushing during the second stage of labor. Even though afferent transmission of sacral nerves S2 to S5 (pelvic floor muscles) is blocked, the ability to push with contractions is maintained, because motor and proprioceptive (dorsal column) functions of the muscles of the abdomen, legs, thighs, and feet are selectively preserved with low-dose CSE and epidural analgesic blockade.

Intermittent Bolus Epidural Analgesia. The traditional technique for maintaining labor analgesia is for the anesthesia provider to administer supplemental epidural doses of local anesthetic on an "as-needed" basis. Many studies have shown that when parturients request supplemental analgesia administration as needed, the mean total consumption of local anesthetic/opioid is reduced compared to analgesia maintenance using continuous infusion techniques.[86] A recent study compared the intermittent bolus technique with PCEA.[87] The latter provided better pain relief during the first and second stages of labor; however, the rate of cesarean delivery was higher in the PCEA group (although the rate of vacuum delivery was lower). This result has not been found in other studies comparing the two techniques. Intermittent "top-up" bolus techniques are as effective as the infusion techniques discussed later.[88] The intermittent bolus technique, however, is associated with more peaks and valleys in terms of analgesia and requires more input from the medical and nursing staffs. Patients tend to be more satisfied with continuous maintenance techniques.

Continuous Epidural Infusion. The most popular anesthetic technique used to maintain epidural analgesia is a CEI of a dilute solution of local anesthetic, usually in combination with a lipophilic opioid (Table 13-4). Potential benefits of this approach include the maintenance of adequate analgesia throughout the labor period,[89] more stable maternal hemodynamics, less need for manual boluses, decreased risk of local anesthetic toxicity, and decreased manpower requirements. Neonatal outcome is the same with bolus or infusion approaches, but less hypotension in the mother is observed when a continuous infusion is used. It should be noted, however, that prolonged labor with a CEI of bupivacaine 0.125% at 10–14 mL/h may cause motor blockade.[90] Infusions of bupivacaine 0.0625% with opioid are associated with less motor blockade while still

providing effective analgesia, but supplemental top-offs may be necessary and higher concentrations may be necessary in some patients.[91] In general, the local anesthetic concentration of the infusion solution should be less than that of a bolus solution in order to provide a similar degree of sensory and motor blockade.

Patient-Controlled Epidural Analgesia.: PCEA combines advantages of both the intermittent bolus and continuous infusion techniques. Analgesia is similar to that provided by intermittent bolus injection and CEI, but maternal satisfaction may be greater.[92] Parturients receiving PCEA require less supplemental manual top-up doses and local anesthetic while reducing side effects and clinician workload.[93] PCEA techniques vary markedly and it is unclear whether this effects analgesia and outcome. At one extreme, there is no background infusion and patients administer a bolus when needed. At the other extreme, a background infusion is administered at a rate that provides analgesia for some or most patients, and patient-controlled bolus doses are administered for breakthrough pain. Even though patient satisfaction is the same with both techniques, bupivacaine consumption may be higher with the background infusion.[87,88] Parturients with background infusions may require outlet forceps for delivery more often than parturients receiving intermittent boluses; midforceps and cesarean delivery rates are similar in both groups.[88] A recent small study found that automated continuous intermittent boluses (CIB) at regular intervals provided longer duration of analgesia, lower pain scores, and a higher sensory block compared to CEI.[94]

Continuous epidural techniques do not obviate the need for frequent assessment of the patient. Patients should be assessed every 1–2 h for maternal blood pressure and FHR tracing, quality of analgesia, sensory level, intensity of motor block, and progress of labor. Low levels of anesthesia may be indicative of catheter migration out of the epidural space, catheter migration into a blood vessel, or administration of an inadequate dose of local anesthetic. A dense motor block may be indicative of catheter migration into the subarachnoid space, or the need to reduce the concentration of local anesthetic, or infusion rate.

To maximize the safety of the continuous epidural technique, the solution of local anesthetic should optimally be prepared by pharmacy personnel under sterile conditions. In practice, however, many anesthesiologists prepare their own infusion bags or syringes. In addition, each labor unit should agree who is responsible for adjusting the rate of epidural infusion. While there is currently some controversy regarding labor nursing assistance with adjustment of infusions, the ACOG in a joint committee opinion with the ASA has recommended that labor nurses should not be restricted from participating in the management of labor pain relief.[38]

Spinal Analgesia

Spinal analgesia (as compared to *anesthesia*) for labor typically involves the subarachnoid administration of an opioid plus or minus a small dose of local anesthetic.

Spinal analgesia can be achieved by performing a single-shot or continuous technique, or as part of a CSE technique (see "Combined Spinal-Epidural Labor Analgesia," below). During the first stage of labor, single-shot subarachnoid injection is not suitable for most parturients because it has a limited duration of action and analgesia cannot be extended. Single-shot subarachnoid injection of an opioid with or without a local anesthetic may be appropriate for women in whom the first stage of labor is expected to be short. It can be followed later by either another spinal injection or initiation of epidural analgesia, if necessary. This technique is used in some parts of the United States where it has gained popularity and has been called "intrathecals."

Spinal analgesia can be initiated with the patient in the lateral decubitus or sitting position and a midline or paramedical approach can be used to enter the subarachnoid space, although many prefer midline in obstetric patients. Techniques for accessing the subarachnoid space are discussed in Chap. 2. Drugs for single-shot spinal mimic those used for CSE analgesia and are discussed later (Table 13-3).

Placement of a catheter in the subarachnoid space allows continuous spinal analgesia/anesthesia by intermittent bolus or continuous infusion. This technique is used more often in high-risk parturients or those patients with difficult placement of an epidural catheter, for example, those with vertebral anatomic abnormalities or morbid obesity.[95] In addition, it is a technique growing in popularity for use following inadvertent dural puncture with an epidural needle (*wet tap*).

Early techniques of continuous spinal analgesia involved the use of large bore needles and catheters. To reduce the high incidence of PDPH, small bore microcatheters were introduced. These were removed from the United States market by the Food and Drug Administration (FDA) in 1992 after several cases of cauda equina syndrome were reported (see Chap. 6). Currently, in the United States, large bore epidural needles and standard epidural catheters are used for continuous spinal anesthesia. If epidural placement was difficult and dural puncture was unanticipated, continuous spinal analgesia can be maintained during labor. Initially, a subarachnoid bolus injection of bupivacaine 1.25–2.5 mg with fentanyl 10–20 µg is administered, followed by the continuous intrathecal infusion of the standard epidural local anesthetic/opioid solution (in the authors' institution bupivacaine 0.0625% with fentanyl 3 µg/mL) at a rate of 1–2 mL/h. Although not adequately studied to make a definitive conclusion, it is possible that threading the epidural catheter intrathecally may decrease the risk of PDPH and leaving it in situ for 24 h may further decrease the incidence (see Chap. 6).[96]

Combined Spinal-Epidural Labor Analgesia

Combined spinal-epidural analgesia is a relatively new technique that has come to replace the traditional epidural for both labor analgesia and surgical (cesarean section) anesthesia at our institution. The anatomy of this block is reviewed in Fig. 2-26. CSE may provide better analgesia than traditional epidural analgesia.[88] Overall, women prefer the faster onset, decreased motor blockade, and feelings of greater self-control that are provided with CSE.[97] In addition, in one study performed in healthy nulliparous women, CSE in early labor was associated with more rapid cervical dilation when compared to epidural analgesia.[98] This finding, however, has not been shown in other studies.

CSE is a two-stage technique that offers the advantages of both epidural and spinal techniques (Box 13-2). The

---

Box 13-2

Advantages and Disadvantages of CSE Technique for Labor Analgesia Compared to Epidural Analgesia

Advantages	Fast onset (2–5 min)
	Immediate sacral block
	Less total maternal and fetal drug exposure
	Minimal or no motor block (opioid-only technique)*
	No acute sympathectomy (opioid-only technique)*
	Decreased incidence of failed epidural analgesia
Disadvantages	Possible increased incidence of fetal bradycardia
	Delayed verification of functioning epidural catheter
	Increased pruritus

*Intrathecal analgesia may be initiated with opioid only or opioid combined with local anesthetic.

subarachnoid injection of opioids, local anesthetics, or a combination of drugs provides almost instant pain relief (within 2–3 min of administration) and is not associated with motor blockade. The onset of sacral analgesia is almost immediate, compared to several hours for lumbar epidural analgesia. This is particularly useful for women in advanced labor. In case labor continues beyond the duration of the subarachnoid block, a low-dose mixture of bupivacaine and fentanyl can be administered through the epidural catheter to maintain analgesia until delivery. If vaginal delivery fails, the epidural catheter can be used to induce anesthesia for operative delivery. Finally, the extra CSF verification step may help decrease the incidence of inadvertent dural puncture.

There are several theoretical concerns associated with CSE analgesia. These include the following:

▶ *Epidural catheter migration through the dural hole.* This risk appears to be minimal following an uncomplicated CSE.[99]

▶ *Potential risk of increased drug leakage through the dural hole, causing unexpectedly high sensory blocks.* This does not appear to be an issue clinically for both CSE labor analgesia and surgical anesthesia.

▶ *Risk of infectious complications with dural hole.* Evidence for an increased risk of infection is not seen.

▶ *Contamination of CSF with metal particles from damaged spinal needle tips during needle-through-needle technique.*[100] Two groups of investigators found no contamination of metallic particles in the intrathecal compartment following the needle-through-needle CSF technique.[101,102]

Additional concerns or disadvantages include the following:

▶ Fetal bradycardia possibly due to uterine hyperstimulation (see "Intrathecal Opioids," this page).

▶ *Unproven epidural catheter.* The epidural catheter is not proven to be functional until several hours after placement, as subarachnoid analgesia is present at the initiation of blockade. This may be a disadvantage for patients at high risk for cesarean delivery (e.g., patient with non-reassuring FHR pattern), or at increased risk for airway complications during general anesthesia should the epidural catheter fail in an emergency.

The technique is described in Chap. 2. It can be initiated in either the lateral or sitting position in laboring women. Patient position may influence the level of sensory blockade, depending of the baricity of injected solutions (see below).

Although the incidence of failed epidural catheters has been shown to be significantly higher with conventional epidural techniques when compared to CSE,[103] some studies have reported technical failures of the spinal component of the CSE technique. The reported incidence of failed CSE analgesia during labor is between 5 and 13%. Riley et al. suggested that failure to obtain CSF from the spinal needle

used in the CSE needle-through-needle technique may be due to inadequate length of the spinal needle.[104] In their study, the longer Gertie Marx needle was always successful in obtaining CSF, and the authors concluded that spinal needles that protrude more than 9 mm beyond the epidural needle tip are necessary to reliably perform the CSE technique. Other explanations for failure of CSF return include lateral deviation of the spinal needle (so it passes to the side of the dural sac), or the "tenting" of the dura mater with the noncutting spinal needle, rather than puncturing it (Fig. 2-28).[105]

The CSE technique may also fail after successful dural puncture because of spinal needle displacement at the time of syringe connection, aspiration of CSF, or injection of the anesthetic. The spinal needle may be easily displaced as it is anchored by only the dura mater.

Early CSE studies advocated letting the spinal analgesia component dissipate prior to initiation of the epidural analgesia. Currently, most clinicians start an epidural infusion soon after the spinal injection so that there is a seamless transition between the spinal and epidural components. Epidural analgesia may be maintained as discussed earlier (intermittent bolus, continuous infusion, or patient-controlled epidural infusion).

Intrathecal Opioids

During the first stage of labor, intrathecal opioids have been shown to reliably produce profound analgesia without motor block (Table 13-5). In the past, morphine was given in doses of 0.5–2.0 mg, but the high incidence of side effects prompted evaluation of different doses and drugs. Administration of very small doses of morphine (as little as 0.25 mg) is associated with a decreased incidence of side effects compared to larger doses.[106] If administered as a sole agent, however, the morphine is associated with a prolonged

Table 13-5

Drugs for Intrathecal Labor Analgesia: Initiation and Maintenance

Drug Solution	Opioid (µg)	Local Anesthetic (mg)
Fentanyl	15–25	–
Sufentanil	5–7.5	–
Bupivacaine-fentanyl	15	1.25–2.5*
Bupivacaine-sufentanil	1.25–2.5	1.25–2.5*

*Lower dose of bupivacaine are associated with shorter duration of analgesia, but less hypotension.

latency unacceptable for labor analgesia. In order to achieve a faster onset of analgesia with fewer side effects, sufentanil and fentanyl have been advocated. When used alone, either of these opioids provides a fast onset (typically 2–5 min) and a duration of analgesia between 60 and 120 min. The ED_{50} of fentanyl for intrathecal labor analgesia was 18.2 μg, and the ED_{50} of sufentanil was 4.1 μg.[107] Therefore, the potency ratio of intrathecal sufentanil to fentanyl for labor analgesia is approximately 4:1. Although the duration of spinal analgesia was longer with intrathecal sufentanil (104 ± 34 min vs. 79 ± 34 min, P = 0.009), one must consider the fact that sufentanil is more expensive and carries a greater risk of dosing error due to its higher potency and concentration.

The ED_{95} of intrathecal fentanyl for labor analgesia is between 20 and 30 μg, and of intrathecal sufentanil is 9 and 15 μg. When fentanyl is used as the sole intrathecal agent for labor analgesia, there appears to be no benefit to increasing the dose beyond 25 μg.[108] The authors routinely use 20 μg of intrathecal fentanyl if used alone, and 15 μg if used with bupivacaine. The intrathecal administration of fentanyl and sufentanil for labor analgesia are off-label uses of the drugs in the United States.

Meperidine may also provide intrathecal labor analgesia. Meperidine possesses weak local anesthetic properties and therefore, has the advantage of providing better somatic analgesia as labor progresses compared to other opioids. It is widely available and inexpensive. The preservative-free formulation should be used. Effective labor analgesia is achieved in 2–12 min, lasting 1–3 h. An additional advantage is that is may reduce the incidence and intensity of shivering.[109] Side effects, however, include an increased incidence of nausea and vomiting. Meperidine has not been associated with delayed respiratory depression but intrathecal doses above 50 mg, or lower doses administered concurrently with other sedatives, might produce this serious side effect.

Serious side effects from lipid-soluble opioid administration in the intrathecal space, although rare, include somnolence, nausea, vomiting, and respiratory depression. While pruritus is relatively common, it is self-limiting and rarely needs to be treated. At the authors' institution less than 1% of parturients who receive intrathecal fentanyl require treatment for pruritus (see "Pruritus," later).

Hypotension following intrathecal opioid injection may occur; therefore, close monitoring of blood pressure is indicated. Fetal bradycardia after intrathecal opioid injection has been observed.[110] A suggested mechanism for fetal bradycardia is the acute decrease in circulating maternal catecholamine concentrations (particularly epinephrine) that occurs after the establishment of analgesia. Since epinephrine is a tocolytic substance, decreased levels may, in turn, cause uterine hypercontractility, decreased uteropla-

cental perfusion, and fetal bradycardia. Therefore, the suggested treatment of fetal bradycardia that occurs shortly after the initiation of neuraxial analgesia is the maternal administration of a tocolytic drug (e.g., nitroglycerine or terbutaline). Usually, uterine hypertonus resolves within 4–8 min and an emergency cesarean delivery is not necessary. At the authors' institution intrathecal fentanyl is used to provide rapid onset of analgesia to approximately 8000 parturients per year with an observed fetal bradycardia rate of less than 1%.

Intrathecal Local Anesthetics

Intrathecal bupivacaine combined with a lipid-soluble opioid has a longer duration of action compared to opioid alone.[111] In addition, the local anesthetic provides somatic analgesia and is therefore, a useful intrathecal component for women in the advanced first and second stage of labor. The incidence of pruritus is lower when intrathecal bupivacaine is combined with fentanyl. Bupivacaine is the most commonly used local anesthetic due to its long duration of analgesia. In a study comparing bupivacaine, ropivacaine, and levobupivacaine, 2.5 mg, bupivacaine was associated with a higher incidence of lower limb motor block compared to the other drugs.[112] The incidence of motor blockade was decreased with ropivacaine 2.5 mg combined with fentanyl (5%), compared to bupivacaine 2.5 mg with fentanyl (40%).[113] Ropivacaine, however, is not approved by the United States FDA for intrathecal injection, so this remains an off-label use of the drug.

Baricity of Intrathecal Analgesic Solutions

All opioid and opioid/local anesthetic combinations used for intrathecal analgesia are hypobaric at 37°C.[114] Therefore, analgesia initiated in the sitting compared to lateral position results in significantly higher maximal cephalad spread of sensory blockade.[115] The addition of dextrose to sufentanil (resulting in a hyperbaric solution) resulted in more limited cephalad spread of sensory blockade compared to dextrose-free sufentanil, but also resulted in less analgesia.[116] Therefore, the routine addition of dextrose to the intrathecal analgesic solution is not recommended.

Ambulation with CSE Analgesia-the "Mobile Epidural"

The approach of using opioid often with the addition of low-dose local anesthetics via the epidural or spinal route can provide a selective sensory block with a minimal motor blockade. This may allow parturients to ambulate during labor—if muscle groups innervated by L5-S1 nerve roots have normal power as assessed by the Bromage scale or related scales.

A test dose of 3 mL of lidocaine 1.5% with epinephrine administered via the epidural catheter may preclude early ambulation. When a conventional epidural test dose was administered after initiation of fentanyl/bupivacaine CSE, motor function was adversely affected for 30–60 min, consistent with the duration of action of epidural lidocaine with epinephrine.[117] Similarly, when a conventional test dose proceeded the epidural administration of 0.125% bupivacaine, 12 mL, with sufentanil 10 µg, ambulation was impaired compared to the same epidural dose without the test dose.[118] While some believe that walking does not enhance or impair active labor,[119] others believe that walking with ambulatory labor analgesia shortens the duration of labor.

COMPLICATIONS AND SIDE EFFECTS OF NEURAXIAL LABOR ANALGESIA

▶ Neurotoxicity

Neurologic complications due to neuraxial anesthesia and analgesia are very rare, especially when compared to the neurologic complications of labor and delivery. However, the injection of medications into the epidural or subarachnoid space has the potential for irritation or damage to neural structures. Therefore, anesthesiologists should take this into consideration and exercise caution when injecting any new agent into the subarachnoid space. Injecting the wrong drug, high concentrations of local anesthetic solutions, or neurotoxic preservatives may be directly toxic to nerve tissue.[120] In addition, direct trauma can be caused by the needle or catheter. To prevent this, a low lumbar level should be chosen as the puncture site, needle advancement should be stopped immediately if the parturient perceives radicular pain, and injection of anesthetic solution should occur only if there is no pain.

Other neurologic complications that have been reported to occur after neuraxial anesthesia include transient neurologic syndrome (TNS), spinal/epidural hematoma, spinal/epidural abscess, and complaints of back pain (see Chap. 6). The relationship between backache and epidural placement does not appear to be causal, but may result from a combination of effective analgesia and stressed posture during labor. There have been no differences in the incidence of long-term back pain between women receiving epidural analgesia and those receiving other forms of pain relief.[121]

▶ Pruritus

Pruritus is the most common side effect of neuraxial opioid administration (see Chap. 6). Its cause remains unclear. Intrathecal opioid administration is associated with a higher incidence of pruritus than epidural administration. The incidence and severity of pruritus can be decreased by administering a lower dose of the opioid and/or the coadministration of a local anesthetic.[122] Intrathecal opioid-induced pruritus appears to be unrelated to histamine release and thus antihistamines are not advocated for treatment. Treatment options include naloxone (0.04–0.08 mg IV) or nalbuphine (2.5–5 mg IV), which act as specific mu-receptor antagonists. Recent evidence demonstrates a close interaction between opioids and the serotoninergic system in the CNS via 5-HT$_3$ receptors.[123] It is believed that serotonin (5-HT) plays a role in pain transmission, and the induction of nausea, and possibly of pruritus, after spinal morphine administration. In a study of parturients experiencing intrathecal morphine-induced pruritus, ondansetron 4 mg effectively treated pruritus 70–80% of the time, versus 30% after placebo (normal saline).[123] Subhypnotic doses of propofol may have an inhibitory effect on the dorsal horn of the spinal cord, decreasing pruritus by causing a generalized reduction in CNS functional activity.[124]

▶ Urinary Retention

The etiology of urinary retention following spinal analgesia is thought to be related to the rapid onset of detrusor muscle relaxation that results from the sacral spinal action of opioids and local anesthetics. It appears to parallel the onset of the analgesia. The clinical significance of urinary retention during labor is unclear.

▶ Delayed Gastric Emptying and Nausea and Vomiting

Both labor and opioid administration (by any route) result in delayed gastric emptying. This may predispose parturients to nausea and vomiting. In addition, delayed emptying may result in greater volume of gastric contents, which increases aspiration risk for patients requiring cesarean delivery, especially in emergency situations that require the induction of general anesthesia. Other causes of nausea and vomiting in the parturient include pregnancy itself and the pain of labor. Nausea may be treated intravenously with metoclopramide or ondansetron. While low-dose droperidol was advocated in the past, concerns regarding cardiac rhythm abnormalities, found to be associated with doses of 10 mg or more, raised questions about its use, and a "black box warning" was issued by the FDA. Subhypnotic doses of propofol (1 mg/kg/h IV) have also been shown to be effective in the prevention of severe nausea.[125]

▶ Postdural Puncture Headache

The incidence of PDPH following dural puncture with a large bore 18-gauge Tuohy needle (while performing epidural, CSE, or continuous spinal analgesia) has been reported to be approximately 50% in the parturient.[126]

The cause of this complication has not been fully identified but CSF leakage with traction on the meninges and intracranial nerves leading to intracranial hypotension is the most likely etiology (see Chap. 6). As previously discussed, the use of noncutting, pencil-point spinal needles has substantially reduced the incidence of PDPH following dural puncture. An advantage of the CSE technique is the ability to use smaller gauge spinal needles to decrease the chances of PDPH. Using the Touhy needle as an introducer allows meticulous puncture of the dura mater with fewer attempts at identifying the subarachnoid space. It is also thought that the decreased chance of PDPH may be related to the fact that as the spinal needle approaches the dura mater, it exits the Touhy needle at an angle, thereby reducing the risk of CSF leakage.[105]

Although several measures have been proposed to decrease the risk of PDPH, none have proved to work with certainty. Some techniques used after unintentional or planned dural puncture include injection of preservative-free saline into the subarachnoid space through the epidural needle or catheter, leaving the catheter in the intrathecal space for a period 12–20 h, and injecting CSF in the epidural syringe back into the subarachnoid space.[127] In a report of seven cases, these measures together decreased the incidence of PDPH to 14%.[127] It has been postulated that leaving the intrathecal catheter in situ, "plugs" the dural tear and causes an inflammatory reaction that will seal the hole by edema and fibrin exudate formation. In an observational study, Ayad et al. found the incidence of PDPH was reduced if a subarachnoid catheter was left in place for 24 h after delivery.[96] Further large-scale studies are needed to confirm the actual benefits of these maneuvers.

Two options exist after inadvertent dural puncture during epidural placement: removal of the epidural needle and placement of an epidural catheter in another interspace, or the placement of an intrathecal catheter through the dural hole. Advantages of the latter include avoidance of the risk of a second dural puncture, and excellent labor analgesia or surgical anesthesia. Extreme care must be taken, however, lest someone mistake the intrathecal catheter for an epidural catheter and inject an epidural dose through the catheter. Placement of an epidural catheter at another interspace avoids this risk. In addition, the catheter may be used for a prophylactic epidural blood patch. A recent randomized study comparing a prophylactic blood patch to a sham patch, however, found no decrease in the incidence of PDPH, although the duration of headache symptoms was decreased.[128]

At the authors' institution the initial and conservative treatment of PDPH consists of a combination of hydration (oral or intravenous), analgesics, and caffeine (500 mg in 1 L lactated Ringer's solution). Caffeine is thought to increase cerebral vascular resistance, decrease cerebral blood flow, and decrease cerebral blood volume. If the headache does not resolve after conservative management, an epidural blood patch is performed.

▶ Fetal Effects

Systemic absorption of opioids and local anesthetics, followed by transplacental transfer, may result in direct effects on the fetus. This may include changes in FHR as well as respiratory depression after delivery. Neonatal respiratory depression occurs more often after intravenous opioid administration during labor.

Epidural administration of opioids has little direct effect on FHR, even if administered by CEI.[129] On the other hand, there have been serious concerns about the fetal bradycardia observed after spinal analgesia (see "Intrathecal Opioids," earlier).

Maternal side effects of opioid administration may affect the fetus indirectly. For example, opioid-induced maternal respiratory depression and hypoxemia may result in fetal hypoxia. The FHR should be monitored while the parturient is undergoing neuraxial labor analgesia. If fetal bradycardia occurs, in utero resuscitation should be undertaken. This includes relief of aortocaval compression, discontinuation of oxytocin, administration of supplemental oxygen, treatment of maternal hypotension, and fetal scalp stimulation. In case of uterine hypertonus, intravenous (60–90 μg) or sublingual (400 μg) nitroglycerin can be used to relax the uterus.[130] If there is no evidence of uterine relaxation within 2 or 3 min, terbutaline (250 μg IV or subcutaneously) can also be administered. Amnioinfusion should also be considered. Emergency delivery is a last resort if fetal bradycardia does not resolve.

NEW AGENTS

New drugs and methods are constantly being evaluated to improve analgesia for labor. Gautier et al.[131] found that the duration of intrathecal labor analgesia can be increased from 104 to 145 min without motor block if clonidine 30 μg is added to intrathecal sufentanil (2.5–5 μg). Other investigators have had similar results when using clonidine alone, with sufentanil, or in addition to bupivacaine and neostigime.[132] Unfortunately, a disadvantage of clonidine is the high incidence of maternal hypotension and sedation. Owen et al.[133] compared intrathecal bupivacaine/fentanyl (BF), BF plus clonidine (BFC), or BFC plus neostigmine (BFCN). The incidence of nausea in the group that received neostigmine was 33%, suggesting that neostigmine is not a useful adjunct for obstetric analgesia. The manufacturer of Duraclon (FDA-approved epidural clonidine formulation) recommends against its use in obstetric patients.

At doses exceeding 100 μg in volunteers, neostigmine was also associated with motor weakness, which may be clinically relevant and may interfere with ambulation. Results from a recent study by Kaya et al. suggest that epidural neostigmine (75–300 μg single bolus) produces modest analgesia and mild sedation without increasing the incidence of maternal nausea.[134] Future studies will need to assess potential adverse effects on uterine tone, uterine activity, and FHR.

Intrathecal administration of medications acting on gamma-aminobutyric acid (GABA) receptors in the spinal cord are now under investigation. Previous animal studies with midazolam suggested the potential for neurotoxicity, but the validity of extrapolating these results to humans has been questioned. Johansen et al.[135] evaluated the potential neurotoxicity of preservative-free midazolam in a sheep model. Continuous infusion of midazolam 5–15 mg/day was well tolerated and did not result in demonstrable histologic neurotoxicity. Preservative-free midazolam 0.03 mg/kg enhanced intrathecal fentanyl labor analgesia with no change in adverse effects.[136] More studies, however, are needed to evaluate the effectiveness and safety of intrathecal midazolam. The formulation of midazolam available in the United States contains preservatives that may be neurotoxic, so at this time commercially available drug should not be administered into the spinal space.

No adjuvant studied to date prolongs the duration of fentanyl or sufentanil/bupivacaine analgesia long enough to avoid the use of epidural maintenance analgesia for most parturients, or eliminates the side effects associated with the current drugs. Therefore, it currently makes little sense to routinely add additional drugs with their added cost, unknown toxicity, and the probable increased risk of errors associated with using multiple drugs.

Spinal microcatheters are being studied and may present a viable and attractive option to produce labor analgesia, if rereleased by the FDA. Data presented by Arkoosh et al. suggest that this technique may offer advantages for labor analgesia compared to current neuraxial techniques.[137]

REFERENCES

1. Halpern SH, Leighton BL. Epidural analgesia and risk of cesarean section. *Lancet* 353:1801, 1999.
2. Zhang J, Yancey MK, Klebanoff MA, et al. Does epidural analgesia prolong labor and increase risk of cesarean delivery? A natural experiment. *Am J Obstet Gynecol* 185:128, 2001.
3. Hawkins JL, Koonin LM, Palmer SK, et al. Anesthesia-related deaths during obstetric delivery in the United States, 1979–1990. *Anesthesiology* 86:277, 1997.
4. Hiltunen P, Raudaskoski T, Ebeling H, et al. Does pain relief during delivery decrease the risk of postnatal depression? *Acta Obstet Gynecol Scan* 83:257, 2004.
5. Melzack R. The myth of painless childbirth (The John J. Bonica Lecture). *Pain* 19:321, 1984.
6. Melzack R, Taenzer P, Feldman P, et al. Labour is still painful after prepared childbirth training. *Can Med Assoc J* 125:357. 1981.
7. Bonica JJ. The nature of pain in parturition. In: Van Zundert A, Ostheimer GW, eds, *Pain Relief and Anesthesia in Obstetrics*. New York: Churchill Livingstone, 1996.
8. Brownridge P. The nature and consequences of childbirth pain. *Eur J Obstet Gynecol Reprod Biol* 59(Suppl):S9, 1995.
9. Berkley KJ, Robbins A, Sato Y. Functional differences between afferent fibers in the hypogastric and pelvic nerves innervating female reproductive organs in the rat. *J Neurophysiol* 69:533, 1993.
10. Siddal PJ, Cousins MJ. Introduction to pain mechanisms: Implications for neural blockade. In: Cousins MJ, Bridenbaugh PO, eds, *Neural Blockade in Clinical Anesthesia and Management of Pain*, 3rd ed. Philadelphia, PA: Lippincott-Raven, 1988, p. 690.
11. Melzack R, Kinch R, Dobkin P, et al. Severity of labour pain: Influence of physical as well as psychologic variables. *Can Med Assoc J* 130:579, 1984.
12. Lowe NK. The pain and discomfort of labor and birth. *J Obstet Gynecol Neonatal Nurs* 25:82, 1996.
13. Fridh G, Kopare T, Gaston-Johansson F, et al. Factors associated with more intense labor pain. *Res Nurs Health* 11:117, 1988.
14. Lowe NK. Differences in first and second stage labor pain between nulliparous and multiparous women. *J Psychosom Obstet Gynecol* 13:243, 1992.
15. Sheiner EK, Sheiner E, Shoham-Vardi I, et al. Ethnic differences influence care giver's estimates of pain during labour. *Pain* 81:299, 1999.
16. Gintzler AR. Endorphin-mediated increases in pain threshold during pregnancy. *Science* 210:193, 1980.
17. Dawson-Basoa ME, Gintzler AR. Estrogen and progesterone activate spinal kappa-opiate receptor analgesic mechanisms. *Pain* 64:608 1996.
18. Casey ML, Smith JW, Nagai K, et al. Progesterone-regulated cyclic modulation of membrane metalloendopeptidase (enkephalinase) in human endometrium. *J Biol Chem* 266:23041, 1991.
19. Eisenach JC, Detweiler DJ, Tong C, et al. Cerebrospinal fluid norepinephrine and acetylcholine concentrations during acute pain. *Anesth Analg* 82:621, 1996.
20. Gordh T Jr, Jansson I, Hartvig P, et al. Interactions between noradrenergic and cholinergic mechanisms involved in spinal nociceptive processing. *Acta Anaesthesiol Scand* 33:39, 1989.
21. Broadbent CR, Maxwell WB, Ferrie R, et al. Ability of anaesthetists to identify a marked lumbar interspace. *Anaesthesia* 55:1122, 2000.
22. Hirabayashi Y, Shimizu R, Fukuda H, et al. Anatomical configuration of the spinal column in the supine position. II. Comparison of pregnant and non-pregnant women. *Br J Anaesth* 75:6, 1995.
23. Hirabayashi Y, Shimizu R, Fukuda H, et al. Effects of the pregnant uterus on the extradural venous plexus in the supine and lateral positions, as determined by magnetic resonance imaging. *Br J Anaesth* 78:317, 1997.
24. Bevacqua BK, Haas T, Brand F. A clinical measure of the posterior epidural space depth. *Reg Anesth* 21:456, 1996.
25. Currie JM. Measurement of the depth to the extradural space using ultrasound. *Br J Anaesth* 56:345, 1984.
26. Westbrook JL, Renowden SA, Carrie LE. Study of the anatomy of the extradural region using magnetic resonance imaging. *Br J Anaesth* 71:495, 1993.

27. Harrison GR, Clowes NWB. The depth of the lumbar epidural space from the skin. *Anaesthesia* 40;685, 1985.

28. Sutton DN, Linter SP. Depth of extradural space and dural puncture. *Anaesthesia* 46:97, 1991.

29. Hogan QH. Epidural anatomy: New observations. *Can J Anaesth* 45:R40, 1998.

30. Hamza J, Smida M, Benhamou D, et al. Parturient's posture during epidural puncture affects the distance from skin to epidural space. *J Clin Anesth* 7:1, 1995.

31. Usubiaga JE, Moya F, Usubiaga LE. . Effect of thoracic and abdominal pressure changes on the epidural space pressure. *Br J Anaesth* 39:612, 1967.

32. Barclay DL, Renegar OJ, Nelson EW Jr. The influence of inferior vena cava compression on the level of spinal anesthesia. *Am J Obstet Gynecol* 101:792, 1968.

33. Datta S, Hurley RJ, Naulty JS, et al. Plasma and cerebrospinal fluid progesterone concentrations in pregnant and nonpregnant women. *Anesth Analg* 65:950, 1986.

34. Sheiner E, Shoham-Vardi I, Sheiner EK, et al. A comparison between the effectiveness of epidural analgesia and parenteral pethidine during labor. *Arch Gynecol Obstet* 263:95, 2000.

35. Shnider SM, Abboud TK, Artal R, et al. Maternal catecholamines decrease during labor after lumbar epidural anesthesia. *Am J Obstet Gynecol* 147:13, 1983.

36. Vahratian A, Zhang J, Hasling J, et al. The effect of early epidural versus early intravenous analgesia use on labor progression: A natural experiment. *Am J Obstet Gynecol* 191:259, 2004.

37. Rogers R, Gilson G, Kammerer-Doak D. Epidural analgesia and active management of labor: Effects on length of labor and mode of delivery. *Obstet Gynecol* 93:995, 1999.

38. Wong CA, Scavone BM, Peaceman AM, et al. The risk of cesarean delivery with neuraxial analgesia given early versus late in labor. *N Engl J Med* 352:655, 2005.

39. American College of Obstetricians and Gynecologists: Obstetric analgesia and anesthesia. *ACOG Practice Bulletin Number* 36. Washington, DC, 2002.

40. American College of Obstetricians and Gynecologists: Pain relief during labor. *ACOG Committee Opinion* 295. Washington, DC, 2004.

41. Pattee C, Ballantyne M, Milne B. Epidural analgesia for labour and delivery: Informed consent issues. *Can J Anaesth* 44:918, 1997.

42. Jackson A, Henry R, Avery N, et al. Informed consent for labour epidurals: What labouring women want to know. *Can J Anaesth* 47:1068, 2000.

43. Practice guidelines for obstetrical anesthesia: A report by the American Society of Anesthesiologists Task Force on Obstetrical Anesthesia. *Anesthesiology* 90:600, 1999.

44. Suonio S, Simpanen AL, Olkkonen H, et al. Effect of the left lateral recumbent position compared with the supine and upright positions on placental blood flow in normal late pregnancy. *Ann Clin Res* 8:22, 1976.

45. Vincent RD, Chestnut DH. Which position is more comfortable for the parturient during identification of the epidural space? *Int J Obstet Anesth* 1:9, 1991.

46. Bahar M, Chanimov M, Cohen ML, et al. The lateral recumbent head-down position decreases the incidence of epidural venous puncture during catheter insertion in obese parturients. *Can J Anaesth* 51:577, 2004.

47. Birnbach DJ, Stein DJ, Murray O, et al. Povidone iodine and skin disinfection before initiation of epidural anesthesia. *Anesthesiology* 88:668, 1998.

48. O'Rourke E, Runyan D, O'Leary J, et al. Contaminated iodophor in the operating room. *Am J Infect Control* 31:255, 2003.

49. Clevenot D, Robert S, Debaene B, et al. Critical review of the literature concerning the comparative use of two antiseptic solutions before intravascular or epidural catheterization. *Ann Fr Anesth Reanim* 22:787, 2003.

50. Schneeberger PM, Janssen M, Voss A. Alpha-hemolytic streptococci: A major pathogen of iatrogenic meningitis following lumbar puncture. *Infection* 24:29, 1996.

51. Panikkar KK, Yentis SM. Wearing of masks for obstetric regional anaesthesia. A postal survey. *Anaesthesia* 51:398, 1996.

52. Trautmann M, Lepper PM, Schmitz FJ. Three cases of bacterial meningitis after spinal and epidural anesthesia. *Eur J Clin Microbiol Infect Dis* 21:43, 2002.

53. Beilin Y, Arnold I, Telfeyan C, et al. Quality of analgesia when air versus saline is used for identification of the epidural space in the parturient. *Reg Anesth Pain Med* 25:596, 2000.

54. Saberski LR, Kondamuri S, Osinubi OY. Identification of the epidural space: Is loss of resistance to air a safe technique? A review of the complications related to the use of air. *Reg Anesth* 22:3, 1997.

55. Dalens B. Gone with the wind-the fate of epidural air. *Reg Anesth* 15:150, 1990.

56. Kennedy TM, Ullman DA, Harte FA, et al. Lumbar root compression secondary to epidural air. *Anesth Analg* 67:1184, 1988.

57. Dickson MA, Moores C, McClure JH. Comparison of single, end-holed and multi-orifice extradural catheters when used for continuous infusion of local anaesthetic during labour. *Br J Anaesth* 79:297, 1997.

58. D'Angelo R, Foss ML, Livesay CH. A comparison of multiport and uniport epidural catheters in laboring patients. *Anesth Analg* 84:1276, 1997.

59. Gadalla F, Lee SH, Choi KC, et al. Injecting saline through the epidural needle decreases the iv epidural catheter placement rate during combined spinal-epidural labour analgesia. *Can J Anaesth* 50:382, 2003.

60. Beilin Y, Bernstein HH, Zucker-Pinchoff B. The optimal distance that a multiorifice epidural catheter should be threaded into the epidural space. *Anesth Analg* 81:301, 1995.

61. Hamilton CL, Riley ET, Cohen SE. Changes in the position of epidural catheters associated with patient movement. *Anesthesiology* 86:778, 1997.

62. Birnbach DJ, Chestnut DH. The epidural test dose in obstetric patients: Has it outlived its usefulness? *Anesth Analg* 88:971, 1999.

63. Moore DC, Batra MS. The components of an effective test dose prior to epidural block. *Anesthesiology* 55:693, 1981.

64. Gaiser RR. The epidural test dose in obstetric anesthesia: It is not obsolete. *J Clin Anesth* 15:474, 2003.

65. Beilin Y, Nair A, Arnold I, et al. A comparison of epidural infusions in the combined spinal/epidural technique for labor analgesia. *Anesth Analg* 94:927, 2002.

66. Polley LS, Columb MO, Naughton NN, et al. Relative analgesic potencies of ropivacaine and bupivacaine for epidural analgesia in labor: Implications for therapeutic indexes. *Anesthesiology* 90:944, 1999.

67. Capogna G, Celleno D, Fusco P, et al. Relative potencies of bupivacaine and ropivacaine for analgesia in labour. *Br J Anaesth* 82:371, 1999.

68. Halpern SH, Breen TW, Campbell DC, et al. A multicenter, randomized, controlled trial comparing bupivacaine with ropivacaine for labor analgesia. *Anesthesiology* 98:1431, 2003.

69. Campbell DC, Zwack RM, Crone LA, et al. Ambulatory labor epidural analgesia: Bupivacaine versus ropivacaine. *Anesth Analg* 90:1384, 2000.

70. Owen MD, Thomas JA, Smith T, et al. Ropivacaine 0.075% and bupivacaine 0.075% with fentanyl 2 microg/mL are equivalent for labor epidural analgesia. *Anesth Analg* 94:179, 2004.

71. Foster RH, Markham A. Levobupivacaine: A review of its pharmacology and use as a local anesthetic. *Drugs* 59:551, 2000. Review.

72. Vercauteren MP, Hans G, De Decker K, et al. Levobupivacaine combined with sufentanil and epinephrine for intrathecal labor analgesia: A comparison with racemic bupivacaine. *Anesth Analg* 93:996, 2001.

73. Bader AM, Tsen LC, Camann WR, et al. Clinical effects and maternal and fetal plasma concentrations of 0.5% epidural levobupivacaine versus bupivacaine for cesarean delivery. *Anesthesiology* 90:1596, 1999.

74. Milaszkiewicz R, Payne N, Loughnan B, et al. Continuous extradural infusion of lignocaine 0.75% vs bupivacaine 0.125% in primiparae: Quality of analgesia and influence on labour. *Anaesthesia* 47:1042, 1992.

75. Abboud TK, Kim KC, Noueihed R, et al. Epidural bupivacaine, chloroprocaine, or lidocaine for cesarean section—maternal and neonatal effects. *Anesth Analg* 62:914, 1983.

76. Grice SC, Eisenach JC, Dewan DM. Labor analgesia with epidural bupivacaine plus fentanyl: Enhancement with epinephrine and inhibition with 2-chloroprocaine. *Anesthesiology* 72:623, 1990.

77. Corke BC, Carlson CG, Dettbarn WD. The influence of 2-chloroprocaine on the subsequent analgesic potency of bupivacaine. *Anesthesiology* 60:25, 1984.

78. Coda B, Bausch S, Haas M, et al. The hypothesis that antagonism of fentanyl analgesia by 2-chloroprocaine is mediated by direct action on opioid receptors. *Reg Anesth* 22:43, 1997.

79. Philipson EH, Kuhnert BR, Syracuse CD. Fetal acidosis, 2-chloroprocaine, and epidural anesthesia for cesarean section. *Am J Obstet Gynecol* 151:322, 1985.

80. Winnie AP, Nader AM. Santayana's prophecy fulfilled. *Reg Anesth Pain Med* 26:558, 2001.

81. Justins DM, Francis D, Houlton PG, et al. A controlled trial of extradural fentanyl in labour. *Br J Anaesth* 54:409, 1982.

82. Polley LS, Columb MO, Naughton NN, et al. Effect of epidural epinephrine on the minimum local analgesic concentration of epidural bupivacaine in labor. *Anesthesiology* 96:1123, 2002.

83. Eisenach JC, Grice SC, Dewan DM. Epinephrine enhances analgesia produced by epidural bupivacaine during labor. *Anesth Analg* 66:447, 1987.

84. Hadzic A, Vloka J, Patel N, et al. Hypertensive crisis after a successful placement of an epidural anesthetic in a hypertensive parturient. Case report. *Reg Anesth* 20:156, 1995.

85. Lysak SZ, Eisenach JC, Dobson CE 2nd. Patient-controlled epidural analgesia during labor: A comparison of three solutions with a continuous infusion control. *Anesthesiology* 72:44, 1990.

86. Ledin Eriksson S, Gentele C, Olofsson CH. PCEA compared to continuous epidural infusion in an ultra-low-dose regimen for labor pain relief: A randomized study. *Acta Anaesthesiol Scand* 47:1085, 2003.

87. Halonen P, Sarvela J, Saisto T, et al. Patient-controlled epidural technique improves analgesia for labor but increases cesarean delivery rate compared with the intermittent bolus technique. *Acta Anaesthesiol Scand* 48:732, 2004.

88. Smedstad KG, Morison DH. A comparative study of continuous and intermittent epidural analgesia for labour and delivery. *Can J Anaesth* 35:234, 1988.

89. Wilson MJ, Cooper G, MacArthur C, et al. Comparative Obstetric Mobile Epidural Trial (COMET) Study Group UK. Randomized controlled trial comparing traditional with two "mobile" epidural techniques: Anesthetic and analgesic efficacy. *Anesthesiology* 97:1567, 2002.

90. Bogod DG, Rosen M, Rees GA. Extradural infusion of 0.125% bupivacaine at 10 ml h-1 to women during labour. *Br J Anaesth* 59:325, 1987.

91. Li DF, Rees GA, Rosen M. Continuous extradural infusion of 0.0625% or 0.125% bupivacaine for pain relief in primigravid labour. *Br J Anaesth* 57:264, 1985.

92. Gambling DR, Huber CJ, Berkowitz J, et al. Patient-controlled epidural analgesia in labour: Varying bolus dose and lockout interval. *Can J Anaesth* 40:211, 1993.

93. Ledin Eriksson S, Gentele C, Olofsson CH. PCEA compared to continuous epidural infusion in an ultra-low-dose regimen for labor pain relief: A randomized study. *Acta Anaesthesiol Scand* 47:1085, 2003.

94. Chua SM, Sia AT. Automated intermittent epidural boluses improve analgesia induced by intrathecal fentanyl during labour. *Can J Anaesth* 51:581, 2004.

95. Smith PS, Wilson RC, Robinson AP, et al. Regional blockade for delivery in women with scoliosis or previous spinal surgery. *Int J Obstet Anesth* 12:17, 2003.

96. Ayad S, Demian Y, Narouze SN, et al. Subarachnoid catheter placement after wet tap for analgesia in labor: Influence on the risk of headache in obstetric patients. *Reg Anesth Pain Med* 28:512, 2003.

97. Collis R. Combined spinal epidural (CSE) analgesia is the preferred technique for labour pain relief. *Acta Anaesthesiol Belg* 53:283, 2002.

98. Tsen LC, Thue B, Datta S, et al. Is combined spinal-epidural analgesia associated with more rapid cervical dilation in nulliparous patients when compared with conventional epidural analgesia? *Anesthesiology* 91:920, 1999.

99. Holmstrom B, Rawal N, Axelsson K, et al. Risk of catheter migration during combined spinal epidural block: Percutaneous epiduroscopy study. *Anesth Analg* 80:747, 1995.

100. Eldor J. Metallic particles in the spinal-epidural needle technique. *Reg Anesth* 19:219, 1994.

101. Holst D, Mollmann M, Schymroszcyk B, et al. No risk of metal toxicity in combined spinal-epidural anesthesia. *Anesth Analg* 88:393, 1999.

102. Herman N, Molin J, Knape KG. No additional metal particle formation using the needle-through-needle combined epidural/spinal technique. *Acta Anaesthesiol Scand* 40:227, 1996.

103. Van de Velde M, Mignolet K, Vandermeersch E, et al. Prospective, randomized comparison of epidural and combined spinal epidural analgesia during labor. *Acta Anaesthesiol Belg* 50:129, 1999.

104. Riley ET, Hamilton CL, Ratner EF, et al. A comparison of the 24-gauge Sprotte and Gertie Marx spinal needles for combined spinal-epidural analgesia during labor. *Anesthesiology* 97:574, 2002.

105. Rawal N, Holmstrom B, Crowhurst JA, et al. The combined spinal-epidural technique. *Anesthesiol Clin North America* 18:267, 2000.

106. Nordberg G, Hedner T, Mellstrand T, et al. Pharmacokinetic aspects of intrathecal morphine analgesia. *Anesthesiology* 60:448, 1984.

107. DeBalli P, Breen TW. Intrathecal opioids for combined spinal-epidural analgesia during labour. *CNS Drugs* 17:889, 2003.

108. Palmer CM, Cork RC, Hays R, et al. The dose-response relation of intrathecal fentanyl for labor analgesia. *Anesthesiology* 88:355, 1998.

109. Roy JD, Girard M, Drolet P. Intrathecal meperidine decreases shivering during cesarean delivery under spinal anesthesia. *Anesth Analg* 98:230, 2004.

110. Van de Velde M, Teunkens A, Hanssens M, et al. Intrathecal sufentanil and fetal heart rate abnormalities: A double-blind, double placebo-controlled trial comparing two forms of combined spinal epidural analgesia with epidural analgesia in labor. *Anesth Analg* 98:1153, 2004.

111. Campbell DC, Camann WR, Datta S. The addition of bupivacaine to intrathecal sufentanil for labor analgesia. *Anesth Analg* 81:305, 1995.

112. Lim Y, Ocampo CE, Sia AT. A comparison of duration of analgesia of intrathecal 2.5 mg of bupivacaine, ropivacaine, and levobupivacaine in combined spinal epidural analgesia for patients in labor. *Anesth Analg* 98:235, 2004.

113. Hughes D, Hill D, Fee JP. Intrathecal ropivacaine or bupivacaine with fentanyl for labour. *Br J Anaesth* 87:733, 2001.

114. Richardson MG, Wissler RN. Densities of dextrose-free intrathecal local anesthetics, opioids, and combinations measured at 37 degrees C. *Anesth Analg* 84:95, 1997.

115. Richardson MG, Thakur R, Abramowicz JS, et al. Maternal posture influences the extent of sensory block produced by intrathecal dextrose-free bupivacaine with fentanyl for labor analgesia. *Anesth Analg* 83:1229, 1996.

116. Ferouz F, Norris MC, Arkoosh VA, et al. Baricity, needle direction, and intrathecal sufentanil labor analgesia. *Anesthesiology* 86:592, 1997.

117. Calimaran AL, Strauss-Hoder TP, Wang WY, et al. The effect of epidural test dose on motor function after a combined spinal-epidural technique for labor analgesia. *Anesth Analg* 96:1167, 2003.

118. Cohen SE, Yeh JY, Riley ET, et al. Walking with labor epidural analgesia: The impact of bupivacaine concentration and a lidocaine-epinephrine test dose. *Anesthesiology* 92:387, 2000.

119. Bloom SL, McIntire DD, Kelly MA, et al. Lack of effect of walking on labor and delivery. *N Engl J Med* 339:76, 1998.

120. Wong CA. Neurologic deficits and labor analgesia. *Reg Anesth Pain Med* 29:341, 2004.

121. Howell CJ, Dean T, Lucking L, et al. Randomised study of long term outcome after epidural versus non-epidural analgesia during labour. *BMJ* 325:357, 2002.

122. Asokumar B, Newman LM, McCarthy RJ, et al. Intrathecal bupivacaine reduces pruritus and prolongs duration of fentanyl analgesia during labor: A prospective, randomized controlled trial. *Anesth Analg* 7:1309, 1998.

123. Charuluxananan S, Somboonviboon W, Kyokong O, et al. Ondansetron for treatment of intrathecal morphine-induced pruritus after cesarean delivery. *Reg Anesth Pain Med* 25:535, 2000.

124. Cavazzuti M, Porro CA, Barbieri A, et al. Brain and spinal cord metabolic activity during propofol anaesthesia. *Br J Anaesth* 66:490, 1991.

125. Numazaki M, Fujii Y. Reduction of emetic symptoms during cesarean delivery with antiemetics: Propofol at subhypnotic dose versus traditional antiemetics. *J Clin Anesth* 15:423, 2003.

126. Choi PT, Galinski SE, Takeuchi L, et al. PDPH is a common complication of neuraxial blockade in parturients: A meta-analysis of obstetrical studies. *Can J Anaesth* 50:460, 2003.

127. Kuczkowski KM, Benumof JL. Decrease in the incidence of post-dural puncture headache: Maintaining CSF volume. *Acta Anaesthesiol Scand* 47:98, 2003.

128. Scavone BM, Wong CA, Sullivan JT, et al. Efficacy of a prophylactic epidural blood patch in preventing post dural puncture headache in parturients after inadvertent dural puncture. *Anesthesiology* 101:1422, 2004.

129. Porter JS, Bonello E, Reynolds F. The effect of epidural opioids on maternal oxygenation during labour and delivery. *Anaesthesia* 51:899, 1996.

130. Mercier FJ, Dounas M, Bouaziz H, et al. Intravenous nitroglycerin to relieve intrapartum fetal distress related to uterine hyperactivity: A prospective observational study. *Anesth Analg* 84:1117, 1997.

131. Gautier PE, De Kock M, Fanard L, et al. Intrathecal clonidine combined with sufentanil for labor analgesia. *Anesthesiology* 88:651, 1998.

132. D'Angelo R, Dean LS, Meister GC, et al. Neostigmine combined with bupivacaine, clonidine, and sufentanil for spinal labor analgesia. *Anesth Analg* 93:1560, 2001.

133. Owen MD, Ozsarac O, Sahin S, et al. Low-dose clonidine and neostigmine prolong the duration of intrathecal bupivacaine-fentanyl for labor analgesia. *Anesthesiology* 92:361, 2000.

134. Kaya FN, Sahin S, Owen MD, et al. Epidural neostigmine produces analgesia but also sedation in women after cesarean delivery. *Anesthesiology* 100:381, 2004.

135. Johansen MJ, Gradert TL, Satterfield WC, et al. Safety of continuous intrathecal midazolam infusion in the sheep model. *Anesth Analg* 98:1528, 2004.

136. Tucker AP, Mezzatesta J, Nadeson R, et al. Intrathecal midazolam II: Combination with intrathecal fentanyl for labor pain. *Anesth Analg* 98:1521, 2004.

137. Arkoosh VA, Palmer CM, Yun E, et al. Continuous spinal labor analgesia: Safety and efficacy. *Anesthesiology* 97:A1561, 2003.

Neuraxial Blockade for Obstetric Surgery

CHAPTER 14

John T. Sullivan

INTRODUCTION

Neuraxial anesthesia for obstetric surgery has become increasingly popular over the last two decades for a variety of reasons. The foremost reason is evidence that neuraxial anesthesia is safer than general anesthesia for most pregnant women. Maternal mortality has declined over this time period and the increased use of neuraxial anesthesia for cesarean delivery is believed to be, in part, responsible.[1] Inability to intubate the trachea and pulmonary aspiration are leading causes of anesthesia-related maternal mortality and both are reduced by the greater use of neuraxial anesthesia in term pregnant patients requiring anesthesia for a surgical procedure. Because of these safety concerns for the mother and fetus, the vast majority of abdominal surgical procedures in the obstetric population in the United States are performed under neuraxial anesthesia.

CESAREAN DELIVERY

Cesarean delivery is the most common major surgical procedure performed in the United States. The choice of anesthetic technique is influenced by many factors, including the safety of the mother and fetus, intra- and postoperative comfort of the mother, need to optimize operative conditions, including muscle relaxation, as well as efficient use of resources. Fortunately, there are a large number of prospective, randomized, double-blinded clinical trials on which to base decisions about neuraxial anesthesia for cesarean delivery.

▶ Spinal Anesthesia

Single-shot spinal anesthesia has the advantage of being simple and rapid. Use of spinal anesthesia for elective, uncomplicated cesarean delivery is more time efficient and cost-effective, and requires less supplemental intravenous anesthesia than epidural anesthesia.[2] The primary disadvantage of spinal anesthesia is that it is not a continuous technique and therefore lacks the flexibility to respond to unanticipated prolongation of surgery. Although the duration of cesarean delivery is typically predictable, there are some circumstances in which it is not, such as a history of multiple abdominal or pelvic surgical procedures, or placental implantation pathology. The administration of supplemental intravenous sedation or conversion to general anesthesia because of inadequate duration of spinal anesthesia places the pregnant patient at greater risk compared to the nonpregnant patient. The increased incidence of a full stomach status, gastroesophageal reflux, and a statistically greater likelihood of difficulty with intubation and mask ventilation, have been implicated in higher maternal morbidity and mortality with deep conscious sedation and general anesthesia in term pregnant patients.

Careful selection of spinal drug(s), dose, and patient position is required before initiating spinal anesthesia for cesarean delivery. The optimal selection of spinal drug(s) is influenced by the value placed on speed of onset, reliability, degree of motor blockade, anesthesia duration, side effect profile, and postoperative analgesia. The risks of converting inadequate spinal anesthesia to general anesthesia in the pregnant patient make this selection more consequential than for many nonobstetric surgical procedures. Additional factors in drug choice include patient-specific conditions, such as comorbidities and body habitus, as well as the skill of the obstetrician.

Local Anesthetic Choice

Bupivacaine is the most widely used local anesthetic for spinal blockade for cesarean delivery in the United States

Table 14-1

Local Anesthetics and Nonopioid Adjuvants for Spinal Anesthesia for Cesarean Delivery

Drug	Dose*	Duration
Local Anesthetic		
Lidocaine	50–90 mg	45–75 min
Mepivacaine	60 mg	60 min
Bupivacaine	7.5–15 mg	60–120 min
Ropivacaine	15–25 mg	60–120 min
Levobupivacaine	7.5–15 mg	60–120 min
Tetracaine	7–10 mg	120–180 min
Adjuvant		
Epinephrine	100–200 µg	
Clonidine	60–150 µg	

*The local anesthetic dose can be decreased by approximately 20–30% with the addition of lipid-soluble opioid (fentanyl or sufentanil, see Table 14-3). Epinephrine prolongs the duration of anesthesia by approximately 30%.

(Table 14-1). There have been extensive clinical trials conducted with spinal bupivacaine and its advantages include established safety, predictability, and cost-effectiveness. Intrathecal bupivacaine (7.5–15 mg) has rapid onset of sensory and motor blockade and intermediate effective duration (90–120 min). Side effects are closely related to the dose and the use of adjuvants.

Lidocaine (50–90 mg) has been used for spinal anesthesia for cesarean delivery with an effective duration of 45–75 min. In an observational study of 50 cesarean patients, plain lidocaine 50 mg resulted in the rapid onset of surgical anesthesia and compete motor blockade.[3] The mean time to complete regression (±SEM) of sensory blockade was 126 ± 7 min. Because of its more rapid regression of sensory blockade compared with bupivacaine, its use should be limited to predictably short procedures.

Spinal anesthesia using ropivacaine has been shown to provide similar duration of sensory blockade with shorter duration of motor blockade compared to bupivacaine. Several clinical investigations have directly compared intrathecal ropivacaine to bupivacaine for cesarean delivery. Both hyperbaric and isobaric ropivacaine solutions have been evaluated. Ropivacaine and bupivacaine are not equipotent, and some investigators have compared equal masses of the two drugs, not equipotent doses. Spinal ropivacaine appears to be about one-half to two-thirds as

potent as spinal bupivacaine.[4,5] Onset time to sensory blockade and peak sensory level are comparable between ropivacaine and bupivacaine. In clinically relevant doses, however, patients who received intrathecal ropivacaine were observed to have resolution of motor blockade approximately 30 min faster than those that received bupivacaine. The impact of earlier regression of motor blockade in terms of patient safety, satisfaction, and economics has not been extensively evaluated in the obstetric population. Whether this particular clinical feature is a benefit in the obstetric population and whether the increased cost compared to bupivacaine is justified, remains to be determined. Ropivacaine is currently not approved by the United States Food and Drug Administration (FDA) for intrathecal use.

Mepivacaine has been used in cesarean delivery and may offer an option for a local anesthetic with a shorter duration of sensory and motor blockade compared to bupivacaine. Meininger et al. reported the blockade characteristics of 100 cesarean delivery patients using hyperbaric mepivacaine 60 mg with and without opioids.[6] Regression of the sensory blockade to T10 was 67 ± 10 min for the opioid-free solution and the duration of motor blockade was 118 ± 20 min. The addition of opioids significantly extended the duration of sensory blockade. However, no controlled studies have compared mepivacaine directly with bupivacaine and the drug is currently not approved by the FDA for intrathecal use.

Levobupivacaine has undergone limited investigation in the pregnant patient. Gautier et al. compared plain bupivacaine, ropivacaine, and levobupivacaine for the intrathecal component of combined spinal-epidural (CSE) anesthesia for cesarean delivery.[7] There were no distinct advantages of levobupivacaine (8 mg) compared with bupivacaine (8 mg) and ropivacaine (12 mg). Duration of levobupivacaine sensory and motor blockade were shorter compared with bupivacaine, and the need for intraoperative augmentation via the epidural catheter were greater (Table 14-2). Levobupivacaine is not approved by the FDA for intrathecal use.

Tetracaine (7–10 mg) has been used extensively for spinal anesthesia for cesarean delivery. Spinal tetracaine and bupivacaine have been compared in the nonobstetric population; sensory and motor blockade are longer with tetracaine. Direct comparisons of these agents in pregnant women are limited. Hauch et al. compared hyperbaric bupivacaine with a mixture of equal volumes of tetracaine 1% and procaine 10% in patients undergoing cesarean delivery.[8] The onset of sensory and motor blockade and adequacy of sensory blockade were similar with the ester local anesthetic mixture compared to bupivacaine. The duration of sensory and motor blockade, however, was longer with the tetracaine-procaine

Table 14-2

A Comparison of Spinal Anesthesia with Plain Bupivacaine, Ropivacaine, and Levobupivacaine for Cesarean Delivery*

	Bupivacaine 8 mg (N = 30)	Ropivacaine 12 mg (N = 30)	Levobupivacaine 8 mg (N = 30)
Time to regression to T10 (min)	122 (75–180)	120 (95–175)	120 (90–150)
Duration of analgesia (min)[†]	145 (90–190)	135 (95–175)	140 (110–270)
Duration motor block (min)[‡]	135 (100–225)	112 (90–165)[§]	120 (75–190)[§]
Need to rescue (%)	3	13	20[§]

*Intrathecal bupivacaine, ropivacaine, and levobupivacaine were compared as part of a CSE anesthesia technique, combined with intrathecal sufentanil 2.5 µg.
[†]Time from intrathecal injection until first analgesia request.
[‡]Time to complete resolution of motor blockade.
[§]Different from bupivacaine, $P < 0.05$.
Data from Ref. 7.

combination, and the sensory level was higher, as was the incidence of hypotension.

Meperidine possesses some local anesthetic properties and can be used alone as an intrathecal injection for cesarean delivery (1 mg/kg).[9] Patients who received meperidine compared to hyperbaric lidocaine (60–70 mg) experienced less hypotension, but more pruritus and sedation. Failure to achieve an adequate sensory and motor blockade was the same (2 out of 25) in each group.

Local Anesthetic Dose

Conclusions about the optimal dose of local anesthetic used for spinal anesthesia for cesarean delivery vary depending on anesthetic technique (patient position, use of adjuvants), surgical technique, and the value placed on speed of onset, duration of blockade, need for motor blockade, tolerance for hypotension, and need for intraoperative anesthetic supplementation. There are numerous dose-response studies addressing the optimal dose of local anesthetic, particularly for bupivacaine. When hyperbaric bupivacaine was used without adjuvants, the optimal dose was 12 mg.[10] With the addition of fentanyl 10 µg, bupivacaine doses as low as 8 mg were used without any need for intraoperative analgesic supplementation. The ED_{50} and ED_{95} of hyperbaric bupivacaine (with fentanyl 10 µg and morphine 200 µg) to establish a T6 level sensory to pinprick in 10 min were 6.7 and 11.0 mg, respectively.[11] However, the ED_{50} and ED_{95} required to eliminate the need for intraoperative epidural bolus supplementation were slightly higher at 7.6 and 11.2 mg, respectively (Fig. 14-1).

Lower doses of spinal bupivacaine have been used for cesarean delivery (bupivacaine 5 mg with fentanyl 25 µg).[12] The principal advantage is less hypotension. The incidence of hypotension was 31% in patients who received plain

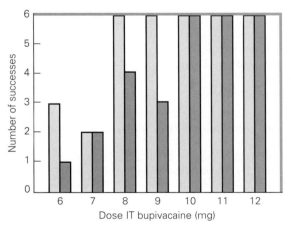

FIGURE 14-1. Successful anesthesia at different doses of intrathecal (IT) bupivacaine combined with fentanyl 10 µg and morphine 200 µg. The graph compares the rate of early successful induction of spinal anesthesia (defined as a T6 sensory level to electrical stimulation 10 min after the intrathecal injection) and rate of late successful spinal anesthesia (T6 sensory level *and* no requirement for supplemental analgesia throughout surgery). There were six patients in each group. There were no early or late failures at bupivacaine doses above 10 mg. Hatched bars = early success; solid bars = late success. *Used with permission from Ginosar Y, Mirikatani E, Drover DR, et al. ED_{50} and ED_{95} of intrathecal hyperbaric bupivacaine coadministered with opioids for cesarean delivery. Anesthesiology 100:676, 2004.*

bupivacaine 5 mg combined with fentanyl 25 µg compared to an incidence of 94% in those who received bupivacaine 10 mg without opioid. Possible limitations of this technique include incomplete motor blockade, short duration sensory blockade, and a greater incidence of intraoperative visceral pain.

Local Anesthetic Volume and Concentration

The roles of local anesthetic volume and concentration in determining cephalad sensory and motor blockade are minor compared to the roles of dose and baricity. This issue is discussed in detail in Chap. 3. Hyperbaric bupivacaine is commonly used in both 0.5 and 0.75% concentrations.

Plain bupivacaine (15 mg) given in higher volume but lower concentration (12 mL of 0.125% vs. 3 mL of 0.5%) yielded a more rapid onset of sensory blockade, but after 5 min in the supine position with left tilt, there were no differences in the peak sensory level compared with patients who received the standard lower volume-higher concentration injectate.[13] Camorcia et al., however, did establish an impact of local anesthetic injectate concentration over a wider volume-concentration range than had previously been studied. They determined the ED_{50} for motor blockade for two concentrations of intrathecal ropivacaine (1.0% vs. 0.1%) using the up-down sequential allocation method as part of a CSE anesthesia for cesarean delivery.[14] The measured baricities of the two solutions were not different. The authors concluded that the ED_{50} required for motor blockade was 50% higher for the 0.1% group compared to the 1.0% concentration group (9.1 mg vs. 6.1 mg).

Anesthetic Baricity and Patient Position

The density of the spinal injectate relative to cerebrospinal fluid (CSF) influences the migration of the drugs relative to patient position (see Chap. 3). The CSF in the term parturient is less dense than that of nonpregnant premenopausal women (Table 3-3). Even though parturients have less dense CSF than nonpregnant individuals, most non-dextrose-containing local anesthetics and combinations of local anesthetic with opioid are hypobaric in this patient population (Table 3-3). It is important to note that many investigations refer to plain, non-dextrose-containing local anesthetic preparations as isobaric when, in fact, they are slightly hypobaric.

Hyperbaric bupivacaine (0.5% or 0.75% in dextrose 80 mg/mL) is widely used in obstetric surgery because of its rapid onset and predictable duration of sensory blockade. Reducing the degree of hyperbaricity does not appear to confer any clinical advantages. In a randomized controlled study of hyperbaric bupivacaine in glucose 80 mg/mL versus glucose 8 mg/mL, there was no difference in onset of sensory block, dose of ephedrine, or maternal satisfaction.[15]

In four direct comparisons of hyperbaric and hypobaric intrathecal bupivacaine for cesarean delivery, three studies showed no differences in latency, blockade height, or duration of the sensory block. Vercauteren et al. concluded that the hyperbaric solutions offered more reliable cephalad sensory spread[16] and Sarvela et al. observed a more rapid onset and regression of motor blockade with hyperbaric bupivacaine.[17] Because almost all solutions injected into the intrathecal space differ in density from CSF, patient position has the potential to alter drug migration, and ultimately sensory blockade. There are additional considerations in positioning a pregnant patient beyond achieving successful anesthesia, including position of the fetus (e.g., presence of a footling breech), uteroplacental perfusion, potential for imminent delivery (e.g., incompetent cervix), and patient comfort. There appears to be no significant impact of the sitting versus the lateral position during initiation of spinal anesthesia with hyperbaric bupivacaine on peak sensory blockade height or time to develop adequate sensory blockade.[18] Baricity influenced the maximum cephalad sensory level and degree of hypotension when analgesia was initiated in the sitting, but not the lateral position.[19]

Investigations comparing the right versus left lateral position for initiation of spinal anesthesia for cesarean delivery demonstrate minimal differences in the clinical characteristics of blockade or the incidence of side effects. Placing a spinal in the left lateral position is associated with a more rapid onset of sensory blockade (higher percentage of patients with a T4 level at 5 min) when compared with the right lateral position.[20] However, at 15 min there is no difference in the maximum block height in the left lateral versus the right lateral position.

Patient Characteristics

It is not an uncommon practice to alter the dose of spinal anesthetics based on patient height. However, several investigations have demonstrated no clear correlation between patient height and maximum sensory level obtained with a single dose of spinal local anesthetic during pregnancy.[21]

Body mass index (BMI) and weight are also not predictive of maximal sensory blockade following a single intrathecal dose of local anesthetic in the pregnant patient (Fig. 14-2).[21] It has been hypothesized that increased abdominal pressure in obese patients results in decreased

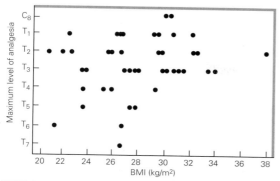

FIGURE 14-2. Spinal anesthesia for cesarean delivery with hyperbaric bupivacaine. There is no correlation between maximum level of analgesia and BMI. ● = one patient, ■ = two patients, ▲ = three patients. *Used with permission from Norris MC. Height, weight, and the spread of subarachnoid hyperbaric bupivacaine in the term parturient. Anesth Analg 67:555, 1988.*

spinal canal CSF volume. This phenomenon has been demonstrated in a magnetic resonance imaging study.[22] The results of these studies suggest that alteration of hyperbaric bupivacaine dose in pregnant patients based on body habitus is not justified.

Speed of Injection

The speed of intrathecal injection may influence maximal height of sensory blockade. Whether injection speed influences the extent of sensory blockade is likely to depend on a host of factors, including density and temperature of the anesthetic solution, patient position, and type of spinal needle. Intrathecal injection of hyperbaric anesthetic solution 4 mL over 120 s while patients were positioned in the left lateral decubitus position resulted in a lower incidence of hypotension compared to injection in under 15 s.[23] In addition, the onset of hypotension was delayed and its severity and duration reduced in the slow injection group.

Intrathecal Adjuvants

Opioids. The addition of opioid to intrathecal local anesthetic has been shown to improve the density of spinal anesthesia,[10] delay sensory blockade recovery without delaying motor blockade recovery,[10,24] allow for reduction in the dose of local anesthetic,[10] and provide postoperative analgesia.[10] The site of action of intrathecal opioids is primarily the mu receptor in the dorsal horn of the spinal cord (see Chap. 3). Systemic and intrathecal spread to

other sites, including the brain, depend on the degree of lipid solubility of the opioid.

Side effects of intrathecal opioids include pruritus, nausea and vomiting, sedation, and respiratory depression (see Chap. 6). Pruritus is common and the incidence is dose dependent. Intraoperative nausea and vomiting is substantially reduced when local anesthetics are supplemented with intrathecal opioids;[24,25] however, the incidence of postoperative nausea and vomiting is increased with long-acting opioids such as morphine. Measurable effects on the neonate are minimal.[24,26] Delayed maternal respiratory depression is primarily associated with hydrophilic opioids such as morphine. Catastrophic respiratory depression is rare in this patient population, but vigilance may also be less rigorous as patients are not routinely nursed in an intensely monitored environment.

Fentanyl is one of the most widely studied and commonly used opioids for spinal anesthesia for cesarean delivery (Table 14-3). When added to intrathecal hyperbaric bupivacaine, intrathecal fentanyl in a dose as low as 6.25 μg improved intraoperative analgesia and extended the time to first request for analgesia and effective analgesia when compared with saline control.[26] Patients were randomized to receive 0, 7.5, 10, 12.5, and 15 μg of intrathecal fentanyl combined with bupivacaine in a dose-response study.[27] Fentanyl 0 or 7.5 μg produced no detectable clinical effect. Intraoperative anesthesia was significantly improved in the 12.5 and 15 μg groups. There appeared to be a ceiling effect at 12.5 μg for postoperative analgesia as the duration of complete and effective analgesia were similar in the 12.5 and 15 μg groups.

Similarly improved intraoperative anesthesia and postoperative analgesia were observed when fentanyl 10 μg was added to a hyperbaric ropivacaine 18 mg[28] and when fentanyl 5 or 10 μg was added to hyperbaric mepivacaine for cesarean delivery.[6] Fentanyl 15 μg combined with hyperbaric lidocaine 80 mg did not affect intraoperative anesthesia but extended the mean duration of anesthesia from 71 to 100 min and reduced the incidence of perioperative nausea and vomiting.[25]

Sufentanil has also been shown to improve intraoperative anesthesia and postoperative analgesia when added to

Table 14-3

Intrathecal Opioids for Spinal Anesthesia for Cesarean Delivery

Opioid	Dose (μg)
Fentanyl	10–20
Sufentanil	2.5–5
Morphine	25–200

local anesthetics for spinal anesthesia. Intrathecal sufentanil 0, 2.5, 5, and 7.5 μg was combined with hyperbaric bupivacaine 12.5 mg in a dose-response study.[29] Onset time of sensory blockade was more rapid in the sufentanil groups. Postoperative analgesia was prolonged in the sufentanil 5 and 7.5 μg groups. The incidence of pruritus and sedation were higher in the sufentanil 7.5 μg group.

Fentanyl 10 μg and sufentanil 2.5 and 5 μg combined with bupivacaine were compared in a randomized trial.[24] Onset of sensory and motor blockade, maximal sensory blockade, and motor blockade resolution were not different from placebo (Table 14-4). Sensory level regression to T10 was longer in the sufentanil groups compared to placebo, and complete and effective analgesia times were significantly prolonged in all opioid groups compared to placebo and in the sufentanil groups compared to fentanyl. Postoperative pruritus was treated significantly more often in the sufentanil 5 μg group.

The addition of preservative-free morphine to hyperbaric bupivacaine improves both intraoperative and postoperative anesthesia and analgesia.[30] Morphine 200 μg reduced the likelihood of intraoperative supplemental analgesia (morphine 41% vs. saline control 82%) and extended the mean duration (±SEM) until first request for analgesia from 2 ± 0.3 to 27 ± 0.7 h. Intrathecal morphine 100–250 μg has been shown to reduce pain scores after cesarean delivery for up to 24 h.[30,31] The use of scheduled nonsteroidal anti-inflammatory medication (NSAIDs) augments intrathecal morphine analgesia and may allow a reduced dose and a decreased incidence of side effects.[32] Patients who received bupivacaine, fentanyl, and intrathecal morphine 100 μg combined with scheduled NSAID

analgesia had similar postoperative pain scores but less pruritus than women who received the same medications with morphine 250 μg.[33]

A dose-response study of intrathecal morphine in combination with oral acetaminophen/hydrocodone suggested that effective postoperative analgesia can be achieved with intrathecal morphine doses as low as 25 μg.[34] The clinical effects of intrathecal morphine do not appear to be influenced significantly by the baricity of the coadministered local anesthetic solution. Morphine 0–0.5 mg was administered with hyperbaric bupivacaine 12.75 mg in a dose-response study.[35] The investigators concluded that there was little benefit to administering intrathecal morphine in doses greater than 0.1 mg (100 μg), as there seemed to be an analgesic ceiling effect at this dose, and pruritus was directly related to dose (Fig. 14-3). There were no differences in the block characteristics, intraoperative discomfort, postoperative systemic morphine use, and side effects in patients who received intrathecal morphine 200 μg in either hypo- or hyperbaric (15 mg) solutions.[36]

Meperidine is unique among opioids in that it has weak local anesthetic qualities following neuraxial injection. It has been used successfully as a single drug for spinal anesthesia for cesarean delivery and tubal ligation.[37] Similar to other intrathecal opioids, meperidine prolongs postoperative analgesia, but unlike other opioids, is associated with a greater incidence of intraoperative nausea and vomiting. Intrathecal meperidine has also been investigated with a primary focus on its antishivering qualities.[38] Although most opioids have been shown to have antishivering qualities, meperidine is superior for the treatment of shivering when

Table 14-4

Intrathecal Hyperbaric Bupivacaine Combined with Opioid*

	Placebo (N = 20)	Fentanyl 10 μg (N = 20)	Sufentanil 2.5 μg (N = 20)	Sufentanil 5 μg (N = 20)
Time to sensory block (min)[†]	7.4 ± 3.4	6.7 ± 2.8	7.1 ± 2.3	7.2 ± 5.7
Maximum block height (dermatome)	T4 (T1-T4)	T3 (T1-T5)	T4 (C6-T5)	T3.5 (T1-T4)
Duration of complete analgesia (min)[‡]	91 ± 13	140 ± 34	175 ± 54[§]	213 ± 76[§,¶]
Time to T10 regression (min)	131 ± 21	148 ± 30	166 ± 40	162 ± 28[§]
Need for postoperative antipruritic agents (n)	1	0	1	9[a]

*Patients were randomized to receive intrathecal hyperbaric bupivacaine 12.5 with placebo, fentanyl 10 μg, or sufentanil 2.5 or 5 μg. Values are mean ± SD or median (range).
[†]Time to sensory blockade at T4.
[‡]Time to VAS ≥ 0.
[§]Different from placebo, $P < 0.05$.
[¶]Different from fentanyl, $P < 0.05$.
[a]Different from placebo, fentanyl, and sufentanil 2.5 μg, $P < 0.05$.
Data from Ref. 24.

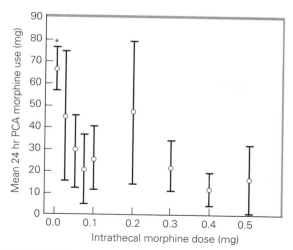

FIGURE 14-3. Mean 24-h patient-controlled intravenous morphine use after intrathecal morphine combined with bupivacaine for postcesarean delivery analgesia (mean ± 95% CI). *P < 0.05 vs. morphine 0.075, 0.1, 0.3, 0.4, and 0.5 mg groups. There appeared to be an analgesic ceiling effect with morphine doses greater than 0.1 mg. *Used with permission from Palmer CM, Emerson S, Volgoropolous D, et al. Dose-response relationship of intrathecal morphine for postcesarean analgesia. Anesthesiology 90:437, 1999.*

injected systemically. Hyperbaric bupivacaine and morphine combined with meperidine (0.2 mg/kg) reduced the incidence and severity of intraoperative and postoperative shivering compared with bupivacaine and morphine without meperidine.[38] There are, however, no studies comparing the antishivering effects of meperidine to other intrathecal opioids.

Diamorphine (heroin) has been used in combination with spinal bupivacaine for cesarean delivery outside of the United States. The ED_{95} of intrathecal diamorphine to prevent intraoperative supplementation is 0.39 mg when combined with hyperbaric bupivacaine 12.5 mg.[39]

Intrathecal nalbuphine (0.8 mg) combined with bupivacaine provided shorter duration analgesia with less pruritus and nausea compared with intrathecal morphine (200 µg) with bupivacaine.[40] Intraoperative analgesia was superior, but the time to first postoperative analgesic intervention was shorter (212 ± 72 min) compared with morphine (585 ± 446 min).

There are conflicting results as to whether the addition of intrathecal fentanyl to morphine substantially improves intraoperative analgesia. One group of investigators reported marginally improved intraoperative analgesia with fentanyl and morphine combined with lidocaine/epinephrine compared with saline and morphine combined with lidocaine/epinephrine.[41] In contrast, the combination of fentanyl and morphine with bupivacaine was no more effective than

morphine and bupivacaine without fentanyl for intraoperative analgesia.[42]

α-Adrenergic Agonists. Intrathecal α-adrenergic agonists, such as epinephrine, neostigmine, and clonidine, combined with local anesthetics, increase the density of sensory and motor blockade, and may prolong duration of blockade. Intrathecal epinephrine, 100–200 µg, reduces the need for intraoperative opioid supplementation,[43] results in more profound motor blockade,[43] and delays the recovery of both the sensory and motor blockade (see Chap. 3).

Intrathecal clonidine, 60–150 µg, combined with hyperbaric bupivacaine 12.5 mg, morphine 100 µg, and fentanyl 15 µg improved the quality and duration of spinal anesthesia but at a cost of increased intraoperative sedation and perioperative vomiting.[44] Clonidine has been associated with sedation which may limit its clinical usefulness in the obstetric population. Intrathecal clonidine is not recommended by the manufacturer for use in pregnancy.

Systemic Adjuvants

Concerns regarding both the maternal (pulmonary aspiration) and neonatal (depression) safety of maternally administered intravenous medications limit their use during cesarean delivery. Most maternally administered systemic analgesics, including opioids, benzodiazepines, and ketamine, are rapidly transmitted to the neonate. Judicious use of these drugs, however, to augment neuraxial blockade or provide anxiolysis, may be justified if the result is avoidance of general anesthesia.

The need for intraoperative systemic opioid supplementation is reduced by adding opioid to the spinal local anesthetic.[24,26,45] In a randomized controlled trial of intrathecal versus systemic fentanyl 12.5 µg during bupivacaine spinal anesthesia, cesarean delivery patients who received intrathecal fentanyl experienced superior intraoperative anesthesia and required less systemic fentanyl supplementation.[45] In addition, the incidence of intraoperative hypotension, and nausea and vomiting was lower, and the duration to first postoperative analgesia request was longer in the intrathecal fentanyl compared to systemic fentanyl group.

Many operative procedures conducted with neuraxial anesthesia, particularly abdominal procedures, are administered with concurrent sedation and anxiolysis. Midazolam used to induce general anesthesia (0.2 mg/kg) negatively impacted neonatal outcomes compared to sodium thiopental.[46] Fentanyl 1 µg/kg and midazolam 0.02 mg/kg administered to the mother at the time of initiation of spinal anesthesia had no apparent adverse neonatal effects or maternal effects.[47] Compared to the control group, there were no differences in maternal amnesia.

Ketamine and nitrous oxide (50% in oxygen) have been used to supplement incomplete anesthesia during neuraxial anesthesia. There is, however, surprisingly little evidence in the literature to support either the safety or efficacy of their use for cesarean delivery.

Complications and Side Effects

Complications and side effects of spinal anesthesia are discussed in detail in Chap. 6. Complications and side effects with specific obstetric implications are discussed below.

Anesthetic Failure. The incidence of failed spinal anesthesia, defined as failure of a single spinal injection to generate adequate sensory blockade for the planned surgical procedure, varies widely depending on technique and the expectations of the patient, anesthesiologist, and obstetrician. It is difficult to investigate anesthetic failure because studies frequently lack objective criteria to determine failure. Meta-analysis of 10 investigations yielded no difference in the failure rate between spinal and epidural anesthesia for cesarean delivery.[48]

Depending on the circumstances (e.g., urgency, condition of the mother or fetus, and risks of alternatives techniques), several options exist. These include repeating spinal anesthesia with a full or partial local anesthetic dose, using epidural anesthesia or CSE anesthesia, supplementation with intravenous or inhalational analgesics, or converting to general anesthesia. In general, intravenous or inhalational anesthetic supplementation is less desirable in the pregnant compared to nonpregnant patient because of the increased incidence of difficult airway and risk of pulmonary aspiration in pregnant women.

Hypotension. Hypotension following spinal anesthesia in the parturient is one of the most common side effects and remains a vexing problem. Because uterine blood flow is not autoregulated, uteroplacental perfusion is directly related to maternal blood pressure. Therefore, a decrease in maternal blood pressure that is tolerated by the mother may not be tolerated by the fetus. The reported incidence of spinal anesthesia-associated hypotension in pregnant women varies depending on the definition of hypotension, but may be as high as 90%.[49] A meta-analysis of studies comparing spinal and epidural anesthesia for cesarean delivery revealed the severity of hypotension is greater with spinal anesthesia (RR 1.23; 95% confidence interval [CI] 1.00–1.51).[48] Another systematic analysis of studies comparing different modes of anesthesia found that spinal anesthesia compared to both general and epidural anesthesia was associated with lower umbilical cord pH and higher base deficit.[50] There is no evidence, however, that this statistical difference in fetal acid-base status results in clinically different neonatal outcome.

Traditional teaching has been the avoidance of spinal anesthesia in severely preeclamptic patients because of the fear that relative hypovolemia secondary to severe hypertension may contribute to severe hypotension after the induction of anesthesia. Recent studies have questioned this teaching. The incidence of hypotension was actually lower in severely preeclamptic patients compared with a healthy cohort in two studies (Fig. 14-4).[51,52] In randomized controlled trials there was no difference in neonatal outcome in severely preeclamptic patients randomized to spinal compared to epidural anesthesia,[53] or CSE, epidural, and general anesthesia.[54] The degree

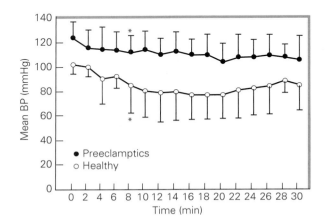

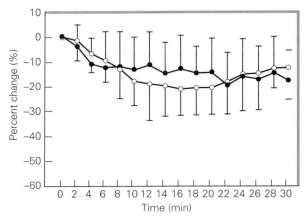

FIGURE 14-4. Changes in mean blood pressure (BP) after spinal anesthesia in preeclamptic and healthy parturients. The top panel shows raw data, whereas percentage changes are shown in the bottom panel. *Time point from which mean BP decreased significantly compared with the corresponding baseline value (*P* < 0.05). In both groups, mean BP decreased significantly from 8 min after the spinal injection until the end of the study period. *Used with permission from Aya AG, Mangin R, Vialles N, et al. Patients with severe preeclampsia experience less hypotension during spinal anesthesia for elective cesarean delivery than healthy parturients: A prospective cohort comparison. Anesth Analg 97:867, 2003.*

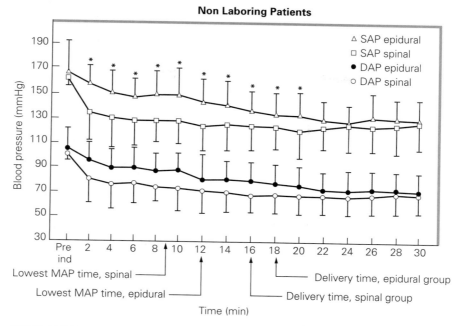

Non Laboring Patients

Legend:
△ SAP epidural
□ SAP spinal
● DAP epidural
○ DAP spinal

Lowest MAP time, spinal
Lowest MAP time, epidural
Delivery time, epidural group
Delivery time, spinal group

Time (min)

FIGURE 14-5. Blood pressure changes after the induction of spinal compared to epidural anesthesia for cesarean delivery in patients with severe preeclampsia. There are significant differences in systolic arterial pressure (SAP) at 1–15 min ($P < 0.001$) and at 16–20 min ($P < 0.005$) and in diastolic arterial pressure (DAP) at 1–15 min ($P < 0.001$) and at 16–20 min ($P < 0.01$) between the two groups. There are no significant differences in SAP and DAP at 22–30 min between groups. Pre ind = the baseline SAP, DAP in preinduction period; delivery time = time from local anesthetic administration to delivery. Data are mean ± SD. *Used with permission from Visalyaputra S, Rodanant O, Somboonviboon W, et al. Spinal versus epidural anesthesia for cesarean delivery in severe preeclampsia: A prospective randomized, multicenter study. Anesth Analg 101:862, 2005.*

of hypotension was similar for spinal compared to epidural anesthesia, although the blood pressure nadir occurred earlier (before delivery) for patients randomized to receive spinal anesthesia (Fig. 14-5).[53] Taken together, these data suggest that spinal anesthesia is safe for women with severe preeclampsia.

Strategies for avoiding hypotension or decreasing its severity following spinal anesthesia for cesarean delivery include vasopressor administration (prophylactic or therapeutic), fluid administration (crystalloid or colloid), lower extremity compression (inflatable boots or stockings), and alterations in spinal anesthetic technique including drug choice and patient position.

Prophylactic vasopressor administration seems logical during spinal anesthesia: a clinical circumstance with a high incidence of hypotension and significant neonatal consequences. Ngan Kee et al. conducted a dose-response study of prophylactic ephedrine during spinal anesthesia.[49] Patients were randomized to receive 0, 10, 20, or 30 mg of intravenous ephedrine 1 min following spinal injection. The incidence of hypotension was 95, 85, 80, and 35%, respectively. Ephedrine 30 mg was the lowest effective dose to reduce the incidence of hypotension. Hypotension was not

eliminated; however, reactive hypertension was reported in 45%. Neonatal outcome as measured by umbilical cord blood gases was not different among groups suggesting that prophylactic ephedrine use has limited clinical utility.

The optimal choice of vasopressor for treatment of hypotension in the term pregnant patients is controversial. Ephedrine, a mixed beta and alpha agonist, has been widely used to treat the hypotension resulting from spinal anesthesia based on data from animal models and has traditionally been the drug-of-choice. Recent randomized clinical trials, however, have challenged this practice. Cooper et al. randomized women scheduled for elective cesarean delivery to bolus administration of phenylephrine 100 μg, ephedrine 3 mg, or both to maintain maternal blood pressure at baseline after induction of spinal anesthesia.[55] The incidence of fetal acidosis was significantly lower in mothers exposed to phenylephrine alone or combined with ephedrine; however, the incidence of maternal nausea was less only in women who received phenylephrine alone.

These data are supported by a meta-analysis of studies comparing ephedrine and phenylephrine for the prevention or treatment of hypotension in women undergoing spinal

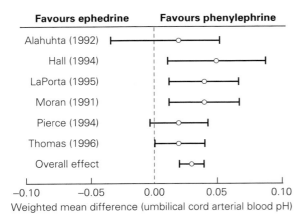

FIGURE 14-6. Meta-analysis of the effect of phenylephrine vs. ephedrine for the treatment of spinal anesthesia-induced hypotension on umbilical cord arterial blood pH. The study's lead author and year of publication are listed in the right column. Data are mean difference with 95% CI. *Used with permission from Lee A, Ngan Kee WD, Gin T. A quantitative, systematic review of randomized controlled trials of ephedrine versus phenylephrine for the management of hypotension during spinal anesthesia for cesarean delivery. Anesth Analg 94:920, 2002.*

anesthesia for cesarean delivery.[56] There were no differences in blood pressure control, but umbilical artery pH was lower after ephedrine compared with phenylephrine (Fig. 14-6). These data suggest that phenylephrine may be as good or better for the treatment of spinal anesthesia-induced hypotension. The studies, however, have only been performed in healthy women undergoing elective cesarean delivery.

A moderate bolus of intravenous crystalloid is a common prophylactic strategy to prevent postspinal hypotension. Rapid crystalloid administration (20 mL/kg) administered immediately after the spinal anesthesia was associated with less vasopressor use than the same volume administered in the 20 min preceding the spinal injection.[57] Although a more expensive strategy, there is evidence that colloid administration either alone or in combination with crystalloid is superior to crystalloid alone for reducing the incidence of hypotension.[58]

A 3-min delay in assuming the supine position after initiation of hyperbaric bupivacaine spinal anesthesia did not result in less hypotension compared to immediately assuming the supine position.[59] Slow intrathecal injection (4 mL in 120 s) compared with faster injection (4 mL in 15 s) did reduce the incidence and severity of hypotension following spinal anesthesia for cesarean delivery, although the incidence of hypotension was still high (68%).[23]

Nausea and Vomiting. Nausea and vomiting are very common during cesarean delivery with spinal anesthesia. Nausea and vomiting are associated with hypotension, visceral pain, and medication administration such as oxytocin.

Hypotension usually occurs within the first 20 min after the induction of spinal anesthesia. Visceral pain occurs when the uterus is exteriorized after delivery or during closure of the fascia. Strategies to prevent and treat nausea and vomiting include pharmacologic prophylaxis and treatment, prompt treatment of hypotension, and other nonpharmacologic treatments.

Intrathecal opioids as part of spinal or epidural anesthesia, with the exception of meperidine, have been shown to substantially reduce the intraoperative use of antiemetics.[24,25] Early administration of ephedrine in response to hypotension has been shown to reduce the incidence of nausea and vomiting.[60] Both therapeutic and prophylactic intravenous ondansetron are effective at reducing the severity of nausea and vomiting.[61,62] In direct comparison, antiserotonergic medications (e.g., ondansetron and granisetron) are more efficacious in preventing nausea and vomiting during cesarean delivery than antidopaminergic medications (e.g., metoclopramide and droperidol).[63,64] One group of investigators has reported that propofol at subhypnotic doses (1 mg/kg/h) was as effective as droperidol or metoclopramide.[65] Antihistamines and dexamethasone have been described as effective antiemetics during cesarean delivery but it is not clear what their relative effectiveness is in comparison with other agents.[66,67] Acupressure during cesarean delivery was an effective nonpharmacologic antiemetic therapy compared to placebo.[68]

Pruritus. The use of intrathecal opioid to improve the density of spinal blockade or provide postpartum analgesia is accompanied by a very high incidence of pruritus. The incidence and severity of pruritus appears to be dose related.[24,29] Strategies to reduce this side effect include using the smallest effective dose for the desired clinical effect. Effective treatment includes the use of opioid antagonists and mixed opioid agonist-antagonists.[69] Subhypnotic doses of propofol were not effective in preventing[70] or treating intrathecal morphine-induced pruritus.[70,71]

Sedation. Sedation following spinal anesthesia has been described with and without intrathecal opioid.[72] The effect may be due to somatic deafferentation, analgesia, anxiolysis, and exhaustion following prolonged labor, in addition to the central effects of opioids. Spinal anesthesia may decrease the minimum anesthetic concentration (MAC) for subsequently administered general anesthesia, and may impact opioid-induced respiratory depression and maternal satisfaction.

High Spinal and Total Spinal Anesthesia. A serious complication of spinal anesthesia is high or total spinal anesthesia requiring acute airway management, and ventilatory and cardiovascular support. Circumstances associated with high spinal anesthesia during cesarean delivery include spinal anesthesia following failed epidural anesthesia[73] and drug error. The mechanism of high or total spinal anesthesia after failed epidural anesthesia is presumed to be either compression of the dura mater by epidural local anesthetic resulting in a decreased CSF volume, leak of local anesthetic from the epidural space (or other paraspinous tissue) through the dural puncture or dura, or a combination of both mechanisms. Strategies to prevent this complication include reducing the intrathecal local anesthetic dose, CSE, continuous spinal, or general anesthesia.

Neurologic Complications. Transient neurologic syndrome (TNS) presents with mild to moderate low back pain presenting several hours following the resolution of otherwise uneventful spinal blockade. The incidence of TNS appears to be lower in the pregnant population. In an observational study of 303 parturients who received spinal anesthesia (232 bupivacaine, 67 lidocaine), none demonstrated any signs of transient radicular syndrome on a standardized postoperative interview (95% CI of incidence of TNS 0–4.5%).[74] In three randomized controlled trials in obstetric patients, the incidence of TNS was 0–7% and did not differ between patients who received intrathecal lidocaine compared to bupivacaine (Table 14-5).[75–77]

The incidence of neurologic complications after spinal anesthesia in obstetric patients appears lower than the general population.[78] Dural puncture, however, appears to be a risk factor for meningitis, perhaps because transient bacteremia is common during childbirth and trauma during dural puncture may cause breach of the blood-brain barrier.[79]

Postdural Puncture Headache. Pregnant women are at high risk for postdural puncture headache (PDPH). Smaller-gauge, noncutting needles are associated with a reduction in the incidence of PDPH and the use of epidural blood patch (see Chap. 2). Attempts to reduce the incidence of PDPH by using ever smaller needles, however, may increase the risk of technical problems. Two hundred and twelve women scheduled for cesarean delivery were randomized to spinal anesthesia with either a 25- or 27-gauge

Whitacre spinal needle.[80] Free flow of CSF was difficult to obtain in eight patients in the 27-gauge group (seven of the eight had subsequent successful spinal placement with a larger needle), compared to none of the patients in the 25-gauge group. PDPH occurred in four patients in the 25-gauge group and none in the 27-gauge group. The authors concluded that choice of spinal needle represents a compromise between improved technical ease and a small risk of PDPH.

Neonatal Effects. Due to the small amount of drugs required for spinal anesthesia there is little direct effect of spinal anesthetic medication on the fetus or neonate. Hypotension and other physiologic effects of spinal anesthesia, however, have the potential to indirectly and adversely affect the fetus. Many variables occurring during cesarean delivery make conclusions about the specific impact of spinal anesthesia difficult to study. These include patient and fetal condition, spinal anesthetic technique, management of blood pressure, use of supplemental oxygen, and time intervals between intrathecal injection, uterine incision, and delivery. There was no difference in neonatal outcome as assessed by umbilical cord blood gases and Apgar scores in healthy women randomized to spinal, epidural, or general anesthesia for elective cesarean delivery.[81] Neurologic and adaptive capacity scores (NACS), however, were higher at 15 and 120 min postpartum in neonates whose mothers had received spinal anesthesia compared with epidural or general anesthesia despite a higher incidence of maternal hypotension in the spinal group. It is unclear if these effects were directly due to anesthetic technique or another clinical variable and if these measures correlate with other broader measures of neonatal outcome.

▶ Epidural Anesthesia

Epidural anesthesia has several advantages compared with spinal anesthesia, including the ability to prolong anesthesia via the indwelling epidural catheter, titrate the extent of sensory blockade, and provide continuous postoperative epidural analgesia. The onset of hypotension is delayed compared to spinal anesthesia. Disadvantages compared

Table 14-5						
Randomized Controlled Trials of TNS after Spinal Anesthesia in Pregnancy						
Study (Year)	*N*	Procedure	TNS Incidence (%)		*P*-value	
			Lidocaine	Bupivacaine		
Aouad (2001)	200	Cesarean delivery	0	0	NS	
Philip (2001)	58	PPTL	3	7	NS	
Beilin (2003)	59	Cervical cerclage	7	0	NS	

with spinal anesthesia include a technically more difficult procedure, greater risk for systemic local anesthetic toxicity, and less sensory and motor blockade. Although it is commonly perceived that epidural anesthesia is associated with a greater need for intraoperative systemic analgesia supplementation compared to spinal anesthesia, this has not been conclusively demonstrated in randomized studies.[82,83]

Local Anesthetic Choice

The choice of local anesthetic for epidural anesthesia for cesarean delivery is primarily based on safety (systemic toxicity), efficacy (speed of onset, density of sensory and motor blockade, and duration), side effects, and cost.

Successful anesthetic blockade for cesarean delivery has been established with most available local anesthetics (Table 14-6). The most commonly used local anesthetics are lidocaine 1.5 or 2%, bupivacaine 0.5%, and 2-chloroprocaine 3%. Bupivacaine 0.75% was associated with higher maternal plasma bupivacaine concentration compared with 0.5% without any benefit in terms of increased sensory or motor blockade.[84] This finding along with reports of maternal cardiac arrest secondary to systemic toxicity with bupivacaine 0.75%[85] have led to the manufacturer's and FDA recommendation that this concentration not be used for cesarean delivery. Epidural ropivacaine has also been studied for cesarean delivery. Although the margin of safety for cardiac toxicity is greater than for bupivacaine, ropivacaine in concentrations higher than 0.5% have not been approved by the FDA for use in obstetrics.

Several investigations have compared the administration of epidural lidocaine 2% with bupivacaine 0.5%.[86,87] Lidocaine is usually administered with epinephrine 1:200,000, as lidocaine without epinephrine does not consistently provide satisfactory surgical anesthesia (see "Adjuvants, α-Adrenergic Agonists," later). Lidocaine with epinephrine results in shorter latency and shorter duration of surgical anesthesia compared to bupivacaine. Neonatal outcomes were not different.

The duration of motor blockade is shorter after ropivacaine epidural anesthesia compared to bupivacaine (duration of Bromage scale 4 motor block 0.9 vs. 2.5 h, $P < 0.05$).[88] There are no differences in onset time of sensory blockade, quality of analgesia, or duration of analgesia between bupivacaine and ropivacaine.[88,89] There were no consistent differences in side effects when equal concentrations were compared. Ropivacaine 0.75% resulted in more severe hypotension[89] and a greater incidence of maternal bradycardia[90] compared with bupivacaine 0.5%, although there were no differences in neonatal outcome.

There does not appear to be an advantage to combining local anesthetics for epidural anesthesia. Two investigations compared the combination of lidocaine 2% and bupivacaine 0.5% to lidocaine 2% or bupivacaine 0.5% alone for the extension of labor epidural analgesia to anesthesia for cesarean delivery. In these studies, there were no differences in the time of onset of sensory blockade or need for intraoperative analgesic supplementation between groups.[91,92]

2-Chloroprocaine is an ester local anesthetic. Its principal advantage for cesarean delivery is its rapid onset time and reduced systemic toxicity secondary to rapid metabolism by plasma esterases. In the setting of nonreassuring fetal status or fetal bradycardia, there may be an advantage to using 2-chloroprocaine. In these circumstances, the rapid onset time may reduce the need for general anesthesia and the reduced toxicity makes the bolus injection of the entire epidural dose (as opposed to incremental injection) safer. Equal volumes of lidocaine 1.5% with epinephrine and 2-chloroprocaine 3%, both alkalinized with sodium bicarbonate, were compared in women requiring urgent cesarean deliveries.[93] The onset time to surgical blockade was faster in the 2-chloroprocaine group (3.1 min vs. 4.4 min) compared to the lidocaine group; however, neonatal outcomes were not different. Lidocaine was detected in some of the neonates of mothers who received it.

Table 14-6

Local Anesthetic Agents for Epidural Anesthesia for Cesarean Delivery*

Drug	Dose (mg)	Onset (min)	Duration (min)
2-Chloroprocaine 3%	450–750	7–17	40–50
Lidocaine 2% with epinephrine 1:200,000	300–500	10–20	75–100
Bupivacaine 0.5%	75–125	10–30	120–180
Ropivacaine 0.5%	75–125	10–30	120–180

*The local anesthetic requirement is higher when epidural blockade is initiated de novo compared to "topping-up" existing epidural labor analgesia. It is helpful to inject 20–25% of the initial dose approximately 15–20 min after the initial dose to "repaint the fence" and make the block denser. The addition of lipid-soluble opioids will also make the block denser (see Table 14-7). The addition of sodium bicarbonate (1 meq/10 mL local anesthetic solution) shortens latency.

Theoretically, 2-chloroprocaine may be safer for the neonate in the setting of fetal acidosis. Fetal acidemia has the potential to increase the proportion of local anesthetic that is in the ionized form (see Chap. 3), preventing its passage back across the placenta into the maternal circulation and thereby contributing to fetal accumulation of the drug. The transfer of 2-chloroprocaine and its metabolite were not influenced by fetal acidosis.[94] Clinical neonatal outcomes, however, were not different between neonates whose mothers received epidural 2-chloroprocaine compared to lidocaine, as discussed in the preceding paragraph.[93] A potential disadvantage of chloroprocaine is its interference with subsequently administered epidural opioids (see "Adjuvants," later).

Levobupivacaine, the S-enantiomer of racemic bupivacaine, is equipotent to bupivacaine, but has less neurologic and cardiac toxicity. Studies comparing epidurally administered levobupivacaine with bupivacaine for cesarean delivery found very little clinical difference between the two drugs.[95] Onset time, quality of sensory and motor blockade, and the duration of sensory blockade were similar between agents.

Local Anesthetic Concentration and Volume

Evaluations of the same local anesthetic dose given in varied concentration and volume suggest that density of the sensory blockade is related to concentration but maximum cephalad sensory blockade and time to maximum blockade are similar between different drug concentrations and are dependent on total dose.[96]

Position

Data are conflicting as to whether patient position influences the speed of onset of sensory blockade with epidural anesthesia. The Trendelenburg position (15 degrees of head-down position) aided the speed of onset of sensory anesthesia with lidocaine epidural anesthesia compared with horizontal position after the lumbar epidural injection of lidocaine 2% with epinephrine and sodium bicarbonate, 20 mL.[97] Ninety-seven percent of patients in the Trendelenburg position achieved a T5 sensory level 10 min after injection compared to 47% of patients in the horizontal position. In contrast, in a smaller study, a 30- to 40-degree head-up position did not influence sacral spread of 2-chloroprocaine compared with the horizontal position.[98] In another study, the extent of left and right sensory blockade was not influenced by whether epidural anesthesia was initiated in the left or right lateral decubitus position.[99] Taken together, these data suggest that patient position during bolus injection of epidural anesthetic solution does not influence the extent of sensory blockade to a clinically significant degree.

Patient Characteristics

Maternal height was a poor predictor of maximal sensory blockade spread with lidocaine epidural anesthesia.[100] BMI was, however, positively correlated with the extend of cephalad sensory blockade spread during bupivacaine epidural anesthesia.[101]

Adjuvants

Opioids. Opioids administered into the epidural space diffuse freely across the dura mater into the CSF and are also absorbed via epidural veins into the systemic circulation (see Chap. 3). Despite evidence of systemic absorption, the primary site of analgesic action of fentanyl administered into the epidural space appears to be mu receptors in the spinal cord. Similar to intrathecal opioid administration in combination with local anesthetics, epidural opioids administered with epidural local anesthetics improve intraoperative and postoperative analgesia (Table 14-7).[102] Onset, duration, and degree of sensory and motor blockade are not altered by the coadministration of opioid, although the quality of intraoperative analgesia is improved. Epidural morphine provides more effective postcesarean analgesia than patient-controlled intravenous morphine or intramuscular morphine administration;[103] however, the incidence of bothersome side effects (e.g., pruritus and nausea and vomiting) may be higher (see "Complications and Side Effects," later). Currently, only morphine and hydromorphone are approved for epidural administration by the FDA, although epidural administration of the lipid-soluble opioids fentanyl and sufentanil are standard of care.

Halonen et al. found that fentanyl 50 μg was as effective as fentanyl 100 μg,[102] Helbo-Hansen et al., however, suggested that fentanyl 75 μg was the minimum effective epidural dose.[104] Combined with bupivacaine 0.5%, fentanyl 75 μg improved the quality of postoperative analgesia for 6 h and increased the interval to first request for supplementary opioid analgesia. The ED_{50} and ED_{95} for epidural fentanyl to reduce postcesarean pain (visual analog score [VAS] less than 10 mm) were 33 and 92 μg, respectively.[105]

Table 14-7	
Epidural Opioids for Cesarean Delivery	
Drug	Dose
Fentanyl	75–100 μg
Sufentanil	10–20 μg
Morphine	3–4 mg
Hydromorphone	0.4–0.75 mg

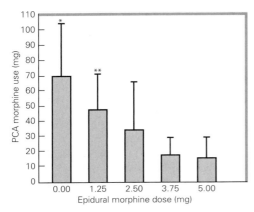

FIGURE 14-7. Dose-response of epidural morphine for postcesarean delivery analgesia: total 24-h PCIA morphine use. Data are mean (±95% CI). *Group 0.0 mg was significantly different from groups 2.5, 3.75, and 5.0 mg; **Group 1.25 was significantly different from groups 3.75 and 5.0 mg (a posteriori, $P < 0.05$). Used with permission from Palmer CM, Nogami WM, Van Maren G, et al. Postcesarean epidural morphine: A dose-response study. Anesth Analg 90:887, 2000.

Sufentanil is also used to supplement epidural anesthesia during cesarean delivery (Table 14-7). Sufentanil significantly reduced the total required epidural ropivacaine dose and pain scores compared to plain ropivacaine epidural anesthesia for cesarean delivery.[106] The ED_{50} and ED_{95} for epidural sufentanil to reduce postcesarean pain (VAS less than 10 mm) were 6.7 and 17.5 µg, respectively.[105]

Morphine provides the longest postcesarean analgesia when compared directly with fentanyl, sufentanil, buprenorphine, or oxymorphone.[107] A dose-response study of epidural morphine for postcesarean delivery analgesia demonstrated that the optimal dose of epidural morphine was 3.75 mg (Fig. 14-7).[108] The incidence of pruritus and nausea and vomiting were not dose related in this study. Epidural hydromorphone (600 µg), another longer-acting neuraxial opioid, offered no benefit compared to epidural morphine 3 mg for postcesarean delivery analgesia.[109] Epidural diamorphine is used for postoperative analgesia in Great Britain, but is not available in the United States.

Data are conflicting as to whether combining lipid-soluble opioids (short latency) with morphine (long latency) improves postoperative analgesia. The results of several studies suggest that epidural fentanyl inhibits the postoperative analgesic qualities of epidural morphine.[110] Acute tolerance is the hypothesized mechanism of this observation.

2-Chloroprocaine may inhibit the efficacy of concurrently or subsequently administered epidural opioids.[111–113] Elective cesarean patients were randomized to receive epidural 2-chloroprocaine 3%, 2-chloroprocaine 3% with epinephrine, or lidocaine 2% with epinephrine anesthesia. All patients subsequently received epidural morphine 5 mg.

Intravenous patient-controlled morphine analgesia requirements over the next 24 h were dramatically less in the lidocaine group compared with the chloroprocaine groups.[111] The analgesia efficacy of epidural fentanyl, but not butorphanol, was less when administered following chloroprocaine compared to lidocaine epidural anesthesia.[112] The mechanism of this observation is not known.

α-Adrenergic Agonists. The addition of α-adrenergic agonists to epidural local anesthetics for cesarean delivery may increase the density of the sensory and motor blockade and improve postoperative analgesia. Epinephrine is usually added to local anesthetic solutions to make a concentration of 1:200,000 (5 µg/mL). Epinephrine added to epidural bupivacaine did not alter the onset or duration of sensory blockade but did improve the efficacy of the block.[114] Systemic uptake of epidural epinephrine in clinical doses does not negatively impact uteroplacental blood flow.[115]

Both clonidine and neostigmine have been studied for postcesarean delivery analgesia; however, their use for this indication is not widespread in the United States and is currently not approved by the FDA.

Sodium Bicarbonate. Alkalinizing epidural local anesthetics (lidocaine, bupivacaine, and mepivacaine) by adding sodium bicarbonate reduces the onset time of sensory and motor blockade and reduces the need for intraoperative analgesic supplementation (see Chap. 3). This technique is also useful when extending labor epidural analgesia to surgical anesthesia. The time to achieve surgical anesthesia with lidocaine 2% plus epinephrine 1:200,000 for cesarean delivery in patients previously receiving epidural bupivacaine/fentanyl for labor analgesia was 5.2 min when alkalinized compared with 9.7 min without pH adjustment.[116]

Complications and Side Effects

Local Anesthetic Toxicity. Albright highlighted the risk of cardiac toxicity when administering a large dose of local anesthetic for cesarean delivery.[85] Even when lower concentration solutions are used, this risk remains a disadvantage of epidural compared with spinal anesthesia. Techniques exist to decrease the risk of toxicity, although none of these techniques by itself is foolproof. The simplest test is aspiration before injection. Aspiration through a multiorifice epidural catheter had a false negative rate of 0.2–0.4% intravascular catheter placement;[117] however, this rate is markedly higher for single-orifice catheters.[118] The lidocaine/ epinephrine test dose has been traditionally used, but may have a higher false positive rate in pregnancy.[119] Alternative tests for intravascular placement include injection of a subtoxic dose of local anesthetic (e.g., lidocaine 100 mg or 2-chloroprocaine 90–100 mg), fentanyl

100 μg, or air. Epidural test doses are discussed in detail in Chap. 2 (Table 2-1). Regardless of the use of a test dose, a judicious strategy is to administer the epidural local anesthetic dose in subtoxic increments and to observe for clinical evidence of intravascular injective for 1–2 min. For urgent or emergency cesarean deliveries when the entire local anesthetic dose needs to be injected quickly without waiting, 2-chloroprocaine is the anesthetic agent of choice, not only because of its rapid onset, but because as an ester local anesthetic, it is rapidly metabolized by plasma esterases. Therefore, an inadvertent intravascular injection of a large dose of 2-chloroprocaine is less consequential than that with amide local anesthetics.

Hypotension. Epidural anesthesia for cesarean delivery is associated with a slower onset and less severe hypotension compared with spinal anesthesia.[48] Strategies for treating hypotension mimic those discussed for spinal anesthesia.

High Spinal and Total Spinal Anesthesia. Inappropriately high level of sensory and motor blockade can occur with epidural anesthesia. In particular, this has been described after the injection through an epidural catheter that is actually in the subdural or subarachnoid space (see Chap. 6), or after the rapid injection of epidural local anesthetic in the presence of a large dural puncture (e.g., previous *wet tap*). Preventative strategies include aspiration of the epidural catheter and incremental injection.

Shivering. Although the exact mechanism remains unknown, epidural anesthesia is associated with a higher incidence of shivering than spinal anesthesia (34% vs. 3%).[120] The incidence of shivering is decreased by the addition of opioid to the epidural local anesthetic.[121]

Pruritus. Pruritus is a common symptom of epidural opioid administration. Strategies to treat pruritus are discussed in Chaps. 6 and 13.

Failed Epidural Anesthesia Following Epidural Labor Analgesia. Epidural catheters previously used for labor analgesia are routinely used to induce anesthesia for cesarean delivery. The failure rate of preexisting labor epidural catheters was 7.1% in a large retrospective study from one institution.[122] Another retrospective analysis identified an increased requirement for supplemental local anesthetic administration to maintain labor analgesia as a risk factor for failed epidural anesthesia for the subsequent cesarean delivery.[123] This suggests that if many supplemental epidural boluses have been required to maintain analgesia, an alternative anesthetic technique should be considered for operative anesthesia (e.g., replace the epidural catheter or initiate of spinal or CSE anesthesia).

Herpes Simplex Virus Recrudescence. The epidural[124] or intrathecal[125] administration of morphine for postcesarean analgesia is associated with an increased incidence of oral herpes simplex virus (HSV) recrudescence. For example, when patients with a history of oral HSV infection were randomized to intrathecal morphine or no intrathecal morphine, 38% of patients in the morphine group had recurrent HSV infection compared to 17% in the control group.[125] The etiology is unknown. Primary neonatal HSV infection has not been reported in any study. There is no evidence the neuraxial morphine increases the risk of recurrent genital herpes infection or that neuraxial fentanyl or sufentanil are associated with recurrent oral HSV infection.

Postdural Puncture Headache. The incidence of inadvertent dural puncture with an epidural needle during attempted initiation of epidural anesthesia or analgesia ranges from 0.04 to 6% in the obstetric population.[126] A meta-analysis of studies in obstetric populations that included approximately 330,000 patients found an incidence of 1.5% (95% CI 1.5–1.5%).[127] The incidence of PDPH after inadvertent dural puncture was 52%. A severe PDPH in the postpartum period is particularly troublesome because it interferes with maternal care of the newborn. Treatment options are the same as for the nonobstetric population and are discussed in Chap. 6.

Neurologic Complications. The most common neurologic complications associated with epidural anesthesia are cranial nerve palsy, epidural abscess and hematoma, anterior spinal artery syndrome, and cranial subdural hematoma.[128] Most neurologic injuries associated with childbirth are intrinsic obstetric palsies.[129] Prospective studies have found an incidence between 0.5 and 1.0%.[129,130] Obstetric patients often present with relative contraindications to neuraxial procedures (e.g., anticoagulation, thrombocytopenia, and infection). These are discussed in detail in Chap. 4. Cesarean delivery, however, is not an elective procedure and often cannot be scheduled to minimize these risks. Therefore, the risks and benefits of general compared to neuraxial anesthesia must be assessed in individual patients.

Neonatal Effects. Conclusions about the impact of epidural anesthesia on the neonate are confounded by many coexisting variables including patient condition, epidural anesthetic technique, blood pressure management, use of supplemental oxygen, and the uterine incision-delivery interval. A randomized trial comparing four different local anesthetic solutions (bupivacaine, chloroprocaine, lidocaine, and lidocaine with epinephrine) for epidural anesthesia for cesarean delivery found no difference in the incidence of maternal hypotension, Apgar scores, umbilical cord acid-base status, or neurobehavioral test scores.[131] Several studies have concluded that the epidural administration of local anesthetics for cesarean delivery does not adversely affect neonatal neurobehavioral scores.[132]

► Combined Spinal-Epidural Anesthesia

Combined spinal-epidural anesthesia offers some of the advantages of both spinal and epidural anesthesia including rapid onset, denser blockade, and the ability to extend the duration of the anesthetic. When compared directly with epidural anesthesia, CSE anesthesia has been shown to be associated with more rapid onset of surgical anesthesia, more intense motor blockade, and greater ephedrine use. Intraoperative assessment of maternal satisfaction was higher and anxiety lower with CSE anesthesia (Fig. 14-8),[82] as was the incidence of intraoperative breakthrough pain and shivering.[120]

Different techniques of CSE anesthesia have been described (Box 14-1). Standard CSE anesthesia involves the intrathecal injection of the standard intrathecal dose (same as single-shot spinal anesthesia). The epidural catheter is sited and secured, but is only used for back-up anesthesia if the initial spinal anesthesia is inadequate or the procedure is prolonged. In sequential CSE anesthesia, a smaller intrathecal dose is injected. For most patients this dose is expected to result in inadequate anesthesia. Fifteen min after the intrathecal injection, epidural local anesthetic is titrated via the epidural

catheter in order to achieve adequate surgical anesthesia.[133] This technique is associated with decreased incidence of hypotension compared to the standard technique,[134] and delayed onset of hypotension,[133] however, the interval from induction of anesthesia to surgical incision is significantly prolonged (18 ± 1 vs. 29 ± 1 [mean ± SEM][133]) compared to single-shot spinal anesthesia. A third variation of CSE anesthesia involves the intrathecal injection of a reduced dose, followed 5 min later by the epidural injection of a standard dose of local anesthetic (regardless of sensory level).[135] Compared to single-shot spinal anesthesia, this technique resulted in a lower incidence of hypotension and less nausea and vomiting without a delay in the onset of surgical anesthesia. CSE anesthesia, however, is technically more complicated than either spinal or epidural anesthesia, and controversy exists within the obstetric anesthesia community as to whether CSE anesthesia should routinely replace single-shot spinal anesthesia for cesarean delivery, or only be used for patients at increased risk for hypotension or the adverse effects of hypotension.

A final CSE technique is epidural volume extension (EVE), wherein the injection of a low intrathecal dose (e.g., bupivacaine 5 mg) is followed by the epidural injection of saline, 5–10 mL. Compression of the dural sac by epidural saline causes the cephalad shift of CSF and cephalad extension of the sensory level (see Chap. 2). Although adequate anesthesia was obtained with this technique without epidural supplementation with local anesthetics, there was no difference in the incidence hypotension.[136] EVE did not decrease the ED_{50}

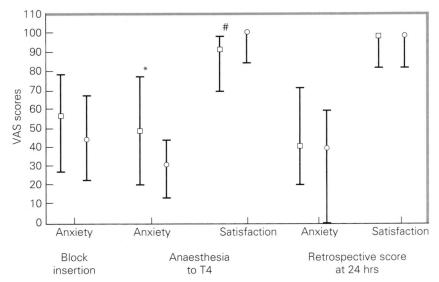

FIGURE 14-8. Randomized, double-blinded study of epidural vs. CSE anesthesia for elective cesarean delivery. Outcomes were assessed using a 100-mm VAS 24 h after delivery. □ = epidural anesthesia, ○ = CSE anesthesia. *$P < 0.01$, #$P < 0.04$. Used with permission from Davies SJ, Paech MJ, Welch H, et al. Maternal experience during epidural or combined spinal-epidural anesthesia for cesarean section: A prospective, randomized trial. Anesth Analg 85:607, 1997.

Box 14-1

Techniques for CSE Anesthesia

	Description of Technique	Advantage/Disadvantage
Standard CSE anesthesia	Intrathecal dose: same as standard spinal dose (bupivacaine 10–12.5 mg)	Advantages: rapid onset of reliable anesthesia
	Epidural dose: none unless needed	Disadvantages: high incidence of hypotension
Sequential CSE anesthesia (titrated epidural injection)	Intrathecal dose: approximately one-half of standard spinal dose (bupivacaine 5 mg)	Advantages: Less hypotension and delayed onset of hypotension compared to spinal anesthesia
	Epidural dose: 15 min after intrathecal dose, 2–3 mL local anesthetic* every 5 min until adequate sensory level	Disadvantages: long induction to delivery interval
CSE anesthesia (empiric epidural injection)	Intrathecal dose: approximately one-half of standard spinal dose (bupivacaine 5–6 mg)	Advantages: rapid onset of reliable anesthesia, less hypotension compared to spinal anesthesia
	Epidural dose: 5 min after intrathecal dose, 10 mL local anesthetic*	Disadvantages: no epidural test dose

*Surgical concentration of local anesthesia (e.g., lidocaine 2% with epinephrine 1:200,000 or bupivacaine 0.5%).

of intrathecal bupivacaine,[137] although duration of motor blockade was shorter.

The usual dose of local anesthesia for sequential CSE anesthesia is approximately one-half the standard single-shot spinal anesthesia dose. Fan et al. investigated the optimal intrathecal hyperbaric bupivacaine dose (2.5, 5, 7.5, or 10 mg) combined with epidural lidocaine 2% with epinephrine titrated to obtain a T4 sensory level, in order to achieve rapid sensory and motor blockade while minimizing hypotension.[134] They concluded that intrathecal bupivacaine 5 mg, combined with an average volume of epidural lidocaine of 10.1 ± 2.0 mL minimized the incidence of hypotension while providing adequate analgesia. Bupivacaine 2.5 mg was associated with inadequate intraoperative analgesia and motor blockade.

CSE anesthesia is technically easier in the sitting patient; however, an additional minute or two is required to site the epidural catheter and this may impact the efficacy and side effects of the technique, particularly when hyperbaric solutions are used. Data are conflicting as to whether the sitting compared to lateral position affects the cephalad distribution of the block and the degree/incidence of hypotension.[138–140] The preponderance of evidence suggests that onset of thoracic sensory blockade is slower and less extensive if the procedure is performed in the sitting compared to lateral position and the incidence of hypotension is lower.[139–141]

Neuraxial Morphine Analgesia

Neuraxial morphine for postoperative analgesia administered as part of a CSE technique can be administered into either the subarachnoid or epidural space. The time to first analgesic request was the same in patients who received epidural morphine 2 mg compared to intrathecal morphine 75 μg, however, patients in the intrathecal morphine group had higher average 24-h pain scores and required more intravenous morphine to treat breakthrough pain.[142] In contrast, the need for rescue medication was the same in patients who received epidural morphine 3 mg compared to intrathecal morphine 200 μg, while rescue analgesia requirements were higher in patients who received intrathecal morphine 100 μg.[143] Conclusions made regarding both of these comparative investigations are limited by assumptions of morphine equipotency between the intrathecal and epidural morphine groups.

▶ Continuous Spinal Anesthesia

Continuous spinal anesthesia combines the advantages of epidural and spinal anesthesia. Currently, the only catheter available for this technique is an epidural catheter. The technique is not widely used because of the high PDPH rate associated with the necessity of puncturing the dura mater with a large-gauge epidural needle. No substantial clinical trials compare this technique to alternative neuraxial anesthetic techniques, although numerous case reports describe its successful employment in unique clinical circumstances. These circumstances include the need for urgent anesthesia in morbidly obese parturients (the rigid epidural needle is technically easier to manipulate than a flimsy spinal needle), or anesthesia for patients with significant cardiac pathology or severe preeclampsia. It is reasonable to initiate continuous spinal anesthesia following inadvertent dural puncture during planned epidural anesthesia. Data are conflicting as to whether the placement of an intrathecal catheter reduces the incidence or severity of subsequent PDPH (see Chap. 6).

▶ Postcesarean Delivery Analgesia

Options for pain management following cesarean delivery include systemic opioid, neuraxial opioid, continuous epidural infusion, local anesthetic wound infiltration, and nonopioid analgesic techniques. The specific details of neuraxial opioid techniques are discussed in the adjuvant opioid sections of spinal and epidural anesthesia in this chapter.

Postcesarean analgesia options involve consideration of the safety, efficacy, and cost of each technique. Respiratory depression is the principal safety concern with the use of postcesarean opioid analgesia; however, it remains poorly understood primarily due to its infrequent occurrence (see Chap. 6). Spinal morphine (100 or 250 μg) has been shown on average to generate less respiratory depression than systemic morphine (8 mg subcutaneous).[144] Clinical circumstances that may generate higher risk of delayed respiratory depression from neuraxial opioids in the obstetric population include underlying pulmonary pathology, concomitantly administered central nervous system depressants, including other opioids, and obesity. Obesity was identified as a potential risk factor for delayed respiratory depression in a prospective observational study of intrathecal morphine.[145] The 24-h postoperative courses of 856 women who received intrathecal morphine 200 μg as part of hyperbaric bupivacaine spinal anesthesia were investigated. Respiratory depression, defined as a SaO_2 less than 85% or a respiratory rate of 10/min or less, was observed in eight women, all of whom were "markedly obese." The obese population represents a group that requires more vigilance during opioid analgesia regardless of the route of administration. Theoretically, patient-controlled intravenous or epidural analgesia (patient-controlled intravenous analgesia [PCIA] or patient-controlled epidural analgesia [PCEA]) may be associated with a lower incidence of respiratory depression compared to single bolus dose, nontitratable neuraxial techniques. The comparative safety of these techniques, however, has not been evaluated for postcesarean delivery analgesia. Regardless of the analgesic technique used, vigilance

remains the primary safety strategy to avoid the complications of respiratory depression.

The use of single dose intrathecal and epidural opioids is associated with more effective analgesia[42,146,147] and higher patient satisfaction[146,147] than systemic opioids following cesarean delivery. Single dose neuraxial opioid administration is a cost-effective postcesarean analgesic technique due to the reduced manpower and equipment needs.[148] Additional options for postcesarean analgesia include the epidural administration of local anesthetics, opioids, or a combination of both. Epidural analgesics can be delivered via a continuous infusion with or without demand PCEA, or demand PCEA alone without an infusion.

Systemic NSAIDs may potentiate neuraxial opioid analgesia and result in improved analgesia. For example, systemic diclofenac combined with epidural morphine provided better analgesia than either drug alone.[149] Although the FDA has not approved ketorolac for use in lactating mothers, it is considered compatible with breastfeeding by the American Academy of Pediatrics.

CERVICAL CERCLAGE

Cerclage for cervical incompetence is one of the most commonly performed procedures in pregnant women. The urgency of the procedure depends on whether it is being performed prophylactically or for premature cervical dilation. The anesthetic considerations for cerclage are altered maternal physiology (consistent with preterm pregnancy), positioning (potential need to avoid the sitting position), extent of sensory blockade (T10 through sacral dermatomes), cervical exposure, and short procedure duration (Box 14-2). If membranes are bulging, avoidance of patient movement and Valsalva maneuver may be necessary to minimize the chance of membrane rupture. Spinal anesthesia with hyperbaric

---

Box 14-2

Anesthetic Considerations for Cervical Cerclage

Altered maternal physiology (2nd trimester pregnancy)

Full stomach (urgent procedure)

Need to maintain supine or Trendelenburg position (bulging membranes)

Need to avoid Valsalva maneuver (risk of rupturing membranes)

Neuraxial anesthesia: T10 (uterus and cervix) through sacral (vaginal) blockade

Short duration procedure (10–20 min)

lidocaine has been widely used for this procedure because of its short duration and excellent sacral anesthesia. Because of concern about TNS associated with the use of spinal lidocaine, Beilin et al. compared spinal anesthesia initiated in the sitting position with plain lidocaine 30 mg and fentanyl 20 μg with hyperbaric bupivacaine 5.25 mg with fentanyl 20 μg.[77] Clinical results, including onset, extent, quality, and resolution of blockade were similar in both groups. If the patient is being nursed in the steep Trendelenburg position because of bulging membranes, hypobaric tetracaine anesthesia (6–8 mg) initiated with the patient in the lateral Trendelenburg position is an alternative.

POSTPARTUM TUBAL LIGATION

The anesthetic requirements for postpartum tubal ligation (PPTL) include the need for a sensory blockade similar to that required for cesarean delivery (T6 or higher), but of shorter duration (20–30 min). This may be achieved by using an in situ epidural catheter placed for labor and delivery analgesia, or initiating spinal or epidural anesthesia. General anesthesia is a less desirable alterative, particularly in the immediate postpartum period. Patients may still be at risk for pulmonary aspiration and airway management may be more difficult than in the nonperipartum patient.

The dose of local anesthesia required for PPTL is similar to that required for cesarean delivery. In a dose-response study of spinal anesthesia for PPTL patients were randomized to receive hyperbaric bupivacaine 5, 7.5, 10, and 12.5 mg in the left lateral position.[150] The investigators concluded that 7.5 mg was the lowest dose that provided adequate intraoperative conditions (1 of 12 patients in the 7.5 mg group required intravenous opioid supplementation despite a T2 sensory level). Bupivacaine 7.5 mg was associated with an earlier return of motor function than 10 and 12.5 mg. The addition of fentanyl 15–25 μg to a low dose of local anesthetic may increase the block success rate. Other alternatives include spinal lidocaine (60–75 mg). There was no difference in the incidence of TNS in patients randomized to intrathecal spinal compared to bupivacaine anesthesia for PPTL.[76]

There is often a delay of many hours after delivery before the tubal ligation procedure is scheduled. It is controversial whether a long delivery-to-surgery interval increases the risk of failed epidural anesthesia in patients with an in situ catheter placed for labor and delivery.[151,152] Certainly, the back and catheter should be inspected before using it after a long interval, as the catheter may become dislodged. 2-Chloroprocaine or lidocaine can be used for epidural anesthesia, although 2-chloroprocaine is more suited to the duration of the surgical procedure.

Local anesthetic requirements decrease during pregnancy. Requirements may return to prepregnancy levels as soon as 1–2 days after delivery and may be as much as 30% higher than intrapartum requirements.[153] Therefore, neuraxial procedures performed on postpartum days 1 and 2 require a higher local anesthetic dose to obtain the same degree of blockade.

Postoperative tubal ligation pain may be underestimated. Intrathecal morphine 50–100 μg[154,155] or epidural morphine 2 mg[156] improved postoperative analgesia and decreased the need for supplemental analgesia compared to control groups.

OOCYTE RETRIEVAL

Transvaginal oocyte retrieval is a frequently performed infertility procedure. It is a short, ambulatory procedure, and the most common anesthetic techniques used are spinal anesthesia and intravenous sedation. In a retrospective review of women who received spinal anesthesia (hyperbaric lidocaine 50–80 mg) versus "heavy" intravenous sedation (alfentanil, midazolam, and propofol) for oocyte retrieval, similar reproductive outcomes were reported, but there was a greater incidence of postprocedural nausea and vomiting (46% vs. 6%) and longer time until recovery room discharge in the patients who received sedation compared with spinal anesthesia.[157]

The addition of fentanyl 10 μg to hyperbaric lidocaine 45 mg for oocyte retrieval resulted in better intra- and postoperative pain scores without any adverse effects.[158] Very low dose bupivacaine (3.75 mg with fentanyl 25 μg) is an alternative to lidocaine spinal anesthesia although prolonged time to voiding and discharged was reported, and 20% of patients required supplemental analgesia.[159]

NONOBSTETRIC ABDOMINAL SURGERY DURING PREGNANCY

Neuraxial anesthesia is a viable alternative to general anesthesia in nonobstetric abdominal surgery during pregnancy. Although laparoscopic abdominal surgery is typically not well tolerated with neuraxial anesthesia, laparotomies for lower abdominal cases such as appendectomy and ovarian cystectomy are successfully performed with spinal or epidural anesthesia during pregnancy.

Uteroplacental perfusion is a primary consideration regardless of anesthetic technique. Additional considerations for nonobstetric surgery during pregnancy depend on the gestational age of the fetus. Teratogenicity and spontaneous fetal loss are concerns early in pregnancy while preterm labor and planning for immediate cesarean delivery are considerations in the latter part of pregnancy (after 24 weeks). The risk of structural teratogenicity is highest during the period of organogenesis (31–71 days after the last menstrual period). No anesthetic agents used in clinically appropriate doses are known teratogens in humans. Severe physiologic aberrations (e.g., hypoxemia and hypercarbia) may be teratogenic or enhance the teratogenicity of other drugs.

Perioperative fetal heart rate monitoring is controversial. Limitations to intraoperative monitoring include technical difficulty obtaining a fetal heart rate during abdominal surgery. During nonobstetric surgery plans for immediate cesarean delivery must be made if the fetus is 24 weeks estimated gestational age or greater.

There are few studies which address neuraxial anesthetic techniques in pregnant patients for nonobstetric surgery. Duration of surgery is less predictable than with other procedures making CSE or epidural anesthesia more attractive techniques than spinal anesthesia. Although many anesthesiologists favor neuraxial anesthesia for surgical procedures performed during pregnancy, there are no data to support a difference in outcome between neuraxial and general anesthesia. The choice of anesthesia ultimately depends on the needs of the surgical procedure along with consideration of altered maternal physiology, gestational age, and expertise of the anesthesiologist with particular techniques.

SUMMARY

The majority of anesthetics for pregnant women are neuraxial. There is convincing evidence for improved safety and outcome for the mother (and ultimately the fetus) for neuraxial compared to general anesthesia for cesarean delivery. Although data do not exist for other surgical procedures performed during pregnancy, neuraxial anesthesia is probably safer for these procedures, too. The primary reason is the ability to avoid airway manipulation, which is more difficult in pregnancy, along with the increased risk of pulmonary aspiration because of altered maternal physiology.

REFERENCES

1. Hawkins JL, Koonin LM, Palmer SK, et al. Anesthesia-related deaths during obstetric delivery in the United States, 1979–1990. *Anesthesiology* 86:277, 1997.
2. Riley ET, Cohen SE, Macario A, et al. Spinal versus epidural anesthesia for cesarean section: A comparison of time efficiency, costs, charges, and complications. *Anesth Analg* 80:709, 1995.
3. Kumar A, Bala I, Bhukal I, et al. Spinal anaesthesia with lidocaine 2% for caesarean section. *Can J Anaesth* 39:915, 1992.
4. McDonald SB, Liu SS, Kopacz DJ, et al. Hyperbaric spinal ropivacaine: A comparison to bupivacaine in volunteers. *Anesthesiology* 90:971, 1999.
5. Camorcia M, Capogna G, Columb MO. Minimum local analgesic doses of ropivacaine, levobupivacaine, and bupivacaine for intrathecal labor analgesia. *Anesthesiology* 102:646, 2005.
6. Meininger D, Byhahn C, Kessler P, et al. Intrathecal fentanyl, sufentanil, or placebo combined with hyperbaric mepivacaine 2% for parturients undergoing elective cesarean delivery. *Anesth Analg* 96:852, 2003.
7. Gautier P, De Kock M, Huberty L, et al. Comparison of the effects of intrathecal ropivacaine, levobupivacaine, and bupivacaine for Caesarean section. *Br J Anaesth* 91:684, 2003.
8. Hauch MA, Hartwell BL, Hunt CO, et al. Comparative effects of subarachnoid hyperbaric bupivacaine and tetracaine-procaine for cesarean delivery. *Reg Anesth* 15:81, 1990.
9. Kafle SK. Intrathecal meperidine for elective caesarean section: A comparison with lidocaine. *Can J Anaesth* 40:718, 1993.
10. Choi DH, Ahn HJ, Kim MH. Bupivacaine-sparing effect of fentanyl in spinal anesthesia for cesarean delivery. *Reg Anesth Pain Med* 25:240, 2000.
11. Ginosar Y, Mirikatani E, Drover DR, et al. ED50 and ED95 of intrathecal hyperbaric bupivacaine coadministered with opioids for cesarean delivery. *Anesthesiology* 100:676, 2004.
12. Ben-David B, Miller G, Gavriel R, et al. Low-dose bupivacaine-fentanyl spinal anesthesia for cesarean delivery. *Reg Anesth Pain Med* 25:235, 2000.
13. Vucevic M, Russell IF. Spinal anaesthesia for caesarean section: 0.125% plain bupivacaine 12 ml compared with 0.5% plain bupivacaine 3 ml. *Br J Anaesth* 68:590, 1992.
14. Camorcia M, Capogna G, Lyons G, et al. The relative motor blocking potencies of intrathecal ropivacaine: Effects of concentration. *Anesth Analg* 98:1779, 2004.
15. Connolly C, McLeod GA, Wildsmith JA. Spinal anaesthesia for Caesarean section with bupivacaine 5 mg mL^{-1} in glucose 8 or 80 mg mL^{-1}. *Br J Anaesth* 86:805, 2001.
16. Vercauteren MP, Coppejans HC, Hoffmann VL, et al. Small-dose hyperbaric versus plain bupivacaine during spinal anesthesia for cesarean section. *Anesth Analg* 86:989, 1998.
17. Sarvela PJ, Halonen PM, Korttila KT. Comparison of 9 mg of intrathecal plain and hyperbaric bupivacaine both with fentanyl for cesarean delivery. *Anesth Analg* 89:1257, 1999.
18. Russell R, Popat M, Richards E, et al. Combined spinal epidural anaesthesia for caesarean section: A randomised comparison of Oxford, lateral and sitting positions. *Int J Obstet Anesth* 11:190, 2002.
19. Hallworth SP, Fernando R, Columb MO, et al. The effect of posture and baricity on the spread of intrathecal bupivacaine for elective cesarean delivery. *Anesth Analg* 100:1159, 2005.
20. Law AC, Lam KK, Irwin MG. The effect of right versus left lateral decubitus positions on induction of spinal anesthesia for cesarean delivery. *Anesth Analg* 97:1795, 2003.
21. Norris MC. Height, weight, and the spread of subarachnoid hyperbaric bupivacaine in the term parturient. *Anesth Analg* 67:555, 1988.
22. Hogan QH, Prost R, Kulier A, et al. Magnetic resonance imaging of cerebrospinal fluid volume and the influence of body habitus and abdominal pressure. *Anesthesiology* 84:1341, 1996.
23. Simon L, Boulay G, Ziane AF, et al. Effect of injection rate on hypotension associated with spinal anesthesia for cesarean section. *Int J Obstet Anesth* 9:10, 2000.
24. Dahlgren G, Hulstrand C, Jakobsson J, et al. Intrathecal sufentanil, fentanyl, or placebo added to bupivacaine for Cesarean section. *Anesth Analg* 85:1288, 1997.
25. Palmer CM, Voulgaropoulos D, Alves D. Subarachnoid fentanyl augments lidocaine spinal anesthesia for cesarean delivery. *Reg Anesth* 20:389, 1995.
26. Hunt CO, Naulty JS, Bader AM, et al. Perioperative analgesia with subarachnoid fentanyl-bupivacaine for cesarean delivery. *Anesthesiology* 71:535, 1989.

27. Chu CC, Shu SS, Lin SM, et al. The effect of intrathecal bupivacaine with combined fentanyl in cesarean section. *Acta Anaesthesiol Sin* 33:149, 1995.

28. Chung CJ, Choi SR, Yeo KH, et al. Hyperbaric spinal ropivacaine for cesarean delivery: A comparison to hyperbaric bupivacaine. *Anesth Analg* 93:157, 2001.

29. Braga Ade F, Braga FS, Poterio GM, et al. Sufentanil added to hyperbaric bupivacaine for subarachnoid block in Caesarean section. *Eur J Anaesthesiol* 20:631, 2003.

30. Abouleish E, Rawal N, Fallon K, et al. Combined intrathecal morphine and bupivacaine for cesarean section. *Anesth Analg* 67:370, 1988.

31. Abboud TK, Dror A, Mosaad P, et al. Mini-dose intrathecal morphine for the relief of post-cesarean section pain: Safety, efficacy, and ventilatory responses to carbon dioxide. *Anesth Analg* 67:137, 1988.

32. Angle PJ, Halpern SH, Leighton BL, et al. A randomized controlled trial examining the effect of naproxen on analgesia during the second day after cesarean delivery. *Anesth Analg* 95:741, 2002.

33. Yang T, Breen TW, Archer D, et al. Comparison of 0.25 mg and 0.1 mg intrathecal morphine for analgesia after Cesarean section. *Can J Anaesth* 46:856, 1999.

34. Gerancher JC, Floyd H, Eisenach J. Determination of an effective dose of intrathecal morphine for pain relief after cesarean delivery. *Anesth Analg* 88:346, 1999.

35. Palmer CM, Emerson S, Volgoropolous D, et al. Dose-response relationship of intrathecal morphine for postcesarean analgesia. *Anesthesiology* 90:437, 1999.

36. Richardson MG, Collins HV, Wissler RN. Intrathecal hypobaric versus hyperbaric bupivacaine with morphine for cesarean section. *Anesth Analg* 87:336, 1998.

37. Camann WR, Bader AM. Spinal anesthesia for cesarean delivery with meperidine as the sole agent. *Int J Obstet Anesth* 1:156, 1992.

38. Roy JD, Girard M, Drolet P. Intrathecal meperidine decreases shivering during cesarean delivery under spinal anesthesia. *Anesth Analg* 98:230, 2004.

39. Saravanan S, Robinson AP, Qayoum Dar A, et al. Minimum dose of intrathecal diamorphine required to prevent intraoperative supplementation of spinal anaesthesia for Caesarean section. *Br J Anaesth* 91:368, 2003.

40. Culebras X, Gaggero G, Zatloukal J, et al. Advantages of intrathecal nalbuphine, compared with intrathecal morphine, after cesarean delivery: An evaluation of postoperative analgesia and adverse effects. *Anesth Analg* 91:601, 2000.

41. Connelly NR, Dunn SM, Ingold V, et al. The use of fentanyl added to morphine-lidocaine-epinephrine spinal solution in patients undergoing cesarean section. *Anesth Analg* 78:918, 1994.

42. Sibilla C, Albertazz P, Zatelli R, et al. Perioperative analgesia for caesarean section: Comparison of intrathecal morphine and fentanyl alone or in combination. *Int J Obstet Anesth* 6:43, 1997.

43. Abouleish EI. Epinephrine improves the quality of spinal hyperbaric bupivacaine for cesarean section. *Anesth Analg* 66:395, 1987.

44. Paech MJ, Pavy TJ, Orlikowski CE, et al. Postcesarean analgesia with spinal morphine, clonidine, or their combination. *Anesth Analg* 98:1460, 2004.

45. Siddik-Sayyid SM, Aouad MT, Jalbout MI, et al. Intrathecal versus intravenous fentanyl for supplementation of subarachnoid block during cesarean delivery. *Anesth Analg* 95:209, 2002.

46. Bland BA, Lawes EG, Duncan PW, et al. Comparison of midazolam and thiopental for rapid sequence anesthetic induction for elective cesarean section. *Anesth Analg* 66:1165, 1987.

47. Frolich MA, Burchfield DJ, Euliano TY, et al. A single dose of fentanyl and midazolam prior to Cesarean section have no adverse neontal effects. *Can J Anaesth* 53:79, 2006.

48. Ng K, Parsons J, Cyna AM, et al. Spinal versus epidural anaesthesia for caesarean section. *Cochrane Database Syst Rev* CD003765, 2004.

49. Ngan Kee WD, Khaw KS, Lee BB, et al. A dose-response study of prophylactic intravenous ephedrine for the prevention of hypotension during spinal anesthesia for cesarean delivery. *Anesth Analg* 90:1390, 2000.

50. Reynolds F, Seed PT. Anaesthesia for Caesarean section and neonatal acid-base status: A meta-analysis. *Anaesthesia* 60:636, 2005.

51. Aya AG, Mangin R, Vialles N, et al. Patients with severe preeclampsia experience less hypotension during spinal anesthesia for elective cesarean delivery than healthy parturients: A prospective cohort comparison. *Anesth Analg* 97:867, 2003.

52. Aya AG, Vialles N, Tanoubi I, et al. Spinal anesthesia-induced hypotension: A risk comparison between patients with severe preeclampsia and healthy women undergoing preterm cesarean delivery. *Anesth Analg* 101:869, 2005.

53. Visalyaputra S, Rodanant O, Somboonviboon W, et al. Spinal versus epidural anesthesia for cesarean delivery in severe preeclampsia: A prospective randomized, multicenter study. *Anesth Analg* 101:862, 2005.

54. Wallace DH, Leveno KJ, Cunningham FG, et al. Randomized comparison of general and regional anesthesia for cesarean delivery in pregnancies complicated by severe preeclampsia. *Obstet Gynecol* 86:193, 1995.

55. Cooper DW, Carpenter M, Mowbray P, et al. Fetal and maternal effects of phenylephrine and ephedrine during spinal anesthesia for cesarean delivery. *Anesthesiology* 97:1582, 2002.

56. Lee A, Ngan Kee WD, Gin T. A quantitative, systematic review of randomized controlled trials of ephedrine versus phenylephrine for the management of hypotension during spinal anesthesia for cesarean delivery. *Anesth Analg* 94:920, 2002.

57. Dyer RA, Farina Z, Joubert IA, et al. Crystalloid preload versus rapid crystalloid administration after induction of spinal anaesthesia (coload) for elective caesarean section. *Anaesth Intensive Care* 32:351, 2004.

58. Riley ET, Cohen SE, Rubenstein AJ, et al. Prevention of hypotension after spinal anesthesia for cesarean section: Six percent hetastarch versus lactated Ringer's solution. *Anesth Analg* 81:838, 1995.

59. Kohler F, Sorensen JF, Helbo-Hansen HS. Effect of delayed supine positioning after induction of spinal anaesthesia for caesarean section. *Acta Anaesthesiol Scand* 46:441, 2002.

60. Datta S, Alper MH, Ostheimer GW, et al. Method of ephedrine administration and nausea and hypotension during spinal anesthesia for cesarean section. *Anesthesiology* 56:68, 1982.

61. Yazigi A, Chalhoub V, Madi-Jebara S, et al. Prophylactic ondansetron is effective in the treatment of nausea and vomiting but not on pruritus after cesarean delivery with intrathecal sufentanil-morphine. *J Clin Anesth* 14:183, 2002.

62. Pan PH, Moore CH. Intraoperative antiemetic efficacy of prophylactic ondansetron versus droperidol for cesarean section patients under epidural anesthesia. *Anesth Analg* 83:982, 1996.

63. Pan PH, Moore CH. Comparing the efficacy of prophylactic metoclopramide, ondansetron, and placebo in cesarean section patients given epidural anesthesia. *J Clin Anesth* 13:430, 2001.

64. Fujii Y, Tanaka H, Toyooka H. Prevention of nausea and vomiting with granisetron, droperidol and metoclopramide during and after spinal anaesthesia for caesarean section: A randomized, double-blind, placebo-controlled trial. *Acta Anaesthesiol Scand* 42:921, 1998.

65. Numazaki M, Fujii Y. Reduction of emetic symptoms during cesarean delivery with antiemetics: Propofol at subhypnotic dose versus traditional antiemetics. *J Clin Anesth* 15:423, 2003.

66. Tzeng JI, Hsing CH, Chu CC, et al. Low-dose dexamethasone reduces nausea and vomiting after epidural morphine: A comparison of metoclopramide with saline. *J Clin Anesth* 14:19, 2002.

67. Nortcliffe SA, Shah J, Buggy DJ. Prevention of postoperative nausea and vomiting after spinal morphine for Caesarean section: Comparison of cyclizine, dexamethasone and placebo. *Br J Anaesth* 90:665, 2003.

68. Stein DJ, Birnbach DJ, Danzer BI, et al. Acupressure versus intravenous metoclopramide to prevent nausea and vomiting during spinal anesthesia for cesarean section. *Anesth Analg* 84:342, 1997.

69. Charuluxananan S, Kyokong O, Somboonviboon W, et al. Nalbuphine versus propofol for treatment of intrathecal morphine-induced pruritus after cesarean delivery. *Anesth Analg* 93:162, 2001.

70. Warwick JP, Kearns CF, Scott WE. The effect of subhypnotic doses of propofol on the incidence of pruritus after intrathecal morphine for caesarean section. *Anaesthesia* 52:270, 1997.

71. Beilin Y, Bernstein HH, Zucker-Pinchoff B, et al. Subhypnotic doses of propofol do not relieve pruritus induced by intrathecal morphine after cesarean section. *Anesth Analg* 86:310, 1998.

72. Marucci M, Diele C, Bruno F, et al. Subarachnoid anaesthesia in caesarean delivery: Effects on alertness. *Minerva Anestesiol* 69:809, 2003.

73. Furst SR, Reisner LS. Risk of high spinal anesthesia following failed epidural block for cesarean delivery. *J Clin Anesth* 7:71, 1995.

74. Wong CA, Slavenas P. The incidence of transient radicular irritation after spinal anesthesia in obstetric patients. *Reg Anesth Pain Med* 24:55, 1999.

75. Aouad MT, Siddik SS, Jalbout MI, et al. Does pregnancy protect against intrathecal lidocaine-induced transient neurologic symptoms? *Anesth Analg* 92:401, 2001.

76. Philip J, Sharma SK, Gottumukkala VN, et al. Transient neurologic symptoms after spinal anesthesia with lidocaine in obstetric patients. *Anesth Analg* 92:405, 2001.

77. Beilin Y, Zahn J, Abramovitz S, et al. Subarachnoid small-dose bupivacaine versus lidocaine for cervical cerclage. *Anesth Analg* 97:56, 2003.

78. Moen V, Dahlgren N, Irestedt L. Severe neurological complications after central neuraxial blockades in Sweden 1990–1999. *Anesthesiology* 101:950, 2004.

79. Reynolds F. Infection as a complication of neuraxial blockade. *Int J Obstet Anesth* 14:183, 2005.

80. Smith EA, Thorburn J, Duckworth RA, et al. A comparison of 25 G and 27 G Whitacre needles for caesarean section. *Anaesthesia* 49:859, 1994.

81. Mahajan J, Singh MM, Anand NK, et al. Anaesthetic technique for elective caesarean section and neurobehavioural status of newborns. *Int J Obstet Anesth* 2:89, 1993.

82. Davies SJ, Paech MJ, Welch H, et al. Maternal experience during epidural or combined spinal-epidural anesthesia for cesarean section: A prospective, randomized trial. *Anesth Analg* 85:607, 1997.

83. Olofsson C, Ekblom A, Skoldefors E, et al. Anesthetic quality during cesarean section following subarachnoid or epidural administration of bupivacaine with or without fentanyl. *Acta Anaesthesiol Scand* 41:332, 1997.

84. Dutton DA, Moir DD, Howie HB, et al. Choice of local anaesthetic drug for extradural caesarean section. Comparison of 0.5% and 0.75% bupivacaine and 1.5% etidocaine. *Br J Anaesth* 56:1361, 1984.

85. Albright GA. Cardiac arrest following regional anesthesia with etidocaine or bupivacaine. *Anesthesiology* 51:285, 1979.

86. Clark V, McGrady E, Sugden C, et al. Speed of onset of sensory block for elective extradural caesarean section: Choice of agent and temperature of injectate. *Br J Anaesth* 72:221, 1994.

87. Paech MJ. Epidural anaesthesia for caesarean section: A comparison of 0.5% bupivacaine and 2% lignocaine both with adrenaline. *Anaesth Intensive Care* 16:187, 1988.

88. Crosby E, Sandler A, Finucane B, et al. Comparison of epidural anaesthesia with ropivacaine 0.5% and bupivacaine 0.5% for caesarean section. *Can J Anaesth* 45:1066, 1998.

89. Bjornestad E, Smedvig JP, Bjerkreim T, et al. Epidural ropivacaine 7.5 mg/ml for elective Caesarean section: A double-blind comparison of efficacy and tolerability with bupivacaine 5 mg/ml. *Acta Anaesthesiol Scand* 43:603, 1999.

90. Kampe S, Tausch B, Paul M, et al. Epidural block with ropivacaine and bupivacaine for elective caesarean section: Maternal cardiovascular parameters, comfort and neonatal well-being. *Curr Med Res Opin* 20:7, 2004.

91. Lucas DN, Ciccone GK, Yentis SM. Extending low-dose epidural analgesia for emergency Caesarean section. A comparison of three solutions. *Anaesthesia* 54:1173, 1999.

92. Howell P, Davies W, Wrigley M, et al. Comparison of four local extradural anaesthetic solutions for elective caesarean section. *Br J Anaesth* 65:648, 1990.

93. Gaiser RR, Cheek TG, Adams HK, et al. Epidural lidocaine for cesarean delivery of the distressed fetus. *Int J Obstet Anesth* 7:27, 1998.

94. Philipson EH, Kuhnert BR, Syracuse CD. Fetal acidosis, 2-chloroprocaine, and epidural anesthesia for cesarean section. *Am J Obstet Gynecol* 151:322, 1985.

95. Bader AM, Tsen LC, Camann WR, et al. Clinical effects and maternal and fetal plasma concentrations of 0.5% epidural levobupivacaine versus bupivacaine for cesarean delivery. *Anesthesiology* 90:1596, 1999.

96. Nakayama M, Yamamoto J, Ichinose H, et al. Effects of volume and concentration of lidocaine on epidural anaesthesia in pregnant females. *Eur J Anaesthesiol* 19:808, 2002.

97. Setayesh AR, Kholdebarin AR, Moghadam MS, et al. The Trendelenburg position increases the spread and accelerates the onset of epidural anesthesia for Cesarean section. *Can J Anaesth* 48:890, 2001.

98. Norris MC, Dewan DM. Effect of gravity on the spread of extradural anaesthesia for caesarean section. *Br J Anaesth* 59:338, 1987.

99. Norris MC, Leighton BL, DeSimone CA, et al. Lateral position and epidural anesthesia for cesarean section. *Anesth Analg* 67:788, 1987.

100. Gambling DR, Mayson K, McMorland GH, et al. Predictability of spread of epidural anesthesia for cesarean section using

incremental doses of lidocaine hydrocarbonate with epinephrine. *Reg Anesth* 14:133, 1989.

101. Hodgkinson R, Husain FJ. Obesity, gravity, and spread of epidural anesthesia. *Anesth Analg* 60:421, 1981.

102. Halonen PM, Paatero H, Hovorka J, et al. Comparison of two fentanyl doses to improve epidural anaesthesia with 0.5% bupivacaine for caesarean section. *Acta Anaesthesiol Scand* 37:774, 1993.

103. Harrison DM, Sinatra R, Morgese L, et al. Epidural narcotic and patient-controlled analgesia for post-cesarean section pain relief. *Anesthesiology* 68:454, 1988.

104. Helbo-Hansen HS, Bang U, Lindholm P, et al. Maternal effects of adding epidural fentanyl to 0.5% bupivacaine for caesarean section. *Int J Obstet Anesth* 2:21, 1993.

105. Grass JA, Sakima NT, Schmidt R, et al. A randomized, double-blind, dose-response comparison of epidural fentanyl versus sufentanil analgesia after cesarean section. *Anesth Analg* 85:365, 1997.

106. Bachmann-Mennenga B, Veit G, Steinicke B, et al. Efficacy of sufentanil addition to ropivacaine epidural anaesthesia for Caesarean section. *Acta Anaesthesiol Scand* 49:532, 2005.

107. Celleno D, Capogna G, Sebastiani M, et al. Epidural analgesia during and after cesarean delivery. Comparison of five opioids. *Reg Anesth* 16:79, 1991.

108. Palmer CM, Nogami WM, Van Maren G, et al. Postcesarean epidural morphine: A dose-response study. *Anesth Analg* 90:887, 2000.

109. Halpern SH, Arellano R, Preston R, et al. Epidural morphine vs hydromorphone in post-caesarean section patients. *Can J Anaesth* 43:595, 1996.

110. Vincent RD, Jr., Chestnut DH, Choi WW, et al. Does epidural fentanyl decrease the efficacy of epidural morphine after cesarean delivery? *Anesth Analg* 74:658, 1992.

111. Karambelkar DJ, Ramanathan S. 2-Chloroprocaine antagonism of epidural morphine analgesia. *Acta Anaesthesiol Scand* 41:774, 1997.

112. Camann WR, Hartigan PM, Gilbertson LI, et al. Chloroprocaine antagonism of epidural opioid analgesia: A receptor-specific phenomenon? *Anesthesiology* 73:860, 1990.

113. Eisenach JC, Schlairet TJ, Dobson CE, et al. Effect of prior anesthetic solution on epidural morphine analgesia. *Anesth Analg* 73:119, 1991.

114. Laishley RS, Morgan BM. A single dose epidural technique for caesarean section. A comparison between 0.5% bupivacaine plain and 0.5% bupivacaine with adrenaline. *Anaesthesia* 43:100, 1988.

115. Alahuhta S, Rasanen J, Jouppila R, et al. Effects of extradural bupivacaine with adrenaline for caesarean section on uteroplacental and fetal circulation. *Br J Anaesth* 67:678, 1991.

116. Lam DT, Ngan Kee WD, Khaw KS. Extension of epidural blockade in labour for emergency Caesarean section using 2% lidocaine with epinephrine and fentanyl, with or without alkalinisation. *Anaesthesia* 56:790, 2001.

117. Norris MC, Fogel ST, Dalman H, et al. Labor epidural analgesia without an intravascular "test dose." *Anesthesiology* 88:1495, 1998.

118. Kenepp NB, Gutsche BB. Inadvertent intravascular injections during lumbar epidural anesthesia. *Anesthesiology* 54:172, 1981.

119. Colonna-Romano P, Nagaraj L. Tests to evaluate intravenous placement of epidural catheters in laboring women: A prospective clinical study. *Anesth Analg* 86:985, 1998.

120. Choi DH, Kim JA, Chung IS. Comparison of combined spinal epidural anesthesia and epidural anesthesia for cesarean section. *Acta Anaesthesiol Scand* 44:214, 2000.

121. Sutherland J, Seaton H, Lowry C. The influence of epidural pethidine on shivering during lower segment caesarean section under epidural anaesthesia. *Anaesth Intensive Care* 19:228, 1991.

122. Pan PH, Bogard TD, Owen MD. Incidence and characteristics of failures in obstetric neuraxial analgesia and anesthesia: A retrospective analysis of 19,259 deliveries. *Int J Obstet Anesth* 13:227, 2004.

123. Riley ET, Papasin J. Epidural catheter function during labor predicts anesthetic efficacy for subsequent cesarean delivery. *Int J Obstet Anesth* 11:81, 2002.

124. Boyle RK. Herpes simplex labialis after epidural or parenteral morphine: A randomized prospective trial in an Australian obstetric population. *Anaesth Intensive Care* 23:433, 1995.

125. Davies PW, Vallejo MC, Shannon KT, et al. Oral herpes simplex reactivation after intrathecal morphine: A prospective randomized trial in an obstetric population. *Anesth Analg* 100:1472, 2005.

126. Berger CW, Crosby ET, Grodecki W. North American survey of the management of dural puncture occurring during labour epidural analgesia. *Can J Anaesth* 45:110, 1998.

127. Choi PT, Galinski SE, Takeuchi L, et al. PDPH is a common complication of neuraxial blockade in parturients: A meta-analysis of obstetrical studies. *Can J Anaesth* 50:460, 2003.

128. Loo CC, Dahlgren G, Irestedt L. Neurological complications in obstetric regional anaesthesia. *Int J Obstet Anesth* 9:99, 2000.

129. Wong CA, Scavone BM, Dugan S, et al. Incidence of postpartum lumbosacral spine and lower extremity nerve injuries. *Obstet Gynecol* 101:279, 2003.

130. Dar AQ, Robinson APC, Lyons G. Postpartum neurologic symptoms following regional blockade: A prospective study with case controls. *Int J Obstet Anesth* 11:85, 2002.

131. Abboud TK, Kim KC, Noueihed R, et al. Epidural bupivacaine, chloroprocaine, or lidocaine for cesarean section—maternal and neonatal effects. *Anesth Analg* 62:914, 1983.

132. Abboud TK, Najappala S, Murakawa K. Comparison of the effects of general and regional anesthesia for cesarean section on neonatal neurologic and adaptive capacity scores. *Anesth Analg* 64:996, 1985.

133. Thoren T, Holmstrom B, Rawal N, et al. Sequential combined spinal epidural block versus spinal block for cesarean section: Effects on maternal hypotension and neurobehavioral function of the newborn. *Anesth Analg* 78:1087, 1994.

134. Fan SZ, Susetio L, Wang YP, et al. Low dose of intrathecal hyperbaric bupivacaine combined with epidural lidocaine for cesarean section—a balance block technique. *Anesth Analg* 78:474, 1994.

135. Choi DH, Ahn HJ, Kim JA. Combined low-dose spinal-epidural anesthesia versus single-shot spinal anesthesia for elective cesarean delivery. *Int J Obstet Anesth* 15:13, 2006.

136. Lew E, Yeo SW, Thomas E. Combined spinal-epidural anesthesia using epidural volume extension leads to faster motor recovery after elective cesarean delivery: A prospective, randomized, double-blind study. *Anesth Analg* 98:810, 2004.

137. Beale N, Evans B, Plaat F, et al. Effect of epidural volume extension on dose requirement of intrathecal hyperbaric bupivacaine at Caesarean section. *Br J Anaesth* 95:500, 2005.

138. Yun EM, Marx GF, Santos AC. The effects of maternal position during induction of combined spinal-epidural anesthesia for cesarean delivery. *Anesth Analg* 87:614, 1998.

139. Coppejans HC, Hendrickx E, Goossens J, et al. The sitting versus right lateral position during combined spinal-epidural anesthesia for cesarean delivery: Block characteristics and severity of hypotension. *Anesth Analg* 102:243, 2006.

140. Rucklidge MW, Paech MJ, Yentis SM. A comparison of the lateral, Oxford and sitting positions for performing combined spinal-epidural anaesthesia for elective Caesarean section. *Anaesthesia* 60:535, 2005.

141. Patel M, Samsoon G, Swami A, et al. Posture and the spread of hyperbaric bupivacaine in parturients using the combined spinal epidural technique. *Can J Anaesth* 40:943, 1993.

142. Duale C, Frey C, Bolandard F, et al. Epidural versus intrathecal morphine for postoperative analgesia after Caesarean section. *Br J Anaesth* 91:690, 2003.

143. Sarvela J, Halonen P, Soikkeli A, et al. A double-blinded, randomized comparison of intrathecal and epidural morphine for elective cesarean delivery. *Anesth Analg* 95:436, 2002.

144. Abboud TK, Dror A, Mosaad P, et al. Mini-dose intrathecal morphine for the relief of post-cesarean section pain: Safety, efficacy, and ventilatory responses to carbon dioxide. *Anesth Analg* 67:137, 1988.

145. Abouleish E, Rashad MN, Rawal N. The addition of 0.2 mg subarachnoid morphine to hyperbaric bupivacaine for cesarean delivery: A prospective study of 856 cases. *Reg Anesth* 16:137, 1991.

146. Swart M, Sewell J, Thomas D. Intrathecal morphine for caesarean section: An assessment of pain relief, satisfaction and side-effects. *Anaesthesia* 52:373, 1997.

147. Rosaeg OP, Lindsay MP. Epidural opioid analgesia after caesarean section: A comparison of patient-controlled analgesia with meperidine and single bolus injection of morphine. *Can J Anaesth* 41:1063, 1994.

148. Vercauteren M, Vereecken K, La Malfa M, et al. Cost effectiveness of analgesia after Caesarean section. A comparison of intrathecal morphine and epidural PCA. *Acta Anaesthesiol Scand* 46:85, 2002.

149. Sun HL, Wu CC, Lin MS, et al. Effects of epidural morphine and intramuscular diclofenac combination in postcesarean analgesia: A dose-range study. *Anesth Analg* 76:284, 1993.

150. Huffnagle SL, Norris MC, Huffnagle HJ, et al. Intrathecal hyperbaric bupivacaine dose response in postpartum tubal ligation patients. *Reg Anesth Pain Med* 27:284, 2002.

151. Vincent RD, Reid RW. Epidural anesthesia for postpartum tubal ligation using epidural catheters placed during labor. *J Clin Anesth* 5:289, 1993.

152. Goodman EJ, Dumas SD. The rate of successful reactivation of labor epidural catheters for postpartum tubal ligation surgery. *Reg Anesth Pain Med* 23:258, 1998.

153. Abouleish EI. Postpartum tubal ligation requires more bupivacaine for spinal anesthesia than does cesarean section. *Anesth Analg* 65:897, 1986.

154. Campbell DC, Riben CM, Rooney ME, et al. Intrathecal morphine for postpartum tubal ligation postoperative analgesia. *Anesth Analg* 93:1006, 2001.

155. Habib AS, Muir HA, White WD, et al. Intrathecal morphine for analgesia after postpartum bilateral tubal ligation. *Anesth Analg* 100:239, 2005.

156. Marcus RJ, Wong CA, Lehor A, et al. Postoperative epidural morphine for postpartum tubal ligation analgesia. *Anesth Analg* 101:876, 2005.

157. Viscomi CM, Hill K, Johnson J, et al. Spinal anesthesia versus intravenous sedation for transvaginal oocyte retrieval: Reproductive outcome, side-effects and recovery profiles. *Int J Obstet Anesth* 6:49, 1997.

158. Martin R, Tsen LC, Tzeng G, et al. Anesthesia for in vitro fertilization: The addition of fentanyl to 1.5% lidocaine. *Anesth Analg* 88:523, 1999.

159. Tsen LC, Schultz R, Martin R, et al. Intrathecal low-dose bupivacaine versus lidocaine for in vitro fertilization procedures. *Reg Anesth Pain Med* 26:52, 2001.

Neuraxial Anesthesia for Pediatric Surgery

CHAPTER 15

Tetsu Uejima
Santhanam Suresh

INTRODUCTION

The current practice of intraoperative regional anesthesia in children has a long history. Spinal anesthesia in children was first reported by Bainbridge and Gray in the early part of the twentieth century. This was soon followed by the first reported use of caudal epidural anesthesia in 1933 by Campbell. As anesthesia developed into a medical specialty of its own, the practice of providing regional anesthesia blossomed. Unfortunately, advances in regional anesthesia in the early half of the twentieth century were not always applied to pediatric patients, perhaps due to a lack of interest and the absence of pediatric anesthesiologists as a subspecialty group.

The last two decades have seen a resurgence of interest in the use of regional anesthesia and postoperative analgesia in adult patients. This trend has extended to the pediatric anesthesia practice where regional anesthesia is routinely performed at tertiary care hospitals as well as community hospitals worldwide. Familiarity of regional anesthetic techniques by parents and surgeons is a large reason for the recent increase in the acceptance of regional techniques in children. An excellent example of this is the use of continuous epidural analgesia for labor and delivery, which has led to a greater acceptance of caudal epidural blockade in infants and children by parents. There is a sense of what to expect from regional anesthesia. Additional information available on the Internet has given parents greater in-depth knowledge prior to accompanying their children to the operating room suite.

Other factors may account for the increased use of regional anesthesia in children. The last two decades has seen a shift from inpatient to ambulatory surgery for many procedures. Although the impetus for this change probably came from third party payers, it has resulted in improved surgical and anesthetic techniques. The intraoperative use of regional anesthetic techniques results in earlier awakening and avoidance of postoperative opioid analgesia, which leads to less postoperative nausea and vomiting,[1] thus facilitating earlier discharge.

The Joint Commission on Accreditation of Hospitals Organization (JCAHO) has recently mandated that pain be viewed as a fifth vital sign. Postoperative pain relief has thus been thrust into the limelight. Intraoperative and postoperative regional anesthesia are excellent means of providing postoperative analgesia in children and offer parents an alternative to traditional means of postoperative analgesia, including patient (or parent)-controlled analgesia (PCA). While postoperative regional anesthesia has its own set of complications, there are some advantages compared to other methods of analgesia. There is no need for the child's cooperation which may be important in very young or developmentally delayed children. There is also less need for nonopioid and opioid analgesics, often resulting in decreased sedation.[2]

There is now a considerable body of literature devoted solely to regional anesthesia in children and considerably more experience and expertise among pediatric anesthesia practitioners. The safety of performing regional anesthesia in these young patients has also improved due to the increased use of peripheral nerve stimulators and better understanding of the pharmacokinetics of local anesthetics in children.

Finally, overall satisfaction by patients, parents, and practitioners appears to be very high. Children may undergo surgical procedures with less postoperative pain, earlier ambulation and discharge, and more rapid recovery than in the past. Parents are less apprehensive when their children are not in pain and may focus their attention on other aspects of their child's recovery. Surgeons have fewer concerns about managing postoperative pain, especially with the ever-increasing presence of acute pain services in pediatric hospitals. A variety of regional blocks may be performed in children. This chapter will focus on spinal, caudal, and epidural blockade in the pediatric population.

RELATIVE CONTRAINDICATIONS, INDICATIONS, AND PATIENT SELECTION

▶ Relative Contraindications

In general, contraindications to neuraxial anesthesia that apply to adult patients also apply to pediatric patients (see Chap. 5). There are, however, contraindications that are unique to the pediatric patient (Box 15-1). Lack of parental consent or child assent (for children over the age of 12 years) is an important contraindication to the performance of neuraxial anesthesia in children. Reasons for refusal include misconceptions about the risks of neuraxial anesthesia, such as the risk of paralysis or unsatisfactory prior experience with neuraxial anesthesia, including postdural puncture headache (PDPH), or incomplete or failed epidural anesthesia. While much can be done by the surgeon and the anesthesiologist to allay parents' concerns, there is often a lack of prospective data in the literature to support the clinical impressions of the advantages of regional anesthesia, especially in the area of major conduction anesthesia.

Most anesthesiologists believe the initiation of neuraxial anesthesia is contraindicated in anesthetized, asleep adults (see Chap. 5). It is commonly accepted that regional blocks may be performed in very young children while they are asleep. There is less consensus as to appropriate practice in older children who may refuse to have the block performed while awake. There is currently heated debate in the anesthesia community regarding the safety of placing thoracic epidural catheters in anesthetized children.[3,4]

Box 15-1

Relative Contraindications to Neuraxial Anesthesia in Children

Lack of parenteral consent

Lack of patient assent (if patient is older than 12 years)

Infection at the puncture site

Anatomic abnormalities (particularly of the spine)

Systemic generalized sepsis

Coagulopathy

Hemodynamic instability

Presence of intracranial shunting devices

Poorly controlled seizures

Difficult airway

Concomitant neuromuscular disease

Other contraindications to neuraxial anesthesia include infection or anatomic deformity at the proposed site, presence of a coagulopathy, poorly controlled seizures, and hemodynamic instability. The presence of a difficult airway is a relative contraindication to neuraxial anesthesia. Airway management is considered by many to be the cornerstone of any pediatric anesthetic practice. Children have limited oxygen reserves and untoward or catastrophic events in children are usually precipitated by airway mishaps, unlike adults, in whom the precipitating event is often cardiovascular in nature.

Several factors should first be considered before performing neuraxial anesthesia in a child with a difficult airway. The first consideration is the nature of the surgical procedure. The anticipated surgical site, the length of the procedure, the surgical position (lateral, prone, supine), and the anticipated degree of postoperative pain are all important considerations. The airway is equally important and potential difficulty with airway management should be clearly identified before the analgesic plan is made. For example, the risks and benefits of performing caudal epidural blockade in a child with a difficult airway undergoing a hernia repair differ from those of a child receiving thoracic epidural analgesia for an intrathoracic procedure. Prior anesthetic records, if available, should be obtained. While the presence of an airway abnormality should not necessarily preclude a child from receiving neuraxial anesthesia, a plan to secure the airway should the need arise must be made prior to proceeding with the anesthetic.

The presence of concurrent neuromuscular disease is a relative contraindication to neuraxial anesthesia. In patients with underlying pulmonary disease, neuraxial anesthesia may be the safest option, but one should always weigh the benefits of neuraxial blockade against the risks of exacerbating the child's neuromuscular symptoms. Parents may attribute postoperative deterioration in the child's medical status to the block and this may become a medicolegal issue.

Prior surgical procedures at the site of the anticipated block procedure may be a relative contraindication. Patients who have spinal dysmorphism repair may be poor candidates for central neuraxial blockade, as well as those with underlying hydrocephalus with indwelling ventriculoperitoneal shunts. Finally, one must consider the capability of the anesthesiologist and the capacity of the institution to conduct and maintain the blockade into the postoperative period. While simple neuraxial blocks, such as single-shot caudal anesthesia/analgesia, may be performed at many institutions, including ambulatory surgical centers, lack of expertise and familiarity with equipment can all lead to poor patient outcomes. A great deal of time, expense, education, and personnel must be invested prior to undertaking an extensive inpatient postoperative acute pain service.

Indications and Patient Selection

The most common indication for neuraxial blockade is to provide or augment postoperative analgesia. This is true whether a single injection or continuous technique is used. Blocks performed prior to the surgical procedure have the added advantage of decreasing general anesthetic requirements which leads to earlier awakening and discharge in ambulatory surgical patients. Preemptive analgesia may also be an important consideration.

Neuraxial anesthesia may be advantageous in the presence of certain medical conditions. Spinal anesthesia in former preterm infants significantly decreases the risk of postoperative apnea in this population of patients.[5] Patients with underlying pulmonary diseases, such as cystic fibrosis, asthma, and bronchopulmonary dysplasia, undergoing lower abdominal or lower extremity procedures, may be good candidates for neuraxial anesthesia. Likewise, patients with underlying neuromuscular diseases may be candidates but may require special considerations as previously discussed. Patients with a family history of malignant hyperthermia are ideal candidates for neuraxial anesthesia in combination with intravenous sedation. Premature infants, while good candidates for neuraxial anesthesia, have a host of medical issues related to their prematurity that should be addressed before making an anesthetic plan.

Parental or patient refusal to allow the administration of a general anesthetic, though rare, is another indication for neuraxial anesthesia. One must realize, however, that neuraxial blockade in infants and young children is often performed in conjunction with general anesthesia and rarely as the sole anesthetic. Older children may undergo surgery with a combination of neuraxial blockade and intravenous sedation. Certain situations in which neuraxial anesthesia is the ideal choice in an adult are virtually impossible to initiate in a young child while he or she was awake.

We must be cognizant that because the overwhelming majority of children who receive neuraxial blockade also receive a general anesthetic, we are potentially placing the child at risk for complications of both anesthetic modalities. When initiating neuraxial blockade in children without general anesthesia, special consideration should be given to administering intravenous sedation to minimize discomfort and psychologic trauma to the patient. Patients should be kept warm during block initiation. There should be a minimum amount of extraneous noise (e.g., conversation and loud music) and the child should be allowed to bring a stuffed animal or a blanket to which he or she is particularly attached. A member of the staff should continue to comfort and reassure the child and to explain each step as the anesthesia team proceeds.

Box 15-2

Differences in Local Anesthetic Pharmacokinetics, Pharmacodynamics, and Toxicity in Children Compared to Adults

Larger volume of distribution

Prolonged elimination half-life

Decreased protein binding

Decreased hepatic metabolism

Decreased toxic plasma concentration

LOCAL ANESTHETICS: PHARMACOKINETCS, PHARMACODYNAMICS, AND TOXICITY

There are several differences in local anesthetic pharmacokinetics and pharmacodynamics in infants and older children (Box 15-2). Larger volumes of distribution in the pediatric population often result in prolonged elimination half-lives.[6] Decreased protein binding, decreased hepatic metabolism, and perhaps, increased sensitivity of sensory nerves due to immature myelination, result in prolonged duration of action, especially in early infancy. Although there is no strong evidence that immaturity of nerve fibers in early infancy increases the sensitivity of sensory fibers to local anesthetics, investigators have reported that the duration of caudal epidural blockade was longer in infants and toddlers than in older children.[7]

Ester Local Anesthetics

Ester local anesthetics are metabolized in the bloodstream by plasma cholinesterase. Plasma cholinesterase activity is decreased in infants during the first 6 months of life resulting in prolonged plasma half-lives of the ester local anesthetics.[8] Despite low cholinesterase activity, chloroprocaine and prilocaine have both been safely used in caudal epidural anesthesia in young children. However, this is of little practical significance. Prilocaine, 2-chloroprocaine, and tetracaine are the three most commonly used ester local anesthetics and of these, only tetracaine is being used with any frequency for spinal anesthesia in infants. On a milligram per kilogram basis these young patients require more tetracaine than their adult counterparts.

Amide Local Anesthetics

The amide local anesthetics lidocaine, bupivacaine, and ropivacaine are much more commonly used than ester local anesthetics for pediatric neuraxial anesthesia. The metabolism of amide local anesthetics depends primarily on the volume of distribution, degree of protein binding, and hepatic metabolism. There are decreased amounts of circulating plasma proteins in the neonate. In particular, the amount of alpha$_1$-acid glycoprotein and albumin are significantly reduced. This results in higher free fractions of bupivacaine and lidocaine in children compared to those found in adults.[9–11]

Amide local anesthetics are metabolized by the microsomal enzyme systems in the liver. Hepatic enzyme systems are immature in early infancy, especially the systems responsible for the metabolism of amide local anesthetics. Mepivacaine, for example, is excreted in the urine virtually unchanged in the neonatal period. The larger volume of distribution in infants and children results in prolonged elimination half-lives of the amide local anesthetics.

Peak plasma levels of local anesthetics occur earlier than in adults[6,11–13] For example, after epidural anesthesia, peak local anesthetic levels occurred after approximately 15 min in children compared to 30 min in adults. Peak plasma levels occur even earlier following intercostal blockade.

These factors predispose the neonate and young infant to local anesthetic toxicity. Moreover, it has been shown that infants manifest signs of cardiovascular depression at serum lidocaine levels that are approximately one-half that of adults.[14] Fortunately, toxicity from single-shot injection of local anesthetics rarely occurs unless the drug is inadvertently administered intravascularly.

▶ Local Anesthetic Toxicity

Two organ systems are affected by local anesthetic toxicity: the central nervous system (CNS) and the cardiovascular system (see Chap. 6). Early CNS toxicity may be manifested by circumoral tingling, lightheadedness, or dizziness. This may be followed by tinnitus and grand mal seizures. Seizures are often short-lived. When serum levels of local anesthetic continue to rise, patients may become comatose and apneic. Long-term sequelae from CNS complications often arise from cerebral anoxia. The seizure threshold can be raised by administering small doses of a benzodiazepam such as midazolam (0.05–0.1 mg/kg IV), diazepam (0.1–0.3 mg/kg IV), or a sedative hypnotic such as thiopental (2–4 mg/kg IV). Hypoventilation should be corrected.

Cardiovascular toxicity initially manifests with hypotension, followed by peripheral vasodilatation and severe myocardial depression. Profound bradycardia may ensue along with ventricular fibrillation that is often refractory to defibrillation. Initial treatment is directed toward maintaining cardiac output by increasing preload, followed by direct peripheral α-adrenergic agents such as phenylephrine. Advanced life support protocols should be instituted in the event of ventricular fibrillation, except that lidocaine should not be used during the resuscitation. Phenytoin sodium

Table 15-1

Local Anesthetic Dosing Guidelines in Children

Local Anesthetic	Maximum Dose (mg/kg)	Duration of action (h)
Lidocaine	7	1.5–2
Bupivacaine	3	3–6
Ropivacaine	3	3–6
Levobupivacaine	3	3–6

(7–10 mg/kg in divided doses) has been reported in the treatment of bupivacaine-induced cardiac dysrhythmias in two newborns after conventional therapy failed.[15]

Local anesthetic toxicity can be prevented by strict adherence to recommended maximum dose guidelines (Table 15-1). As a general rule, the lowest concentration of local anesthetic should be used to: (1) minimize potential for toxicity; (2) minimize the incidence of motor blockade; and (3) maximize the total volume of drug which may be administered. Epinephrine may be added to local anesthetic solutions to: (1) maximize the duration of action of the block; (2) act as a marker for accidental intravascular injection; and (3) decrease surgical blood loss by providing local vasoconstriction. Injections should be given slowly and incrementally at all times, especially in those sites which result in high serum levels, such as intercostal and caudal blocks. Frequent aspiration will help to detect possible inadvertent injection of local anesthetics.

Intravascular Test Dose

Many regional blocks are performed in children while they are under general anesthesia. While nerve stimulators are useful in identifying peripheral nerves, the accidental intravascular injection of local anesthetics during caudal, lumbar, or thoracic epidural anesthesia in an anesthetized child may be difficult to detect. The keys to preventing this complication are frequent aspiration, administration of small aliquots at a time, and the addition of a marker such as epinephrine to the local anesthetic solution. The standard epinephrine dilution for epidural anesthesia is 1:200,000 (5 μg/mL).

Epinephrine is a reliable marker for accidental intravascular injection in adults. The recommended criterion for heart rate increase in adults is 20 bpm. Investigators, however, have demonstrated that this criterion is not always reliable in detecting intravascular injections during halothane anesthesia.[16] Reliability was increased by pretreatment with intravenous atropine 10 μg/kg. An increase in the heart rate of greater than 10 bpm was observed in nearly all, but not all

> **Box 15-3**
>
> ### Intravascular Epinephrine Test Dose in Children
>
> Epinephrine (0.5–0.75 µg/kg)
>
> Reliability increased with atropine pretreatment (10 µg/kg)
>
> Positive intravenous test dose
>
> Increase in heart rate of 10 bpm
>
> Alteration in T-wave amplitude > 25%

of the study patients who received atropine. Sensitivity of the test was improved in patients pretreated with atropine compared to those who were not. During isoflurane anesthesia and after pretreatment with atropine, a heart rate increase greater than or equal to 20 bpm had a sensitivity of approximately 50% for intravascular epinephrine injection.[17] However, a heart rate increase greater than or equal to 10 bpm had 90% sensitivity after epinephrine 0.5 µg/kg and 100% sensitivity after epinephrine 0.75 µg/kg.[17] Similar results were obtained during sevoflurane anesthesia in children,[18] suggesting that an intravascular test dose of epinephrine (0.5–0.75 µg/kg) should follow atropine pretreatment and 10 bpm increase in heart rate should be used as a cut-off value (Box 15-3).

Isoproterenol has been found to reliably precipitate heart rate changes after intravascular injections.[19] However, uncertainty regarding potential neurotoxicity has prevented its use as a marker of intravascular injection.

Several groups of investigators have reported that T-wave amplitude changes of greater than 25% were associated with intravascular injections of epinephrine.[19–21] In conclusion, heart rate changes induced with an epinephrine test dose containing epinephrine 0.5–0.75 µg/kg is a highly reliable, but not 100% sensitive marker, for intravascular injection. However, the sensitivity can be increased by also measuring changes in blood pressure and T-wave amplitude.

SPINAL ANESTHESIA

Spinal anesthesia has been used in children since the early twentieth century, although it was seldom used in general practice during the early and midtwentieth century. Spinal anesthesia gained popularity following the report by Abajian et al. in 1984 of spinal anesthesia in high-risk infants.[22] The authors suggested that postoperative apnea was less likely in former preterm infants who received spinal compared to general anesthesia. Subsequent reports confirmed the safety and efficacy of spinal anesthesia in this population.[23,24] The overwhelming majority of children who receive spinal

anesthesia today are former preterm infants or young term infants. Lower abdominal, peri-inguinal, urologic, and lower extremity procedures of appropriate duration may be performed under spinal anesthesia.

▶ Postoperative Apnea

Apnea may occur following general anesthesia in former preterm infants.[25] There are a number of small studies in the literature examining postoperative apnea in preterm infants. There is disagreement as to the incidence of apnea and the conceptual age at which a former preterm infant may safely undergo general anesthesia on an outpatient basis. This is probably due to the small number of patients in each study, variations in methodology used to detect apnea, and lack of uniformity in anesthetic techniques.

Coté et al. performed a meta-analysis of eight studies comprising 255 patients investigating postoperative apnea in former preterm infants after general anesthesia.[25] Overall, the risk of apnea was independently related to both gestational age and conceptual age. Additional risk factors for postoperative apnea were hematocrit less than 30% and continued apneic episodes at home. The authors stratified patients into two risk groups: a 5% risk group and a 1% risk group. The risk of postoperative apnea did not fall below 5% with 95% statistical confidence until patients reached a postconceptual age of 48 weeks with a gestational age of 35 weeks. The risk of apnea did not fall below 1% with 95% statistical confidence until infants reached 54 weeks conceptual age with a gestational age of 35 weeks or postconceptual age of 56 weeks with a gestational age of 32 weeks (Table 15-2).

Because of the significant risk of apnea in former preterm infants, heightened monitoring is indicated after anesthesia in these patients. The most conservative recommendations are from Kurth et al.[26] They recommend former preterm infants be at least 60 weeks conceptual age and demonstrate 12 apnea-free hours postoperatively as criteria for early discharge.

Table 15-2

Risk of Apnea: Conceptual and Gestational Age*

Risk of Apnea (%)[†]	Gestational Age (week)	Postconceptual Age (week)
<1	>32	>56
<1	>35	>54
<5	>35	>48

*Nonanemic patients.
[†]Upper limit of 95% confidence interval.
Data from Ref. 25.

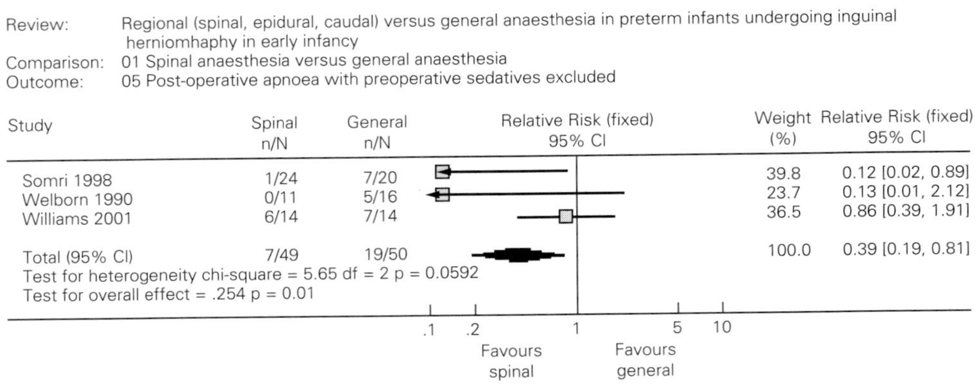

Review: Regional (spinal, epidural, caudal) versus general anaesthesia in preterm infants undergoing inguinal herniomhaphy in early infancy
Comparison: 01 Spinal anaesthesia versus general anaesthesia
Outcome: 05 Post-operative apnoea with preoperative sedatives excluded

Study	Spinal n/N	General n/N	Relative Risk (fixed) 95% CI	Weight (%)	Relative Risk (fixed) 95% CI
Somri 1998	1/24	7/20		39.8	0.12 [0.02, 0.89]
Welborn 1990	0/11	5/16		23.7	0.13 [0.01, 2.12]
Williams 2001	6/14	7/14		36.5	0.86 [0.39, 1.91]
Total (95% CI)	7/49	19/50		100.0	0.39 [0.19, 0.81]

Test for heterogeneity chi-square = 5.65 df = 2 p = 0.0592
Test for overall effect = .254 p = 0.01

.1 .2   1   5   10
Favours spinal   Favours general

FIGURE 15-1. Systematic review of spinal (without sedation) vs. general anesthesia for risk of postoperative apnea in formerly preterm infants. *Used with permission from Craven PD, Badawi N, Henderson-Smart DJ, et al. Regional (spinal, epidural, caudal) versus general anaesthesia in preterm infants undergoing inguinal herniorrhaphy in early infancy. Cochrane Database Syst Rev CD003669, 2003.*

The incidence of postoperative apnea following general anesthesia can be significantly reduced by the administration of intravenous caffeine 10 mg/kg after the induction of anesthesia.[27] Caffeine is a methylxanthine derivative similar to theophylline but it has a much wider therapeutic and safety window. Caffeine may be administered as a single bolus injection without concerns over CNS or cardiovascular side effects.

Several small studies and anecdotal experience suggest that the incidence of postoperative apnea may also be significantly decreased, but not eliminated, with the use of spinal or other regional anesthesia techniques in at-risk infants (Fig. 15-1).[24] It should be noted that the concomitant use of ketamine and spinal anesthesia in these patients may actually increase the incidence of postoperative apnea beyond that found in patients who undergo general inhalation anesthesia.[5] Very little information is available regarding other potential advantages of spinal anesthesia over general anesthesia in this population. A small randomized study of former preterm infants who received spinal anesthesia showed a decrease in the incidence of postoperative desaturation and bradycardia compared with those who received general anesthesia for inguinal herniorrhaphy.[28] An observational study of over 250 former preterm infants found a 4.9% incidence of postoperative apnea after spinal anesthesia for inguinal herniorrhaphy.[29] The mean gestational age in the infants with postoperative apnea was 28 weeks, with a mean conceptual age of 42.9 weeks. Eight infants exhibited self-limited episodes of postoperative bradycardia. A prospective study from France reported no incidences of postoperative apnea in a subset of 30 former preterm infants who received spinal anesthesia.[30]

▶ Spinal Cord Anatomy

There are anatomic differences in neonates and infants compared to adults which are important to the technique of

spinal anesthesia in children. The spinal cord in neonates and infants terminates at a much lower level than in adults (Fig. 15-2). The conus medullaris may extend as low as the L3 vertebral body and does not terminate at the average

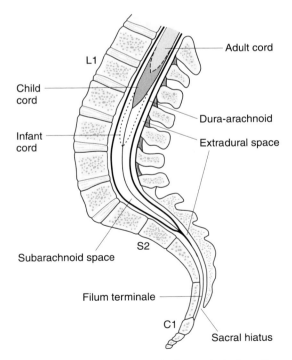

FIGURE 15-2. Sagittal view of the lumbar vertebral column. The end of the spinal cord is at the L3 level in an infant. *Used with permission from Kleinman W, Mikhail M. Spinal, epidural, and caudal blocks. In: Morgan GE, Mikhail MS, Murray M, eds, Clinical Anesthesiology, 4th ed. New York: McGraw-Hill, 2006, p. 289.*

adult level of L1 until the end of the first year of life. In order to avoid injury to the spinal cord, subarachnoid blockade should be performed at the L4-L5 or L5-S1 interspace in neonates and young infants.

In adults, it is common to perform spinal anesthesia at the interspace immediately above a line drawn between the two superior aspects of the iliac crests (intercristal or Tuffier's line, see Chap. 1). This usually represents the L3-L4 interspace. The pelvis is proportionately smaller in neonates than in adults and the sacrum is located higher relative to the iliac crests. Therefore, the intercristal line crosses the midline at the L5-S1 interspace in neonates and this traditional landmark may safely be used in these patients.[31] Similar to the conus medullaris, the dural sac terminates at a lower level in newborns; approximately at the S3 level. The terminal sac rises to the adult level of S1-S2 by the end of infancy, along with the spinal cord.

Compared to their adult counterparts, infants and young children have much more cerebrospinal fluid (CSF) on a milligram per kilogram basis. This finding may account for the larger doses of local anesthetic, on a milligram per kilogram basis, that are required for spinal anesthesia in infants and children.

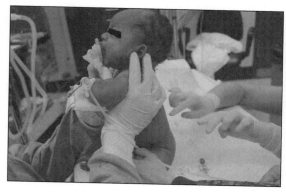

FIGURE 15-3. The sitting position for spinal anesthesia in a neonate or infant. Note that the head is maintained in the neutral position by an assistant to prevent airway obstruction.

▶ Technique for Performing Spinal Anesthesia in Infants

Preparation

Similar to all regional anesthetic techniques, successful spinal anesthesia in infants depends on thorough preparation (Box 15-4). The operating room should be warm prior to bringing the patient into the room. If necessary, warm blankets and radiant heating lamps should be available to prevent hypothermia while the block is being performed. Standard monitors (electrocardiogram, pulse oximeter, blood pressure cuff) should be placed prior to positioning the infant in either the lateral decubitus or sitting position. Special care should be taken to insure that the infant's airway is not obstructed as may occur with flexion of the neck.[32] The decision whether to initiate spinal anesthesia in the lateral or sitting position is based on the baricity of the anesthetic solution and desired distribution of the spinal anesthetic solution, as well as the personal preference of the anesthesiologist. If the sitting position is chosen, the infant's head should be supported in a manner that will maintain a patent airway by an assistant (Fig. 15-3). Neck flexion is not necessary in order to perform spinal anesthesia.

Fluid loading prior to the spinal anesthetic is not necessary. It is exceedingly rare to observe hypotension or bradycardia. Hemodynamic stability during spinal anesthesia is well documented in these patients.[33] The authors believe that intravenous access should be obtained prior to initiating spinal anesthesia. However, some practitioners advocate obtaining venous access in a lower extremity after the spinal anesthetic has been administered.

Technique

The L4-L5 or L5-S1 interspace should be identified and the area prepared in a sterile fashion and draped accordingly. Local anesthesia or EMLA cream (eutectic mixture of local anesthetic cream) may be administered at the skin puncture site. A short 22- or 25-gauge styleted spinal needle (2.5 cm for neonates and infants, 6.4–7.6 cm for older children) is used for the procedure. A midline approach is recommended over the paramedian approach, as the subarachnoid space is shallow and easily approached from the midline.

Box 15-4

Spinal Anesthesia in Infants

Prevent hypothermia

    Warm OR prior to induction

    Radiant heat lamps

    Warm blankets

Place monitors prior to initiating spinal block

Sitting or lateral position

Beware of airway obstruction (especially when sitting position is used)

Fluid loading not necessary

Avoid head-down position after the block initiation

Often very little resistance is encountered when entering the ligamentum flavum and no distinct "pop" is felt with dural puncture. Once CSF is seen exiting the needle, the local anesthetic is injected slowly, over a period of approximately 1 min, into the subarachnoid space. It should be noted that the total volume of drug to be given may be very small, depending on the weight of the baby.

The level of sensory blockade is assessed by observing the infant's response to pinprick or by using a cold stimulus (e.g., an alcohol swab), as well as by observing the rate and pattern of ventilation. A rapidly ascending level of blockade after injection of a hyperbaric solution may be curbed by placing the patient in a slight reverse Trendelenburg position. It is crucial that the baby's head not be lowered below the torso to prevent cephalad spread of the local anesthetic leading to total spinal anesthesia.

Drugs

A variety of local anesthetic agents and doses have been used to provide spinal anesthesia in infants, including lidocaine, tetracaine, and bupivacaine (Table 15-3). Tetracaine has been used most commonly in doses varying from 0.5 to 1 mg/kg in a hyperbaric solution. Most pediatric practitioners use doses in this range although there are no data to support this. At the high end of the dose range, sensory blockade to T2 to T4 is commonly achieved with little or no ventilatory or cardiovascular compromise. Bupivacaine has been used in a similar dose range as both plain and glucose-containing solutions. There may be a slightly higher success rate in non-infant children with hyperbaric solutions. Hyperbaric lidocaine 2–3 mg/kg with 1:200,000 epinephrine may be employed for very short procedures.

The duration of surgical anesthesia in infants following a single spinal injection of tetracaine or bupivacaine averages 60–90 min. Anesthesia rarely exceeds 120 min. Recovery of motor function is significantly faster in infants compared to adults. When taking into account the relatively large doses of local anesthetic that are required, this is a short duration of action. Several factors may explain this phenomenon. There

is a relatively larger CSF volume on a milligram per kilogram basis, with infants averaging 4 mL/kg and adults approximately 2 mL/kg. Additionally, the diameter and surface areas of the spinal cord and nerve roots, as well as the rate of CSF absorption, are different, and this may contribute to a relatively shorter duration of spinal anesthesia.

Little information is available in the literature regarding the use of spinal anesthesia in children. Scattered reports in this age group have used lower local anesthetic doses than those recommended in infants.[33,34] Lidocaine 1 mg/kg has been successfully used in young children 3–10 years of age.[33] Likewise, tetracaine 0.3–0.4 mg/kg has been successfully employed in children 12 weeks to 2 years of age and 0.2–0.3 mg/kg in older children.[35]

▶ Ventilatory and Cardiovascular Effects of Spinal Anesthesia

Relatively larger doses of local anesthetic are required in infants in order to reliably achieve a satisfactory level of neuraxial blockade. With the doses previously cited, it is not unusual to achieve a level of sensory and motor blockade as high as T2 to T4. Infants tend to maintain their tidal volumes without an increase in respiratory rate in spite of high levels of spinal blockade.[36] Young infants, in particular, are pure diaphragmatic breathers and perhaps this is the reason why these patients manifest little clinical compromise despite high levels of blockade. One should, however, always be vigilant for changes in ventilation in these patients and be prepared to intervene immediately should there be any ventilatory compromise.

Hypotension and bradycardia are exceedingly rare complications in neonates, infants, and young children. Dohi et al. found no hypotension in children less than 5 years of age receiving spinal anesthesia without prior fluid loading.[33] Frumiento et al. reported four episodes of bradycardia associated with high spinal blocks in a series of 247 high-risk infants with only 2 patients requiring vagolytic therapy.[29] Oberlander et al. reported that former preterm infants exhibit remarkably little change in their overall autonomic response to spinal anesthesia.[37] After high spinal anesthesia infants respond by reflexly withdrawing vagal parasympathetic tone to the heart, thereby minimizing changes in heart rate and, presumably, blood pressure. Infants also have parasympathetic dominance due to immaturity of the still-developing sympathetic nervous system. Therefore, high sympathetic blockade may have less vasodilatory and cardiovascular effects in infants.

▶ Complications

Failure rates of approximately 5% have been reported in the hands of experienced practitioners.[29,35] Reasons for failed

Table 15-3

Local Anesthetic Solutions for Spinal Anesthesia in Infants

5% lidocaine in dextrose	1–3 mg/kg
1% tetracaine in dextrose	0.5–1 mg/kg
0.75% bupivacaine in dextrose	0.5–1 mg/kg
0.5% bupivacaine (isobaric)	0.5–1 mg/kg
0.5% ropivacaine (isobaric)	0.5 mg/kg

spinal anesthesia include practitioner inexperience, anatomic variations, infant movement, or poor positioning. In the event of failed or incomplete spinal anesthesia, the options are to attempt another spinal anesthetic, supplement the anesthetic with intravenous drugs, attempt the procedure under local anesthesia, or convert to general anesthesia. Special attention should be paid to the infant's airway when supplementing spinal anesthesia with anything other than local anesthesia. Repeating the spinal block may result in a very high or total spinal blockade. Supplementation of spinal blockade with intravenous agents may predispose at-risk former preterm infants to intraoperative and postoperative apnea. Another option is to initiate caudal blockade after failed spinal anesthesia. This usually provides adequate analgesia/anesthesia for the duration of operative procedure without the risks of sedation or general anesthesia.

The incidence of PDPH after spinal anesthesia is unknown in infants and preverbal children, and unclear in older children, though the overall incidence appears to be quite low. Pediatricians have employed large-gauge beveled spinal needles for diagnostic lumbar punctures for many years with a seemingly low incidence of headache. A prospective study in pediatric oncology patients using a 20-gauge beveled spinal needle reported headache to be a rare complication in children under 13 years of age compared to older children.[38] A prospective French study reported no headache in a series of 506 spinal anesthetics performed in all pediatric age groups.[30] Others, however, have reported a low incidence of PDPH after dural puncture in children. Slater reported a 2% incidence of PDPH in patients 2–17 years of age employing either 20- or 22-gauge spinal needles.[39] Kokki et al. reported a 4% incidence of PDPH in children with the use of 25- or 27-gauge cutting or pencil-point needles.[40] None of the patients required an epidural blood patch. It is unclear why the incidence of PDPH in children is low. One theory is that the low CSF pressure in children diminishes CSF leakage and this may protect the patient from developing a PDPH.

The overall incidence of backache following spinal anesthesia in children has not been well investigated. One study reported a 5% incidence of backache and a 1.5% incidence of transient neurologic syndrome.[40] Infection at the puncture site is a rare complication. The potential risk of introducing a small "plug" of epidermoid tissue into the spinal canal, resulting in epidermoid tumors, is a theoretical complication involving the use of nonstyleted needles.[41] While it is difficult to prove cause and effect, it may be prudent to avoid using non-styleted spinal needles.

Several factors may contribute to total spinal anesthesia in infants. First, the dose of local anesthetic required in a neonate on a milligram per kilogram basis is much higher relative to an adult. Individual neonatal variation using the standard doses may cause total or very high spinal blockade in some patients. Rapid injection of the local anesthetic may

also be a contributing factor. Should the block be initiated in the lateral decubitus position, care should be taken to insure that the operating room table is indeed horizontal to the floor. Slight degrees of Trendelenburg position (head-down position) may lead to total spinal blockade. Total spinal blockade may occur when the lower extremities are raised in order to place an electrocautery pad on the infant's back. Once the local anesthetic has been administered, care should be taken to keep the infant in the supine position. The pad can be placed immediately after the spinal has been administered or, if necessary, the entire baby should be lifted in a flat supine manner in order to expose the back.

Total or high spinal blockade is remarkably well tolerated without hemodynamic compromise. Neonates rarely exhibit hypotension or bradycardia (see "Ventilatory and Cardiovascular Effects of Spinal Anesthesia" above).[22,23,33] Hypotension and bradycardia after total spinal anesthesia in infants, however, have been reported and may require pharmacologic intervention.[42] Apnea will universally occur with total spinal blockade, but ventilatory support may not be required in neonates with a high spinal blockade. Vigilance is of the essence as these patients are uncommunicative and have marginal ventilatory reserve.

EPIDURAL ANESTHESIA

Several epidural anesthetic techniques are used in children. Lumbar and thoracic epidural anesthesia may be administered as in the adult population with virtually identical indications and contraindications. One significant difference in the pediatric population is the common use of the caudal epidural route in either a "single-shot" fashion or via an indwelling catheter. As in spinal anesthesia, hypotension and bradycardia are rarely observed in infants and children during epidural anesthesia and intravascular fluid loading is generally not necessary.

▶ Single-Shot Caudal Epidural Anesthesia

Indications and Advantages

Caudal epidural anesthesia in children was first reported by Campbell in 1933. In the last two to three decades, caudal epidural anesthesia has become a routine part of anesthetic plans, particularly for infants and young children undergoing procedures below the lower abdomen. Caudal blockade is the most frequently performed regional procedure in children today. Many common procedures such as inguinal herniorrhaphy, orchidopexy, circumcision, hypospadias repair, and distal orthopedic procedures are amenable to caudal analgesia. In addition, upper abdominal, flank, and even thoracic procedures may be amenable to caudal anesthesia in select patients in specific circumstances.

Caudal epidural analgesia is popular for infants and children because: (1) landmarks are easily identifiable; (2) the procedure is technically easy to master; (3) there is a low incidence of complications; (4) acceptance rate by parents is high, probably due to the common use of epidural analgesia for labor and delivery; (5) the technique is versatile and abdominal and thoracic sensory blockade can be achieved in infants; and (6) the block is generally associated with hemodynamic stability.

Most caudal blocks are performed in conjunction with light general anesthesia. The block allows a lighter plane of anesthesia resulting in more rapid emergence and discharge. The use of low concentrations of local anesthetics permits early ambulation while maintaining satisfactory postoperative analgesia. Opioid requirements and the incidence of postoperative vomiting are significantly reduced with the use of caudal blockade. Single-shot or continuous caudal epidural anesthesia may also be used as the sole anesthetic in former preterm and high-risk infants undergoing peri-inguinal procedures.

Anatomic Considerations

The anatomy of the sacrum is significantly different in infants and in young children compared to adults. The sacral plate is a triangularly shaped bone located between the coccyx and the lumbar vertebrae. The plate is formed by fusion of the five sacral vertebrae; however, ossification is usually incomplete until the child reaches 8 years of age. The caudal epidural space can be accessed through the sacral hiatus (Fig. 1-2). The sacral hiatus forms due to the failure of fusion of the fifth sacral vertebral arch and is covered by the sacrococcygeal membrane. The important landmarks are the sacral cornua. The absence of a sacral fat pad in young pediatric patients makes these landmarks easy to identify. Many techniques have been advocated to locate the sacral cornua. The authors find it easiest to initially identify the coccyx and continue to palpate in the midline in a cephalad fashion. The first two bony prominences that are palpated on either side of the midline approximately 1 cm apart are the sacral cornua. There are a myriad number of variations of sacral anatomy that are described in standard anesthesia textbooks.

The sacral nerves, vessels, and lymphatics are located within the sacral triangle. The sacral hiatus in infants is located more cephalad compared to adults and the dura may end more caudad, increasing the risk of inadvertent dural puncture in this age group. The epidural fat is less densely packed and offers less resistance to drug administration than in adults. This facilitates more cephalad spread of drugs, as well as the more distal placement of catheters cephalad to the caudal epidural space.

Technique

The patient is placed in the prone or lateral decubitus position (Fig. 15-4). A roll should be placed under the hips in the prone position or the knees drawn up to the chest when the lateral decubitus position is used. The patient's back or abdomen may face the practitioner depending on his or her preference. Following sterile preparation, the sacral cornua are identified as described. The index of the second and third fingers of the practitioner's nondominant hand may be used to palpate the two cornua. One may elect to wear sterile gloves or to palpate the two cornua through an alcohol swab to maintain sterility.

A variety of needles are available for single-shot caudal blockade. The authors prefer a short B-bevel caudal needle with a stylet (22-gauge, 3.8 cm) to allow better tactile feedback when the sacrococcygeal membrane is punctured, and to decrease the likelihood of inadvertent dural or vascular puncture, or intraosseous placement of the needle tip. As in spinal anesthesia, a styleted needle is preferred to avoid the possibility of introducing epidermoid tissue into the caudal epidural space. The needle should be inserted in the midline at an angle of 45–60 degrees to the plane of the skin. The ulnar aspect of the hand should be placed on the patient's back for better control and stability. Once the skin is punctured, the needle is advanced until a distinctive "pop" is palpated when the sacrococcygeal membrane is punctured. The angle of the needle is decreased to 20–30 degrees and the needle is advanced 2–4 mm into the caudal canal. Advancing the needle farther increases the possibility of an inadvertent dural puncture.

Aspiration of the needle should reveal the absence of blood or CSF. A test dose of 0.1 mL/kg of a local anesthetic solution containing 1:200,000 epinephrine should be used

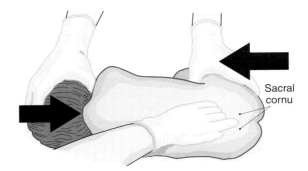

FIGURE 15-4. Positioning an infant or young child for caudal anesthesia. *Used with permission from Kleinman W, Mikhail M. Spinal, epidural, and caudal blocks. In: Morgan GE, Mikhail MS, Murray M, eds, Clinical Anesthesiology, 4th ed. New York: McGraw-Hill, 2006, p. 289.*

as a test dose as discussed early in this chapter. This dose of epinephrine is quite sensitive in producing an increase in heart rate even while the patient is under general anesthesia. Following the test dose, the remaining dose of local anesthetic should be administered in small increments with aspiration of the syringe between each increment. The total dose is usually divided into four to six increments. There should be little resistance with injection. Subcutaneous injection should be suspected when there is resistance to injection, crepitance over the sacral plate, or fullness over the skin just cephalad to the injection site. A technique using a nerve stimulator has been described which may offer a better indication of placement in the caudal space.[43]

The choice of whether to perform a single-shot caudal or to insert a caudal catheter depends on several factors. The first is the need for prolonged postoperative analgesia. Another factor to consider is the length of the procedure. For the overwhelming majority of pediatric surgical cases in ambulatory surgical patients, a single-shot caudal will provide sufficient analgesia. For surgical procedures lasting longer than 2 h, however, some consideration should be given to adapting the anesthetic to maximize the duration of postoperative analgesia. The following options may be considered.

1. A caudal catheter may be inserted.

2. A single-shot caudal blockade may be performed prior to the procedure and the block repeated prior to emergence. The disadvantage of this option is that the second block may not be effective. There is a low, but not insignificant, failure rate of 4–11% associated with single-shot caudal blocks.[44,45] Failures occur more often in children over 7 years of age, most likely due to differences in anatomy at this age.

3. An adjuvant drug may be added to the local anesthetic, in addition to epinephrine, to prolong the duration of blockade. Many drugs have been studied; however, fentanyl and clonidine are the most popular additives (see "Adjuvants," later).

4. High-risk infants undergoing long procedures may be managed using a combined spinal-caudal anesthesia technique. Spinal anesthesia is induced, followed by insertion of a caudal epidural catheter without general anesthesia.

Drug Choices and Dose

Drugs and doses used for caudal anesthesia in infants and children are summarized in Box 15-5. Bupivacaine and ropivacaine are the two most commonly used local anesthetics in children. Lidocaine is not commonly used

---

Box 15-5

Caudal Anesthetic Drugs in Infants and Children

Outpatient procedures

  0.125% bupivacaine with epinephrine 1:200,000

  0.2 % ropivacaine with epinephrine 1:200,000

  1 mL/kg provides approximately T10 level

  Larger volumes may provide higher levels in infants and young children

  Clonidine or fentanyl (1–2 μg/kg) may prolong the duration of the block

---

because of its short duration of action. Ropivacaine causes less motor blockade than bupivacaine and its therapeutic index is higher (see Chap. 3).[46,47] It is, however, also considerably more expensive than bupivacaine. Most studies comparing ropivacaine to bupivacaine for single-shot caudal blockade report similar clinical profiles. The authors prefer to use bupivacaine in their practice. They have had nearly two decades of experience with bupivacaine with very few adverse events, and none have been life threatening. There have been some recent studies using levobupivacaine, the S(-)-enantiomer of racemic bupivacaine.[67] It appears to be a viable alternative to bupivacaine; however, this drug is no longer available in the United States.

Local anesthetic concentration and volume are important factors in determining the density and sensory level of blockade. In general, the lowest concentration of local anesthetic required to achieve the desired effect should be used. Most pediatric patients receive regional anesthesia in conjunction with a light general anesthetic. The main purpose of regional anesthesia in most children is to provide intraoperative and postoperative analgesia. Total drug dose is important in avoiding local anesthetic toxicity. The use of high concentrations of local anesthetics produces more motor blockade and limits the volume of local anesthetic which may be administered. For these reasons, the authors generally avoid using high concentrations of local anesthetics such as 0.5% bupivacaine or 0.5% ropivacaine.

A second consideration is recovery of motor function in ambulatory surgical patients. Using concentrations higher than 0.2% bupivacaine or 0.2% ropivacaine may cause an unacceptably high incidence of motor blockade. For children undergoing minor outpatient surgical procedures, a single-shot caudal epidural is commonly performed.

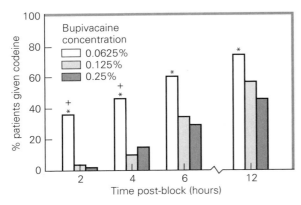

FIGURE 15-5. Percent infants and children requiring supplemental oral codeine analgesia after single-shot caudal block analgesia with bupivacaine 0.0625, 0.125, and 0.25%. *$P < 0.05$ for 0.0625% vs. 0.25%, +$P < 0.05$ for 0.0625% vs. 0.125%. There was no difference between 0.125 and 0.25% at any time. *Used with permission from Wolf AR, Valley RD, Fear DW, et al. Bupivacaine for caudal analgesia in infants and children: The optimal effective concentration. Anesthesiology 69:102, 1988.*

Caudal bupivacaine 0.125% was as effective as 0.25% for postoperative analgesia (Fig. 15-5).[48] In the authors' experience, 0.125% bupivacaine or 0.2% ropivacaine with 1:200,000 epinephrine provides reliable postoperative analgesia for 4–6 h without significant motor blockade.

Higher concentrations of local anesthetics may be used in patients undergoing major surgical procedures. To increase the margin of safety, some practitioners believe that the maximum allowable dosage of bupivacaine should be reduced from a dose of 3 mg/kg in adults to 2.5 mg/kg in infants.[48,49] When using bupivacaine concentrations higher than 0.25% special care should be taken to calculate the total dose of local anesthetic administered in order to insure that recommended upper dose limits are not exceeded. Although the authors advocate using lower maximum allowable doses in infants, practitioners have reported the successful use of 0.375% bupivacaine as a single-shot caudal anesthetic (3.75 mg/kg) in high-risk infants undergoing major intra-abdominal procedures.[50]

A variety of formulas have been advocated for calculating the volume of local anesthetic necessary based on the patient's age, weight, height, and desired level of sensory blockade. Regardless of which formula is used, it is prudent to use one that is simple to remember and which reliably provides the desired level of block with a minimum risk of local anesthetic toxicity. Takasaki et al. found body weight, rather than patient age, to better predict spread of local anesthetic following a caudal block.[51] The authors prefer to administer doses on a weight basis and for most procedures administer 1.0 mL/kg of a dilute solution such as 0.125% bupivacaine to a maximum volume of 30 mL.

This dose will reliably result in T10 sensory blockade and this concentration is well below maximum levels recommended in the literature. Higher doses such as 1.25 mL/kg, or even 1.5 mL/kg, may be administered should more cephalad blockade be desired, again without the risk of local anesthetic toxicity.

Adjuvants. Adjuvants may be used to prolong the duration of blockade, particularly for single-shot caudal epidural blockade.[52] Epinephrine in a concentration of 1:200,000 is the most commonly used adjuvant for caudal anesthesia. The rational for its use in epidural anesthesia is discussed in Chap. 3. Epinephrine has the added benefit of serving as a marker for inadvertent intravascular injection.

Opioids are added to caudal epidural blocks in order to improve the quality of sensory blockade and prolong duration. Morphine administered through the caudal route has been successfully used for postoperative pain management in patients undergoing open heart surgery.[53] Adverse effects of morphine administered in the caudal space include pruritus, nausea, vomiting, urinary retention, and delayed respiratory depression. Respiratory depression may be a significant problem in infants and hence we avoid caudal morphine administered either as a bolus dose or via continuous infusions in infants.[54,55] Fentanyl has been used in the epidural space in adults for a number of years. Literature is rather sparse regarding the use and efficacy of fentanyl as an additive in children undergoing single-shot caudal blockade and the data are conflicting as to whether there is benefit.[56,57] One study found an increased incidence of nausea and vomiting following fentanyl administered as of component of caudal anesthesia compared to groups without fentanyl.[57] The authors' interpretation of the literature is that no definitive conclusion can yet be reached regarding fentanyl and single-shot caudal blockade. At the authors' institution fentanyl 2 μg/kg is used as an adjunct to single-shot caudal anesthesia, although its use is usually reserved for more extensive or painful procedures or in patients who have a urinary catheter in the postoperative period.

Clonidine is an alpha$_2$ agonist which can improve the quality of single-shot caudal blockade as well as prolong its duration of action without the unwanted side effects of epidural opioids (Fig. 15-6).[57] Clonidine acts by stimulating descending noradrenergic medullospinal pathways which in turn inhibit the release of nociceptive neurotransmitters in the dorsal horn of the spinal cord (see Chap. 3). Bolus doses of 1–5 μg/kg have been recommended;[58,59] clonidine 1–2 μg/kg is commonly used. Higher doses are associated with sedation and hemodynamic instability in the form of hypotension and bradycardia,[59] although doses as low as 2 μg/kg have been associated with postoperative sedation. Epidural clonidine blunts the ventilatory response to CO_2. Although respiratory depression does not

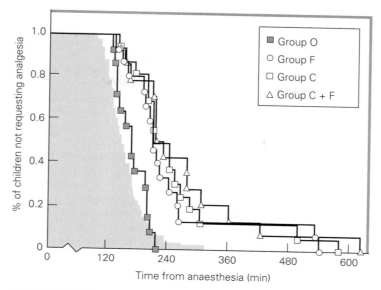

FIGURE 15-6. Addition of fentanyl and clonidine to single-shot caudal bupivacaine/ lidocaine for caudal anesthesia in children: time from injection to first request for analgesia. O = local anesthesia alone, F = local anesthetic plus fentanyl, C = local anesthetic plus clonidine, C + F = local anesthetic plus fentanyl and clonidine. The time is significantly longer in the three groups that received fentanyl, clonidine, or both compared to local anesthetic alone ($P = 0.035$). Shaded area = duration of surgical procedure. *Used with permission from Constant I, Gall O, Gouyet L, et al. Addition of clonidine or fentanyl to local anaesthetics prolongs the duration of surgical analgesia after single shot caudal block in children. Br J Anaesth 80:294, 1998.*

appear to be a common problem,[60] apnea has been reported in a term neonate who received a caudal block consisting of 0.2% ropivacaine 1 mL/kg with clonidine 2 µg/kg.[61] The authors use clonidine 1–2 µg/kg as an adjunct to single-shot caudal epidural anesthesia in children over the age of 1 year.

▶ **Continuous Caudal Epidural Anesthesia**

Continuous caudal epidural anesthesia offers the same advantages that a single-shot technique offers without limitation on the duration of the procedure. An added advantage is continuous postoperative analgesia. While the overwhelming majority of caudal epidural catheters are inserted in anesthetized infants and children, continuous caudal anesthesia may be used effectively as the sole anesthetic in awake neonates and young infants.[62]

The authors usually use caudal epidural catheters in infants or in young preschool age children, and lumbar or thoracic epidural catheters in older children. A variety of methods have been described for inserting caudal catheters. A standard Crawford needle may be placed in the caudal epidural space and a standard epidural catheter inserted through it. Others prefer using a 18- or 16-gauge intravenous catheter as an introducer and passing the epidural catheter through the intravenous catheter once it has been placed in the caudal epidural space. Regardless of the technique used, the same guidelines that apply to the placement of epidural catheters in adults should be used with caudal catheters in children. Adult epidural catheters are used in older children. In young children there may be an advantage to using styleted catheters when advancing the catheter tip to more cephalad vertebral levels.

Catheters should be advanced to the appropriate segmental level when possible. In infants it is often possible to advance catheters up to the thoracic level via the caudal route. This mode of analgesia is routinely offered to parents of infants and children undergoing abdominal and thoracic procedures at the authors' institution. Caudal epidural catheters advanced to the thoracic level have been used in neonates undergoing repair of esophageal atresia.[63] Gunter and Eng demonstrated that catheters could be passed to thoracic segments via a caudal approach in patients as old as 10 years of age.[64] In general, studies demonstrate a higher success rate of thoracic catheter placement via the caudal approach in infants compared to older children and a higher success rate with styleted epidural catheters. There are some risks to advancing catheters a long distance from the insertion site. The catheters may become kinked or knotted or pass into a dural sleeve. Indeed, coiled catheters have been reported in several series.[64]

Several methods other than pinprick or cold stimuli have been described to more precisely ascertain the vertebral level of the catheter tip. One method is to inject a small dose of contrast dye under fluoroscopy. A second is to use a plain radiograph to confirm position of a radiopaque catheter. A third technique involves using a nerve stimulator in a saline-filled catheter and stimulating the catheter to elicit a motor response. This technique is highly sensitive and specific.

▶ Complications of Caudal Anesthesia

The overall complication rate from single-shot caudal injections (Box 15-6) is difficult to quantify. Technical difficulties in identifying the anatomic landmarks may result in the local anesthetic being injected subcutaneously or intraosseously. The authors observe this routinely in their institution where 40–60 residents are trained annually. A common error is to misidentify the sacral cornua. A second common error is to puncture the skin too far caudally from the cornua. Subcutaneous injection of even small volumes of local anesthetic will obliterate the cornua making subsequent identification of the caudal epidural space difficult, if not impossible. Intraosseous injection is more likely to occur when very sharp needles are used. Injection of local anesthetics into the sacral marrow will result in systemic toxicity.[65] Sharp needles or the use of excessive force can cause injury to pelvic organs. For these reasons, the authors recommend using blunt short-bevel needles. These needles also allow for better tactile feedback.

Motor weakness is unusual when low concentrations of local anesthetics are used for single-shot injections. Concentrations higher than 0.2% bupivacaine or 0.2% ropivacaine will often result in some degree of motor blockade. Because 0.125% bupivacaine has been shown to be just as effective as 0.25% bupivacaine in providing postoperative pain relief,[48] the authors recommend limiting the bupivacaine concentration to 0.125% or less in children undergoing ambulatory surgery.

Box 15-6

Complications of Caudal Anesthesia

Subcutaneous injection

Intraosseous injection

Intravascular injection

Subarachnoid injection

Delayed micturition

Urinary retention

Back pain

Neonates and very young infants are at greater risk for local anesthetic toxicity due to a variety of reasons discussed early in this chapter. Overt seizures have been reported in children receiving continuous infusions of local anesthetics.[66,67] The current recommendation is to limit the infusion rate of bupivacaine to 0.2 mg/kg/h in neonates and young infants, and 0.4 mg/kg/h in older infants and children.[49,68] Larsson et al. measured plasma bupivacaine levels in neonates receiving continuous epidural infusions and found that in five of nine infants, plasma levels were still increasing after 48 h.[65] The authors recommended using dilute solutions of local anesthetics (less than and equal to 0.125% bupivacaine) for postoperative analgesia to avoid this potential complication.

Delayed micturition may occur, but the exact incidence is unknown. True urinary retention has been reported to occur but is an exceedingly rare complication if low concentrations of local anesthetics are used. Vomiting may occur but the incidence has been shown to be significantly less in children receiving caudal blockade compared to those receiving intravenous morphine.[69]

Unilateral blockade is rarely observed after single-shot caudal blockade, especially in infants and young children. Septation of the epidural space and density of epidural fat tissue increases with advancing age.[44] Prolonged blockade following a single-shot injection is most likely due to inadvertent use of a high concentration of local anesthetic or a dural puncture. Dural puncture may occur with sharp-tipped needles or when the needle is advanced too far in a cephalad direction, resulting in puncture of the distal end of the dura and subsequent spinal anesthesia.

Intravascular injection into epidural vessels is another possible complication. This is more likely to occur when the needle is advanced too far into the caudal canal or when sharp-tipped needles are used compared to blunt-tipped needles.[70] Blood may not always be aspirated prior to injection. Special attention is required since most blocks are performed under general anesthesia in children. Factors reported to influence the incidence of vascular puncture are operator inexperience, use of a sharp-tipped needle, and difficulty in locating the sacral hiatus.[45]

Catheter knotting or kinking may occur when long catheter lengths are passed into the epidural space, as discussed previously. There is some concern regarding catheter infection with the prolonged use of caudal catheters compared to lumbar epidural catheters due to the proximity of the sacral hiatus to the rectum. While the overall infection rate associated with caudal epidural catheters appears to be quite low, there have been isolated case reports of infections related to epidural catheters in children.[71] Kost-Byerly et al. prospectively examined bacterial colonization and infection rates after caudal catheter insertion compared with lumbar epidural catheter insertion.[72] Bacterial colonization rates were similar at both insertion sites. Children less than 3 years of age were more likely to have colonized caudal catheters compared to those older than 3 years of age (41% vs. 31%). There were no serious infections after short-term (3 days) caudal or lumbar epidural catheter placement. In contrast to these results, McNeely et al. prospectively examined the same issue and found the bacterial colonization rate to be five times higher in caudal compared to lumbar epidural catheters (20% vs. 4%).[73] However, the mean age of their patient population was younger. Again, no serious infections were identified.

Permanent neurologic injury following single-shot caudal or caudal epidural catheter placement appears to be exceedingly low. There are no large prospective studies and the retrospective studies report almost no permanent neurologic complications. In truth, the real incidence is not known. Nonetheless, extensive experience among hundreds of pediatric practitioners around the world for the last several decades seems to support the clinical impression of an extremely low neurologic complication rate.

▶ Lumbar and Thoracic Epidural Anesthesia

The first report of continuous epidural anesthesia in infants and children was by Ruston in 1954. Since that time, lumbar and thoracic epidural catheters have been used with increasing frequency both intraoperatively in conjunction with general anesthesia, and to provide postoperative analgesia following major orthopedic, abdominal, and thoracic surgical procedures in all age groups.[74–77] In the authors' practice lumbar epidural catheters are favored over caudal epidural catheters in children over 3 years of age. The standard of care regarding insertion, care, and management of lumbar and thoracic epidural catheters applies equally to children and adults.

Lumbar insertion of epidural catheters may be performed in awake, sedated, or anesthetized children. It is common practice to insert lumbar epidural catheters in young children after induction of general anesthesia. While there is some contention in the literature regarding the risk-benefit ratio of inserting thoracic epidural catheters in children under general anesthesia, this does not appear to be the case for lumbar epidural catheters.[3] Two points should be noted regarding epidural catheter insertion in children:

1. The ligamentum flavum is extremely soft and a distinctive "pop" may not be felt when penetrating this layer.

2. The distance from the skin to the epidural space may be very shallow. Several formulae for determining the skin to epidural space distance have been recommended, primarily based on the child's weight.[78–80] One study recommended a simple formula for patients between 6 months and 10 years of age: depth (mm) = weight (kg).[79] There

was poor correlation with this formula and the best fit regression line in patients under 6 months of age and over 10 years of age. Differences in technique and the angle of insertion of the epidural needle may account for significant variation in depth. Regardless of which formula is used, one should be cognizant of the wide variation in skin-epidural space distance in individual patients. The practitioner should check for loss of resistance shortly after skin puncture, especially in neonates and young infants, as the distance may be very short (less than 10 mm).

Similar to caudal epidural catheters, lumbar epidural catheters may be advanced cephalad to thoracic vertebral levels, but with significantly less success than via the caudal route in infants. Differences in the density of epidural fat in older children, as well as changes that occur in lumbosacral spine lordosis once children begin to walk, may account for the low success rate. The success rate of reaching the thoracic segments may be improved by using styleted catheters, inserting the catheter in the upper lumbar interspaces, and using a more cephalad angle when inserting the epidural needle.

Thoracic epidural catheters are being used more commonly at tertiary care centers for procedures such as thoracotomies and repair of pectus excavatum. Placement of thoracic epidural catheters in children evokes heated debate as to whether to place the catheters in awake or anesthetized children. The debate intensified following a report by Bromage and Benumof in which a 62-year-old woman suffered permanent paraplegia following placement of a thoracic epidural catheter while under general anesthesia.[81] Several aspects of this case deserve mentioning. The insertion site at T12 was immediately adjacent to a scar from a prior lumbar laminectomy. Multiple attempts were made by more than one anesthesiologist with air being injected with each pass in order to identify the epidural space. This debate was very elegantly summarized in an editorial by Krane et al.[3] In general, if the child is old enough to safely cooperate while awake, an awake placement of a thoracic epidural catheter is preferred.

Epidural catheters may be placed intraoperatively under direct vision by the surgeon to provide postoperative analgesia following spine surgery. One and two catheter techniques have been described using intermittent boluses or continuous infusions.[82] The authors have used a single catheter technique with the tip of the catheter placed at approximately T6-T7 with good success.

Several groups of investigators have reported on the use of nerve stimulation to verify epidural catheter placement.[83,84] Goobie et al. found that this technique did not provide any advantage over conventional techniques (e.g., cutaneous landmarks) for confirmation of lumbar or thoracic epidural catheter placement in 30 pediatric patients.[83]

Incidence of Complications

There are no definitive data regarding the risk-benefit ratio of placing lumbar or thoracic catheters in anesthetized children. There is a large body of experience with the safe use of lumbar epidural catheters and very few complications have been reported in the literature. A large prospective study by the French-Language Society of Pediatric Anesthesiologists summarized data from over 15,000 central blocks in children.[30] Of these, 50% were single-shot caudal blocks. Another 9.4% consisted of caudal, lumbar, and thoracic epidural catheters. The investigators concluded that the incidence of complications was very low and no patient in the study suffered permanent neurologic injury. These results are in stark contrast to a large retrospective report published in 1995 analyzing complications in over 24,000 epidural blocks in children.[85] These investigators reported three infant deaths and two other infants had paraplegia and quadriplegia. It is impossible to ascertain why there are conflicting results in these two large series. Isolated case reports of neurologic complications have also appeared in the literature.

▶ Management of Postoperative Pain Using Epidural Catheters

Fentanyl can improve the quality and prolong the duration of the blockade and may be superior to morphine when administered in the epidural space for postoperative pain relief in children.[86] The introduction of pain management services has widely expanded anesthesiologists' input into patient care outside of the operating room. This gives anesthesiologists an opportunity to carefully design a well thought-out plan for providing postoperative pain relief. The introduction of PCA, along with the use of epidural catheters in adult patients, has increased the awareness of the potential for use of epidural catheters in children. Although early reports of epidural catheters in children were published in the 1980s,[74] the widespread use of epidural analgesia as a modality of pain relief in children did not occur until the late 1990s. Postoperative epidural analgesia is appropriate for major lower extremity and spine orthopedic procedures, and open abdominal and thoracic procedures.

The authors' practice of epidural analgesia is summarized in Box 15-7. The epidural catheter is inserted close to the vertebral level of the incision. Choice of local anesthetic with additives is based on surgical procedure. The usual choice of intraoperative local anesthetic is 0.125% bupivacaine with fentanyl 2–5 µg/kg, or clonidine 1–2 µg/kg. Postoperatively, a solution of 0.1% bupivacaine is used. A basal rate of 0.2–0.4 mg/kg/h is used. If the patient has the cognitive ability to understand pain (usually school-age

---

> **Box 15-7**
>
> ### Continuous Caudal Epidural Analgesia in Children
>
> Place catheter tip as close to the incision dermatome as possible
>
> Avoid using high concentrations of local anesthetics (>0.125% bupivacaine)
>
> Infuse 0.1% bupivacaine at 0.2–0.4 mg/kg/h
>
> Use lower infusion rates in neonates and infants
>
> Consider adding fentanyl 1–2 µg/kg/h for painful procedures
>
> Consider PCEA in older children (>6 years of age)

children), patient-controlled epidural analgesia (PCEA) is used.[87] Fentanyl 1–2 µg/kg/h may be added as necessary. The catheter is left in place for approximately 72 h, although in certain instances the catheter may be left for as long as 5 days. Care should be taken to visualize the catheter insertion site. If the patient has a hip spica cast, every effort should be made to create a window at the catheter insertion site.[88]

Patients should be provided adequate systemic analgesia before the epidural infusion is discontinued. This will ensure analgesia once the effect of the local anesthetic solution resolves. Most children will experience some degree of motor blockade. Hence, they should be physically supported when walking during epidural blockade. The heels should be padded so that pressure sores do not develop. Pulse oximetry is required at the authors' institution for all children with continuous blockade.

SUMMARY

Central neuraxial anesthesia in the form of spinal and epidural anesthesia is becoming increasingly popular among pediatric anesthesiologists. The advantages of intraoperative neuraxial anesthesia include decreased use of volatile agents, earlier awakening, earlier ambulation and discharge, a lower incidence of postoperative nausea and vomiting, and lower requirements for postoperative opioids. Single-shot caudal epidural blockade remains the most popular block performed in infants and children. This is due to its technical ease, high degree of efficacy, and low complication rate.

Continuous epidural catheters have also become more widely used in recent years, primarily in conjunction with general anesthesia in the operating room, but also for postoperative pain management. A great deal of controversy exists regarding the placement of epidural catheters in anesthetized children, particularly at thoracic levels. While the incidence of serious complications appears to be quite low, serious complications have been reported, particularly in infants.

Enthusiasm for the opportunity to provide a pain-free perioperative course for children must, however, be tempered by our current lack of prospective data demonstrating an advantage of postoperative neuraxial anesthesia over systemic opioid analgesia. A recent insightful editorial explored this issue.[89] While the authors' clinical impression is that many children benefit from postoperative epidural analgesia, the paucity of prospective data makes it difficult to make concrete judgments and to provide parents with statistical information regarding its efficacy and complication rates. Patient safety should always be the first and foremost concern. Cost, the necessity for staff education, failed analgesia, parental and surgeon acceptance, and the additional time required for catheter placement in the operating room are additional factors to consider.

The authors strongly advocate the use of regional anesthesia and analgesia in their practice, realizing fully the lack of information that is currently available. Single-shot caudal epidural blockade has a long history of efficacy and a very low complication rate. The block is technically simple to perform and has proven benefits to the patient in the postoperative period. While the same cannot be said for continuous epidural analgesia via epidural catheters, the authors believe that, in experienced hands children can undergo major surgical procedures with better pain control and few complications with intraoperative and postoperative epidural analgesia. It is their hope, that with future studies and advances, children may indeed undergo surgical procedures with minimal discomfort and a very low risk of complications. Utilization of central neuraxial blockade in children, including using more sophisticated techniques for placement of epidural catheters, such as ultrasonography, may improve safety over conventional methods of analgesia and placement of epidural catheters. The decision whether to use central neuraxial blockade in any child should be decided on a case-by-case basis, based on the child's baseline health status, the planned surgical procedure, and anticipated need for postoperative analgesia. Peripheral nerve blocks may be an alternative to neuraxial blockade for some procedures, as they may offer a long duration and improved analgesia without the untoward side effects of central neuraxial blockade.

REFERENCES

1. Suresh S, Barcelona SL, Young NM, et al. Postoperative pain relief in children undergoing tympanomastoid surgery: Is a regional block better than opioids? *Anesth Analg* 94:859, 2002.
2. Hannallah RS, Broadman LM, Belman AB, et al. Comparison of caudal and ilioinguinal/iliohypogastric nerve blocks for control of post-orchiopexy pain in pediatric ambulatory surgery. *Anesthesiology* 66:832, 1987.
3. Krane EJ, Dalens BJ, Murat I, et al. The safety of epidurals placed during general anesthesia. *Reg Anesth Pain Med* 23:433, 1998.
4. Suresh S. Thoracic epidural catheter placement in children: Are we there yet? *Reg Anesth Pain Med* 29:83, 2004.
5. Welborn LG, Rice LJ, Hannallah RS, et al. Postoperative apnea in former preterm infants: Prospective comparison of spinal and general anesthesia. *Anesthesiology* 72:838, 1990.
6. Ecoffey C, Desparmet J, Berdeaux A, et al. Pharmacokinetics of lignocaine in children following caudal anaesthesia. *Br J Anaesth* 56:1399, 1984.
7. Warner MA, Kunkel SE, Offord KO, et al. The effects of age, epinephrine, and operative site on duration of caudal analgesia in pediatric patients. *Anesth Analg* 66:995, 1987.
8. Zsigmond EK, Downs JR. Plasma cholinesterase activity in newborns and infants. *Can Anaesth Soc J* 18:278, 1971.
9. Ala-Kokko TI, Partanen A, Karinen J, et al. Pharmacokinetics of 0.2% ropivacaine and 0.2% bupivacaine following caudal blocks in children. *Acta Anaesthesiol Scand* 44:1099, 2000.
10. Bricker SR, Telford RJ, Booker PD. Pharmacokinetics of bupivacaine following intraoperative intercostal nerve block in neonates and in infants aged less than 6 months. *Anesthesiology* 70:942, 1989.
11. Ecoffey C, Desparmet J, Maury M, et al. Bupivacaine in children: Pharmacokinetics following caudal anesthesia. *Anesthesiology* 63:447, 1985.
12. Eyres RL. Local anaesthetic agents in infancy. *Paediatr Anaesth* 5:213, 1995.
13. Rothstein P, Arthur GR, Feldman HS, et al. Bupivacaine for intercostal nerve blocks in children: Blood concentrations and pharmacokinetics. *Anesth Analg* 65:625, 1986.
14. Mirkin BL. Developmental pharmacology. *Annu Rev Pharmacol* 10:255, 1970.
15. Maxwell LG, Martin LD, Yaster M. Bupivacaine-induced cardiac toxicity in neonates: Successful treatment with intravenous phenytoin. *Anesthesiology* 80:682, 1994.
16. Desparmet J, Mateo J, Ecoffey C, et al. Efficacy of an epidural test dose in children anesthetized with halothane. *Anesthesiology* 72:249, 1990.
17. Sethna NF, Sullivan L, Retik A, et al. Efficacy of simulated epinephrine-containing epidural test dose after intravenous atropine during isoflurane anesthesia in children. *Reg Anesth Pain Med* 25:566, 2000.
18. Tanaka M, Nishikawa T. Simulation of an epidural test dose with intravenous epinephrine in sevoflurane-anesthetized children. *Anesth Analg* 86:952, 1998.
19. Tanaka M, Kimura T, Goyagi T, et al. Evaluating hemodynamic and T wave criteria of simulated intravascular test doses using bupivacaine or isoproterenol in anesthetized children. *Anesth Analg* 91:567, 2000.
20. Freid EB, Bailey AG, Valley RD. Electrocardiographic and hemodynamic changes associated with unintentional intravascular injection of bupivacaine with epinephrine in infants. *Anesthesiology* 79:394, 1993.
21. Fisher QA, Shaffner DH, Yaster M. Detection of intravascular injection of regional anaesthetics in children. *Can J Anaesth* 44:592, 1997.
22. Abajian JC, Mellish RW, Browne AF, et al. Spinal anesthesia for surgery in the high-risk infant. *Anesth Analg* 63:359, 1984.
23. Harnik EV, Hoy GR, Potolicchio S, et al. Spinal anesthesia in premature infants recovering from respiratory distress syndrome. *Anesthesiology* 64:95, 1986.

24. Craven PD, Badawi N, Henderson-Smart DJ, et al. Regional (spinal, epidural, caudal) versus general anaesthesia in preterm infants undergoing inguinal herniorrhaphy in early infancy. *Cochrane Database Syst Rev* CD003669, 2003.

25. Coté CJ, Zaslavsky A, Downes JJ, et al. Postoperative apnea in former preterm infants after inguinal herniorrhaphy. A combined analysis. *Anesthesiology* 82:809, 1995.

26. Kurth CD, Spitzer AR, Broennle AM, et al. Postoperative apnea in preterm infants. *Anesthesiology* 66:483, 1987.

27. Welborn LG, de Soto H, Hannallah RS, et al. The use of caffeine in the control of post-anesthetic apnea in former premature infants. *Anesthesiology* 68:796, 1988.

28. Krane EJ, Haberkern CM, Jacobson LE. Postoperative apnea, bradycardia, and oxygen desaturation in formerly premature infants: Prospective comparison of spinal and general anesthesia. *Anesth Analg* 80:7, 1995.

29. Frumiento C, Abajian JC, Vane DW. Spinal anesthesia for preterm infants undergoing inguinal hernia repair. *Arch Surg* 135:445, 2000.

30. Giaufre E, Dalens B, Gombert A. Epidemiology and morbidity of regional anesthesia in children: A one-year prospective survey of the French-Language Society of Pediatric Anesthesiologists. *Anesth Analg* 83:904, 1996.

31. Busoni P, Messeri A. Spinal anesthesia in children: Surface anatomy. *Anesth Analg* 68:418, 1989.

32. Gleason CA, Martin RJ, Anderson JV, et al. Optimal position for a spinal tap in preterm infants. *Pediatrics* 71:31, 1983.

33. Dohi S, Naito H, Takahashi T. Age-related changes in blood pressure and duration of motor block in spinal anesthesia. *Anesthesiology* 50:319, 1979.

34. Kokki H, Hendolin H. Hyperbaric bupivacaine for spinal anaesthesia in 7-18 yr old children: Comparison of bupivacaine 5 mg ml-1 in 0.9% and 8% glucose solutions. *Br J Anaesth* 84:59, 2000.

35. Blaise GA, Roy WL. Spinal anaesthesia for minor paediatric surgery. *Can Anaesth Soc J* 33:227, 1986.

36. Pascucci RC, Hershenson MB, Sethna NF, et al. Chest wall motion of infants during spinal anesthesia. *J Appl Physiol* 68:2087, 1990.

37. Oberlander TF, Berde CB, Lam KH, et al. Infants tolerate spinal anesthesia with minimal overall autonomic changes: Analysis of heart rate variability in former premature infants undergoing hernia repair. *Anesth Analg* 80:20, 1995.

38. Bolder PM. Postlumbar puncture headache in pediatric oncology patients. *Anesthesiology* 65:696, 1986.

39. Slater HM, Stephen CR. Hypobaric pontocaine spinal anesthesia in children. *Anesthesiology* 11:709, 1950.

40. Kokki H, Tuovinen K, Hendolin H. Spinal anaesthesia for paediatric day-case surgery: A double-blind, randomized, parallel group, prospective comparison of isobaric and hyperbaric bupivacaine. *Br J Anaesth* 81:502, 1998.

41. Shaywitz BA. Epidermoid spinal cord tumors and previous lumbar punctures. *J Pediatr* 80:638, 1972.

42. Wright TE, Orr RJ, Haberkern CM, et al. Complications during spinal anesthesia in infants: High spinal blockade. *Anesthesiology* 73:1290, 1990.

43. Tsui BC, Tarkkila P, Gupta S, et al. Confirmation of caudal needle placement using nerve stimulation. *Anesthesiology* 91:374, 1999.

44. Dalens B, Hasnaoui A. Caudal anesthesia in pediatric surgery: Success rate and adverse effects in 750 consecutive patients. *Anesth Analg* 68:83, 1989.

45. Veyckemans F, Van Obbergh LJ, Gouverneur JM. Lessons from 1100 pediatric caudal blocks in a teaching hospital. *Reg Anesth* 17:119, 1992.

46. Da Conceicao MJ, Coelho L, Khalil M. Ropivacaine 0.25% compared with bupivacaine 0.25% by the caudal route. *Paediatr Anaesth* 9:229, 1999.

47. Ivani G, Lampugnani E, Torre M, et al. Comparison of ropivacaine with bupivacaine for paediatric caudal block. *Br J Anaesth* 81:247, 1998.

48. Wolf AR, Valley RD, Fear DW, et al. Bupivacaine for caudal analgesia in infants and children: The optimal effective concentration. *Anesthesiology* 69:102, 1988.

49. Berde CB. Convulsions associated with pediatric regional anesthesia. *Anesth Analg* 75:164, 1992.

50. Cucchiaro G, De Lagausie P, El-Ghonemi A, et al. Single-dose caudal anesthesia for major intraabdominal operations in high-risk infants. *Anesth Analg* 92:1439, 2001.

51. Takasaki M, Dohi S, Kawabata Y, et al. Dosage of lidocaine for caudal anesthesia in infants and children. *Anesthesiology* 47:527, 1977.

52. Cook B, Grubb DJ, Aldridge LA, et al. Comparison of the effects of adrenaline, clonidine and ketamine on the duration of caudal analgesia produced by bupivacaine in children. *Br J Anaesth* 75:698, 1995.

53. Rosen KR, Rosen DA. Caudal epidural morphine for control of pain following open heart surgery in children. *Anesthesiology* 70:418, 1989.

54. Attia J, Ecoffey C, Sandouk P, et al. Epidural morphine in children: Pharmacokinetics and CO2 sensitivity. *Anesthesiology* 65:590, 1986.

55. Karl HW, Tyler DC, Krane EJ. Respiratory depression after low-dose caudal morphine. *Can J Anaesth* 43:1065, 1996.

56. Campbell FA, Yentis SM, Fear DW, et al. Analgesic efficacy and safety of a caudal bupivacaine-fentanyl mixture in children. *Can J Anaesth* 39:661, 1992.

57. Constant I, Gall O, Gouyet L, et al. Addition of clonidine or fentanyl to local anaesthetics prolongs the duration of surgical analgesia after single shot caudal block in children. *Br J Anaesth* 80:294, 1998.

58. Ivani G, Bergendahl HT, Lampugnani E, et al. Plasma levels of clonidine following epidural bolus injection in children. *Acta Anaesthesiol Scand* 42:306, 1998.

59. Ivani G, De Negri P, Conio A, et al. Ropivacaine-clonidine combination for caudal blockade in children. *Acta Anaesthesiol Scand* 44:446, 2000.

60. Penon C, Ecoffey C, Cohen SE. Ventilatory response to carbon dioxide after epidural clonidine injection. *Anesth Analg* 72:761, 1991.

61. Breschan C, Krumpholz R, Likar R, et al. Can a dose of 2microg.kg(-1) caudal clonidine cause respiratory depression in neonates? *Paediatr Anaesth* 9:81, 1999.

62. Broadman LM. Use of spinal or continuous caudal anesthesia for inguinal hernia repair in premature infants: Are there advantages? *Reg Anesth* 21(6S):108, 1996.

63. Bosenberg AT, Bland BA, Schulte-Steinberg O, et al. Thoracic epidural anesthesia via caudal route in infants. *Anesthesiology* 69:265, 1988.

64. Gunter JB, Eng C. Thoracic epidural anesthesia via the caudal approach in children. *Anesthesiology* 76:935, 1992.

65. Larsson BA, Lonnqvist PA, Olsson GL. Plasma concentrations of bupivacaine in neonates after continuous epidural infusion. *Anesth Analg* 84:501, 1997.

66. Agarwal R, Gutlove DP, Lockhart CH. Seizures occurring in pediatric patients receiving continuous infusion of bupivacaine. *Anesth Analg* 75:284, 1992.

67. Auroy Y, Narchi P, Messiah A, et al. Serious complications related to regional anesthesia: Results of a prospective survey in France. *Anesthesiology* 87:479, 1997.

68. Berde CB. Toxicity of local anesthetics in infants and children. *J Pediatr* 122:S14, 1993.

69. Jensen BH. Caudal block for post-operative pain relief in children after genital operations. A comparison between bupivacaine and morphine. *Acta Anaesthesiol Scand* 25:373, 1981.

70. McGown RG. Caudal analgesia in children. Five hundred cases for procedures below the diaphragm. *Anaesthesia* 37:806, 1982.

71. Emmanuel ER. Post-sacral extradural catheter abscess in a child. *Br J Anaesth* 73:548, 1994.

72. Kost-Byerly S, Tobin JR, Greenberg RS, et al. Bacterial colonization and infection rate of continuous epidural catheters in children. *Anesth Analg* 86:712, 1998.

73. McNeely JK, Trentadue NC, Rusy LM, et al. Culture of bacteria from lumbar and caudal epidural catheters used for postoperative analgesia in children. *Reg Anesth* 22:428, 1997.

74. Ecoffey C, Dubousset AM, Samii K. Lumbar and thoracic epidural anesthesia for urologic and upper abdominal surgery in infants and children. *Anesthesiology* 65:87, 1986.

75. Dalens B, Tanguy A, Haberer JP. Lumbar epidural anesthesia for operative and postoperative pain relief in infants and young children. *Anesth Analg* 65:1069, 1986.

76. Kart T, Walther-Larsen S, Svejborg TF, et al. Comparison of continuous epidural infusion of fentanyl and bupivacaine with intermittent epidural administration of morphine for postoperative pain management in children. *Acta Anaesthesiol Scand* 41:461, 1997.

77. Desparmet J, Meistelman C, Barre J, et al. Continuous epidural infusion of bupivacaine for postoperative pain relief in children. *Anesthesiology* 67:108, 1987.

78. Hasan MA, Howard RF, Lloyd-Thomas AR. Depth of epidural space in children. *Anaesthesia* 49:1085, 1994.

79. Bosenberg AT, Gouws E. Skin-epidural distance in children. *Anaesthesia* 50:895, 1995.

80. Yamashita M. Mathematical formulae for assessing the depth of the epidural space in children. *Anaesthesia* 52:94, 1997.

81. Bromage PR, Benumof JL. Paraplegia following intracord injection during attempted epidural anesthesia under general anesthesia. *Reg Anesth Pain Med* 23:104, 1998.

82. Tobias JD. A review of intrathecal and epidural analgesia after spinal surgery in children. *Anesth Analg* 98:956, 2004.

83. Goobie SM, Montgomery CJ, Basu R, et al. Confirmation of direct epidural catheter placement using nerve stimulation in pediatric anesthesia. *Anesth Analg* 97:984, 2003.

84. Tsui BC, Gupta S, Finucane B. Confirmation of epidural catheter placement using nerve stimulation. *Can J Anaesth* 45:640, 1998.

85. Flandin-Blety C, Barrier G. Accidents following extradural analgesia in children. The results of a retrospective study. *Paediatr Anaesth* 5:41, 1995.

86. Lejus C, Roussiere G, Testa S, et al. Postoperative extradural analgesia in children: Comparison of morphine with fentanyl. *Br J Anaesth* 72:156, 1994.

87. Birmingham PK, Wheeler M, Suresh S, et al. Patient-controlled epidural analgesia in children: Can they do it? *Anesth Analg* 96:686, 2003.

88. Suresh S, Birmingham PK, Trombino LJ. Visualization of lumbar epidural catheters in patients with a hip spica cast. *Anesth Analg* 78:605, 1994.

89. Chalkiadis G. The rise and fall of continuous epidural infusions in children. *Paediatr Anaesth* 13:91, 2003.

Postoperative Neuraxial Analgesia

CHAPTER 16

Honorio T. Benzon
Kenneth D. Candido
Cynthia A. Wong

HISTORY

Pert and Snyder, in 1973, identified saturable, stereoselective receptors for opioids and naloxone.[1] In 1975, Hughes et al. isolated and characterized endogenous opioids.[2] These two discoveries laid the foundations for neuraxial opioid administration. Autoradiographic mapping of opioid receptor distribution was achieved in 1977, wherein the highest densities were shown to be located in the substantia gelatinosa of the spinal cord, medullary dorsal horn, and periaqueductal gray matter.[3] Also in 1977, Yaksh and Rudy demonstrated prolonged, dose-dependent, stereospecific, naloxone-reversible analgesia after intrathecal morphine administration in the rat.[4] Shortly thereafter, in 1979, Wang et al. reported the first use of subarachnoid morphine in humans in a double-blinded, placebo-controlled, crossover study in eight cancer patients. Seventy-five percent (6/8) of the patients had complete relief of pain without side effects.[5] The technique of neuraxial administration of opioid analgesics, without concomitant sensory, sympathetic, or motor blockade attendant to the use of neuraxial local anesthetics was clinically established. The potential for patients to ambulate without developing orthostatic hypotension or motor incoordination associated with parenteral opioids or epidural local anesthetics is another advantage. In this chapter, we will discuss the clinical practice of intrathecal and epidural opioid analgesia, either alone, or in combination with other drugs.

INTRATHECAL OPIOID ANALGESIA

Intrathecal analgesia with opioids and adjuvant agents is often employed for the treatment of acute postoperative and chronic pain. The technique is used for a number of common surgical procedures. Advantages of the technique include prolonged analgesia with a single injection, particularly if morphine is used, minimal hemodynamic changes, and no motor blockade. Disadvantages include frequent bothersome and rare serious side effects.

▶ Mechanisms and Pharmacology

Drugs injected into cerebrospinal fluid (CSF) diffuse across the pia mater into the spinal cord. The primary site of action is the spinal cord. Physical and chemical properties of the drug determine analgesia latency, site of action, duration of analgesia, and side effects (see Chap. 3).

Opioids are the class of drugs most commonly employed for intrathecal postoperative analgesia. Opioid receptors are located in Rexed laminae I, II, and V of the dorsal horn of the spinal cord.[6] Blockade of mu- and kappa-opioid receptors in the spinal cord modulate primary afferent transmission of nociceptive information responsible for pain. Intrathecal opioids inhibit C-fiber nociceptive transmission more easily than A-delta fiber transmission; therefore, opioids more effectively inhibit transmission of dull compared to sharp pain.

Analgesia speed of onset is directly related to lipid solubility, whereas dermatomal spread and duration of action are inversely related to lipid solubility. Highly lipid-soluble drugs such as fentanyl and sufentanil have a fast onset and short duration of action (Table 16-1).[7] The drugs are quickly redistributed to the spinal cord near the level of injection and the CSF concentration is barely detectable shortly after intrathecal injection.[8] Little drug circulates in CSF to spinal cord levels cephalad or caudad to the injection site, and analgesia is segmentally localized. Fentanyl and sufentanil are commonly used to supplement intraoperative spinal anesthesia. They may provide short-term postoperative analgesia (several hours), but are impractical for

Table 16-1

Characteristics of Intrathecal Opioids

Opioid	Oil-Water Partition Coefficient	pK_a	Typical Adult Dose	Latency (min)	Duration of Analgesia (min)
Morphine	1.4	7.9	0.05–0.25 mg	30–60	480–1440
Meperidine	8.5	39	10–100 mg	2–12	60–400
Fentanyl	813	8.4	10–50 µg	5–10	30–120
Sufentanil	1778	8.0	2.5–12.5 µg	3–6	60–180

Source: Data from Refs. 6, 7.

long-term postoperative analgesia unless administered using a continuous intrathecal catheter technique.

Morphine is the prototype drug for intrathecal analgesia. Because it is hydrophilic, morphine penetrates the spinal cord very slowly, resulting in a longer latency and longer duration of action than the lipid-soluble opioids (Table 16-1). Relatively high concentrations remain in the CSF, serving as a morphine depot for many hours after injection. Morphine circulates in CSF to more cephalad spinal cord levels and the brain stem, resulting in increased dermatomal spread and a different side effect profile. Meperidine is the only opioid that has local anesthetic properties in clinical doses and therefore, unlike the other opioids, can be used alone to provide surgical anesthesia.[9] Analgesia is longer lasting than fentanyl, but significantly shorter than morphine. Intrathecal diamorphine is used for postoperative analgesia in Great Britain.[10]

▷ Advantages of Intrathecal Opioids

Intrathecal opioid analgesia has several advantages compared to systemic and epidural opioid administration. A single dose of morphine can provide many hours of analgesia without the peaks and valleys associated with systemic opioid administration. The analgesic dose of intrathecal opioids, particularly for morphine, is much lower than the systemic or epidural dose. Serum opioid levels following intrathecal injection are barely detectable, and this minimizes side effects such as sedation.[6] Cannulation of the subarachnoid space is more reliable and technically easier than cannulation of the epidural space. There is no necessity to maintain an epidural catheter. A single-shot technique with a small needle may be safer in patients for whom pharmacologic anticoagulation will be initiated immediately after surgery. The issue of timing of epidural catheter removal is avoided. Intrathecal opioids administered before surgery improve intraoperative analgesia.[11]

Intrathecal opioids do not block the sympathetic nervous system, as do neuraxial local anesthetics. Therefore, they are not associated with adverse hemodynamic consequences. In addition, opioids do not cause motor or sensory blockade. Ambulation may be safer compared to neuraxial analgesic techniques using local anesthetics because sympathetic blockade-induced orthostatic hypotension is avoided, as is muscle weakness and altered proprioception. Finally, intrathecal opioids may be used as adjuncts to intrathecal or epidural local anesthetics, thus lowering the concentration of local anesthetic required for analgesia, and mitigating the undesirable side effects of neuraxial local anesthetics.

▷ Adjuvants to Intrathecal Opioid Analgesia

Adjuvants are added to intrathecal opioids in an attempt to prolong analgesia, lower the necessary dose of opioid, and perhaps decrease side effects. Several studies have suggested that epinephrine (0.1–0.2 mg) potentiates intrathecal morphine.[12,13] Clonidine is the most studied adjuvant to intrathecal opioid analgesia.

Clonidine

Clonidine is an α_2-adrenergic receptor agonist that increases the antinociceptive threshold by activating descending noradrenergic pathways in the spinal cord, resulting in inhibition of substance P release (see Chap. 3). The clinical data on whether clonidine potentiates intrathecal opioid analgesia are equivocal. Clonidine has been administered in combination with intrathecal morphine by both the oral and intrathecal routes for many surgical procedures. Patients treated with clonidine have a higher incidence of hypotension and sedation.

Oral clonidine 5 µg/kg enhanced intrathecal morphine (0.2 mg) analgesia after abdominal hysterectomy,[14] but clonidine 3 µg/kg with morphine 5 µg/kg after radical prostatectomy did not improve analgesia compared to morphine alone.[15] Similarly, intrathecal clonidine, 25–75 µg, improved intrathecal morphine analgesia after cardiac[16] and total knee arthroplasty procedures,[17] but not after hip arthroplasty.[18] Review of the current data suggests that clonidine may play a role when combined with low-dose intrathecal morphine. Lower doses (15–30 µg) are probably equally efficacious and are associated with less hypotension and sedation.

▶ Disadvantages and Side Effects of Intrathecal Opioids

Intrathecal opioid analgesia is commonly used as a single-shot technique. Therefore, the drug dose cannot be titrated or repeated. Side effects are usually dose dependent and may be merely bothersome or potentially fatal (see Chap. 6).

Pruritus

Pruritus is the most common side effect of intrathecal opioids and occurs at a higher rate after intrathecal compared to systemic administration. The mechanism is unclear, but is likely related to rostral migration of the opioid and interaction with opioid receptors in the trigeminal nucleus on the superficial surface of the medulla.[19] The time course of pruritus onset after intrathecal morphine appears to parallel the rostral spread of the drug.[20] Pruritus is not a result of histamine release. Facial pruritus in the distribution of the trigeminal nerve is common, but the itching may be generalized. The reported incidence of pruritus after intrathecal opioids ranges from 30 to 100% with an average reported rate of 58% after intrathecal morphine.[21,22] This wide range probably reflects whether investigators specifically asked if pruritus was present. The incidence appears to be higher in obstetric patients,[21] although few patients actually require treatment.[20] The incidence and severity of pruritus appear to be dose dependent.[10,20,23]

A number of therapies have been studied for the prevention and treatment of intrathecal opioid-induced pruritus. Naloxone, naltrexone, nalbuphine, and droperidol were identified as efficacious in the prevention of pruritus in a systematic review.[22] Data are conflicting as to whether prophylactic intravenous ondansetron is effective in reducing the incidence of pruritus associated with intrathecal morphine. Ondansetron 0.1 mg/kg was more effective in preventing pruritus after intrathecal morphine in obstetric patients compared to placebo and diphenhydramine in one study,[24] and was more effective than placebo, but less effective than nalbuphine in another obstetric study.[25] In contrast, after major orthopedic surgery, ondansetron did not prevent pruritus compared to placebo control.[26] Drugs found not to be effective in the prevention of pruritus include intravenous propofol,

intrathecal epinephrine, intramuscular hydroxyzine,[22] and celecoxib.[27]

There are few studies evaluating the treatment of established pruritus. Nalbuphine was more effective than propofol[28] or diphenhydramine.[29] Although antihistamines are commonly used to treat pruritus, and may be effective,[20] the likely mechanism is sedation, rather than direct antagonism of pruritus. Studies are conflicting as to whether low-dose intravenous propofol (10–20 mg) has a beneficial effect.[21] Ondansetron (8 mg) was more effective than placebo after intrathecal or epidural morphine in orthopedic patients.[30] Many practitioners administer low-dose naloxone or nalbuphine for the treatment of pruritus. A continuous infusion of naloxone may be required for ongoing relief. Dose ranges for drugs used to treat pruritus are listed in Table 6-11.

Nausea and Vomiting

Nausea and vomiting occur after intrathecal morphine injection. The reported incidence is between 20 and 40%, and is comparable to the incidence associated with intravenous and epidural opioid administration. Meperidine appears to be associated with the highest incidence of nausea and vomiting, whereas fentanyl and sufentanil are associated with the lowest risk.[31] Intrathecal morphine-induced nausea and vomiting appear to be dose related.[32] Limited data suggest that the incidence of nausea and vomiting does not differ between epidural and intrathecal opioid administration.[31] Intrathecal clonidine is not associated with an increased incidence of nausea and vomiting; however, intrathecal neostigmine is associated with a significant risk of nausea and vomiting and this may limit its clinical usefulness as an analgesic adjunct.

Intrathecal opioid-induced nausea and vomiting are most likely the results of cephalad migration of the opioid in CSF to opioid receptors in the area postrema and chemotactic trigger zone in the medulla.[19] Significant morphine concentrations in the medulla oblongata occur 5–6 h after the intrathecal injection of morphine and this corresponds to the time of peak nausea and vomiting.[31] Low-dose opioid antagonists are effective in treating nausea without reversing analgesia.[22] In a recent study in orthopedic and endoscopic urologic procedure, patients found that intramuscular haloperidol 1 or 2 mg decreased the incidence of postoperative nausea and vomiting after intrathecal morphine.[33] Drugs used to treat neuraxial opioid-induced nausea and vomiting are listed in Table 6-7.

Urinary Retention

Urinary retention after intrathecal opioid administration is much more common than after equivalent systemic doses.[19] It is more likely to occur in males. The probable mechanism involves the interaction of opioids with sacral opioid receptors. This leads to inhibition of sacral parasympathetic outflow which causes detrusor muscle relaxation. Naloxone is an effective treatment for urinary retention, but analgesia may be reversed. Bladder catheterization may be necessary.

Oral Herpes Simplex Reactivation

Oral herpes simplex virus reactivation has been reported after intrathecal morphine. The 30-day incidence of herpes simplex 1 reactivation was 38% in a group of women who received intrathecal and systemic morphine analgesia, compared to 17% in those who received only systemic morphine analgesia after spinal anesthesia for cesarean delivery.[34] A possible mechanism is the cephalad migration of morphine in CSF to opioid receptors in the trigeminal nucleus, where the virus is known to reside in latent form. An alternative mechanism involves opioid-induced facial pruritus, itching, and subsequent reactivation of latent virus.

Respiratory Depression

Respiratory depression is the most feared complication of intrathecal opioid analgesia. The risk of respiratory depression is dose dependent. The incidence of respiratory depression requiring intervention appears to be approximately 1%, which is not different from the risk following epidural or systemic opioid analgesia.[19] The degree of lipophilicity determines the timing of respiratory depression. Early respiratory depression (within several minutes to an hour of administration) does not occur after intrathecal morphine and is rare after intrathecal sufentanil and fentanyl. It is more common after epidural administration of sufentanil and fentanyl, and this may be related to systemic absorption of the drugs. In contrast, the respiratory depression associated with intrathecal morphine commonly occurs 6–12 h after administration. This parallels the rostral spread of morphine in the CSF to opioid receptors in the respiratory center in the ventral medulla.

Factors associated with an increased risk of respiratory depression include high doses of intrathecal morphine (more than 0.5 mg), concomitant administration of sedatives or other central nervous system depressants, advanced age, obesity, and sleep apnea. Clinical signs and symptoms are not sensitive indicators of respiratory depression.[35] Respiratory rate and pupil size did not predict respiratory depression as measured by ventilatory response to carbon dioxide in volunteers. The most reliable sign appears to be depressed level of consciousness, presumably caused by hypercarbia.[19] Supplemental oxygen prevents hypoxemia, but not hypercarbia.

Protocols for monitoring respiratory depression after intrathecal morphine vary from institution to institution.

Some institutions require care in a monitored unit. Others monitor respiratory rate and sedation on a regular basis for 12–24 h after opioid injection. Since intrathecal morphine doses less than 0.4 mg are associated with a low risk of respiratory depression that is not different from other routes of opioid administration, special monitoring does not seem warranted for these patients. Patients at increased risk of respiratory depression should receive more intensive monitoring.

Respiratory depression associated with intrathecal morphine can be reversed with naloxone. The respiratory depression may recur after a single dose of naloxone, therefore, repeated bolus administration or a continuous infusion may be necessary. In a nonemergency situation small bolus doses of naloxone (40–80 µg) can be titrated to effect. In an emergency, a larger dose (0.2–0.4 mg) should be administered.

▶ Clinical Applications of Intrathecal Postoperative Analgesia

Intrathecal opioids, primarily morphine, provide excellent analgesia after a variety of surgical procedures, including cardiothoracic, orthopedic, gynecologic, and obstetric procedures. Adequate dose-response studies are lacking for most procedures. Suggested intrathecal morphine doses for specific surgical procedures have been summarized in Table 16-2.

Obstetric Surgery

Intrathecal morphine has been most often studied for postoperative cesarean delivery analgesia (see Chap. 14). One group of investigators randomized patients to nine doses of intrathecal morphine between 0 and 0.5 mg and concluded that there was no reason to use more than 0.1 mg.[36] Higher doses were associated with a greater incidence of side effects with no additional analgesia benefit. A systematic review of all randomized studies comparing intrathecal morphine to saline placebo reached the same conclusion.[32] The authors noted that for every 100 women who receive 0.1 mg intrathecal morphine, 43 will experience pruritus and 10 will experience nausea that they would not have experienced without treatment. A much lower dose of intrathecal morphine, 0.025 mg, provided satisfactory analgesia with minimal side effects when combined with a regular dose of a systemic nonsteroidal anti-inflammatory drug.[37] A small study compared intrathecal diamorphine 0.2 mg to morphine 0.2 mg. Analgesia was similar between the two groups, but there was a higher incidence of drowsiness and pruritus in the diamorphine patients.[38] Intrathecal morphine 0.1 mg improved postoperative analgesia after spinal anesthesia for postpartum tubal ligation with an

Table 16-2		
Recommended Intrathecal Doses of Opioids		
Type of Surgical Procedure	Suggested Intrathecal Morphine Dose (µg)	Reference no.
Cesarean delivery	25–100*	32, 36, 37
Laparoscopic abdominal surgery	75–200	43, 44
Open cholecystectomy	60–120	42
Total knee arthroplasty	100–200[†]	46, 47
Total hip arthroplasty	200	46
Lumbar spine with fusion	300	48
Lumbar spine with instrumentation, multilevel	20 µg/kg	49
Coronary artery bypass grafting	250–500 µg	52, 53
Off-pump coronary artery bypass grafting	5 µg/kg	54
Thoracotomy	200–500[‡]	56, 57
Transurethral resection of the prostate	50	59

*Combined with diclofenac.
[†]Age > 65 years.
[‡]Combined with sufentanil 20–50 µg.

acceptable side effect profile compared to intravenous morphine patient-controlled analgesia (PCA).[39]

Abdominal and Pelvic Surgery

Several studies have addressed intrathecal morphine in gynecologic patients (see Chap. 12). Patients were randomized to morphine 0, 0.1, 0.3, or 0.5 mg for postoperative abdominal hysterectomy analgesia. The authors noted inadequate analgesia after 0.1 mg and recommended 0.3 mg as the optimal dose with fewest side effects. Investigators in Thailand compared intrathecal morphine 0.2, 0.25, and 0.3 mg and found that doses higher than 0.2 mg provided no added analgesia efficacy, but were associated with an increased incidence of side effects.[40]

Intrathecal morphine 0.3 mg plus PCA provided better analgesia at the cost of an increased incidence of nausea and vomiting in patients undergoing major abdominal surgery.[41] Lower morphine doses were not studied. Lower doses of morphine (0.06–0.12 mg) were effective for postoperative open cholecystectomy analgesia.[42] Following laparoscopic abdominal surgery, intrathecal morphine 0.075–0.2 mg provided improved analgesia compared to placebo without an increase in the incidence of nausea and vomiting.[43,44] Although intrathecal morphine and sufentanil provided profound analgesia following abdominal aortic surgery, investigators studying 217 patients found no difference in the combined incidence of cardiac, respiratory, or renal complications compared to patients in a control group without intrathecal opioid.[45]

Orthopedic Surgery

Intrathecal morphine has been used for both total joint arthroplasty and major spinal surgery (see Chap. 7). Total knee arthroplasty is more painful than total hip arthroplasty. Patients undergoing both joint procedures were randomized to receive morphine 0, 0.1, 0.2, or 0.3 mg.[46] Supplemental morphine use was less in hip arthroscopy patients who received intrathecal morphine, but not in knee arthroplasty patients. However, patients undergoing both procedures were more satisfied with their pain relief after intrathecal morphine 0.2 or 0.3 mg and there was no increase in the incidence of nausea, vomiting, or oxygen desaturation. The authors concluded that morphine 0.2 mg provides good to excellent pain control in most patients after knee or hip arthroplasty. In patients older than 65 years of age undergoing hip arthroplasty, morphine 0.1 mg was found to best balance efficacy and side effects.[47]

Patients undergoing lumbar spinal fusion surgery were randomized to receive intrathecal morphine 0.2, 0.3, or 0.4 mg.[48] Pain control was better with the higher doses, but 0.4 mg was associated with more respiratory depression. After elective multilevel posterior spinal instrumentation, intrathecal morphine 20 µg/kg provided better pain relief and was associated with fewer respiratory complications and shorter intensive care unit (ICU) stays compared to 10 µg/kg or no morphine.[49]

Cardiac Surgery

Many small studies describe the use of intrathecal morphine in cardiac surgery patients. Although there is a theoretical concern about the risk of spinal-epidural hematoma because of heparin administration during cardiac surgery, this complication has not been reported. Investigators have studied intrathecal morphine alone, or intrathecal morphine in combination with sufentanil and clonidine. Most studies are small and many are not blinded. Early blinded studies in coronary artery bypass grafting patients used high-dose morphine (e.g., morphine 10 µg/kg[50] or 4.0 mg[51]) combined with a moderate- to high-dose intraoperative opioid anesthetic technique. Postoperative analgesic requirements were markedly less in the intrathecal morphine groups, but time to extubation was delayed. Other investigators have combined lower doses of intrathecal morphine (0.25–0.5 mg) with lower dose, or shorter-acting intraoperative opioid anesthetic techniques without adversely effecting time to extubation, even in fast-track cardiac surgery patients.[52,53] Intrathecal morphine has also been used successfully in off-pump coronary artery bypass grafting patients.[54]

Thoracic Surgery

Epidural analgesia has been shown to reduce pulmonary morbidity after thoracotomy.[55] There are only a few studies of intrathecal morphine combined with sufentanil in thoracotomy patients.[56,57] Both studies found that intrathecal analgesia markedly reduced systemic analgesic requirements. The studies were too small to assess differences in other outcomes and no study has compared continuous thoracic epidural analgesia to single-shot intrathecal morphine analgesia. One study compared epidural analgesia with bupivacaine and fentanyl to intermittent intrathecal morphine combined with cyclooxygenase-1 and cyclooxygenase-2 (COX-1 and COX-2) inhibitors. Intrathecal morphine with a COX-2 inhibitor was associated with superior analgesia, highest patient satisfaction, and least reduction in peak expiratory flow rate (PEFR) compared to the other groups.[58]

Urologic Surgery

Low-dose intrathecal morphine (0, 0.05, or 0.1 mg) was studied in patients undergoing transurethral resection of the prostate.[59] Morphine 0.05 mg was associated with improved analgesia without an increased risk of nausea or vomiting.

EPIDURAL OPIOID ANALGESIA

▶ Dural Transport

The physical characteristics and mechanism of action of epidural opioids are discussed in detail in Chap. 3. The transport of opioids through the dura mater explains the divergent clinical effects of different opioids. In an elegant study, Bernards et al. investigated the epidural, CSF, and plasma pharmacokinetics of epidural opioids.[60] They found a significant correlation between the hydrophobicity of the opioid and the mean residence time both in the extracellular fluid of the lumbar epidural space and in the epidural venous plasma. The hydrophobicity of the opioid was linearly related to the terminal elimination half-life of the opioid in the lumbar epidural space. The authors postulated that hydrophobic opioids are more sequestered in the lipoidal environments surrounding the epidural space compared to the hydrophilic opioids. The slow release of the sequestered opioid back into the extracellular fluid of the epidural space results in a prolonged elimination half-life and an increase in the mean residence time of the hydrophobic opioid. This prolonged residence time of hydrophobic opioids in the epidural space explains the spinal mechanism of analgesic effect of morphine compared to the minimal spinal analgesic effect of fentanyl, alfentanil, and sufentanil after injection into the lumbar epidural space. The terminal elimination half-life in the thoracic epidural space correlated with the molecular weight of the opioid, not hydrophobicity. The authors theorized that the terminal elimination half-life of the opioid in the thoracic epidural space may be dependent on the rate at which the opioid spreads rostrally rather than the rate at which the opioids are eliminated from the thoracic epidural space.[60]

CSF opioid kinetics differ from epidural space kinetics.[60] There were no differences in the mean residence time and terminal elimination half-lives of the different opioids in the intrathecal space after epidural administration. Also, there was no correlation between the pharmacokinetic parameters and the hydrophobic character or molecular weight of the opioid. It appears that diffusion through the multiple meningeal barriers is the rate-limiting step that controls the terminal elimination half-lives of neuraxial opioids. The terminal elimination half-life of morphine is longer in the intrathecal space than in the epidural space, resulting in its greater bioavailability. The dose-normalized concentration of morphine in the CSF is significantly greater than that of fentanyl, alfentanil, or sufentanil and predicts a significantly greater morphine content in the spinal cord.[61] These findings are consistent with clinical studies that showed that epidural morphine produces analgesia via a spinal mechanism, in contrast to fentanyl and sufentanil (see "Clinical Aspects," next).

Table 16-3

Epidural Opioids: Common Doses, Onset Time, and Duration of Analgesic Effects

Drug	Single Dose	Onset (min)	Duration (h)	Infusion Solution (µg/mL)	Continuous Infusion
Fentanyl	50–100 µg	5–10	2.5–4	5–10	25–100 µg/h
Sufentanil	10–50 µg	5	2–4	1	10–20 µg/h
Meperidine*	20–50 mg	5–15	6 (4–20)	2500	10–30 mg/h
Methadone	2–8 mg	10	6–10	10–15	0.1–0.3 mg/h
Hydromorphone	0.5–1 mg	10–15	10–12	5–10	0.05–0.1 mg/h
Morphine	1–5 mg	30–60	18	10	0.05–0.1 mg/h

*Several hospitals have discontinued the use of meperidine because of its side effect profile and accumulation of active metabolites.

▶ Clinical Aspects

Epidural opioids can be given as a single dose or as a continuous infusion. Commonly used epidural opioids include morphine, hydromorphone, and fentanyl. Epidural methadone and buprenorphine have been studied. Epidural opioids vary as to their latency and duration of analgesia (Table 16-3) and these differences are clinically important. Epidural fentanyl is more appropriate for outpatient surgery and morphine for inpatient procedures where its side effects can be appropriately monitored. Dilution of epidural fentanyl with 10 mL of preservative-free saline may shorten the onset and prolong the duration of analgesic effect of fentanyl.[62] A combination of a lipophilic opioid such as sufentanil and a hydrophilic opioid such as morphine may take advantage of the short onset time of the lipophilic opioid and the prolonged analgesic duration of the hydrophilic opioid.[63]

The infusion of opioids provides continuous analgesia for at least the duration of the infusion. Clinically useful opioid concentrations are listed in Table 16-3. The mechanism of analgesic action of the opioid infusion has been the subject of controversy. The current consensus is that lipophilic opioids act primarily via a supraspinal or systemic mechanism.[64–67] Several studies showed no differences in the pain scores, plasma concentrations, and side effects between patients who received either epidural or intravenous infusions of fentanyl. Hydrophilic opioid infusions, on the other hand, produce analgesia primarily via a spinal mechanism.[68] Studies have shown that continuous epidural morphine infusion provides better analgesia compared to systemic opioids.[69–71] In contrast to lipophilic opioids, hydrophilic opioids provide effective analgesia when epidural catheter placement is not congruent with the surgical incision (see below).

The addition of dilute local anesthetic to epidural opioid is usually recommended since laboratory and clinical studies show synergism of effect when the drugs are administered in combination.[72–74] Not all studies, however, have found an additive analgesic effect when epidural local anesthetics and opioids are combined.[75–78] Furthermore, 2-chloroprocaine, with or without epinephrine, appeared to interfere with epidural morphine analgesia in patients who had cesarean delivery.[79]

The addition of local anesthetic affords several advantages. These include blockade of cardiac sympathetic outflow resulting in decreased heart rate, lower blood pressure, and reduced myocardial oxygen consumption; reflex inhibition of phrenic nerve and diaphragmatic activity; improved gastrointestinal motility; and decreased hypercoagulability and thrombotic events. The addition of a local anesthetic, however, necessitates more vigilant hemodynamic and neurologic (especially in the presence of anticoagulation) monitoring.

The vertebral level of placement of the epidural catheter is clinically important. Wu and Thomsen emphasized the congruency of the catheter placement with the site of surgical incision.[80,81] This implies placement of the epidural catheter in the midthoracic level for thoracic surgery, mid-to low-thoracic placement for upper intra-abdominal procedures, low-thoracic placement for lower abdominal and hip surgeries, and high-lumbar placement for lower extremity surgery (Table 16-4). When placing the catheter, it is

Table 16-4

Epidural Catheter Location and Surgical Site

Surgical Site	Epidural Catheter Insertion Site
Thoracic	T4 to T7
Upper abdominal	T5 to T8
Lower abdominal	T9 to T11
Hip	T12 to L2
Knee	L2 to L4
Perineum	L3 to L5

important to recognize the level at which spinal nerves actually exit the vertebral canal (see Chap. 1). For example, the fourth lumbar nerve root exits the vertebral canal through the intervertebral foramen between the L4 and L5 vertebral bodies. The actual spinal cord origin of the L4 nerve root is higher, at approximately the T11 to T12 level of the vertebral column. This is due to the differential growth of the spinal cord and the vertebral column during maturation. This is of greater clinical significance in the lumbar region and less important for thoracic catheters. Most clinicians continue to place catheters at the vertebral level where a given nerve root exits the intervertebral foramen. While this is acceptable and standard practice, the catheter should theoretically be placed at the level where a given nerve originates from the spinal cord. This consideration may be relevant for individuals in whom a reduction in drug doses is essential.

Doses of analgesic agents should be tailored not only to the surgical site, but also to the age and physical status of the patient. The standard single-shot bolus doses typically used at the authors' institution for providing postoperative neuraxial analgesia for two of the most commonly used epidural opioids, morphine and hydromorphone, are shown in Table 16-5. These doses are routinely administered between 30 and 45 min prior to the completion of the surgical procedure. Sterile, preservative-free drug preparations are used. After patients have arrived in the postanesthesia care unit (PACU), continuous infusions of local anesthetic and opioid may be initiated, usually after patients demonstrate recovery of motor function.

Table 16-5

Patient Age and Initial Epidural Bolus Dose of Morphine and Hydromorphone

Age (years)	Morphine Dose (mg)	Hydromorphone Dose (mg)
Thoracic Catheter		
15–44	4	1.0
45–65	3	1.0
66–75	2	0.5
>75	1	0.5
Lumbar Catheter		
15–44	5	1.0
45–65	3–4	1.0
66–75	2–2.5	0.5–1.0
>75	1.5–2.0	0.5

▶ Adjuvants to Epidural Opioid Analgesia

A number of adjuvants have been combined with opioid-only or local anesthetic-opioid analgesic solutions. The advantage of adjuvants is that lower doses of drugs can be used, thus minimizing side effects. Analgesia may be improved because the use of different drugs takes advantage of differing mechanisms of analgesia. Adjuvants and epidural dosing guidelines are summarized in Table 16-6. With the exception of clonidine and epinephrine, these drugs have not been approved by the United States Food and Drug Administration for epidural administration, and therefore, administration by this route is an off-label use of the drug.

Clonidine

Clonidine is an α_2-adrenoceptor agonist that may be used as an adjuvant for neuraxial analgesia (see Chap. 3). Several studies have demonstrated efficacy of epidural clonidine for postoperative analgesia. Compared to intravenous clonidine 8 µg/kg administration, epidural clonidine after major spine surgery provided better analgesia, less sedation, and less hypotension.[82] The analgesia from epidural clonidine analgesia is comparable, if not superior to, epidural sufentanil analgesia.[83] Clonidine potentiates the analgesia from epidural sufentanil.[84] This potentiation is more pronounced with epidural, compared to systemic, clonidine administration. In one study, clonidine added to epidural sufentanil not only improved postoperative analgesia, but also reduced intraoperative isoflurane requirements.[85] Intraoperative epidural clonidine infusion resulted in dose-dependent control of hemodynamic changes associated with major abdominal surgical procedures during general anesthesia maintained with an intravenous propofol.[86] In addition, the higher infusion rate (8 µg/kg bolus followed by 2 µg/kg/h infusion) provided more predictable analgesia. Following abdominal gynecologic surgery, postoperative thoracic epidural clonidine infusions of 20 µg/h added to epidural fentanyl and bupivacaine provided better analgesia, but were associated with more pronounced hemodynamic changes compared to infusion rates of 10 or 15 µg/h.[87]

Several studies have attempted to find the ideal combination of epidural clonidine, bupivacaine, and fentanyl for optimal postoperative analgesia. The combinations of drugs that provide the best analgesia with fewest side effects for abdominal[88] and major orthopedic knee and hip surgery[89] are detailed in Table 16-7.

Armand et al. attempted to perform a meta-analysis of epidural clonidine studies published between 1985 and 1997.[90] All but 16 studies suffered from serious design flaws. The data from these 16 studies were difficult to interpret

Table 16-6

Adjuncts to Epidural Analgesia

Adjunct	Dose	Comment
Clonidine	Bolus: 75–800 µg, 1–8 µg/kg Infusion: 10–50 µg/h, 0.3–2 µg/kg/h	Usually combined with local anesthetic, opioid, or both Side effects: sedation, hypotension, bradycardia
Ketamine	Bolus: 20–30 mg, 0.5–1 mg/kg Infusion: 0.5–1 mg/h	Administered with epidural morphine. Minimal side effects
Epinephrine	Bolus and infusion: 1.5–5 µg/mL local anesthetic solution	Dose < 1.5 µg/mL did not improve analgesia
Midazolam	Bolus: 0.05 mg/kg in 5–10 mL saline Infusion: 0.8–1.6 mg/h	Administered with bupivacaine Side effects: sedation, amnesia
Droperidol	Bolus: 1.25–5 mg Infusion: 2.5 mg over 24 h	Administered with bupivacaine and fentanyl Less sedation than IV route
Neostigmine	Bolus: 1–4 µg/kg, 60 µg	Administered with morphine
Naloxone	Infusion: 0.21 µg/kg/h	Administered with bupivacaine and fentanyl Analgesia maintained with faster return of bowel function

because of variation in clonidine dose, method and vertebral level of administration, type of surgery, and rescue drugs. This precluded any meta-analysis and the authors concluded that further well-designed, dose-response studies

Table 16-7

Optimal Combinations of Epidural Bupivacaine, Fentanyl, and Clonidine

Major Abdominal Procedure	Rate*		
Bupivacaine dose (mg/h)	9	8	13
Fentanyl dose (µg/h)	21	30	25
Clonidine dose (µg/h)	5	0	0
Infusion rate (mL/h)	7	9	9
Major Orthopedic Procedure	**Drug Concentration†**			
Bupivacaine (mg/mL)	1.0	0.9	0.6	0.5
Fentanyl (µg/mL)	1.4	3.0	2.5	2.4
Clonidine (µg/mL)	0.5	0.3	0.8	1.0

*Optimal combinations of thoracic epidural bupivacaine, fentanyl, and clonidine (infusion rate) for postoperative analgesia following major abdominal surgery are listed within a column.
†Optimal drug concentration combinations of lumbar (L3 to L4) epidural bupivacaine, fentanyl, and clonidine for postoperative analgesia following major orthopedic hip and knee procedures are listed within a column. Infusion rates were initiated at 7 mL/h. Nurses administered a 5 mL bolus (60 min lockout) for breakthrough pain, and increased infusion rate by 2 mL/h to a maximum of 15 mL/h.
Source: Data from Refs. 88, 89.

are necessary to optimally define the role of epidural clonidine for postoperative analgesia.

In children, a clear dose-response relationship was identified for continuous infusions of epidural clonidine combined with epidural ropivacaine for postoperative analgesia following repair of hypospadias in young boys.[91] Clonidine dosages between 0.08 and 0.12 µg/kg/h, combined with ropivacaine 0.16 mg/kg/h, provided optimal postoperative analgesia with an acceptable side effect profile (Fig. 16-1).

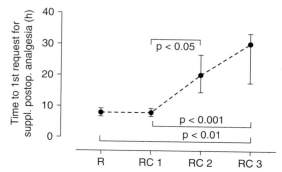

FIGURE 16-1. Time to first request for supplemental analgesia: dose-response of epidural clonidine combined with an epidural ropivacaine infusion for postoperative analgesia in 60 boys after repair of hypospadias. R = ropivacaine 0.2 mg/kg/h, RC1 = ropivacaine 0.16 mg/kg/h plus clonidine 0.04 µg/kg/h, RC2 = ropivacaine 0.16 mg/kg/h plus clonidine 0.08 µg/kg/h, and RC3 = ropivacaine 0.16 mg/kg/h plus clonidine 0.12 µg/kg/h. *Used with permission from De Negri P, Ivani G, Visconti C, et al. The dose-response relationship for clonidine added to a postoperative continuous epidural infusion of ropivacaine in children. Anesth Analg 93:71, 2001.*

The superiority of combined epidural clonidine (0.02 µg/kg/h) and ropivacaine (0.2 mg/kg/h) over epidural clonidine alone was shown in another pediatric study.[92]

Ketamine

Ketamine, an *N*-methyl-D-aspartate receptor channel blocker, has been studied almost as extensively as clonidine for postoperative neuraxial analgesia. Ketamine alone appears to provide no significant analgesia, but the combination of ketamine 10 mg and morphine 0.5 mg provided better analgesia than morphine alone.[93] The epidural administration of ketamine 30 mg, before or after skin incision, prolonged the time to first analgesic use and reduced postoperative PCA consumption after hysterectomy.[94] Several studies have shown that the addition of ketamine improves analgesia from epidural morphine,[95] morphine/bupivacaine,[96] and epidural ropivacaine.[97] A systematic review of randomized, double-blinded clinical trials on epidural ketamine added to opioid analgesics found that five of eight controlled studies demonstrated beneficial effects without prohibitive adverse effects.[98] Epidural ketamine appears to have no preemptive analgesic effect.[99]

Epinephrine

Epinephrine is frequently used as an adjuvant in regional anesthesia and neuraxial analgesia techniques. The addition of epinephrine to thoracic epidural infusions of fentanyl or fentanyl/bupivacaine resulted in improved analgesia, increased sensory blockade, lower sedation scores, and lower infusion rates.[100–102] These findings imply that coadministration of epidural fentanyl with epinephrine slows systemic fentanyl absorption and results in fewer systemic side effects of fentanyl.[101] The thoracic administration of epinephrine appears to be more effective than lumbar administration. This is probably related to the greater distance from the lumbar injection site to the α_2-adrenergic receptors in the spinal cord. An epinephrine concentration of 1.5 µg/mL is the minimum effective concentration when combined with bupivacaine and fentanyl for thoracic epidural analgesia.[103]

Other Epidural Analgesia Adjuvants

Midazolam has been shown to have an analgesic effect by single-shot epidural administration as well as by continuous infusion. Epidural midazolam (0.8 and 1.6 mg/h) combined with bupivacaine resulted in better analgesia compared to bupivacaine alone, but was associated with more sedation and amnesia when administered following gastrectomy.[104] Midazolam combined with bupivacaine results in excellent analgesia and amnesia.[105] Diluent volumes of 5–10 mL appear to be ideal for midazolam (0.05 mg/kg) injected into a thoracic epidural catheter following upper abdominal surgery.[106]

Droperidol, a butyrophenone, is used as an antiemetic agent in the perioperative setting. The data are conflicting, but some investigators have found that intravenous and epidural droperidol decrease the incidence and severity of epidural morphine-induced pruritus. Epidural administration may be associated with less sedation. Epidural droperidol 1.25, 2.5, and 5 mg reduced pruritus associated with epidural morphine 2 mg.[107] Compared to epidural butorphanol 2 mg, epidural droperidol 2.5 mg had a better analgesia/side effect profile when combined with fentanyl/bupivacaine in 40 mL infused over 24 h.[108] In a direct comparison of intravenous and epidural droperidol, epidural administration was superior in reducing pruritus, nausea, and vomiting after epidural morphine.[109]

Neostigmine has also been administered with local anesthetics for potentiation of neuraxial analgesia. Epidural neostigmine, in doses of 1–4 µg/kg, produced dose-dependent analgesia when administered as part of a combined spinal-epidural anesthetic; the analgesia persisted up to 8 h.[110] Epidural neostigmine, but not intra-articular neostigmine, resulted in postoperative analgesia.[111] The addition of 60 µg neostigmine to epidural morphine resulted in prolonged analgesia and fewer side effects compared to control groups with epidural saline, morphine alone, or neostigmine alone.[112]

Naloxone, an opioid antagonist, has been successfully coadministered with morphine into the epidural space. Patients who had naloxone (0.208 µg/kg/h), in addition to epidural morphine and bupivacaine, had a shorter onset time to first passage of flatus and feces and equivalent analgesia compared to epidural morphine/bupivacaine. Naloxone appears to reduce morphine-induced intestinal hypomotility without antagonizing the analgesic properties of morphine.[113]

▶ Side Effects, Complications, and Technical Failures

The side effects of epidural opioids are similar to those associated with systemic and intrathecal opioids and include nausea and vomiting, pruritus, and respiratory depression (see Chap. 6). The incidence of side effects is summarized in Table 16-8. Hypotension is rarely associated with epidural opioid administration. However, blood pressure may decrease after epidural opioid administration, presumably secondary to the indirect effects of complete analgesia. This is especially true in hypovolemic patients.

The incidence of nausea and vomiting is 20–50% after a single dose of epidural opioid[19,114,115] and 45–80% after

Table 16-8

Incidence of Side Effects of Epidural Opioid Analgesia

Side Effect	Epidural Opioid	Systemic Opioid	Dose Dependent	Treatment
Nausea and vomiting	20–50% (single dose) 45–80% (infusion)	9–38%	Yes	Naloxone, naltrexone, nalbuphine, droperidol
Pruritus	7–38%	15–18%	Not clear	Naloxone, naltrexone, nalbuphine
Urinary retention	70–80%	18%	No	Naloxone (low dose)
Respiratory depression	0.1–0.9%	Same	Yes	Naloxone

continuous epidural opioid infusions.[116,117] The incidence appears to be dose dependent. Treatments include naloxone, metoclopramide, droperidol, dexamethasone, subhypnotic doses of propofol, and transdermal scopolamine (Table 6-7).

Pruritus is not related to peripheral histamine release.[19] It is probably secondary to activation of an "itch center" in the medulla, interaction with opioid receptors in the trigeminal nucleus or nerve roots, or changes in the sensory modulation of the trigeminal nerve and upper cervical spinal cord.[118] The incidence of pruritus associated with epidural opioids ranges from 7 to 38%[81] and can be as high as 60%.[22,119,120] This is in contrast to an incidence of 15–18% following systemic opioid administration.[22,119,120] Treatments includes nalbuphine, naloxone, or naltrexone (Table 6-11).[22]

Urinary retention is related to spinal opioid receptor activation, resulting in a decrease in detrusor muscle contraction[19] and is not dose dependent.[121] The incidence of urinary retention after epidural opioids is 70–80% compared to 18% with systemic opioids.[19,119] Treatment includes low-dose naloxone; however, this may reverse analgesia.[122]

Respiratory depression is the most feared complication of neuraxial opioids. It is dose dependent and the incidence ranges from 0.1 to 0.9%.[123–127] It should be noted that this incidence is not higher than that seen after systemic opioids.[126,127] The incidence and timing of respiratory depression differs for lipophilic and hydrophilic opioids. Respiratory depression from lipophilic opioids usually occurs within 2 h of administration.[118] These drugs are rapidly absorbed from the epidural venous plexus into the systemic circulation and reach the respiratory centers relatively quickly. Hydrophilic opioids, in contrast, reach the brain stem slowly via rostral migration in CSF. This may take as many as 12 h after injection, but usually occurs 6–12 h after lumbar epidural administration.

Factors that increase the risk of respiratory depression include concomitant use of systemic opioids and sedatives, higher vertebral levels of epidural injection, presence of comorbidities (patients with sleep apnea or chronic obstructive pulmonary disease), increased age, and an opioid-naive state. The respiratory rate of the patient is not a reliable sole predictor of impending respiratory depression.[128] Sedation status is as important. Treatment of respiratory depression includes naloxone in 0.1–0.2 mg increments followed by a continuous infusion at 0.5–5 µg/kg/h.[127]

The placement of an epidural catheter that is "incision congruent" results in a lower incidence of analgesic drug-induced side effects, such as pruritus, nausea, vomiting, and lower extremity motor block.[80] Thoracic epidural local anesthetic-opioid infusions, compared to lumbar infusions, result in a lower incidence of hypotension, lower extremity weakness, and urinary retention.[129–131] The incidence of hypotension from local anesthetic-based epidural regimens ranges from 0.7 to 3%[124,130] to as high as 8–14%,[81] while the incidence of lower extremity motor blockade ranges from 1 to 3%.[57,81] It should be noted that lower extremity numbness and weakness may be a sign of epidural hematoma.[132]

Technical failures include unsuccessful placement of the epidural catheter in the epidural space, unilateral blockade, missed segments, and premature catheter dislodgement. The rate of technical failure of a thoracic epidural catheter has been reported as high as 19% in the first 72 h.[133] A review of published studies on the management of acute postoperative pain estimated the incidence of premature epidural catheter dislodgement at 5.7% (95% confidence interval [CI]: 4.0–7.4%).[134]

▶ Effects of Neuraxial Analgesia on Postoperative Pain

The efficacy of postoperative epidural analgesia in relieving acute postoperative pain has been the subject of numerous studies.[81,134,135] Two recent publications summarized the results of studies done in this area. Dolin et al.[134] reviewed the literature between 1966 and 1999, including a MED-LINE search and hand search of four anesthesiology journals. From 800 original papers, they identified 165 publications with usable data. The investigators pooled the data on pain scores and compared the incidence of moderate-severe and severe pain after major surgery with three analgesic techniques: intramuscular analgesia, PCA, and epidural analgesia. The overall mean incidence (95% CI) of moderate-severe pain and severe pain with the three techniques were 29.7% (26–33%) and 10.9% (8.4–13.4%), respectively. The investigators concluded that epidural analgesia was the most efficacious technique of pain relief after major surgery. The data for the three analgesic techniques are summarized in Table 16-9. Also of note, between 1973 and 1999, the overall incidence of moderate-severe pain at rest fell significantly by 1.9% per annum.[134]

Block et al.[81] performed a meta-analysis of the efficacy of postoperative epidural analgesia. The investigators analyzed 100 studies published between 1966 and April 2002 that met inclusion criteria. Included studies compared postoperative analgesia in adult patients randomized to epidural versus parenteral opioids where pain was measured with a visual analog scale (VAS) or numeric rating scale. There were no differences in mean VAS among intravenous PCA, intramuscular, and subcutaneous opioid administration. However, epidural analgesia provided better postoperative analgesia compared with parenteral opioids for postoperative days 1 through 4 (Fig. 16-2). For all types of surgery (thoracic, abdominal, pelvic, and lower extremity surgery) and pain measurements, all forms of epidural analgesia (thoracic or lumbar, local anesthetic or opioid, or combinations) provided significantly better postoperative analgesia compared with parenteral opioid analgesia.[81]

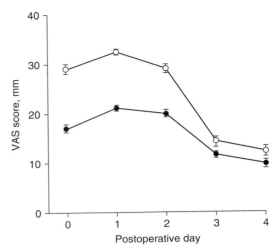

No. of patient-observations

Parenteral opioids	1104	2635	1496	794	536
Epidural analogesia	1010	2618	1527	822	566

○ Parenteral opioids   ● Epidural analgesia

FIGURE 16-2. Mean VAS and 95% CI for acute postoperative pain on postoperative days 0 through 4: epidural compared to parenteral opioid analgesia. $P < 0.001$ for all days after Bonferroni correction for multiple comparisons. *Used with permission from Block BM, Liu SS, Rowlingson AJ, et al. Efficacy of postoperative epidural analgesia: A meta-analysis. JAMA 290:2455, 2003.*

▶ Outcomes

"Outcomes research" involves the assessment of the effectiveness of a health-care intervention on various aspects of patient care.[136] In addition to clinical outcomes, outcomes research includes functional health status, patient satisfaction, and economic measurements. This section will address clinical outcomes after neuraxial analgesia.

Major Morbidity and Mortality: Initial Studies

The landmark study by Yeager et al.[137] showed a significant beneficial effect of epidural anesthesia and postoperative epidural analgesia, compared to general anesthesia and systemic analgesia, on the operative outcome in high-risk surgical patients who underwent intra-abdominal, thoracic, and major vascular surgery. Patients randomized to the epidural anesthesia/analgesia group had significantly lower incidences of mortality, cardiovascular failure, major infections, and overall complications (Table 16-10). The investigators also found that urinary cortisol concentration, a marker of the stress response, was significantly diminished in the first 24 h in the patients who had epidural anesthesia

Table 16-9

Effectiveness of Postoperative Pain Management

	Intramuscular	PCA	Epidural
	Moderate-Severe Pain		
Number of studies	29	45	62
Percent with pain (95% CI)	67 (58–76)	36 (31–40)	21 (18–24)
	Severe Pain		
Number of studies	21	27	30
Percent with pain (95% CI)	29 (19–39)	10 (8–13)	8 (6–10)

Source: Data from Ref. 134.

Table 16-10

Randomized Controlled Trials in Patients Undergoing Abdominal Surgery: Epidural Anesthesia/Analgesia Compared to General Anesthesia/Systemic Analgesia

	Yeager	Park	Rigg
Type of surgery	Abdominal	Abdominal	Abdominal
Number of patients	53	1021	888
Study groups	Epidural-general anesthesia/epidural analgesia vs. general anesthesia/systemic analgesia		
Findings			
Mortality	Epidural: decreased	Same	Same
Cardiovascular morbidity	Epidural: decreased	Same	Same
Infection	Epidural: decreased	Same	Same
Respiratory morbidity	ND	ND	Epidural: decreased
Length of stay	ND	Epidural: shorter ICU stay (aortic surgery patients)	ND
ICU stay	ND	Epidural: shorter*	ND
Hospital stay	ND	Same	ND
Comment	Study terminated early	Epidural: shorter intubation time*	Epidural: less respiratory failure

*In aortic surgery patients. ND = No Data
Source: Data from Refs. 137, 153, 154.

and postoperative epidural analgesia. The interpretation of the study results, however, was controversial, as the study was not blinded, analgesia in the control group was poor, and the study was terminated early. The results of other trials are shown in Table 16-10.

A study by Tuman et al.[138] in patients undergoing major vascular surgery produced similar results: the rates of infection and overall postoperative complications, and the duration of ICU stay were significantly reduced in patients randomized to receive combined general-epidural anesthesia followed by epidural analgesia, compared to general anesthesia followed by systemic opioid analgesia.[138] In addition, the general-epidural anesthesia/analgesia technique attenuated the state of hypercoagulability present in vascular surgical patients. This resulted in a lower incidence of thrombotic events, including peripheral arterial graft and coronary artery or deep venous thrombosis.

The beneficial effect of epidural anesthesia/analgesia compared to general anesthesia/systemic analgesia was also found in patients who underwent lower extremity vascular surgery.[139] Two of 49 patients in the epidural group required regrafting or thrombolectomy compared to 11 of 51 patients in the general anesthesia group. In contrast, the incidence of cardiac morbidity and mortality (myocardial

ischemia or infarction, unstable angina, or cardiac death) and the rate of major infection, renal failure, and pulmonary complications, were similar between groups.

Postoperative arterial thrombosis may be related to preoperative levels of plasminogen activator inhibitor-1 (PAI-1). PAI-1 levels increased in the first 24 h after surgery in patients who had general anesthesia,[140] while remaining unchanged in the patients who had epidural anesthesia/epidural opioid analgesia. In summary, early studies[137–139] showed conflicting results as to whether perioperative epidural anesthesia/analgesia has beneficial effects in reducing major morbidity and mortality after surgery. In addition, it is difficult to tease out the effects of epidural *anesthesia* versus epidural *analgesia*, as well as the effects of epidural local anesthetics compared to epidural opioids.

Other prospective randomized studies addressed the effects of perioperative neuraxial anesthesia/analgesia on perioperative mortality and morbidity.[141–143] Baron et al.[141] compared intraoperative thoracic epidural anesthesia combined with light general anesthesia with standard "balanced" general anesthesia. There were no differences between the groups in terms of cardiovascular morbidity, myocardial ischemia or infarction, or respiratory morbidity.[141] However, the authors could not exclude the possibility that postoperative epidural analgesia may favorably influence outcome, as the postoperative pain regimen in both groups was left to the responsibility of the attending anesthesiologist. Patients in both groups received subcutaneous morphine, epidural fentanyl, or epidural bupivacaine.[141]

The roles of intraoperative neuraxial anesthesia and postoperative epidural analgesia were better defined in a double-blinded study of patients undergoing abdominal aortic procedures.[143] Norris et al. compared four treatment groups: combined general-thoracic epidural anesthesia or general anesthesia alone, with either postoperative intravenous or epidural PCA. Postoperative outcomes were similar among the four groups with respect to death, myocardial infarction and ischemia, reoperation, pneumonia, and renal failure. Epidural PCA was associated with a significantly shorter time to extubation. However, the length of hospital stay and medical costs were similar among the four treatment groups.[143]

Similar findings were noted when epidural or spinal anesthesia was compared with general anesthesia in patients who underwent peripheral vascular surgery.[142] Postoperative pain control in the three groups was similar and not controlled by study protocol: intravenous morphine while the patients were in the ICU and either subcutaneous morphine, intravenous meperidine, or oral analgesics when the patients were in the hospital wards. Cardiovascular morbidity and overall mortality rates were not significantly different among the three groups.

Meta-Analysis: Effects of Neuraxial Analgesia on Cardiac, Pulmonary, and Gastrointestinal Outcomes

Most studies on the effects of perioperative epidural analgesia were underpowered as the cost of conducting large prospective, controlled studies is prohibitive. To compensate for inadequate numbers in individual studies, meta-analyses are often performed. The results of meta-analyses of studies comparing neuraxial to general anesthesia are summarized in Table 16-11.

Rodgers et al. analyzed studies that compared neuraxial anesthesia (spinal or epidural) with general anesthesia.[144] The analysis included 141 studies (9559 patients) published before 1997. Overall mortality rate was decreased by approximately one-third in the neuraxial group (103 deaths/4871 patients vs. 144 deaths/4688 patients, $P = 0.006$). Neuraxial blockade also reduced the odds of deep vein thrombosis by 44%, pulmonary embolism by 55%, transfusion requirements by 50%, pneumonia by 39%, and respiratory depression by 59% (all $P < 0.001$). There were no differences in the incidence of cardiac deaths between the techniques. The analysis suggested that the improved

---

Table 16-11

Summary of Meta-analyses: Epidural Anesthesia/Analgesia Compared to General Anesthesia/Systemic Analgesia

	Rodgers	Beattie	Ballantyne
Number of papers reviewed	141	11	48
Dates	Before 1997	1996–1998	1966–1995
Number of patients	9559	1173	Not stated
Comparisons	Neuraxial vs. general anesthesia	Postoperative epidural vs. systemic analgesia	Effect of systemic, epidural (local anesthetic and opioid), nerve block, and infiltration analgesic techniques on postoperative pulmonary function*
Significant differences favoring epidural anesthesia*	Mortality (103/4871 vs. 144/4688) Deep vein thrombosis, pulmonary embolism, transfusion requirements, pneumonia, respiratory depression	Mortality rate same Postoperative myocardial infarction	Epidural local anesthetics: decreased infection and overall pulmonary complications Epidural opioids: decreased incidence of atelectasis

*See text for details.
Source: Data from Refs. 55, 144, 145.

outcome was secondary to the use of neuraxial blockade rather than the avoidance of general anesthesia.[144]

A subsequent meta-analysis specifically analyzed the effect of epidural analgesia on postoperative myocardial infarction.[145] Studies published between 1966 and 1998 in which postoperative epidural analgesia (extended for at least 24 h after surgery) was compared to parenteral analgesia were included (1173 patients). The overall postoperative myocardial infarction rate was 6.3%, with lower rates in the epidural group (rate difference −3.8%; 95% CI, −7.4% to −0.2%; $P = 0.049$). Subgroup analysis comparing patients with thoracic epidural to systemic analgesia found a significant reduction in postoperative myocardial infarction (rate difference −5.3%; 95% CI, −9.9% to −0.7%; $P = 0.04$). There was no difference in the frequency of in-hospital death. The authors urged caution in the interpretation of their conclusions, as they had difficulty in determining cardiac risk within the study populations and because none of the reviewed trials was double-blinded.

A third meta-analysis looked at the effects of postoperative analgesic therapies on pulmonary outcome.[55] Forty-eight randomized trials published between 1996 and 1995 were included. The effects of several analgesic techniques on postoperative pulmonary function following a variety of surgical procedures were assessed: systemic opioid, epidural opioid, epidural local anesthetic, epidural opioid with local anesthetic, thoracic versus lumbar epidural opioid, intercostal nerve block, wound infiltration with local anesthetic, and intrapleural local anesthetic. Compared with systemic opioids, epidural opioids decreased the incidence of pulmonary atelectasis and had a weak tendency to reduce the incidence of pulmonary infections, and overall pulmonary complications. Epidural local anesthetics increased PaO_2 and decreased the incidence of pulmonary infections and overall pulmonary complications compared with systemic opioids. Intercostal nerve blocks tended to improve measures in pulmonary outcome (incidence of atelectasis and incidence of pulmonary complications overall) but the differences did not reach statistical significance. There were no significant differences in the surrogate measures of pulmonary function (forced expiratory volume in 1 s [FEV1], forced vital capacity [FVC], and PEFR). Together, the results of these meta-analyses support the use of epidural analgesia to reduce postoperative pulmonary morbidity (Table 16-11).

The pulmonary benefits of epidural analgesia may be secondary to blockade of the reflex inhibition of the phrenic nerve and diaphragmatic activation that occurs after major surgery.[146,147] Ballantyne et al.[55] noted that not all the studies that demonstrated superior analgesia with the experimental treatments (i.e., epidural analgesia) demonstrated improvements in pulmonary function. This suggests that factors other than pain are important in the etiology of postoperative pulmonary impairment.

Steinbrook reviewed the effects of epidural anesthesia on gastrointestinal motility.[148] If the epidural catheter was placed above T12, gastrointestinal function recovered significantly more rapidly in the patients who received epidural compared to systemic analgesia. Lumbar epidural catheters were not as consistently effective as thoracic catheters. Local anesthetics and local anesthetic-opioid mixtures seem to be more effective and have fewer side effects than epidural opioids alone.[148,149] The mechanisms by which thoracic epidural anesthesia promotes gastrointestinal motility includes blockade of thoracolumbar sympathetic efferent nerves, unopposed parasympathetic efferent nerve activity, blockade of nociceptive afferent impulses, reduced need for postoperative opioids, increased gastrointestinal blood flow, and systemic absorption of the local anesthetic.[148] Therefore, the congruency of the site of the vertebral level of epidural catheter placement to the site of abdominal incision, and the inclusion of local anesthetic in the epidural analgesia technique, are important in reducing postoperative ileus.

Subsequent Randomized Studies

Meta-analyses should be confirmed by large prospective, randomized studies.[150–152] Recently published large, randomized studies have not confirmed beneficial effects of perioperative epidural analgesia.[153–155] In a multicenter Veterans Affairs study of 1021 patients who underwent intra-abdominal aortic, gastric, biliary, or colon operations, there were no differences in mortality or morbidity between the epidural group (epidural plus light general anesthesia and postoperative epidural morphine analgesia) and the control group (general anesthesia and postoperative parenteral opioid analgesia) (Table 16-10).[153] In a secondary analysis, the investigators found that the patients randomized to the epidural group for aortic surgery had shorter intubation times and ICU stays.

A large ($n = 888$) multicenter Australian study, called the Multicentre Australian Study of Epidural Anesthesia or MASTER trial, compared combined general-epidural anesthesia/epidural analgesia and general anesthesia/intravenous opioid analgesia for major abdominal surgery in high-risk patients.[154] Inclusion criteria for high-risk patients included the presence of one of the following risk factors: morbid obesity, diabetes mellitus, chronic renal failure, respiratory insufficiency, major hepatocellular disease, myocardial ischemia, acute myocardial infarction, cardiac failure, age over 75 years; or two of the following risk factors: hypertension, cardiac dysrhythmia, moderate obesity, frailty, or previous myocardial infarction. The endpoints in the MASTER trial included perioperative death, cardiovascular event, renal failure, gastrointestinal failure, hepatic and hematologic failure, and the incidence of inflammation or sepsis.

Although postoperative analgesia was superior in the epidural group, there were no differences in mortality or the incidence of major morbidity between the groups, except the incidence of respiratory failure was lower in the epidural group (23% vs. 30%, $P = 0.02$) (Table 16-10). To determine if perioperative epidural analgesia resulted in beneficial effects in selected categories of high-risk patients (e.g., high-risk for respiratory or cardiac event, or aortic surgery), a predetermined subset of patients in the MASTER trial were analyzed separately.[155] There was a small reduction in the duration of postoperative ventilation in the epidural group, however, there was no difference in morbidity or mortality between the two groups, or in the length of ICU or hospital stay. Several criticisms have been leveled at the MASTER study.[156] These include the lack of clarity in the study protocol, such as whether the epidural catheter placement was congruent with the presumed site of nociceptive impulses, confirmation of epidural placement, duration of the intraoperative local anesthetic infusions and the postoperative local anesthetic-opioid infusions, establishment of criteria for extubation or length of stay in the ICU or hospital, and the presence of observer bias due to the lack of sham epidural placements.

The inability of large, prospective, randomized, and controlled studies to confirm the conclusions of the meta-analyses of smaller studies may be due to several reasons. These include the inclusion of older, outdated studies,[150] inclusion of studies with duplicated data, and publication bias in the meta-analyses studies. Publication biases may be secondary to the exclusion of non-English language trials and unpublished data.[136] Meta-analyses that include mainly small trials can overestimate the effect of treatment.[157] The assimilation of incidental data from studies that were primarily designed to examine other endpoints may increase the possibility of false positive findings. The conclusions of meta-analyses are based on nonoriginal data from studies that may vary in study design, subject population, and outcomes criteria.[136] Finally, it is entirely possible that the incremental advances in perioperative care will make it difficult to demonstrate major differences in outcome from any treatment modality.[155]

▶ Conclusions on Outcomes Research

The benefits of perioperative epidural analgesia in decreasing morbidity and mortality have not been completely proven. In a review written in 2000, Wu and Fleisher[136] concluded that the physiologic and analgesic benefits of postoperative epidural analgesia are influenced by the level of epidural catheter placement (catheter-incision congruent vs. incongruent placement), type of analgesic agent (whether local anesthetic was added in the infusion), and the duration of epidural analgesia. They noted that perioperative (intraoperative and postoperative) epidural anesthesia and analgesia may reduce postoperative mortality and morbidity and that the use of perioperative neuraxial anesthesia reduces overall mortality by approximately 30%. Thoracic, but not lumbar, epidural analgesia significantly decreases the incidence of postoperative myocardial infarction. High-thoracic epidural analgesia with local anesthetic blocks cardiac sympathetic outflow, attenuating increases in heart rate, blood pressure, inotropy, and myocardial oxygen consumption.[80,158] The administration of a neuraxial technique with local anesthetic diminishes perioperative hypercoagulability by increasing peripheral blood flow, decreasing blood viscosity, preserving fibrinolytic activity, and attenuating increases in coagulation factors. These factors result in lower vaso-occlusive and thromboembolic events postoperatively. Perioperative neuraxial anesthesia decreases the incidence of atelectasis and respiratory complications[55] and perioperative epidural analgesia facilitates postoperative extubation and shorter length of stay in the ICU in high-risk patients who underwent thoracic surgery.[133,159] The salutary effect of neuraxial anesthesia is secondary to the preservation of hypoxic pulmonary vasoconstriction in poorly ventilated segments of the lung, attenuation of the reflex inhibition of diaphragmatic activity, and decreased use of systemic opioids because of effective analgesia. Earlier return of gastrointestinal function occur when the catheter is incision-congruent.[80,149] Studies that limited epidural analgesia for less than 24 h showed no benefit in regard to the return of gastrointestinal function. A decreased incidence of postoperative myocardial infarction occurred when the epidural analgesia was used during the postoperative, but not intraoperative period alone.[80]

REFERENCES

1. Pert CB, Snyder SH. Opiate receptor: Demonstration in nervous tissue. *Science* 179:1011, 1973.
2. Hughes J, Smith TW, Kosterlitz HW, et al. Identification of two related pentapeptides from the brain with potent opiate agonist activity. *Nature* 258:577, 1975.
3. Lord JA, Waterfield AA, Hughes J, et al. Endogenous opioid peptides: Multiple agonists and receptors. *Nature* 267:495, 1977.
4. Yaksh TL, Rudy TA. Studies on the direct spinal action of narcotics in the production of analgesia in the rat. *J Pharmacol Exp Ther* 202:411, 1977.
5. Wang JK, Nauss LA, Thomas JE. Pain relief by intrathecally applied morphine in man. *Anesthesiology* 50:149, 1979.
6. Cousins MJ, Mather LE. Intrathecal and epidural administration of opioids. *Anesthesiology* 61:276, 1984.
7. Richman JM, Wu CL. Intrathecal opioid injections for postoperative pain. In: Benzon HT, Raja SN, Molloy RE, et al., eds, *Essentials of Pain Medicine and Regional Anesthesia*. Philadelphia, PA: Elsevier, 2005, p. 239.
8. Hansdottir V, Hedner T, Woestenborghs R, et al. The CSF and plasma pharmacokinetics of sufentanil after intrathecal administration. *Anesthesiology* 74:264, 1991.

9. Ngan Kee WD. Epidural pethidine: Pharmacology and clinical experience. *Anaesth Intensive Care* 26:247, 1998.

10. Kelly MC, Carabine UA, Mirakhur RK. Intrathecal diamorphine for analgesia after caesarean section. A dose finding study and assessment of side-effects. *Anaesthesia* 53:231, 1998.

11. Abouleish E, Rawal N, Fallon K, et al. Combined intrathecal morphine and bupivacaine for cesarean section. *Anesth Analg* 67:370, 1988.

12. Goyagi T, Nishikawa T. The addition of epinephrine enhances postoperative analgesia by intrathecal morphine. *Anesth Analg* 81:508, 1995.

13. Abouleish E, Rawal N, Tobon-Randall B, et al. A clinical and laboratory study to compare the addition of 0.2 mg of morphine, 0.2 mg of epinephrine, or their combination to hyperbaric bupivacaine for spinal anesthesia in cesarean section. *Anesth Analg* 77:457, 1993.

14. Goyagi T, Nishikawa T. Oral clonidine premedication enhances the quality of postoperative analgesia by intrathecal morphine. *Anesth Analg* 82:1192, 1996.

15. Mayson KV, Gofton EA, Chambers KG. Premedication with low dose oral clonidine does not enhance postoperative analgesia of intrathecal morphine. *Can J Anaesth* 47:752, 2000.

16. Lena P, Balarac N, Arnulf JJ, et al. Intrathecal morphine and clonidine for coronary artery bypass grafting. *Br J Anaesth* 90:300, 2003.

17. Sites BD, Beach M, Biggs R, et al. Intrathecal clonidine added to a bupivacaine-morphine spinal anesthetic improves postoperative analgesia for total knee arthroplasty. *Anesth Analg* 96:1083, 2003.

18. Grace D, Bunting H, Milligan KR, et al. Postoperative analgesia after co-administration of clonidine and morphine by the intrathecal route in patients undergoing hip replacement. *Anesth Analg* 80:86, 1995.

19. Chaney MA. Side effects of intrathecal and epidural opioids. *Can J Anaesth* 42:891, 1995.

20. Slappendel R, Weber EW, Benraad B, et al. Itching after intrathecal morphine. Incidence and treatment. *Eur J Anaesthesiol* 17:616, 2000.

21. Szarvas S, Harmon D, Murphy D. Neuraxial opioid-induced pruritus: A review. *J Clin Anesth* 15:234, 2003.

22. Kjellberg F, Tramer MR. Pharmacological control of opioid-induced pruritus: A quantitative systematic review of randomized trials. *Eur J Anaesthesiol* 18:346, 2001.

23. Wong CA, Scavone BM, Loffredi M, et al. The dose-response of intrathecal sufentanil added to bupivacaine for labor analgesia. *Anesthesiology* 92:1553, 2000.

24. Yeh HM, Chen LK, Lin CJ, et al. Prophylactic intravenous ondansetron reduces the incidence of intrathecal morphine-induced pruritus in patients undergoing cesarean delivery. *Anesth Analg* 91:172, 2000.

25. Charuluxananan S, Kyokong O, Somboonviboon W, et al. Nalbuphine versus ondansetron for prevention of intrathecal morphine-induced pruritus after cesarean delivery. *Anesth Analg* 96:1789, 2003.

26. Szarvas S, Chellapuri RS, Harmon DC, et al. A comparison of dexamethasone, ondansetron, and dexamethasone plus ondansetron as prophylactic antiemetic and antipruritic therapy in patients receiving intrathecal morphine for major orthopedic surgery. *Anesth Analg* 97:259, 2003.

27. Lee LH, Irwin MG, Lim J, et al. The effect of celecoxib on intrathecal morphine-induced pruritus in patients undergoing Caesarean section. *Anaesthesia* 59:876, 2004.

28. Charuluxananan S, Kyokong O, Somboonviboon W, et al. Nalbuphine versus propofol for treatment of intrathecal morphine-induced pruritus after cesarean delivery. *Anesth Analg* 93:162, 2001.

29. Alhashemi JA, Crosby ET, Grodecki W, et al. Treatment of intrathecal morphine-induced pruritus following caesarean section. *Can J Anaesth* 44:1060, 1997.

30. Borgeat A, Stirnemann HR. Ondansetron is effective to treat spinal or epidural morphine-induced pruritus. *Anesthesiology* 90:432, 1999.

31. Borgeat A, Ekatodramis G, Schenker CA. Postoperative nausea and vomiting in regional anesthesia: A review. *Anesthesiology* 98:530, 2003.

32. Dahl JB, Jeppesen IS, Jorgensen H, et al. Intraoperative and postoperative analgesic efficacy and adverse effects of intrathecal opioids in patients undergoing cesarean section with spinal anesthesia: A qualitative and quantitative systematic review of randomized controlled trials. *Anesthesiology* 91:1919, 1999.

33. Parlow JL, Costache I, Avery N, et al. Single-dose haloperidol for the prophylaxis of postoperative nausea and vomiting after intrathecal morphine. *Anesth Analg* 98:1072, 2004.

34. Davies PW, Vallejo MC, Shannon KT, et al. Oral herpes simplex reactivation after intrathecal morphine: A prospective randomized trial in an obstetric population. *Anesth Analg* 100:1472, 2005.

35. Bailey PL, Rhondeau S, Schafer PG, et al. Dose-response pharmacology of intrathecal morphine in human volunteers. *Anesthesiology* 79:49, 1993.

36. Palmer CM, Emerson S, Volgoropolous D, et al. Dose-response relationship of intrathecal morphine for postcesarean analgesia. *Anesthesiology* 90:437, 1999.

37. Cardoso MMSC, Carvalho JCA, Amaro AR. Small doses of intrathecal morphine combined with systemic diclofenac for post operative pain control after cesarean delivery. *Anesth Analg* 86:538, 1998.

38. Husaini SW, Russel IF. Intrathecal diamorphine compared with morphine for postoperative analgesia after Caesarean section under spinal anaesthesia. *Br J Anaesth* 81:135, 1998.

39. Campbell DC, Riben CM, Rooney ME, et al. Intrathecal morphine for postpartum tubal ligation postoperative analgesia. *Anesth Analg* 93:1006, 2001.

40. Rodanant O, Sirichotewithayakorn P, Sriprajittichai P, et al. An optimal dose study of intrathecal morphine in gynecological patients. *J Med Assoc Thai* 86(Suppl 2):S331, 2003.

41. Devys JM, Mora A, Plaud B, et al. Intrathecal + PCA morphine improves analgesia during the first 24 hr after major abdominal surgery compared to PCA alone. *Can J Anaesth* 50:355, 2003.

42. Yamaguchi H, Watanabe S, Motokawa K, et al. Intrathecal morphine dose-response data for pain relief after cholecystectomy. *Anesth Analg* 70:168, 1990.

43. Motamed C, Bouaziz H, Franco D, et al. Analgesic effect of low-dose intrathecal morphine and bupivacaine in laparoscopic cholecystectomy. *Anaesthesia* 55:118, 2000.

44. Kong SK, Onsiong SM, Chiu WK, et al. Use of intrathecal morphine for postoperative pain relief after elective laparoscopic colorectal surgery. *Anaesthesia* 57:1168, 2002.

45. Fleron MH, Weiskopf RB, Bertrand M, et al. A comparison of intrathecal opioid and intravenous analgesia for the incidence of cardiovascular, respiratory, and renal complications after abdominal aortic surgery. *Anesth Analg* 97:2, 2003.

46. Rathmell JP, Pino CA, Taylor R, et al. Intrathecal morphine for postoperative analgesia: A randomized, controlled, dose-ranging study after hip and knee arthroplasty. *Anesth Analg* 97:1452, 2003.

47. Murphy PM, Stack D, Kinirons B, et al. Optimizing the dose of intrathecal morphine in older patients undergoing hip arthroplasty. *Anesth Analg* 97:1709, 2003.

48. Boezaart AP, Eksteen JA, Spuy GV, et al. Intrathecal morphine. Double-blind evaluation of optimal dosage for analgesia after major lumbar spinal surgery. *Spine* 24:1131, 1999.

49. Urban MK, Jules-Elysee K, Urquhart B, et al. Reduction in postoperative pain after spinal fusion with instrumentation using intrathecal morphine. *Spine* 27:535, 2002.

50. Chaney MA, Furry PA, Fluder EM, et al. Intrathecal morphine for coronary artery bypass grafting and early extubation. *Anesth Analg* 84:241, 1997.

51. Chaney MA, Smith KR, Barclay JC, et al. Large-dose intrathecal morphine for coronary artery bypass grafting. *Anesth Analg* 83:215, 1996.

52. Vanstrum GS, Bjornson KM, Ilko R. Postoperative effects of intrathecal morphine in coronary artery bypass surgery. *Anesth Analg* 67:261, 1988.

53. Alhashemi JA, Sharpe MD, Harris CL, et al. Effect of subarachnoid morphine administration on extubation time after coronary artery bypass graft surgery. *J Cardiothorac Vasc Anesth* 14:639, 2000.

54. Jara FM, Klush J, Kilaru V. Intrathecal morphine for off-pump coronary artery bypass patients. *Heart Surg Forum* 4:57, 2001.

55. Ballantyne JC, Carr DB, deFerranti S, et al. The comparative effects of postoperative analgesic therapies on pulmonary outcome: Cumulative meta-analyses of randomized, controlled trials. *Anesth Analg* 86:598, 1998.

56. Mason N, Gondret R, Junca A, et al. Intrathecal sufentanil and morphine for post-thoracotomy pain relief. *Br J Anaesth* 86:236, 2001.

57. Liu N, Kuhlman G, Dalibon N, et al. A randomized, double-blinded comparison of intrathecal morphine, sufentanil and their combination versus IV morphine patient-controlled analgesia for postthoracotomy pain. *Anesth Analg* 92:31, 2001.

58. McCrory C, Diviney D, Moriarty J, et al. Comparison between repeat bolus intrathecal morphine and an epidurally delivered bupivacaine and fentanyl combination in the management of post-thoracotomy pain with or without cyclooxygenase inhibition. *J Cardiothorac Vasc Anesth* 16:607, 2002.

59. Sakai T, Use T, Shimamoto H, et al. Mini-dose (0.05 mg) intrathecal morphine provides effective analgesia after transurethral resection of the prostate. *Can J Anaesth* 50:1027, 2003.

60. Bernards CM, Shen DD, Sterling ES, et al. Epidural, cerebrospinal fluid, and plasma pharmacokinetics of epidural opioids (part 1): Differences among opioids. *Anesthesiology* 99:455, 2003.

61. Ummenhofer WC, Arends RH, Shen DD, et al. Comparative spinal distribution and clearance kinetics of intrathecally administered morphine, fentanyl, alfentanil, and sufentanil. *Anesthesiology* 92:739, 2000.

62. Birnbach DJ, Johnson MD, Arcario T, et al. Effect of diluent volume on analgesia produced by epidural fentanyl. *Anesth Analg* 68:808, 1989.

63. Dottrens M, Rifat K, Morel DR. Comparison of extradural administration of sufentanil, morphine and sufentanil-morphine combination after caesarean section. *Br J Anaesth* 69:9, 1992.

64. Loper KA, Ready LB, Downey M, et al. Epidural and intravenous fentanyl infusions are clinically equivalent after knee surgery. *Anesth Analg* 70:72, 1990.

65. Sandler AN, Stringer D, Panos L, et al. A randomized, double-blind comparison of lumbar epidural and intravenous fentanyl infusions for postthoracotomy pain relief. Analgesic, pharmacokinetic, and respiratory effects. *Anesthesiology* 77:626, 1992.

66. Guinard JP, Mavrocordatos P, Chiolero R, et al. A randomized comparison of intravenous versus lumbar and thoracic epidural fentanyl for analgesia after thoracotomy. *Anesthesiology* 77:1108, 1992.

67. Salomaki TE, Laitinen JO, Nuutinen LS. A randomized double-blind comparison of epidural versus intravenous fentanyl infusion for analgesia after thoracotomy. *Anesthesiology* 75:790, 1991.

68. de Leon-Casasola OA, Lema MJ. Postoperative epidural opioid analgesia: What are the choices? *Anesth Analg* 83:867, 1996.

69. Loper KA, Ready LB. Epidural morphine after anterior cruciate ligament repair: A comparison with patient-controlled intravenous morphine. *Anesth Analg* 68:350, 1989.

70. Rauck RL, Raj PP, Knarr DC, et al. Comparison of the efficacy of epidural morphine given by intermittent injection or continuous infusion for the management of postoperative pain. *Reg Anesth* 19:316, 1994.

71. Malviya S, Pandit UA, Merkel S, et al. A comparison of continuous epidural infusion and intermittent intravenous bolus doses of morphine in children undergoing selective dorsal rhizotomy. *Reg Anesth Pain Med* 24:438, 1999.

72. Chestnut DH, Owen CL, Bates JN, et al. Continuous infusion epidural analgesia during labor: A randomized, double-blind comparison of 0.0625% bupivacaine/0.0002% fentanyl versus 0.125% bupivacaine. *Anesthesiology* 68:754, 1988.

73. George KA, Wright PM, Chisakuta A. Continuous thoracic epidural fentanyl for post-thoracotomy pain relief: With or without bupivacaine? *Anaesthesia* 46:732, 1991.

74. Dahl JB, Rosenberg J, Hansen BL, et al. Differential analgesic effects of low-dose epidural morphine and morphine-bupivacaine at rest and during mobilization after major abdominal surgery. *Anesth Analg* 74:362, 1992.

75. Badner NH, Reimer EJ, Komar WE, et al. Low-dose bupivacaine does not improve postoperative epidural fentanyl analgesia in orthopedic patients. *Anesth Analg* 72:337, 1991.

76. Badner NH, Komar WE. Bupivacaine 0.1% does not improve post-operative epidural fentanyl analgesia after abdominal or thoracic surgery. *Can J Anaesth* 39:330, 1992.

77. Parker RK, Sawaki Y, White PF. Epidural patient-controlled analgesia: Influence of bupivacaine and hydromorphone basal infusion on pain control after cesarean delivery. *Anesth Analg* 75:740, 1992.

78. Benzon HT, Wong CA, Wong HY, et al. The effect of low-dose bupivacaine on postoperative epidural fentanyl analgesia and thrombelastography. *Anesth Analg* 79:911, 1994.

79. Karambelkar DJ, Ramanathan S. 2-Chloroprocaine antagonism of epidural morphine analgesia. *Acta Anaesthesiol Scand* 41:774, 1997.

80. Wu C, Thomsen R. Effect of postoperative epidural analgesia on patient outcomes. *Tech Reg Anesth Pain Manag* 7:140, 2003.

81. Block BM, Liu SS, Rowlingson AJ, et al. Efficacy of postoperative epidural analgesia: A meta-analysis. *JAMA* 290:2455, 2003.

82. Bernard JM, Kick O, Bonnet F. Comparison of intravenous and epidural clonidine for postoperative patient-controlled analgesia. *Anesth Analg* 81:706, 1995.

83. De Kock M, Famenne F, Deckers G, et al. Epidural clonidine or sufentanil for intraoperative and postoperative analgesia. *Anesth Analg* 81:1154, 1995.

84. Vercauteren MP, Saldien V, Bosschaerts P, et al. Potentiation of sufentanil by clonidine in PCEA with or without basal infusion. *Eur J Anaesthesiol* 13:571, 1996.

85. Samso E, Valles J, Pol O, et al. Comparative assessment of the anaesthetic and analgesic effects of intramuscular and epidural clonidine in humans. *Can J Anaesth* 43:1195, 1996.

86. De Kock M, Wiederkher P, Laghmiche A, et al. Epidural clonidine used as the sole analgesic agent during and after abdominal surgery. A dose-response study. *Anesthesiology* 86:285, 1997.

87. Paech MJ, Pavy TJ, Orlikowski CE, et al. Postoperative epidural infusion: A randomized, double-blind, dose-finding trial of clonidine in combination with bupivacaine and fentanyl. *Anesth Analg* 84:1323, 1997.

88. Curatolo M, Schnider TW, Petersen-Felix S, et al. A direct search procedure to optimize combinations of epidural bupivacaine, fentanyl, and clonidine for postoperative analgesia. *Anesthesiology* 92:325, 2000.

89. Sveticic G, Gentilini A, Eichenberger U, et al. Combinations of bupivacaine, fentanyl, and clonidine for lumbar epidural postoperative analgesia: A novel optimization procedure. *Anesthesiology* 101:1381, 2004.

90. Armand S, Langlade A, Boutros A, et al. Meta-analysis of the efficacy of extradural clonidine to relieve postoperative pain: An impossible task. *Br J Anaesth* 81:126, 1998.

91. De Negri P, Ivani G, Visconti C, et al. The dose-response relationship for clonidine added to a postoperative continuous epidural infusion of ropivacaine in children. *Anesth Analg* 93:71, 2001.

92. Klamt JG, Garcia LV, Stocche RM, et al. Epidural infusion of clonidine or clonidine plus ropivacaine for postoperative analgesia in children undergoing major abdominal surgery. *J Clin Anesth* 15:510, 2003.

93. Wong CS, Liaw WJ, Tung CS, et al. Ketamine potentiates analgesic effect of morphine in postoperative epidural pain control. *Reg Anesth* 21:534, 1996.

94. Abdel-Ghaffar ME, Abdulatif MA, al-Ghamdi A, et al. Epidural ketamine reduces post-operative epidural PCA consumption of fentanyl/bupivacaine. *Can J Anaesth* 45:103, 1998.

95. Tan PH, Kuo MC, Kao PF, et al. Patient-controlled epidural analgesia with morphine or morphine plus ketamine for postoperative pain relief. *Eur J Anaesthesiol* 16:820, 1999.

96. Chia YY, Liu K, Liu YC, et al. Adding ketamine in a multimodal patient-controlled epidural regimen reduces postoperative pain and analgesic consumption. *Anesth Analg* 86:1245, 1998.

97. Himmelseher S, Ziegler-Pithamitsis D, Argiriadou H, et al. Small-dose S(+)-ketamine reduces postoperative pain when applied with ropivacaine in epidural anesthesia for total knee arthroplasty. *Anesth Analg* 92:1290, 2001.

98. Subramaniam K, Subramaniam B, Steinbrook RA. Ketamine as adjuvant analgesic to opioids: A quantitative and qualitative systematic review. *Anesth Analg* 99:482, 2004.

99. Subramaniam B, Subramaniam K, Pawar DK, et al. Preoperative epidural ketamine in combination with morphine does not have a clinically relevant intra- and postoperative opioid-sparing effect. *Anesth Analg* 93:1321, 2001.

100. Baron CM, Kowalski SE, Greengrass R, et al. Epinephrine decreases postoperative requirements for continuous thoracic epidural fentanyl infusions. *Anesth Analg* 82:760, 1996.

101. Niemi G, Breivik H. Adrenaline markedly improves thoracic epidural analgesia produced by a low-dose infusion of bupivacaine, fentanyl and adrenaline. A randomised, double-blind, cross-over study with and without adrenaline. *Acta Anaesthesiol Scand* 42:897, 1998.

102. Sakaguchi Y, Sakura S, Shinzawa M, et al. Does adrenaline improve epidural bupivacaine and fentanyl analgesia after abdominal surgery? *Anaesth Intensive Care* 28:522, 2000.

103. Niemi G, Breivik H. The minimally effective concentration of adrenaline in a low-concentration thoracic epidural analgesic infusion of bupivacaine, fentanyl and adrenaline after major surgery. A randomized, double-blind, dose-finding study. *Acta Anaesthesiol Scand* 47:439, 2003.

104. Nishiyama T, Yokoyama T, Hanaoka K. Midazolam improves postoperative epidural analgesia with continuous infusion of local anaesthetics. *Can J Anaesth* 45:551, 1998.

105. Nishiyama T, Matsukawa T, Hanaoka K. Effects of adding midazolam on the postoperative epidural analgesia with two different doses of bupivacaine. *J Clin Anesth* 14:92, 2002.

106. Nishiyama T, Hanaoka K. Effect of diluent volume on post-operative analgesia and sedation produced by epidurally administered midazolam. *Eur J Anaesthesiol* 15:275, 1998.

107. Horta ML, Ramos L, Goncalves ZR. The inhibition of epidural morphine-induced pruritus by epidural droperidol. *Anesth Analg* 90:638, 2000.

108. Kotake Y, Matsumoto M, Ai K, et al. Additional droperidol, not butorphanol, augments epidural fentanyl analgesia following anorectal surgery. *J Clin Anesth* 12:9, 2000.

109. Nakata K, Mammoto T, Kita T, et al. Continuous epidural, not intravenous, droperidol inhibits pruritus, nausea, and vomiting during epidural morphine analgesia. *J Clin Anesth* 14:121, 2002.

110. Lauretti GR, de Oliveira R, Reis MP, et al. Study of three different doses of epidural neostigmine coadministered with lidocaine for postoperative analgesia. *Anesthesiology* 90:1534, 1999.

111. Lauretti GR, de Oliveira R, Perez MV, et al. Postoperative analgesia by intraarticular and epidural neostigmine following knee surgery. *J Clin Anesth* 12:444, 2000.

112. Omais M, Lauretti GR, Paccola CA. Epidural morphine and neostigmine for postoperative analgesia after orthopedic surgery. *Anesth Analg* 95:1698, 2002.

113. Lee J, Shim JY, Choi JH, et al. Epidural naloxone reduces intestinal hypomotility but not analgesia of epidural morphine. *Can J Anaesth* 48:54, 2001.

114. Wang JJ, Tzeng JI, Ho ST, et al. The prophylactic effect of tropisetron on epidural morphine-related nausea and vomiting: A comparison of dexamethasone with saline. *Anesth Analg* 94:749, 2002.

115. Tzeng JI, Hsing CH, Chu CC, et al. Low-dose dexamethasone reduces nausea and vomiting after epidural morphine: A comparison of metoclopramide with saline. *J Clin Anesth* 14:19, 2002.

116. White MJ, Berghausen EJ, Dumont SW, et al. Side effects during continuous epidural infusion of morphine and fentanyl. *Can J Anaesth* 39:576, 1992.

117. Gedney JA, Liu EH. Side-effects of epidural infusions of opioid bupivacaine mixtures. *Anaesthesia* 53:1148, 1998.

118. Casey Z, Wu CL. Epidural opioids for postoperative pain. In: Benzon HT, Raja S, Molloy RE, et al., eds, *Essentials of Pain Medicine and Regional Anesthesia*. New York: W.B. Saunders, 2005, p. 246.

119. Walder B, Schafer M, Henzi I, et al. Efficacy and safety of patient-controlled opioid analgesia for acute postoperative pain. A quantitative systematic review. *Acta Anaesthesiol Scand* 45:795, 2001.

120. Bucklin BA, Chestnut DH, Hawkins JL. Intrathecal opioids versus epidural local anesthetics for labor analgesia: A meta-analysis. *Reg Anesth Pain Med* 27:23, 2002.

121. O'Riordan JA, Hopkins PM, Ravenscroft A, et al. Patient-controlled analgesia and urinary retention following lower limb joint replacement: Prospective audit and logistic regression analysis. *Eur J Anaesthesiol* 17:431, 2000.

122. Wang J, Pennefather S, Russell G. Low-dose naloxone in the treatment of urinary retention during epidural fentanyl causes excessive reversal of analgesia. *Br J Anaesth* 80:565, 1998.

123. Ready LB, Loper KA, Nessly M, et al. Postoperative epidural morphine is safe on surgical wards. *Anesthesiology* 75:452, 1991.

124. de Leon-Casasola OA, Parker B, Lema MJ, et al. Postoperative epidural bupivacaine-morphine therapy. Experience with 4,227 surgical cancer patients. *Anesthesiology* 81:368, 1994.

125. de Leon-Casasola OA, Parker BM, Lema MJ, et al. Epidural analgesia versus intravenous patient-controlled analgesia. Differences in the postoperative course of cancer patients. *Reg Anesth* 19:307, 1994.

126. Etches RC. Respiratory depression associated with patient-controlled analgesia: A review of eight cases. *Can J Anaesth* 41:125, 1994.

127. Mulroy MF. Monitoring opioids. *Reg Anesth* 21:89, 1996.

128. Bailey PL, Rhondeau S, Schafer PG, et al. Dose-response pharmacology of intrathecal morphine in human volunteers. *Anesthesiology* 79:49, 1993.

129. Chisakuta AM, George KA, Hawthorne CT. Postoperative epidural infusion of a mixture of bupivacaine 0.2% with fentanyl for upper abdominal surgery. A comparison of thoracic and lumbar routes. *Anaesthesia* 50:72, 1995.

130. Liu SS, Allen HW, Olsson GL. Patient-controlled epidural analgesia with bupivacaine and fentanyl on hospital wards: Prospective experience with 1,030 surgical patients. *Anesthesiology* 88:688, 1998.

131. Magnusdottir H, Kirno K, Ricksten SE, et al. High thoracic epidural anesthesia does not inhibit sympathetic nerve activity in the lower extremities. *Anesthesiology* 91:1299, 1999.

132. Horlocker TT, Wedel DJ, Benzon H, et al. Regional anesthesia in the anticoagulated patient: Defining the risks (the second ASRA Consensus Conference on Neuraxial Anesthesia and Anticoagulation). *Reg Anesth Pain Med* 28:172, 2003.

133. Stenseth R, Bjella L, Berg EM, et al. Effects of thoracic epidural analgesia on pulmonary function after coronary artery bypass surgery. *Eur J Cardiothorac Surg* 10:859, 1996.

134. Dolin SJ, Cashman JN, Bland JM. Effectiveness of acute postoperative pain management: I. Evidence from published data. *Br J Anaesth* 89:409, 2002.

135. Benzon HT, Wong HY, Belavic AM Jr, et al. A randomized double-blind comparison of epidural fentanyl infusion versus patient-controlled analgesia with morphine for postthoracotomy pain. *Anesth Analg* 76:316, 1993.

136. Wu CL, Fleisher LA. Outcomes research in regional anesthesia and analgesia. *Anesth Analg* 91:1232, 2000.

137. Yeager MP, Glass DD, Neff RK, et al. Epidural anesthesia and analgesia in high-risk surgical patients. *Anesthesiology* 66:729, 1987.

138. Tuman KJ, McCarthy RJ, March RJ, et al. Effects of epidural anesthesia and analgesia on coagulation and outcome after major vascular surgery. *Anesth Analg* 73:696, 1991.

139. Christopherson R, Beattie C, Frank SM, et al. Perioperative morbidity in patients randomized to epidural or general anesthesia for lower extremity vascular surgery. Perioperative Ischemia Randomized Anesthesia Trial Study Group. *Anesthesiology* 79:422, 1993.

140. Rosenfeld BA, Beattie C, Christopherson R, et al. The effects of different anesthetic regimens on fibrinolysis and the development of postoperative arterial thrombosis. Perioperative Ischemia Randomized Anesthesia Trial Study Group. *Anesthesiology* 79:435, 1993.

141. Baron JF, Bertrand M, Barre E, et al. Combined epidural and general anesthesia versus general anesthesia for abdominal aortic surgery. *Anesthesiology* 75:611, 1991.

142. Bode RH Jr, Lewis KP, Zarich SW, et al. Cardiac outcome after peripheral vascular surgery. Comparison of general and regional anesthesia. *Anesthesiology* 84:3, 1996.

143. Norris EJ, Beattie C, Perler BA, et al. Double-masked randomized trial comparing alternate combinations of intraoperative anesthesia and postoperative analgesia in abdominal aortic surgery. *Anesthesiology* 95:1054, 2001.

144. Rodgers A, Walker N, Schug S, et al. Reduction of postoperative mortality and morbidity with epidural or spinal anaesthesia: Results from overview of randomised trials. *BMJ* 321:1493, 2000.

145. Beattie WS, Badner NH, Choi P. Epidural analgesia reduces postoperative myocardial infarction: A meta-analysis. *Anesth Analg* 93:853, 2001.

146. Manikian B, Cantineau JP, Bertrand M, et al. Improvement of diaphragmatic function by a thoracic extradural block after upper abdominal surgery. *Anesthesiology* 68:379, 1988.

147. Pansard JL, Mankikian B, Bertrand M, et al. Effects of thoracic extradural block on diaphragmatic electrical activity and contractility after upper abdominal surgery. *Anesthesiology* 78:63, 1993.

148. Steinbrook RA. Epidural anesthesia and gastrointestinal motility. *Anesth Analg* 86:837, 1998.

149. Hodgson PS, Liu SS. Thoracic epidural anesthesia and analgesia for abdominal surgery: Effects on gastrointestinal function and perfusion. *Baillieres Clin Anaesthesiol* 13:9, 1999.

150. LeLorier J, Gregoire G, Benhaddad A, et al. Discrepancies between meta-analyses and subsequent large randomized, controlled trials. *N Engl J Med* 337:536, 1997.

151. Myles PS. Why we need large randomized studies in anaesthesia. *Br J Anaesth* 83:833, 1999.

152. Rigg JR, Jamrozik K, Myles PS, et al. Design of the multicenter Australian study of epidural anesthesia and analgesia in major surgery: The MASTER trial. *Control Clin Trials* 21:244, 2000.

153. Park WY, Thompson JS, Lee KK. Effect of epidural anesthesia and analgesia on perioperative outcome: A randomized, controlled Veterans Affairs cooperative study. *Ann Surg* 234:560, 2001.

154. Rigg JR, Jamrozik K, Myles PS, et al. Epidural anaesthesia and analgesia and outcome of major surgery: A randomised trial. *Lancet* 359:1276, 2002.

155. Peyton PJ, Myles PS, Silbert BS, et al. Perioperative epidural analgesia and outcome after major abdominal surgery in high-risk patients. *Anesth Analg* 96:548, 2003.

156. de Leon-Casasola OA. When it comes to outcome, we need to define what a perioperative epidural technique is. *Anesth Analg* 96:315, 2003.

157. Pogue J, Yusuf S. Overcoming the limitations of current meta-analysis of randomised controlled trials. *Lancet* 351:47, 1998.

158. Liu S, Carpenter RL, Neal JM. Epidural anesthesia and analgesia. Their role in postoperative outcome. *Anesthesiology* 82:1474, 1995.

159. Turfrey DJ, Ray DA, Sutcliffe NP, et al. Thoracic epidural anaesthesia for coronary artery bypass graft surgery. Effects on postoperative complications. *Anaesthesia* 52:1090, 1997.

Neuraxial Techniques for Management and Prevention of Chronic Pain

Antoun M. Nader
Robert E. Molloy

This chapter considers the use of neuraxial techniques for the prevention and management of chronic pain. With this goal in mind, four chronic pain syndromes are discussed: lumbar radiculopathy, complex regional pain syndrome (CRPS), postherpetic neuralgia (PHN), and phantom limb pain. In each instance, epidural injection or analgesia may play an important role in pain management or prevention.

LUMBAR RADICULOPATHY AND EPIDURAL STEROID INJECTION

Epidemiology

The International Association for the Study of Pain defines pain as "an unpleasant sensory and emotional experience associated with actual or potential tissue damage, or described in terms of such damage."[1] Back pain (estimated life time prevalence of 60–90%[2]) has very serious physical, social, and economic consequences. Acute low back pain is the fifth most common reason for a visit to the physician and nonsurgical low back pain is the fourth most common admission diagnosis for patients over age 65.[3,4] Chronic back pain (3–6 months) is the second most frequent chronic pain problem for which patients seek medical help, and it is the most common cause of work-related disability in people under 45 years of age. Acute back pain resolves spontaneously in 90% of cases. However, more than half of the patients will have another episode within a few years.[5] In addition, when the pain complaints persist (10%), back pain evolves into a chronic pain syndrome with physical (patient deconditioning), behavioral, and neurophysiologic ramifications. Therefore, appropriate treatment and follow-up are very important, and neuraxial injections have become an accepted tool to increase function and decrease pain, especially when there is an associated radicular component (pain along the distribution of a nerve root). Lumbar radiculopathy may have a favorable response to epidural steroid injections with a mild to moderate improvement in leg pain, improvement in sensory deficits, and reduction in the need for analgesics (see below).[6]

Clinical Features

Lumbar radicular pain is usually described as sharp, stabbing, and radiating from the lower back to the affected extremity. It is often severe, and is exaggerated by sitting, coughing, and sneezing. The onset is abrupt, and the patient usually has a difficult time finding a position of comfort. More than 95% of lumbar radicular symptoms occur in the L4, L5, or S1 distribution. Involvement of the L4 nerve root results in diminished patellar reflex, weakness of knee extension, hip flexion, hip adduction, and sensory loss in the medial leg (Table 17-1). Involvement of the L5 nerve root results in weakness of the great toe extensors and dorsiflexors of the foot, and sensory loss on the dorsum of the foot and in the first web space. Involvement of the S1 nerve root results in a diminished ankle reflex, weakness of the plantar flexors, and sensory loss of the posterior calf and lateral foot. With a large central disc herniation, compression of the cauda equina may result in bilateral radicular signs and sphincter disturbances. L1 to L3 radiculopathies refer pain to the groin and anterior thigh and often do not radiate beyond the knee. Lumbar radicular pain is associated with an antalgic gait (trunk shift), a reduced range of spinal movement, a reduced straight leg raise (less than 45 degrees), and a positive neural stretch test.

It is important to inquire about any recent trauma (possibility of a fracture); any signs that may indicate serious spinal pathology (red flags) such as spinal cord tumor (Box 17-1); and for psychosocial factors that are indicative of chronicity and disability (Box 17-2).[7]

Table 17-1

Clinical Findings in Lumbosacral Radiculopathies

Root Affected	Pain Distribution	Sensory Distribution	Motor Distribution	Reflexes
S1	Posterior thigh Posterior leg Lateral foot	Posterolateral leg Lateral foot	Foot/toe plantar flexion Knee flexion Hip extension	Achilles
L5	Posterolateral thigh Lateral leg Medial foot	Lateral leg Dorsal foot Great toe	Foot/toe dorsiflexion Knee flexion Hip extension	
L4	Anterior thigh Medial leg	Medial leg Medial malleolus	Knee extension Hip flexion Hip adduction	Patellar
L3	Anterior thigh Knee	Distal anteromedial thigh	Knee extension Hip flexion Hip adduction	Patellar Thigh adductors
L2	Inguinal region Anterior thigh	Anterior thigh	Hip flexion Hip adduction	Cremasteric Thigh adductors

Data from Ref. 2.

The diagnosis is usually based on history, physical examination, and review of available studies. Magnetic resonance imaging (MRI) is the most helpful diagnostic imaging test in identifying spinal pathology; electromyography and nerve conduction velocity (EMG/NCV) studies are helpful if peripheral neuropathy, peripheral nerve entrapment, or nerve injury is suspected. Flexion/extension films are requested if spinal instability is suspected. Computerized tomography (CT) and myelography are helpful when MRI is not available. The differential diagnosis of lumbar radicular pain is listed in Box 17-3. There is a wealth of information that can be obtained from imaging of the spine prior to an intervention. However, an MRI is not required in every patient. Imaging of the spine should be reserved for cases when there is a diagnostic dilemma or in the presence of red flags (Box 17-2).

▶ Treatment

In the absence of serious spinal pathology, acute back pain and radiculopathy should be treated conservatively with oral analgesics, short-term oral steroid use and/or epidural steroid injections, and adjunct physiotherapy. The patient is

Box 17-1

Indicators for Serious Spinal Pathology (Red Flags) with Complaint of Lower Back Pain

- Fever
- Unexplained weight loss
- Bladder and bowel dysfunction
- Rapidly progressing neurologic deficit
- Saddle anesthesia
- Abnormal gait
- History of cancer (carcinoma)
- Abnormal presentation (thoracic pain)
- Associated comorbidities and older age

Box 17-2

Psychosocial Factors Suggesting Chronicity and Disability with Lower Back Pain

- Depression
- Social withdrawal
- Reduced activity level
- Secondary gain
- Negative attitude toward treatment

Box 17-3

Differential Diagnosis of Lumbar Radicular Pain

▸ Herniated nucleus propulsus

▸ Demyelinating conditions

▸ Extraspinal nerve entrapment

▸ Trochanteric bursitis

▸ Piriformis muscle syndrome

▸ Thoracic and intraspinal pathology

▸ Cauda equina syndrome

Box 17-4

Proposed Mechanisms of Action of Steroids in the Treatment of Herniated Nucleus Pulposus

▸ Prostaglandin synthesis inhibition

▸ Membrane stabilization

▸ Inhibition of neuropeptide synthesis and action

▸ Inhibition of phospholipase A2 activity

▸ Inhibition of the vasoneurium vascular response

▸ Anesthetic-like action (C fibers)

---

usually advised to resume normal activity as appropriate (guided by pain restriction) as soon as possible. In a systematic review of randomized controlled trials of conservative treatment of sciatica, Vroomen et al.[8] considered traction, exercise therapy, and drug therapy, concluding that none of these interventions was unequivocally effective. However, they reported that epidural steroid injection may be beneficial in a subgroup of patients with nerve compression. Although the majority of patients with back pain have a favorable course, patients with intractable leg pain, recurrent episodes of radiculopathy, perianal numbness, motor loss or severe single nerve root paralysis, progressive neurologic deficit, cauda equina syndrome, urinary retention, or prolonged symptoms (12 weeks) should be referred to a multidisciplinary pain clinic for immediate evaluation.

▸ Epidural Steroid Injection

Rationale

A possible chemical mechanism for radicular pain was first hypothesized in 1977. After intervertebral disc injury, the enzyme phospholipase A2 is released from the disc. Phospholipase A2 in turn releases arachidonic acid into the epidural space, propagating an inflammatory response, mediated through leukotrienes and prostaglandins. In addition, after noxious stimulation of the dorsal root ganglia, neuropeptides (such as substance P and calcitonin gene-related peptide) are released, which potentiate the inflammatory response. Corticosteroids have known anti-inflammatory properties related to the inhibition of prostaglandin synthesis. Other possible mechanisms of action include membrane stabilization, inhibition of neuropeptide synthesis or action, blocking phospholipase A2 activity, and blocking the endoneural increase in vascular permeability induced by the released inflammatory substances.[9] Corticosteroids also have an anesthetic-like action, in that they block the nociceptive C fibers independent of their anti-inflammatory properties (Box 17-4).

Clinical Indications

Basic science evidence and practical experience support lumbar epidural steroid injection as a valid treatment component for lumbosacral radicular pain syndromes resulting from disc herniation.[10] A meta-analysis of this literature was published by Watts and Silagy in 1995.[11] Efficacy was defined as pain relief (at least 75% improvement) in the short (60 days) and long term (1 year). Epidural steroid injection increased the odds ratio of pain relief to 2.61 in the short term and to 1.87 in the long term. Efficacy was independent of the route of administration (i.e., caudal or lumbar). Also, epidural steroid injection may be beneficial for some discogenic axial pain syndromes caused by an annular tear. Steroid injection is especially beneficial in the early stages of treatment or when the patient is suffering a flare up, as it is associated with relatively prolonged pain relief without excessive opioid intake. Additional injections should be deferred for at least 1 week to allow time to assess therapeutic effect of the corticosteroid. Suppression of the hypothalamic-pituitary-adrenal axis may persist for 3 weeks, although plasma levels of steroid are not detected.

Injection of the Steroid

Corticosteroids may be administered orally. However, injection of steroids in the epidural space theoretically may yield a higher concentration of agent in the target area. It is less likely to be affected by local blood flow, which is frequently impaired in compressive lesions. The route of epidural steroid injection may also affect the target site concentration; caudal or interlaminar epidural steroid injections are affected by the presence of scar tissue in the epidural space, especially in postlaminectomy syndromes. Although epidural steroid injection for the treatment of radicular pain is a widely used procedure, some inconsistency exists in the literature as to the type of steroid injected, the volume of the injectate, and the requirement for fluoroscopic guidance.

> **Box 17-5**
>
> ## Interlaminar Vs. Transforaminal Epidural Steroid Injection
>
> | Interlaminar | Transforaminal |
> | --- | --- |
> | May be done without radiologic guidance | Radiologic guidance necessary |
> | Posterior epidural space | Anterior epidural-radicular space |
> | Bilateral spread | Diagnostic value (nerve root block) |
> | Affected by the presence of scar tissue | Therapeutic for foraminal and extraforaminal herniations |

Data are conflicting as to the success rate of blind (performed without radiologic guidance) epidural steroid injection techniques. The results of some studies suggest that the blind performance of epidural steroid injection is associated with misplacement of the steroid up to 40% of the time with the caudal technique and up to 30% of the time with the interlaminar technique.[12–14] Traditionally, radiologists have reported low success rates with blind injection of epidural steroid (48–62% success[13]) but a 99% success rate using fluoroscopy and radiologic contrast material.[15] However, anesthesiologists reported a 99% success rate in providing epidural anesthesia using a blind loss-of-resistance (LOR) technique and a 17-gauge Tuohy needle without image guidance.[16] Even in patients with previous back surgery, success rates of 88–91% have been reported.[17] Using a 20-gauge epidural needle, Liu et al.[18] reported that the sensitivity of the LOR technique for identification of the epidural space is 99% with a positive predictive value of 92%. The reported specificity of the LOR was 92% with a negative predictive value of 75%.

Fluoroscopy is an essential component of the transforaminal approach to the epidural space, which has the advantage of placing the agent in the anterior epidural space, closer to the site of pathology (Box 17-5). This route of administration is also of diagnostic value. Injection of a small volume (up to 3 mL) of local anesthetic with steroids, at a single segmental level is used to determine whether a particular nerve root is responsible for the radicular symptoms. In addition, this route of administration may have a theoretical advantage in foraminal or extraforaminal disc herniations. A theoretical advantage of transforaminal epidural steroid injection for radicular pain has been proposed but not clearly demonstrated in clinical studies.[10,19]

The caudal approach to epidural steroid injection may be preferred when spread of injectate to sacral nerves is desired. However, spread to the level of lumbar nerve roots is unpredictable, particularly in patients with previous back surgery. A radiopaque catheter may be inserted to better target a specific nerve root.

Cervical epidural steroid injection has been used to treat cervical radicular pain as well as head and neck pain. Anatomic studies have demonstrated high rates of discontinuity of the ligamentum flavum in the cervical region. This may predispose to a higher rate of false positive identification of the epidural space. In addition, the consequence of unrecognized intrathecal or intravascular injection during blind cervical epidural steroid injection may lead to severe neurologic sequelae. The use of fluoroscopic guidance and contrast epidurography is strongly suggested.[20] Cervical transforaminal epidural steroid injection may be associated with increased risk of serious neurologic sequelae.[20]

The general consensus is that fluoroscopic guidance is usually helpful. If the first injection is done without fluoroscopy and is ineffective, a second injection should be done with fluoroscopy to ensure proper positioning and diffusion. Further injections are not warranted if there is not a favorable response after two injections.

The risks and benefits of the procedure should be discussed with the patient and informed consent obtained. Epidural steroid injections are performed using sterile technique in a room equipped for resuscitation. The procedure (Box 17-6)

> **Box 17-6**
>
> ## Summary of Epidural Steroid Injection Technique
>
> - Preprocedure—detailed history and physical examination
>   - Informed consent
>   - Patient preparation (e.g., need for sedation and antibiotic prophylaxis)
> - Procedure—standard monitoring (heart rate, blood pressure, pulse oximetry)
>   - Surface anatomy marking
>   - Sterile technique
>   - Subcutaneous local anesthesia infiltration
>   - Needle placement (20 g Tuohy needle)
>   - Needle position confirmation
>   - Injection of steroids (e.g., 80 mg DepoMedrol in 5 mL saline)
> - Postprocedure—patient reevaluation (e.g., no new neurologic finding)
>   - Discharge when vital signs are stable (30 min)
>   - Postprocedure discharge instructions

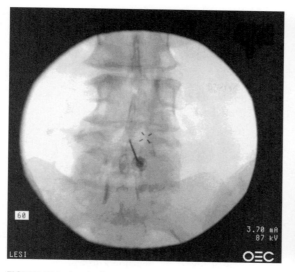

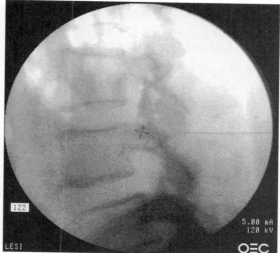

FIGURE 17-1. Interlaminar approach to epidural steroid injection. (A) Anteroposterior view. Radiographic confirmation of needle position at L4-L5. Nerve roots are delineated bilaterally. (B) Lateral view. Radiographic confirmation of needle position L4-L5 and contrast in posterior epidural space.

may be done in the sitting, lateral, or prone positions. Standard anesthesia monitors should be applied. A 20-gauge epidural needle is usually selected for the single injection technique. The epidural space is usually identified using LOR to air technique. Alternative methods, such as LOR to saline or hanging-drop technique, have been described. The needle tip position is confirmed under fluoroscopic and radiographic guidance (Figs. 17-1 and 17-2). The syringe is removed, and

the needle opening is inspected for blood or spinal fluid. Contrast is injected to confirm epidural spread to the desired target site. In the lumbar area, 80 mg of methylprednisolone (40–120 mg)[21–23] in 3–8 mL of saline or local anesthetic (e.g., 1% lidocaine) is the usual steroid injected. Triamcinolone (40–80 mg)[24,25] or betamethasone (18 mg)[26] have been used to decrease the incidence of ischemic injury, should accidental intra-arterial injection occur, particularly with transforaminal

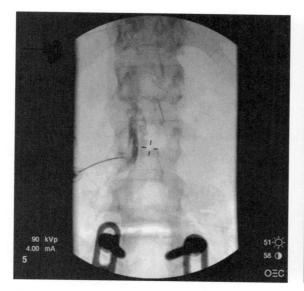

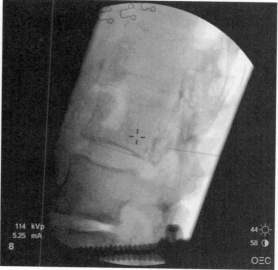

FIGURE 17-2. Transforaminal approach to epidural steroid injection. (A) Anteroposterior view. Radiographic confirmation of needle placement at left L2-L3 level, with delineation of left L2 nerve root and unilateral epidural spread of contrast. (B) Lateral view. Confirmation of needle location at L2-L3 level with anterior and posterior spread of the dye.

injection. The medications are injected slowly to reduce the incidence of injection pain and prevent a rapid increase in cerebrospinal fluid (CSF) pressure which may lead to neurologic sequelae. The needle is flushed with sterile saline, the stylet is replaced, and the needle is removed. The patient is observed until satisfactory recovery (i.e., stable vital signs and absence of unexpected neurologic deficits). A follow-up visit is scheduled in 1–2 weeks.

Complications

Epidural steroid injection is usually considered a low-risk procedure. Complications can be related either to the steroid effects or to the procedure itself (Box 17-7). Complications related to the steroids are usually dose dependent. The most common adverse reactions reported after epidural steroid injections include insomnia, facial flushing, fever (less than 37.8°C), nonpositional headache, transient worsening of pain, and nausea. Botwin et al.[27] reported the incidence of complications of fluoroscopically guided caudal epidural steroid injection was 15.6%. Fluid retention, mood swings, local fat atrophy, depigmentation of the skin, minor changes in serum glucose, Cushing syndrome, and suppression of the pituitary-adrenal axis have been reported.

The most common procedure-related complication is a vasovagal response. Other complications include misplacement of the medication, dural puncture with subsequent positional headache (up to 5% in the intralaminar vs. 0.6% in the caudal approach),[33] and exacerbation of the radicular pain (greater than 4%).[28–30] This symptom may be avoided by slow injection. Intrathecal administration of steroid preparations has come under investigation after reports of arachnoiditis following intrathecal methylprednisolone injections. However, subsequent studies failed to demonstrate adverse effects on neural tissue with methylprednisolone acetate,[31] triamcinolone,[32] or betamethasone acetate.[33] Rare complications such as spinal infections, hematoma formation, nerve root injury, myopathy, retinal hemorrhage, and transient paralysis have been reported. Idiosyncratic reactions are extremely rare. The total complication rate in most series is between 5 and 15%, and the complications are almost always transient.

Absolute contraindications include infection at the injection site, the use of anticoagulants and antiplatelet agents, bleeding disorder, rapidly progressive neural deficit, cauda equina syndrome, uncontrolled diabetes, and congestive heart failure. Psychosocial barriers to recovery and the presence of symptoms for more than a year are associated with poor outcome (Box 17-8).

COMPLEX REGIONAL PAIN SYNDROME

▶ Definition

"Complex regional pain syndrome" is a pain disorder in which the pain is disproportionate to the initial patient injury (Box 17-9). The disorder is complex because it

Box 17-10

Criteria for Diagnosis of CRPS

CRPS Type I	CRPS Type II
Noxious event	Nerve injury
Allodynia or hyperalgesia	Allodynia or hyperalgesia
Edema, sweating abnormalities, trophic changes	Edema, sweating abnormalities, trophic changes
No clear identifiable condition that accounts for the pain	No clear identifiable condition that accounts for the pain

Box 17-12

Trophic Abnormalities in CRPS

Site	Early Stage	Late Stage
Limb	Edema	Atrophy Muscle and joint contracture
Skin	Dry, hot, pink Increased perfusion	Blue, cold, sweaty Decreased perfusion Thin, glossy skin Fragile, uneven, curled hair Ridged, brittle, discolored nail
Bone	Increased uptake on bone scan	Demineralization, Osteoporosis

involves multiple organ systems with abnormal blood flow, sweating abnormalities, trophic changes, and fine motor impairment. The pain distribution tends to be regional (not dermatomal), and is not limited to the area initially affected.[34–39] The pathophysiology of CRPS is not entirely understood. The pain can be sympathetically maintained (SMP—responsive to sympathetic blocking interventions) or sympathetically independent (SIP).[40,41] The diagnosis is excluded by the presence of a condition that would otherwise account for the degree of pain and dysfunction.

According to the International Association for the Study of Pain,[42] CRPS is divided into two categories based on the absence or presence of an identifiable nerve injury: CRPS type I, formerly known as reflex sympathetic dystrophy, and CRPS type II, formerly known as causalgia (Box 17-10).

▶ Clinical Features

Sensory Abnormalities

Pain is the essential feature of CRPS. It is characteristically disproportionate to the initiating event with no spatial relation to an individual nerve (Box 17-11). It is frequently reported as a burning sensation, usually spontaneous,[43]

mostly felt at the distal extremity in the dependent position. Typically, joint movements exacerbate the pain. Mechanical and thermal allodynia (cold more often than heat) and hyperalgesia are frequently present.[44–47] In addition, 50% of patients with chronic CRPS type I develop hypoesthesia and hypoalgesia in the same body quadrant or the half body of the affected site[48] with increased mechanical and thermal threshold on the affected side. These patients have a longer period of illness, greater pain intensity, and a higher tendency to develop somatomotor changes.[49,50] The pain can be described as SMP or SIP based on the positive or negative effect of selective blockade of the sympathetic nervous system or blockade of adrenergicreceptors. Therefore, SMP is a symptom in a subset of patients and is not essential for the diagnosis of CRPS.[40,41]

Autonomic and Trophic Abnormalities

Autonomic abnormalities and trophic changes are present at some time during the course of the disease (Box 17-12). Swelling is found in almost all patients. Symptoms are usually exacerbated by evoked pain. Sudomotor abnormalities,

Box 17-11

Pain Characteristics in CRPS Type I

Quality	Intensity	Location	Duration
Spontaneous burning Allodynia, mechanical Allodynia, thermal Regional hypoesthesia	Severe Disproportionate to noxious event	Distal part Deep somatic	Unremitting Worsens with time Disproportionate to inciting event

frequently hyperhidrosis, are very common.[51,52] Limb temperature asymmetry of more than 1 degree is present in 30–80% of patients. Three distinct vascular regulation patterns are identified in relation to the duration of the disorder. In the early acute stage, the affected limb is usually warmer, skin perfusion values are higher, and norepinephrine concentrations in the venous effluent from the affected area are low. In addition, sympathetic vasoconstrictor neurons are difficult to activate.[53] In the intermediate stage, temperature and skin perfusion tests may be either high or low depending on the sympathetic activity. In the chronic stage, the limb is colder, skin perfusion test values are low, and norepinephrine concentrations remain low in the affected side. Passing into the chronic stage, the edema resolve; and the limb atrophies with muscle contracture, constriction of the tendon sheaths, and joint stiffness. Abnormal skin (thin, glossy), nail (brittle and discolored), and hair growth (fragile, uneven, curled) may be present. Bone involvement is frequent. Initially, increased isotope uptake on bone scanning is found. Later, there is rapid and profound bone loss with patchy demineralization. Fractures are uncommon.[53]

Somatomotor Abnormalities

Motor symptoms, although not included in the definition, are frequently present. Weakness of all muscles in the affected area is present in 70% of patients. In addition, patients may present with postural or action tremor (50%) and dystonia (10%). Typically, small, precise movements are impaired. Except in the chronic stages, nerve conduction studies are usually normal.[54]

Psychologic Abnormalities

Most patients have a normal psychologic profile. An association with previous psychologic stress, however, has been noted. A low pain threshold, emotional lability, and depression may be present.

PATHOPHYSIOLOGY

A number of hypothetical mechanisms for the disease have been described (Fig. 17-3).[55,56] In the peripheral nervous system, the continuous barrage of noxious stimuli sensitizes the small polymodal A-delta and C fibers, leading to hyperalgesia. In the spinal cord, there may be sensitization of the wide dynamic range neurons that occurs after intense peripheral stimulation of A-delta and C fibers.[57] In addition, the activity of the low-threshold A-beta mechanoreceptor fibers is altered, which may induce a state of hyperalgesia and allodynia.[58] There is also growing evidence that the sympathetic nervous system is involved, especially when the

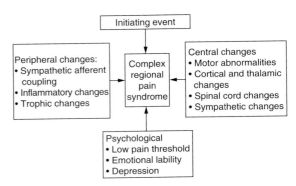

FIGURE 17-3. Pathophysiology of CRPS.

pain or autonomic components are relieved by sympathetic blocks. In the acute stage of the syndrome, there is functional inhibition of cutaneous sympathetic vasoconstrictor activity. In the chronic stage, after the initial inhibition, secondary end-organ supersensitivity is manifested by increased vasoconstriction, reduced skin temperature, and enhanced sudomotor activity. The SMP may be maintained by pathologic coupling of sympathetic and afferent activity either in the periphery, between sympathetic fibers and C fibers, or in the dorsal root ganglia.[54] Central nervous system (CNS) alterations, probably in the cortex and thalamus,[48] may also play a role in CRPS, especially in patients with extensive sensory deficits; however it is not clear whether changes in the CNS are primary abnormalities or secondary to pain.

▶ Treatment

Treatment of CRPS should be immediate and directed toward restoration of extremity function and rehabilitation.[59] Treatment includes pain relief, mobilization, and desensitization of the affected extremity (Fig. 17-4).[58] Movement phobia should be overcome, and physical therapy should be facilitated. A combination of analgesic and adjuvant drugs, including tricyclic antidepressants, anticonvulsants, membrane stabilizers, and α_1-, and α_2-adrenoreceptor agonists are employed to help accomplish the above therapeutic goals. Randomized controlled trials support the use of steroids, amitriptyline, and gabapentin. In addition, regional and neuraxial techniques play an important role in diagnosis as well as treatment, especially in SMP. As discussed earlier, the diagnosis of SMP is established by determining the magnitude of pain relief achieved with an appropriate sympathetic block. However, the results of local anesthetic blocks should be interpreted with caution[60] as the adequacy of the sympathetic block in SMP must be demonstrated simultaneously with the degree of pain relief obtained.[53] The adequacy of sympathetic block is assessed by measuring

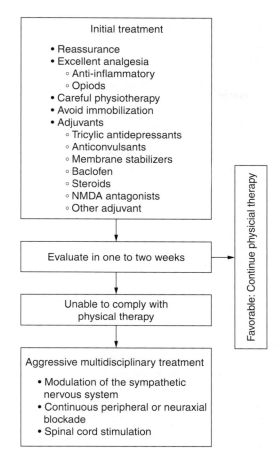

FIGURE 17-4. Treatment of CRPS.

after which neuromodulation should be considered.[62] An epidural catheter should be implanted under strict sterile technique. Fluoroscopic guidance is helpful, especially if unilateral catheter placement is favored. Bupivacaine in low concentration (0.1–0.25%) titrated to provide analgesia, is the preferred drug by virtue of its ability to interrupt nociception while preferentially sparing motor function and proprioception. The addition of opioids to the epidural infusion (morphine or hydromorphone) allows for a decreased local anesthetic concentration and decreased motor block, which might interfere with functional restoration. Clonidine administered in the epidural space may potentiate hypotension, but has demonstrated efficacy in CRPS.[63] A short period of hospitalization may be necessary to identify the most effective dose. Regional anesthesia should provide the analgesic effects and the sympatholysis necessary to promote functional restoration. Central neuraxial infusions help manage allodynia and this contributes to the restoration of joint movement. The vertebral level of epidural catheter placement is important; T2 to T3 for the upper extremity and T12 for the lower extremity.

Infection is the most feared complication of long-term catheter implantation. Infection, if it occurs, is usually local and is superficial to the deep fascia. It therefore readily responds to antibiotic treatment.[39] If a spinal or paraspinous infection is suspected, the catheter should be removed and neurologic consultation and spine imaging are required.

Other therapies for CRPS that have been used with varying degrees of success include transcutaneous nerve stimulation, peripheral nerve stimulation, spinal cord stimulation,[64] and intrathecal baclofen[65] (Fig. 17-4).

HERPES ZOSTER AND POSTHERPETIC NEURALGIA

▶ Epidemiology

Herpes zoster (shingles) is caused by a reactivation of latent herpes virus (varicella zoster), which lies dormant in the dorsal root or cranial nerve ganglia. The primary childhood infection with herpes virus causes varicella (chickenpox), usually a mild, benign, contagious disease. A varicella vaccine became available in 1994, and many children are now vaccinated against the disease. By adulthood, over 90% of the population is seropositive for varicella[66] and is at risk for developing herpes zoster with a lifetime prevalence estimated at 10–20%. The most common complication of herpes zoster is PHN. About 22% of the patients who develop herpes zoster continue to have pain and/or abnormal sensations 3 months after the rash appearance. At 1 year, 5–10% of patients still have PHN, and

changes in skin blood flow, skin temperature, or skin resistance. This is especially important when the goal is diagnosis of SMP. However, when therapy is the intended purpose, local anesthetics can be administered intrathecally, epidurally, or in proximity to the sympathetic nervous system. Observational studies suggest that about 85% of patients report acute relief after regional block techniques, and about 60% experience long-term pain relief.[39] In addition, one prospective study[61] showed that perioperative sympathetic (stellate ganglion) blockade, prior to an operation on the limb affected with CRPS, reduced the postoperative recurrence of the disease.

In order to achieve sustained pain relief, a series of injections, or the placement of a catheter for long-term infusion, may be required. Common sites for continuous block include the epidural space, the subarachnoid space, peripheral plexuses and nerves, and sympathetic plexuses and nerves. Continuous nerve or plexus block can be used for up to 6 weeks, and an epidural catheter can be retained for up to 6 months,

Table 17-2

Herpes Zoster Dermatomal Involvement

Thoracic	46.1%
Cervical	21.74%
Lumbar	14.86%
Trigeminal	11.15%
Sacral	5.4%
Geniculate ganglion	0.75%

Data from Ref. 68.

Box 17-13

Pain and Abnormal Sensation Categories in PHN

1. Constant, spontaneous burning pain
2. Brief recurrent, shooting, electric shock-type pain
3. Tactile allodynia (burning pain evoked by light touch)
4. Reduced skin sensitivity and/or itching, prickling, and other abnormal sensations

usually further resolution is limited.[67] Other neurologic complications include zoster sine herpete (the presence of severe pain and hyperesthesia in a dermatomal distribution without evidence of a rash), encephalitis, myelitis, and postinfectious polyneuritis.

▶ Clinical Manifestations

Herpes Zoster: Acute Stage

Herpes zoster reactivation is preceded by a prodrome, characterized by headache, photophobia, and malaise, which is followed by localized abnormal skin sensations (itching, tingling pain) for 1–5 days. A maculopapular rash, which progresses to vesicular eruption, pustulation, ulceration, and crusting, usually clustered in one to three dermatomal distributions, characterizes the acute stage. The thoracic dermatomes are most commonly affected, followed by the cervical and lumbar area and the face (Table 17-2). The first and second branches of the trigeminal nerve are the most common cranial nerves involved, and this can be associated with zoster keratitis. Other branches of the trigeminal nerve, the facial nerve, and sacral areas can also be affected.[68] The cutaneous eruption is almost always unilateral and does not cross the midline. Over a period of 2–4 weeks, the skin lesions heal, often with scaring and pigmentation in the affected area. Advanced age is the most significant predisposing factor for acute herpes zoster. An additional risk factor for shingles is immune suppression, either disease or drug induced.

Postherpetic Neuralgia

The most commonly accepted definition of PHN is the presence of significant pain or abnormal sensations 3 months after rash healing.[69] However, this definition is not universally accepted. Other authors have defined PHN as pain persisting beyond the crusting of lesions, or pain lasting more than 1–6 months after the acute infection.[69] Pain is usually described as constant burning or as an intermittent electric shock-type discomfort. It can be associated with allodynia, hyperesthesia, or hypoesthesia (Box 17-13). Age is the most significant predisposing factor with an estimated 10% increase in the incidence of PHN with each 1-year increment in age.[70] Other predisposing factors include severe prodromal pain and severe pain accompanying the rash. The incidence of PHN is higher in women than men. Well-established PHN may lead to a severe physical and social disability.

Following recovery from an initial varicella infection, the virus is usually quiescent in the dorsal root ganglia. During the acute phase of herpes zoster infection, the virus is reactivated and spreads from the dorsal root ganglion along the peripheral nerve, leading to inflammation of these neural structures and resulting in skin rash.[71] There is limited inflammation with minimal or no damage to the ganglia, posterior roots, or nerve endings in case of complete recovery. However, in case of widespread inflammation and damage, there is continuous nociceptor excitation and an efflux of pain signals from damaged tissues, nociceptors, and C fibers to the dorsal horn, which leads to and maintains central (dorsal horn) sensitization and hyperexcitability. In addition, in another subset of patients, especially when central sensitization is accompanied by C fiber degeneration, there may be sprouting of large diameter, mechanoreceptor A-beta fibers from the deeper layers of the substantia gelatinosa into the more superficial layers usually occupied by the C fibers with resultant mechanical allodynia.[72] The damage may also spread to the dorsal horn leading to a subclinical inflammation of the spinal cord. In addition, the activation of the sympathetic nervous system may play a role in pain by causing severe neural ischemia from intense perineural vascular constriction. Furthermore, a coupling between the efferent sympathetic system and afferent sensory innervation may maintain and potentiate pain. Damaged C fibers may acquire a hypersensitivity to α_1-adrenergic fibers, which respond to sympathetic activation. In the chronic stage, there is evidence of sprouting of the sympathetic nervous system in the dorsal root ganglia, which may affect the primary afferent neurons in their cell bodies.[73]

▶ Treatment

Therapeutic strategies for managing acute herpes zoster should include treatment of the acute episode as well as prevention of PHN and its consequences. Medical treatments have varying beneficial effects and include antiviral agents (acyclovir, valacyclovir, famciclovir), mild analgesics, opioids, antidepressants, membrane stabilizers, gabapentin, and a lidocaine patch. In addition, central neuraxial, peripheral, and sympathetic nerve blocks have been used extensively to treat pain in acute herpes zoster, to prevent PHN, and to treat PHN.

Epidural Local Anesthetics and Steroids

Many observational studies suggest that epidural local anesthetics have a beneficial effect in the treatment of herpes zoster infection and prevention of PHN.[74–77] For example, in a descriptive review of 2300 patients with acute herpes zoster or PHN, Dan[78] concluded that a continuous epidural infusion of local anesthetics is effective in relieving moderate to severe acute herpetic pain, decreasing allodynia, and shortening the duration of acute herpetic pain and PHN. The author infused 0.5% bupivacaine at 0.3–0.7 mL/h for at least 12–14 days, along with the administration of antiviral drugs for 5 days in a subset of patients. Patients with the epidural infusion achieved more rapid hospital discharge (when 90% pain relief was achieved) and complete pain relief than historical control patients treated with bolus injections of 1% mepivacaine 4–6 mL, three to four times daily, in combination with antiviral drugs for 5 days.

Local anesthetics may block axonal transport and axonal spread of the virus.[79] Thus, in addition to providing short-term pain relief, they may prevent PHN.[68] In addition, the axonal transport blocking capacity of the local anesthetic drugs has been demonstrated at concentrations lower than those used in clinical settings. Treatment should begin as early as possible for best efficacy.[74–76,80] Epidural injections are more effective if performed within 10–15 days after the onset of symptoms. The local anesthetic volume is determined based on the dermatomal level of herpes zoster lesions and the total number of spinal segments involved. Cervical epidural injections may be used for lesions located in the trigeminal area. Steroids (methylprednisolone 40–80 mg)[77,80,81] are frequently added to the epidural local anesthetic injection because of their anti-inflammatory and lysosomal protection properties, although no data exist as to whether this improves outcomes.[82]

When possible, continuous epidural catheter techniques are preferred to repeated single-shot epidural injections, although this has not been well studied. In a randomized prospective trial of 600 patients with acute herpes zoster, Pasqualucci et al.[68] concluded that continuous epidural anesthetic block in combination with steroids was more effective than treatment with intravenous acyclovir and steroids in preventing PHN at 1, 3, 6, and 12 months (Table 17-3). Reported complications in the epidural group ($n = 255$) included displacement of epidural catheter (9 patients), frequent sweating and fainting spells (2 patients), neck pain (1 patient), leg paresis and oliguria (1 patient), dural puncture and catheter repositioning (16 patients). The incidence of pain after 1 year was 22.2% in the acyclovir and steroid group compared to 1.6% in the epidural local anesthetic and steroid group. The recommended initial concentration of bupivacaine, 0.25%, should be titrated to provide effective analgesia, in a volume that covers the involved dermatomes.[68]

Sympathetic Blocks

The role of sympathetic nerve block in the treatment of herpes zoster infection is controversial, mainly because of the lack of well-controlled studies of early sympathetic nerve blockade. Tenicela et al.,[83] in a prospective randomized controlled trial of herpes zoster treatment in 20 patients, concluded that sympathetic nerve blocks with bupivacaine are effective in treating acute pain in herpes zoster when

---

Table 17-3

Prevention of PHN: Effect of Systemic Vs. Epidural Treatment on Complete Recovery

	Systemic Treatment* Complete Recovery (%) ($N = 230$)	Epidural Treatment† Complete Recovery (%) ($N = 255$)
1 month	14	45.9
3 months	57.3	87.1
6 months	65.1	91.0
1 year	65.6	94.1

*Systemic treatment: intravenous acyclovir (10 mg/kg, four times daily for 10 days) and intravenous prednisolone (60 mg/day for 9 days, then decreasing doses of oral prednisone up to day 21).
†Epidural treatment: bupivacaine 0.25% (6–12 mL bolus dose, every 8–12 h for 7–21 days, within 7 days of rash onset) and oral methylprednisolone (40 mg, every 3–4 days). Mean time to initiation of treatment: 4.3 ± 2.3 days.
Data from Ref. 68.

compared to placebo blocks. Winnie and Hartwell[84] compared sympathetic blockade performed within the first 2 weeks of rash onset to sympathetic blockade performed 6 months after onset in 122 patients with herpes zoster. Eighty-six percent of patients experienced lasting pain relief after the early block compared to only 21% in the late group. After reviewing the literature, Wu et al.[85] concluded that there is support for the efficacy of sympathetic block in reducing the duration of acute herpes pain. The reviewers, however, did not find compelling support for the use of sympathetic nerve blocks, administered early in acute herpes zoster, to prevent PHN. Long-standing PHN does not appear to respond to local anesthetic sympathetic blockade. The current evidence suggests that early treatment with epidural local anesthetics in combination with steroids is effective in the management of severe acute herpes zoster pain and may prevent PHN, but that early sympathetic blockade does not prevent PHN.

PHANTOM LIMB PAIN

▶ Definition and Epidemiology

Following amputation, persistent limb sensation can occur with an incidence ranging from 5 to 90%.[86] Nonpainful sensations are very common in the year after amputation and are seldom distressing (Box 17-14). In addition, virtually all amputees experience immediate postamputation stump pain. The pain may be localized to the residual limb (stump pain) or present as abnormal pain sensation in the distribution of the missing limb part (phantom limb pain).

Initially, following amputation, the phantom limb resembles the preamputation limb in shape and length. However, over time, the proximal part fades; the remaining phantom is compromised of the distal portion with the greatest representation in the somatosensory cortex. This gradual change in length is referred to as telescoping, where the distal phantom is gradually felt to approach the residual limb (amputation site).

Box 17-14	
Definitions of Postamputation Sensory Phenomena	
Phantom sensation	Any sensation of the missing limb except pain
Residual limb pain or stump pain	Pain at the site of an extremity amputation
Phantom limb pain	Painful sensations referred to the absent limb

Persistent limb pain after the normal healing period occurs in about 5–22% of amputees.[87] Parkes[88] reported a 50% incidence of residual limb pain in the first few weeks after amputation, but this declined to 13% at 13 months follow-up. Stump pain may be multifactorial in origin; local pathology such as ischemia, infection, neuroma formation, bone spurs, scar tissue formation, and an ill-fitting prosthesis may be involved.

In contrast to the literature on phantom sensation and stump pain, there is wide variability in the reported prevalence of phantom pain among the amputee population. Sternbach et al.[89] reported an incidence of 0.5–10%, while Sherman et al.[90] were able to detect a much higher incidence (85%). It is likely that the difference in the prevalence is a function of the amputee's reluctance to report his or her experience to the health-care provider. In contrast to stump pain, the pathophysiology of phantom limb pain is very complex in nature; multiple elements may be involved, including the peripheral nervous system, the spinal cord, and the brain. Stump pain and phantom limb pain may coexist, with a higher prevalence of phantom limb pain in patients who have stump pain.[91]

▶ Clinical Features

Phantom sensation is usually reported as mild tingling or tightness, or described as pins and needles (Box 17-15).[92] Most amputees retain the sense of position of the phantom limb. Stump pain is usually described as stabbing, shocking, or burning. It is usually localized at the lower end of the stump, close to the scar. It can occur spontaneously or in response to light stimulation. Occasionally, very intense pain, referred to as nerve storm, can occur; it is often associated with spontaneous movement, sweating, cold sensation, and reduced blood flow to the stump.

Phantom limb pain is predominantly localized at the distal portion of the missing limb; it is primarily felt in the fingers and palm of the hand, and in the toes and feet of the lower extremity. It is described as burning, cramping, shooting, stabbing, throbbing, or a numb sensation.[86] Many patients report sensations similar in quality and intensity to preamputation pain. It tends to be intermittent in nature, rarely constant. The pain is more common in the elderly, and rarely occurs in the young population. It is also more frequent in proximal thigh, above knee amputations. Other predisposing factors include severe preoperative pain or amputation of a dominant hand.[93] Most of these patients develop phantom limb pain within a week; however, there are case reports of phantom limb pain occurring after several years.[94] The pain can be severe enough to hinder life style. Characteristically, over years, phantom limb pain tends to decrease in intensity and

Box 17-15

Comparative Clinical Features of Postamputation Sensory Phenomena

	Prevalence	Localization	Quality
Phantom sensation	Virtually 100%	Initially: resembles preamputation Over time: telescoping	Tingling, tightness
Residual limb or stump pain	Initially: 50–60% 1–2 years: 10–20%	Lower end of stump	Stabbing, shocking, burning
Phantom limb pain	Varies: 0.5–85%	Distal amputated portion	Burning, cramping

location; its spatial distribution is diminished in a telescopic manner with the pain sensation disappearing from proximal to distal.

▶ Pathophysiology

Both peripheral and central factors are involved in the pathophysiology of the phantom limb sensations and phantom limb pain. In addition, psychologic factors may affect the severity and course of the pain experience (Fig. 17-5).

Peripheral Factors

There is a high correlation between the presence of residual stump pain and phantom limb pain, which suggests that peripheral factors may play a role in phantom limb pain.[95] In the residual stump, there is regenerative sprouting of the injured axons and neuroma formation, with enlarged and disorganized endings of C fibers and demyelinated A fibers. This may result in an increased rate of spontaneous activity and in increased sensitivity to mechanical and chemical stimulation. In addition, there may be ectopic discharges from the dorsal root ganglia.[96] Local anesthetic block of a stump neuroma may eliminate the stump nerve activity but not the dorsal root ganglia discharge.[95]

Central Factors

Increased activity in peripheral nociceptors may lead to an increase in the excitability of dorsal horn neurons and a reduction in the nervous system transmission inhibitory processes. Peripheral nerve injury may lead to a sprouting of A-beta fibers into lamina II, an area normally innervated by C fibers. The incoming A fiber input may be interpreted as a painful stimulation.[72] In addition, there is an expansion of the receptive field in the areas adjacent to the deafferented limb, which may lead to an invasion of the spinal cord area representing the deafferented limb. Supraspinal areas, including the somatosensory and motor cortex, thalamus, reticular formation, and limbic system, are also involved. Melzack[97] suggested that an amputation might alter the sensory input from the periphery to these areas, which may lead to an altered neurosignature (neuromatrix theory) and the experience of a phantom. In addition, other studies have showed that changes in the functional and structural architecture of the primary somatosensory cortex may occur after amputation.[98–100]

▶ Treatment

Phantom limb sensation is rarely distressing; in fact, the sensation may help the amputee adapt to the new prosthesis. Although immediate postoperative stump pain may be easy to treat, treatment of phantom limb pain may be challenging;[95] therefore, prevention may play an important role. Furthermore, in the light of the high prevalence of preoperative limb pain and postamputation stump pain, continuous pre- and postoperative pain control should be beneficial. More specifically, perioperative epidural analgesia may be effective in decreasing the incidence of phantom limb pain.[101]

Many pharmacologic and nonpharmacologic treatments have been tried with variable success. Box 17-16 lists commonly used treatments for phantom limb pain that are supported by at least one controlled study demonstrating a beneficial effect. Mechanism-based treatments are usually the most effective. Perineural injection of lidocaine was

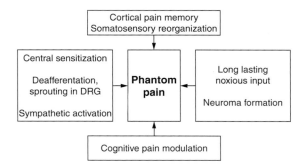

FIGURE 17-5. Etiology of phantom limb pain.

Box 17-16

Phantom Limb Pain Treatments with Positive Effect

Pharmacologic	Anesthetic	Psychologic	Others
Opioids, Ketamine	Lidocaine stump infiltration	Sensory discrimination training	Transcutaneous electric nerve stimulation (TENS)

shown to be effective in patients with neuroma.[102] Other noninterventional pain treatments may be helpful. These include tricyclic antidepressants, sodium channel blockers, anticonvulsants, calcitonin, N-methyl-D-aspartate (NMDA) receptor antagonists, and opioids. In addition, noninvasive techniques such as transcutaneous electrical stimulation, vibration technique, acupuncture, hypnosis, and biofeedback have been tried with limited success.[95]

Prevention of Phantom Limb Pain

Preemptive analgesia has been effective in preventing phantom limb pain; however, results have not been consistent. In a study by Bach et al.,[101] 25 patients were randomized to receive either preoperative continuous epidural analgesia for 3 days (with bupivacaine and/or morphine), sufficient to render them pain free, or a traditional systemic analgesic regimen. All 11 patients who received an epidural infusion were pain free 6 months after the amputation, whereas 5 out of 14 who received systemic narcotic treatment had phantom limb pain at 6 months. In a nonrandomized study by Jahangiri et al.,[103] 24 patients with preoperative pain were divided into two groups. A study group received an epidural infusion of bupivacaine, diamorphine, and clonidine 24–48 h preoperatively and continued for 3 days postoperatively; and a control group received on-demand systemic opioid analgesia. All patients received general anesthesia for surgery. At 1-year follow-up, 1 out of 13 patients in the study group had pain, whereas 8 patients out of 11 in the control group had pain. Other studies[104,105] of patients undergoing limb amputation have shown that epidural infusions started before surgery and continued for the duration of surgery, and for several days after amputation, confer the most protection for long-term relief. By contrast, Nikolajsen et al., in a blinded and placebo controlled trial, initiated epidural infusions of either bupivacaine and morphine, or epidural saline with systemic opioid, within 1 day of amputation. Both groups received similar epidural analgesia in the postoperative period. The incidence and intensity of phantom pain were similar in both groups.[106] The authors concluded that it is impossible to prevent phantom limb pain using an epidural block for a short duration.

Katz and Melzack[107] have suggested that both implicit and explicit pain memories should be treated. Therefore, they suggested that combined general and spinal anesthesia are needed for amputation surgery. Again, however, combined general and spinal anesthesia have not been consistently effective in preventing phantom limb pain.

In conclusion, post amputation patients may experience a wide range of symptoms ranging from nonpainful limb sensation to severe stump and phantom pain. There is a high correlation between severe preamputation pain and phantom and stump pain. Postoperative epidural analgesia is effective in treating postamputation stump pain. Preoperative epidural analgesia beginning more than 3 days before the amputation may decrease the incidence of phantom limb pain.

SUMMARY

Epidural injections are useful adjuncts in the treatment of several chronic pain syndromes, including acute lumbar radiculopathy, CRPS, PHN, and phantom limb pain. Epidural steroid injections are effective for the treatment of acute radicular pain resulting from disc herniation, and may also be useful in the treatment of discogenic axial pain syndromes caused by an annular tear. Short- or long-term local anesthetic neuraxial blockade may be useful for the diagnosis of CRPS and as part of multimodal CRPS therapy. Continuous local anesthetic epidural infusions are beneficial in the treatment of acute herpes zoster pain, as well as for the prevention and treatment of PHN. Epidural analgesia is an effective therapy for postamputation stump pain. Further research is required to define the role of epidural techniques in these chronic pain syndromes.

REFERENCES

1. Mersky H, Bogduk N. *Classification of Chronic Pain*, 2nd ed. Seattle: IASP Press, 1994.
2. Devereaux MW. Neck and low back pain. *Med Clin North Am* 87:643, 2003.
3. Anderson G. Epidemiological features of chronic low-back pain. *Lancet* 354:581, 1999.
4. Hart LG, Deyo RA, Cherkin DC. Physician office visits for low back pain: Frequency, clinical evaluation, and treatment patterns from a U.S. national survey. *Spine* 20:11, 1995.
5. Bigos S, Bowyer O, Braen G, et al. Acute Low Back Pain Problems in Adults. Clinical Practice Guideline, Quick Reference Guide Number 14. U.S. Department of Health and Human Services,

Public Health Service, Agency for Health Care Policy and Research. AHCPR Pub. No. 95-0643, December 1994.

6. Carette S, Leclaire R, Marcoux S, et al. Epidural corticosteroid injections for sciatica due to herniated nucleus pulposus. *N Engl J Med* 336:1634, 1997.

7. Samanta J, Kendall J, Samanta A. Chronic low back pain. *BMJ* 326:535, 2003.

8. Vroomen P, De Krom M, Slofstra P, et al. Conservative treatment of sciatica: A systematic review. *J Spinal Disord* 13:463, 2000.

9. Byrod G, Otani K, Brisby H, et al. Methylprednisolone reduces the early vascular permeability increase in spinal nerve roots induced by epidural nucleus pulposus application. *J Orthop Res* 18:983, 2000.

10. Weinstein S, Herring S. Lumbar epidural steroid injections. *Spine J* 3:37S, 2003.

11. Watts RW, Silagy CA. A meta-analysis on the efficacy of epidural corticosteroids in the treatment of sciatica. *Anaesth Intensive Care* 23:564, 1995.

12. Dreyfuss P. Epidural steroid injections: A procedure ideally performed with fluoroscopic control and contrast media. *ISIS Newsletter,* Vol. 1, 1993, p. 34.

13. Renfrew DL, Moore TE, Kathol MH, et al. Correct placement of epidural steroid injections: Fluoroscopic guidance and contrast administration. *Am J Neuroradiol* 12:1003, 1991.

14. White AH, Derby R, Wynne G. Epidural injection for the diagnosis and treatment of low-back pain. *Spine* 5:78, 1980.

15. Johnson BA, Schellhaus KP, Pollei SR. Epidurography and therapeutic epidural injections: Technical considerations and experience with 5334 cases. *Am J Neuroradiol* 20:697, 1999.

16. Sharrock NE, Urquhart B, Mineo R. Extradural anaesthesia in patients with previous lumbar spine surgery. *Br J Anaesth* 65:237, 1990.

17. Fredman B, Nun MB, Zohar E, et al. Epidural steroids for treating "failed back surgery syndrome": Is fluoroscopy really necessary? *Anesth Analg* 88:367, 1999.

18. Liu S, Melmed P, Klos J, et al. Prospective experience with a 20-gauge Tuohy needle for lumbar epidural steroid injections: Is confirmation with fluoroscopy necessary? *Reg Anesth Pain Med* 26:143, 2001.

19. Vad VB, Bhat AL, Lutz GE, Cammisa F. Transforaminal epidural steroid injections in lumbosacral radiculopathy: A prospective randomized study. *Spine* 27:11, 2002.

20. Stojanovic MP, Vu T-H, Caneris O, et al. The role of fluoroscopy in cervical epidural steroid injections. *Spine* 27:509, 2002.

21. Beliveau P. A comparison between epidural anaesthesia with and without corticosteroid in the treatment of sciatica. *Rheumatol Phys Med* 11:40, 1971.

22. Cuckler JM, Bernini PA, Wiesel SW, et al. The use of epidural steroids in the treatment of lumbar radicular pain. *J Bone Joint Surg Am* 67:63, 1985.

23. Mathews JA, Mills SB, Jenkins VM, et al. Back pain and sciatica: Controlled trials of manipulation, traction, sclerosant, and epidural injections. *Br J Rheumatol* 26:416, 1987.

24. Bush K, Hillier S. A controlled study of caudal epidural injections of triamcinolone plus procaine for the management of intractable sciatica. *Spine* 15:572, 1991.

25. Rocco AG, Frank E, Kaul AF, et al. Epidural steroids, epidural morphine, and epidural steroids combined with morphine in the treatment of postlaminectomy syndrome. *Pain* 36:297, 1989.

26. Riew KD, Yin Y, Gilula L, et al. The effect of nerve-root injections on the need for operative treatment of lumbar radicular pain. *J Bone Joint Surg* 82A:1589, 2000.

27. Botwin KP, Gruber RD, Bouchlas CG, et al. Complications of fluoroscopically guided caudal epidural injections. *Am J Phys Med Rehabil* 80:416, 2001.

28. Gilly R. Essai de traitement de 50 cas de sciatiques et de radiculalgies lombaires par le celestene chronodose en infiltrations paradiculaire [French]. *Mars Med* 107:341, 1970.

29. Burn JMB, Langdon L. Lumbar epidural injection for the treatment of chronic sciatica. *Rheumatol Phys Med* 10:368, 1970.

30. Snoek W, Weber H, Jorgensen B. Double blind evaluation of extradural methylprednisolone for herniated lumbar discs. *Acta Orthop Scand* 48:635, 1977.

31. Boas RA, Synek BJL. Histopathological responses to spinal depot steroid injections in sheep. Presented at the 115th session of the National Health and Medical Research Council, June 1993.

32. Delaney RJ, Rowlingson JC, Carron H, et al. Epidural steroid effects on nerves and meninges. *Anesth Analg* 58:610, 1980.

33. Latham JM, Fraser RD, Moore RJ, et al. The pathologic effect of intrathecal betamethasone. *Spine* 22:1558, 1997.

34. Baron R, Janig W. Pain syndromes with causal participation of the sympathetic nervous system. *Anaesthesist* 47:4, 1998.

35. Baron R, Wasner G. Complex regional pain syndromes. *Curr Pain Headache Rep* 5:114, 2001.

36. Baron R, Fields HL, Janig W, et al. National Institutes of Health Workshop: Reflex sympathetic dystrophy/complex regional pain syndromes: State-of-the-science. *Anesth Analg* 95:1812, 2002.

37. Janig W, Baron R. Complex regional pain syndrome is a disease of the central nervous system. *Clin Auton Res* 12:150, 2002.

38. Harden RN, Baron R, Janig W. *Complex Regional Pain Syndrome.* Seattle: IASP Press, 2001.

39. Wasner G, Schattschneider J, Binder A, et al. Complex regional pain syndrome. Diagnostic mechanisms, CNS involvement and therapy. *Spinal Cord* 41:61, 2003.

40. Arner S. Intravenous phentolamine test: Diagnostic and prognostic use in reflex sympathetic dystrophy. *Pain* 46:17, 1991.

41. Raja SN, Treede RD, Davis KD, et al. Systemic alpha-adrenergic blockade with phentolamine: A diagnostic test for sympathetically maintained pain. *Anesthesiology* 74:691, 1991.

42. Belmonte C, Cervero F. *Neurobiology of Nociceptors.* Oxford: Oxford University Press, 1996.

43. Baron R, Wasner G. Complex regional pain syndromes. *Curr Pain Headache Rep* 5:114, 2001.

44. Maleki J, LeBel AA, Bennett GJ, et al. Patterns of spread in complex regional pain syndrome, type I (reflex sympathetic dystrophy). *Pain* 88:259, 2000.

45. Price DD, Long S, Huitt C. Sensory testing of pathophysiological mechanisms of pain in patients with reflex sympathetic dystrophy. *Pain* 49:163, 1992.

46. Sieweke N, Birklein F, Riedl B, et al. Patterns of hyperalgesia in complex regional pain syndrome. *Pain* 80:171, 1999.

47. Woolf CJ, Mannion RJ. Neuropathic pain: Aetiology, symptoms, mechanisms, and management. *Lancet* 353:1959, 1999.

48. Rommel O, Malin JP, Zenz M, et al. Quantitative sensory testing, neurophysiological and psychological examination in patients with complex regional pain syndrome and hemisensory deficits. *Pain* 93:279, 2001.

49. Rommel O, Gehling M, Dertwinkel R, et al. Hemisensory impairment in patients with complex regional pain syndrome. *Pain* 80:95, 1999.

50. Thimineur M, Sood P, Kravitz E, et al. Central nervous system abnormalities in complex regional pain syndrome (CRPS): Clinical and quantitative evidence of medullary dysfunction. *Clin J Pain* 14:256, 1998.

51. Wasner G, Heckmann K, Maier C, et al. Vascular abnormalities in acute reflex sympathetic dystrophy (CRPS I); complete inhibition of sympathetic nerve activity with recovery. *Arch Neurol* 56:613, 1999.

52. Low PA, Amadio PC, Wilson PR, et al. Laboratory findings in reflex sympathetic dystrophy: A preliminary report. *Clin J Pain* 10:235, 1994.

53. Atkins RM. Aspects of current management. Complex Regional Pain Syndrome. *J Bone Joint Surg* 85(B):1100, 2003.

54. Janig W, Baron R. Complex regional pain syndrome: Mystery explained? *Lancet* 2:687, 2003.

55. Stanton-Hicks M. Complex regional pain syndrome: Controversies. *Clin J Pain* 16(Suppl):S33, 2000.

56. Stanton-Hicks M. Spinal cord stimulation for the management of complex regional pain syndromes. *Neuromodulation* 2:193, 1999.

57. Gracely RH, Lynch SA, Bennett GJ. Painful neuropathy: Altered central processing maintained dynamically by peripheral input. *Pain* 51:175, 1992.

58. Stanton-Hicks M. Complex regional pain syndrome. *Anesthesiol Clin North America* 21:733, 2003.

59. Stanton-Hicks M, Baron R, Boas R, et al. Complex regional pain syndromes: Guidelines for therapy. *Clin J Pain* 14:155, 1998.

60. Treede R-D, Davis KD, Campbell JN, et al. The plasticity of cutaneous hyperalgesia during sympathetic ganglionic blockade in patients with neuropathic pain. *Brain* 115:607, 1992.

61. Reuben SS, Rosenthal EA, Steinberg RB. Surgery on the affected upper extremity of patients with a history of complex regional pain syndrome: A retrospective study of 100 patients. *J Hand Surg [Am]* 25:1147, 2000.

62. Kumar K, Nath RK, Toth C. Spinal cord stimulation is effective in the management of reflex sympathetic dystrophy. *Neurosurgery* 40:503, 1997.

63. Rauch RL, Eisenach JC, Jackson K, et al. Epidural clonidine for refractory reflex sympathetic dystrophy. *Anesthesiology* 79:1163, 1993.

64. Kemler MA, Barendse GA, van Kleef M, et al. Spinal cord stimulation in patients with chronic reflex sympathetic dystrophy. *N Engl J Med* 343:618, 2000.

65. vanHilten BJ, van de Beek WJ, Hoff JI, et al. Intrathecal baclofen for the treatment of dystonia in patients with reflex sympathetic dystrophy. *N Engl J Med* 343:625, 2000.

66. John G, Richard W. Herpes zoster. *N Engl J Med* 347:340, 2002.

67. Johnson RW. The future of predictors, prevention, and therapy in postherpetic neuralgia. *Neurology* 45(Suppl)8:S70, 1995.

68. Pasqualucci A, Pasqualucci V, Galla F, et al. Prevention of postherpetic neuralgia: Acyclovir and prednisolone versus epidural local anesthetic and methylprednisolone. *Acta Anaesthesiol Scand* 44:910, 2000.

69. Dworkin RH, Portenoy RK. Proposed classification of herpes zoster pain (letter). *Lancet* 343:1648, 1994.

70. Choo PW, Galil K, Donahue JG, et al. Risk factors for postherpetic neuralgia. *Arch Intern Med* 157:1217, 1997.

71. Penfold MET, Armati P, Cunningham AL. Axonal transport of herpes simplex virions to epidermal cells: Evidence for a specialized mode of virus transport and assembly. *Proc Natl Acad Sci USA* 91:6529, 1994.

72. Woolf CJ, Shortland P, Coggeshall RE. Peripheral nerve injury triggers central sprouting of myelinated afferents. *Nature* 355:75, 1992.

73. Janig W, Levine JD, Michaelis M. Interactions of sympathetic and primary afferent neurons following nerve injury and tissue trauma. *Prog Brain Res* 113:161, 1996.

74. Colding A. The effect of regional sympathetic blocks in treatments of herpes Zoster. *Acta Anaesthesiol Scand* 13:133, 1969.

75. Manabe H, Dan K, Higa K. Continuous epidural infusion of local anesthetics and shorter duration of acute zoster-associated pain. *Clin J Pain* 11:220, 1995.

76. Wicks MA, Gomez FAR. The use of epidural blocks and trigeminal ganglion in acute herpes zoster for the prevention of post herpetic neuralgia. Pain in Europe, Congress of European Federation of IASP Chapters. Verona, Italy, May 18–21, 1995, p. 153A.

77. Whitley RJ, Weiss H, Gnann JW Jr, et al. Acyclovir with and without prednisolone for the treatment of herpes zoster. A randomized, placebo-controlled trial. The National Institute of Allergy and Infectious Diseases Collaborative Antiviral Study Group. *Ann Intern Med* 125:376, 1996.

78. Dan K. Nerve block therapy and postherpetic neuralgia. *Crit Rev Phys Rehab Med* 7:93, 1995.

79. Lavoie PA, Khazen T, Filion PR. Mechanism of the inhibition of fast axonal transport by local anesthetics. *Neuropharmacology* 28:175, 1989.

80. Wood MJ, Johnson RW, McKendrick MW, et al. A randomized trial of acyclovir for 7 days or 21 days with and without prednisolone for treatment of acute herpes zoster. *N Engl J Med* 330:896, 1994.

81. Pernak J, Erdmann W, Bryant JD. Acute herpes zoster of the trigeminal nerve and its treatment. *J Pain Therapy* 3:101, 1993.

82. Moesker A, Boersma EP. The effect of extradural administration of corticosteroids as pain treatment of acute herpes zoster and prevention of postherpetic neuralgia. *Pain Clinic* 1:273, 1975.

83. Tenicela R, Lovasik D, Eaglestein W. Treatment of herpes zoster with sympathetic blocks. *Clin J Pain* 1:63, 1985.

84. Winnie AP, Hartwell PW. Relationship between time of treatment of acute herpes Zoster with sympathetic blockade and prevention of post-herpetic neuralgia: Clinical support for a new theory of the mechanism by which sympathetic blockade provides therapeutic benefit. *Reg Anesth* 18:277, 1993.

85. Wu C, Marsh A, Dworkin R. The role of sympathetic nerve blocks in herpes zoster and postherpetic neuralgia. *Pain* 87:121, 2000.

86. Hill A. Phantom limb pain: A review of the literature on attributes and potential mechanisms. *J Pain Symptom Manage* 17:125, 1999.

87. Cohen SP, Christo PJ, Maroz L. Pain management in trauma patients. *Am J Phys Med Rehabil* 83:142, 2004.

88. Parkes CM. Factors determining the persistence of phantom pain in the amputee. *J Psychosom Res* 17:97, 1973.

89. Sternbach T, Nadvrona H, Arazi D. A five year follow-up study of phantom limb pain in post-traumatic amputees. *Scand J Rehabil Med* 14:203, 1982.

90. Sherman RA, Sherman CJ, Parker L. Chronic phantom and stump pain among American veterans: Results of a survey. *Pain* 18:83, 1984.

91. Katz J. Prevention of phantom limb pain by regional anaesthesia. *Lancet* 349:519, 1997.

92. Haber WB. Effects of loss of limb on sensory functions. *J Psychol* 40:115, 1995.

93. Loeser JD. Pain after amputation: Phantom limb and stump pain. In: Loeser JD, Butler SH, Chapman CR, et al., eds, *Bonica's Management of Pain*, 3rd ed. Philadelphia, PA: Lippincott Williams and Wilkins, 2001, p. 412.

94. Nikolajsen L, Ilkjaer S, Jensen TS. Effect of preoperative extradural bupivacaine and morphine on stump sensation in lower limb amputees. *Br J Anaesth* 81:348, 1998.

95. Flor H. Phantom-limb pain: Characteristics, causes, and treatment. *Lancet Neurol* 1:182, 2002.

96. Devor M, Seltzer Z. Pathophysiology of damaged nerves in relation to chronic pain. In: Wall PD, Melzack RA, eds, *Textbook of Pain*, 4th ed. New York: Churchill-Livingstone, 1999, p. 128.

97. Melzack RA. Phantom limbs and the concept of a neuromatrix. *Trends Neurosci* 13:88, 1990.

98. Pons TP, Garrahty PE, Ommaya AK, et al. Massive cortical reorganization after sensory deafferentation in adult macaques. *Science* 252:1857, 1991.

99. Flor H, Elbert T, Knecht S, et al. Phantom limb pain as a perceptual correlate of cortical reorganization following arm amputation. *Nature* 357:482, 1995.

100. Birbaumer N, Lutzenberger W, Montoya P, et al. Effects of regional anesthesia on phantom limb pain are mirrored in changes in cortical reorganization. *J Neurosci* 17:5503, 1997.

101. Bach S, Noreng MF, Tjellden NU. Phantom limb pain in amputees during the first 12 months following limb amputation, after preoperative lumbar epidural blockade. *Pain* 33:297, 1988.

102. Chabal C, Jacobson L, Russell LC, et al. Pain response to perineuromal injection of normal saline, epinephrine, and lidocaine in humans. *Pain* 49:9, 1992.

103. Jahangiri M, Bradley JWP, Jayatunga AP, et al. Prevention of phantom pain after major lower limb amputation by epidural infusion of diamorphine, clonidine and bupivacaine. *Ann R Coll Surg Engl* 76:324, 1994.

104. Shug SA, Burrell R, Payne J, et al. Preemptive epidural analgesia may prevent phantom limb pain. *Reg Anesth* 20:256, 1995.

105. Katsuly-Liapis I, Georgakis P, Tierry C. Preemptive extradural analgesia reduces the incidence of phantom pain in lower limb amputees. *Br J Anaesth* 76:125, 1996.

106. Nikolajsen L, Ilkjaer S, Christensen JH, et al. Randomized trial of epidural bupivacaine and morphine in prevention of stump and phantom pain in lower-limb amputation. *Lancet* 350:1353, 1997.

107. Katz J, Melzack R. Pain 'memories' in phantom limbs: Review and clinical observations. *Pain* 43:319, 1990.

INDEX

Page numbers followed by *f* or *t* indicate figures or tables, respectively.